Quantitative EEG, Event-Related Potentials and Neurotherapy

Quantitative EEG, Event–Related Potentials and Neurotherapy

Juri D. Kropotov

AMSTERDAM • BOSTON • HEIDELBERG • LONDON • NEW YORK • OXFORD
PARIS • SAN DIEGO • SAN FRANCISCO • SINGAPORE • SYDNEY • TOKYO
Academic Press is an imprint of Elsevier

Academic Press is an imprint of Elsevier
525 B Street, Suite 1900, San Diego, CA 92101-4495, USA
30 Corporate Drive, Suite 400, Burlington, MA 01803, USA
32 Jamestown Road, London NW1 7BY, UK

First edition 2009

Notice
No responsibility is assumed by the publisher for any injury and/or damage to persons
or property as a matter of products liability, negligence or otherwise, or from any use
or operation of any methods, products, instructions or ideas contained in the material
herein. Because of rapid advances in the medical sciences, in particular, independent
verification of diagnoses and drug dosages should be made

Library of Congress Cataloging-in-Publication Data
A catalog record for this book is available from the Library of Congress

British Library Cataloguing in Publication Data
A catalogue record for this book is available from the British Library

ISBN: 978-0-12-374512-5

For information on all Academic Press publications
visit our website at www.elsevierdirect.com

Typeset by Charon Tec Ltd., A Macmillan Company. (www.macmillansolutions.com)

Printed and bound in the United Kingdom
Transferred to Digital Printing, 2011

To my sons Maxim and Ivan (Vania) with love, hope, and faith.

Contents

PART I

EEG Rhythms

1   *Slow, Infra-Slow Potentials, and Delta Rhythms*

2   *Alpha Rhythms*

3 Beta Rhythms

4 Frontal Midline Theta Rhythm

5 Paroxysmal Events

6 QEEG Endophenotypes

7 QEEG During Sleep

8 *Methods of Analysis of Background EEG*

9 Practice

PART II

Event–Related Potentials

10 Sensory Systems

11 *Attention Networks*

13 *Affective System*

14 *Memory Systems*

15 *Methods: Neuronal Networks and Event-Related Potentials*

16 Practice: ERP analysis

PART III

Disorders of the Brain Systems

17 Attention Deficit Hyperactivity Disorder

18   *Schizophrenia*

19   *Addiction*

Conclusion

Preface

The idea to write this book first appeared in December 2002 in a beautiful resort near Lisbon where Jay Gunkelman and the author were holding a workshop on "Basic Principles of QEEG and Neurofeedback." The workshop was the first event sponsored by the European Chapter of the International Society for Neuronal regulation. The students kept asking us where they could find the material we were teaching and what kind of a textbook we would recommend. To our disappointment we could not answer those questions. The impact to make action was made by Sara Purdy – a publishing Editor for behavioral neurosciences – who noticed that one of our papers (Kropotov et al., 2005) published in *International Journal of Psychophysiology* was one of the most heavily down-loaded papers of the Journal. The interest to this field is growing and the field itself needs handbooks.

Jay and the author decided to make an equal contribution to the textbook with Jay orienting to technical issues and the author covering the theoretical part of the textbook. But when 2 years ago I started to write the manuscript it turned out that theoretical ideas which I was going to present and which were based on 30 years of my experience in neuroscience and neurotherapy might not be necessarily shared by Jay and other people in the field. So, besides common facts and ideas that dominate currently in the field, the manuscript was going to include many personal experimental findings, theoretical considerations, and views on new developments in the filed that might stay aside from the mainstream. Moreover, I strongly felt that my attempt to simplify quite complicated issues of the brain functioning and dysfunctioning will be met with criticism from many scholars in the field. That is why, with all my appreciation of Jay Gunkelman's contribution to QEEG and neurotherapy and with a strong hesitation I decided to write the book on my own. The reader has to decide whether it was the right idea or not.

In writing the book, several intentions were driving the author:

1. To provide a *holistic picture of the quantitative EEG and event-related potentials as a recently emerged unified scientific field*. Quantitative EEG (QEEG) and event-related potentials (ERPs) constitute quite different "windows" for looking at the brain physiology. Those two "windows" are associated with different neuronal mechanisms and reflect different functions of the neuronal networks: (a) modulation of information flow for the background EEG oscillations (QEEG) on the one hand and (b) manifestation of stages

of information flow for ERPs on the other hand. With this aim the book includes two separate parts: Part I EEG Rhythms and Part II ERPs. Because the book is oriented to a broad range of readers only the breakthrough experimental facts and theoretical inferences made on these facts are presented. In almost all chapters of Part I and Part II the reader will find a simplified neuronal model that explains existing data and that can be used for further basic research as well as for understanding general ideas of diagnostic tools exemplified in QEEG and ERPs. In this respect the book differs from other books which consider QEEG and ERPs separately while usually confined with description of existing facts and methods.

2. To present *a unified description of the methods of quantitative EEG and ERPs*. During the last few years new methods emerged in the field such as (a) low resolution electromagnetic tomography (LORETA) with a new standardized version named s-LORETA, (b) spatial filtration of artifacts from the raw EEG, (c) decomposition of the background EEG and EEG responses into power–time–frequency representations by means of wavelet analysis, (d) extraction of so-called event related de/synchronization as a parameter reflecting reactivity of certain EEG rhythms, (e) decomposition of ERPs into independent components with different spatial–temporal characteristics and different functional meanings. The description of those new methods together with description of conventional methods is presented in separate chapters called Methods of Part I and Part II. In this respect the book is a unique one because it describes all methods from a single theoretical point of view. Moreover, the description of the methods is simplified so that even non-mathematically educated people could read these parts of the book and hopefully get a feeling of understanding why these methods work and what new information they provide to the basic science and to the diagnostics of brain disorders.

3. To give *a scientifically based overview of all existing approaches in the field of neurotherapy* including conventional EEG-based neurofeedback and recently emerged methods of the brain–computer interface (BCI) such as ERP-based BCI, fMRI-based BCI, as well as methods of electrical stimulation of the brain such as transcranial direct current stimulation (tDCS), transcranial magnetic stimulation (TMS) and some others. This overview is presented in Part III of the book. And again the book differs from other books published on the topic of neurofeedback not only by considering non-conventional methods of neurotherapy but also by providing a theoretical basis of practical applications of old and new methodological approaches.

4. To provide the reader with *a practical knowledge* which will be helpful both for beginners in the field, and for experienced practitioners. Part I and Part II of the book include chapters called Practice. These chapters are equipped with educational software. The software is stored in a zipped form and are provided via a web site created and hosted by Elsevier, and

accessed through this one common URL: www.elsevierdirect.com/
companions/9780123745125. Readers will have access to the educational
software and some EEG files recorded in healthy subjects and patients. The
software also includes a part of the normative database so that the reader
will be able not only to analyze EEG spectra and components of ERPs
but also to compare the corresponding EEG/ERPs parameters with the
normative data. In this respect the book is a unique one and seems to be
the first in the field to help the reader to practice the conventional methods
that existed in the field since 1960 (such as spectral analysis) and to try new
methods of QEEG/ERPs analysis that emerged during the last few years.

In accordance with these intentions the book it oriented to a broad audience:

to students in neurosciences who want to get a holistic view of brain functioning
and to learn how some aspects of brain functioning are reflected in the
background EEG oscillations and components of ERPs;

to neurologists and psychiatrists who would like to add new diagnostic and
treatment tools to their traditional methods;

to psychologists and neuropsychologists who are looking for new brain techniques
for assessing brain functioning and dysfunctioning;

to school psychologists who want to know about alternative methods for
correcting behavioral problems in children;

to experts in rehabilitation medicine who want to learn about advanced methods
in monitoring and correcting stroke and traumatic brain injuries;

and, finally, to all others including those who are in the field *of neurocomputing,
computer engineering, technical vision, robotics*…who are interested in the
organization of the human brain, the living device that equips us with
emotions, reasoning, planning, memories, speech…, and who would like to
implement these qualities in technical devices.

The book is illustrated by four types of figures:

1. Schematic representations of ideas presented in the book. These figures
are actually visual images of the text and, in most cases, reflect common
thoughts and models dominated in the field.
2. Schematic representations of results obtained in one or several experimental
papers. These figures in a schematic form display the main results of the
corresponding papers in a form common to all other illustrations of the
book.
3. Results of intracranial recording of local field potentials in neurologic and
psychiatric patients. Those were patients who did not respond to other
forms of treatment and to whom electrodes were stereotactically implanted
for diagnostic and therapeutic purposes. These results were obtained in
the author's laboratory of the Institute of the Human Brain of Russian

Academy of Sciences. Most of the results were published in English in international journals. However some results (especially in 1970s) were published only in Russian.

4. Results of various types of analysis of 19-channel EEG recordings in healthy subjects and in different groups of patients. The results were obtained in the author's laboratories of the Institute of the Human Brain of Russian Academy of Sciences and of the Norwegian University of Science and Technology, as well as in other centers in Switzerland, England, and Holland. These centers explore the methodology developed in the Institute of the Human Brain. We will refer to the data in healthy subjects as the Human Brain Institute (HBI) Normative Database.

Acknowledgments

My first thanks are to my Teacher Professor Natalia Bechtereva – a grand daughter of famous Russian psychiatrist Vladimir Bechterev[1]. In 1972 she invited me, a post-graduate student of Leningrad State University with the major in quantum mechanics[2], to join her team[3]. The main idea of Professor Bechtereva was to search for "neuronal code of human mental activity"[4]. Those were years when, on the one hand, researchers were not satisfied by results of previous studies of the human EEG, and on the other hand, euphoria for new possibilities opened by recordings spike activity of single neurons occupied scientific minds. Unfortunately, these hopes never came true. However, the studies of human neuronal reactions performed in our group showed that neurons of subcortical structures were involved not only in motor actions, but also in sensory and cognitive functions. In 1980s three of us (Yury Gogolitsyn, Sergei Pakhomov, and me) developed the first version of hardware/software system[5] for recording and analyzing electrophysiological data.

In 1990s, the science horizons were once more widened due to introduction of new methods such as positron emission tomography (PET) and magnetic resonance imaging (MRI). The institute of the Human Brain (director Sviatoslav Medvedev) was the first one in the Soviet Union that built up a PET center[6]. And

---

[1]According to some unchecked rumors he examined Stalin in 1927 and made diagnose "paranoia" after which he was murdered by KGB agents. We do not know whether it is true or not, but at least it shows how powerful was Bechterev in those days.

[2]During all my young years I was interested in physics and mathematics and graduated the most prestigious high school in Leningrad with profound teaching in physics and mathematics (Lyceum/School 239). Studying at Leningrad State University I was inspired by Professor Boris Pavlov who taught me a broad view to mathematics that helped me later in modeling neuronal networks and in applying sophisticated EEG methods of analysis.

[3]Meeting Professor Bechtereva made a difference in my life: with her supervision in 2 years I defended my first dissertation (equivalent to PhD) and in 10 years I became a head of laboratory in her Department, named Department of Human Neurophysiology of the Institute of Experimental Medicine of USSR Academy of Medical Sciences and shortly after that in 1985 I was awarded the USSR State Prize – the most prestigious award in Science and Technology in the former USSR.

[4]These ideas were in turn inspired by pioneering work by Grey Walter from Neurological Institute in Bristol.

[5]The system was based on a French mini-computer named Plurimat-S and was programmed in Assembler and Fortran languages.

[6]The money was given to us directly due to decision of Michael Gorbachev and who was in those days the General Secretary of the Communist Party of the Soviet Union.

once more an initial euphoria was replaced by deep disappointment: no qualitatively new data have been obtained.

All this happened before "perestroika" proclaimed by Michael Gorbachev became a real disaster. In 1991 the Soviet Union was broken down and with its collapsing the funding of science in the former USSR ceased. To earn the leaving people in my laboratory started to bargain tea packages and did a lot of other "business-like" enterprises. Most of the researchers from my laboratory left the Soviet Union for a better life to the West. Yury Gogolitsyn immigrated to England, Andrey Sevastianov and Michael Kuznetzov went to the United States, Aleksander Popov – to Australia, Oleg Korzukov – to Finland. In 1992–1993 I myself was working with Peter Kugler, Helen Crowford, and Karl Pribram from Brain Research Center at Radford University in Virginia on mathematical simulation of realistic neural networks. I am very grateful for their help and their friendship. Perestroika and the fall down of the iron curtain opened new opportunities in collaboration with other universities in the west. Here I want to mention our joint research with a Nobel Prize Winner Ilia Prigogine[7] and a joint research with Risto Näätänen, an outstanding Finnish psychologist.

Meanwhile, in cooperation with the Television Institute which in those days belonged to the USSR Military–Industrial Complex we created a company (Director Nikolai Brinken) called "Potential" with the aim to manufacture electroencephalographs. At the beginning we were working in collaboration with Don Tucker, a Professor of University of Oregon and the founder of the EGI company. In those years a student of mine Valery Ponomarev became involved in programming software for EEG recording and analysis[8].

In 2000 I met Barry Sterman at his workshop in 2000 in Ulvik – a small town in the South West of Norway. The workshop was organized by Jonelle Villar and Geir Flatabo. They were the first who introduced this field to Norwegian medical and scientific community. Several years later Knut Hestad invited me to organize an EEG lab and to lecture QEEG and neurotherapy at Norwegian University of Science and Technology.

I would unable to write the book without help from many other people who dedicated their lives to the field of quantitative EEG and neurotherapy. First of all I want to mention Valery Ponomarev, a programmer and senior research fellow in my laboratory who wrote most of the software I presented in the book. Andeas Mueller from Switzerland was the first who accepted the methodology developed in my laboratory and helped tremendously in collecting data for the Human Brain Institute Normative Database. Many other researchers and clinicians from different countries helped me in collecting the clinical data. They are

---

[7]He was a second generation Russian immigrant of the post-October revolution time.

[8]His first attempt of programming was re-writing the software package that Gogolitsyn, Pakhomov, and me created for analyzing impulse activity of neurons in 1980–1981. Valery further on became a co-author of most of my papers.

Leonid Chutko, Inna Nikeshina, Elena Yaovenko, Vera Grin-Yatsenko, and Katia Beliakova from my own laboratory, Jay Gunkelman and Curtis Cripe from the United States, Andreas Mueller, Marietta Chatzigeorgiou, and Stefan Sakellaridis from Switzerland, Knut Hestad, Venke Arntsberg, Stig Hollup, and Jan Bruno from Norway, Beverly and Tony Steffert from England, Wytze van der Zwaag from Holland and many, many others.

Studies in my laboratory during the last 15 years were supported by grants from different agencies such as Soros Foundation, Russian Foundation for Fundamental Research, Russian Humanitarian Science Foundation, USA National Science Foundation ... The grant from Austrian Academy of Sciences was given to Susan Etlinger and me to write a book on Neuroinformatics. Susan taught me not only English language but also a more careful attitude to details.

Here I especially want to thank Doug Richards, the President of Foundation of Dreamers, for financial support of my research during the last several years. Being a romantic personality he believed in my ideas and helped me enormously to finish some of my projects.

I did not mention many other people who taught me at school and university, with whom I worked in the Institute of Experimental Medicine, Institute of the Human Brain in St. Petersburg, Radford University, University of Oregon in the USA, and in Norwegian University of Science in Trondheim, and whose ideas and experience formed my own views to the field of electrophysiology of the human brain.

August 2008, St. Petersburg

Introduction: Basic Concepts of QEEG and Neurotherapy

The human brain is the most sophisticated substrate on the earth. Functioning of this anatomical substrate determines the whole complexity of the human behavior. During last 80 years basic science discovered several methods to study functioning of the human brain. These methods include invasive approaches, such as electrical recording of impulse activity of single and multi-neurons, recording local field potentials and intracranial event-related potentials (ERPs), as well as polarographic recordings of brain tissue oxygen. The invasive approaches require implantation of electrodes in the human (for clinical purposes) or animal (for experimental purposes) brain. The non-invasive approaches include magnetic resonance imaging (MRI), positron emission tomography (PET), magneto-encephalography (MEG) and electroencephalography (EEG). Both, invasive and non-invasive methods provide us with several overlapping but still different windows that enable us to look at what is happening in the living brain from different points of view. EEG is only one of many methods!

In Introduction we are going (1) to give the reader a general overview of the methods for assessment the brain functioning, (2) to show the differences and similarities between EEG and other methods, (3) to briefly indicate the potential power of EEG for revealing individual peculiarities in the normal brain and endophenotypes of the diseased brain, (4) and, finally, to impose the basic idea that feeding back the known electro- and metabolic parameters might enable the healthy subjects and patients voluntarily (when the parameter is just presented through sensory modalities) or involuntarily (when the electrical currents are injected into the brain) to control their brain functioning.

I. GLOSSARY

Action potential (sometimes called neuronal spike) *of a neuron* is a discharge of a neuron that is associated with fast (around millisecond) opening and closing of Na^+ and K^+ ion channels in the neuronal membrane. The discharge takes place if depolarization of the membrane reaches a threshold. The action potential is considered as a simplest event of information processing in neuronal networks associated with transferring of a "bit" of information from one neuron to others.

Biochemistry is a branch of science that studies chemical properties of complex molecules in the living organism.

Brain imaging is a recently emerged discipline within *medicine* and *neuroscience*. Brain imaging falls into two broad categories – structural imaging and functional imaging. *Structural imaging* deals with 3D parameters characterizing the anatomical or biochemical structure of the brain. *Functional imaging* deals with dynamics of the brain parameters. MRI, PET, and EEG are examples of functional imaging.

Deep brain stimulation a continuous application of short current pulses via implanted electrodes that is supposed to lead to functional blockade of the stimulated neuronal networks.

Electroencephalogram (EEG) is brain-related electrical potentials recorded from the scalp.

Electroencephalography is a set of methods of measurement and analysis of the EEG.

Electrophysiology is a branch of *physiology* that studies the flow of *ions* in biological tissues and uses electrophysiological methods for recording these currents.

Endophenotypes are heritable quantitative traits (such as EEG power in specific frequency bands or components of event-related potentials) that index an individual's liability to develop or manifest a given disease or behavioral trait.

Event-related potentials (ERPs) are local field potentials or EEG recorded during a psychological task (such as ODDBALL or GO/NOGO) and averaged over trials of the same category. In the course of averaging, spontaneous positive and negative fluctuations cancel each other, leaving averaged potentials associated with stages of information processing in the brain.

Functional MRI (fMRI) is a method of measuring inhomogeneity of hydrogen atoms due to a complex processes associated with blood oxygenation, oxygen consumption, and activation of neuronal network.

Gene functionally is the unit of *heredity* and structurally consists of a long strand of *DNA*. Gene contains a *promoter*, which controls the activity of a gene, and a coding sequence, which determines what the gene produces.

Genotype is the specific genetic structure of a subject in a form of *DNA*. The terms genotype and phenotype represent two extreme levels of human organization: molecular level at DNA and holistic level at behavior. Genotype and phenotype are not directly correlated: some genes may express a given phenotype only in a certain environment, while some phenotypes may be the result of multiple genotypes.

Local field potentials are potentials recorded by micro and macro electrodes inserted into brain tissue. These potentials are generated by membranes of local neurons and glia.

Magnetic resonance imaging (MRI) is a method of measuring the density of some elemental magnets (such as hydrogen atoms) placed in the strong magnetic field by recording the response of these magnets to radio signals. The response is called a magnetic resonance.

Magneto-encephalography (MEG) is a non-invasive technique for detecting magnetic fields that are associated with brain activity. As the magnetic fields of the brain are weak, extremely sensitive magnetic detectors which work at very low, superconducting temperatures are used to pick up the signal.

Molecular genetics a branch of science that studies molecular basis of DNA, RNA, and related molecular structures in the living organs.

Multi unit activity is a sequence of action potentials of a group of neurons that surround an electrode placed into the brain tissue. Multi unit activity is recorded extracellularly by micro (around few microns in diameter) or macro (up to 100 microns) electrodes.

Neuroscience is a branch of science that studies the brain and its relationship with the mind.

Neurotherapy is a set of neurophysiologically based methods for modifying brain function. The methods include neurofeedback, transcranial direct current stimulation and transmagnetic stimulation.

Phenotype of a subject is either his/her specific *behavior*, a manifestation of a *trait* or a total physical appearance such as size, *eye color*... Many phenotypes are determined by multiple *genes* and influenced by *environmental* factors. Because phenotypes are much easier to observe than genotypes modern medicine such as neurology and psychiatry uses behavioral phenotypes for classification and diagnosis of brain diseases.

Polarographic method of oxygen measurement is based on the fact that the voltage of −0.63V applied to a polarizable electrode (such as a gold wire inserted into a brain tissue) creates a current that is proportional to the concentration of oxygen in the brain tissue.

Psychology is a branch of science that studies behavior using specific methods for description behavior patterns and inferring brain mechanisms from this description ("black box" approach in brain studies).

QEEG, quantitative EEG − a collection of quantitative methods designed to process EEG signals. QEEG includes spectral and wavelet analysis of EEG.

Single unit activity is a sequence of action potentials of a single neuron recorded by electrode inserted into the neuron (intracellular recording) or placed nearby the neuron (extracellular recording). The duration of a spike is about 1 ms. Consequently, amplifiers for single unit recordings usually have a frequency band of 100 Hz–10,000 Hz.

Stereotactic neurosurgery is a microsurgical intervention in deep brain structures for lesion, biopsy, or implantation that is based on a 3D coordinate system established with the help of neuroimaging.

II. THE PLACE OF EEG IN NEUROSCIENCE AND MEDICINE

A. Goals of Neuroscience

Human behavior is conventionally divided into two main categories: normal behavior, that covers behavioral patterns of healthy subjects, and abnormal behavior, that is associated with brain disorders. Normal behavior is mainly studied by basic

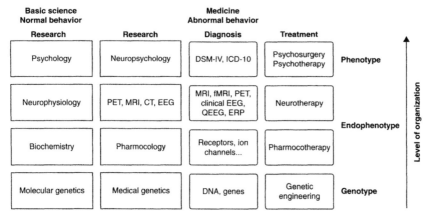

FIGURE I.1   The place of QEEG and neurotherapy in the basic and medical sciences. Studies of normal behavior are carried out by psychology, physiology, biochemistry and molecular genetics. Studies of abnormal behavior are carried out by neuropsychology, pathophysiology, pharmacology and medical genetics. Diagnosis is made on the basis of description of behavior according to DSM-IV or ICD-10 manuals. In modern medicine there is a strong tendency to search for so called endophenotypes – objective diagnostic parameters specific for a given disorder. Treatment is provided at four different levels of brain/behavior organization by psychotherapy, psychosurgery, neurotherapy and pharmacotherapy.

sciences, usually united under the name "neuroscience," while abnormal behavior is a subject of medical science. Neuroscience explores the brain and its relationship with mind (see Fig. I.1). Studying the human brain besides the reasons of pure curiosity has two ultimate goals. The first goal is associated with neurology, psychiatry, psychotherapy, and medical psychology[1] and is to help (1) understanding anatomical and physiological markers of brain diseases and (2) treating brain disorders.

B. Goals of Psychiatry and Neurology

One of the main tasks of psychiatry and neurology is associated with objective assessment of brain dysfunction. Currently, the only way for diagnosis brain disease remains a verbal description of abnormality of behavior in specific terms, defined by manuals such as Diagnostic Statistical Manual in the USA (DSM–IV) or International Classification of Disorders in Europe (ICD-10) (Fig. I.1). According

---

[1]The second goal of neuroscience is to mimic the brain in various applications. This goal is associated with mathematical simulation of neuronal networks and building up electronic devices, called neurocomputers, based on principles of information processing in the brain. The scope of the book is confined by the first goal. We are going to present the experimental data, theoretical knowledge, and methodological tools that enable neurologists, psychiatrists, psychologists, psychotherapists, and health care practitioner to assess brain dysfunctions and on the basis of this assessment to provide the optimal treatment for their patients.

to these manuals all brain dysfunctions are separated into distinct categories, called diseases. Each disease is labeled by a name (such as Parkinson's disease or schizophrenia) and considered as a separate entity defined by symptoms (elemental abnormal behavioral patterns) and/or by syndromes (groups of symptoms). An example of a description of symptoms of a particular brain disease is given by the list of behavioral patterns of attention deficit hyperactivity disorder (ADHD)[2].

C. Phenotype and Genotype

A significant role in neuronal network functioning belongs to mediators and receptors that determine dynamical properties of synaptic connections in neuronal networks. Studying the subcellular processes and molecular mechanisms of synaptic functioning is a scope of biochemistry in the basic science and pharmacology[3] in medicine. The production of neuronal mediators, ion channels, and receptors is controlled by genes. Genes form a genotype of a human subject. The term "phenotype" reflects actual anatomical and physiological properties of the subject and as the consequence of these properties – the subject's behavior. The genotype is the largest influencing factor in the development of the phenotype, but it is not the only one. Normal as well as abnormal human behavioral patterns are shaped by complex interactions of environmental and genetic factors. The mechanisms of such gene–environment interactions are still poorly understood[4].

The number of studies in neuroscience has been exponentially increasing and the knowledge obtained in the last 10–20 years dramatically changed our understanding of the brain. These changes prompted a new cycle in developing clinical applications of EEG. However EEG is not the only method that neuroscience provides to clinical practice. The most known of them are MEG, PET, and MRI. All these methods are usually united under the common name "neuroimaging." Each of the methods deals with a specific neuroanatomical or neurophysiological

---

[2]See, for example, Wikipedia, a *multilingual, web-based, free content encyclopedia* project. Wikipedia is *written* collaboratively by volunteers from all around the world. With rare exceptions, its articles can be *edited* by anyone with access to the Internet, simply by clicking the *edit this page link*. The name Wikipedia is a *portmanteau* of the words *wiki* (a type of collaborative website) and *encyclopedia*. Since its creation in 2001, Wikipedia has grown rapidly into one of the largest reference web-sites. The description of ADHD and its symptoms you can find on: http://en.wikipedia.org/wiki/Attention-Deficit_Hyperactivity_Disorder.

[3]Although the use of *psychoactive drugs* was known thousand years ago, psychopharmacology as a science started in 1950s when drugs affecting schizophrenia and depression were accidentally found.

[4]Complexity of the brain is a major factor that makes it difficult to elucidate the genotype–phenotype relationship. The point is that cells in the brain are different from each other revealing different properties in different brain systems while their interactions are subject to change depending on environmental factors. As a consequence, complex interactions of genes and environment define impairment in neuronal systems and operations they perform.

parameter and provides a small "window" to the brain. The relationships of these methods and electroencephalography are briefly presented below.

D. MEG as a Complementary Method to EEG

EEG in humans was discovered around 80 years ago by a German scientist Hans Berger. During these years periods of flourishing and enthusiasm were mixed with periods of decay and ignorance. Periods of flourishing were associated with appearance of new technology in recording and analyzing EEG data while periods of ignorance took place when some alternative methods of brain imaging appeared. Now we know that EEG is a sum of microdipoles representing pyramidal cells oriented perpendicular to the surface of the head. The orientation of electrical dipoles actually means that EEG is the most sensitive to radial sources. In addition to electric fields neurons generate magnetic fields[5]. MEG is a sum of magnetic fields arising from the network of current dipoles. These dipoles correspond to currents in bundles of pyramidal neurons that are parallel to the surface of the head and consequently located in the sulci of the cortex. Thus, MEG and EEG can be considered as supplementary methods: the most effect in MEG is generated by tangential currents, that is, currents in sulci, while the most effect in EEG is generated by radial currents, in particular, currents in gyri near the surface (Fig. I.2). In contrast to the electric currents in EEG, the magnetic fields are not distorted by the scalp[6].

E. MRI

The MRI method is based on physical phenomenon known as magnetic resonance. Many organic elements like hydrogen atoms are elementary magnets. In their common state, any of these tiny magnets is oriented randomly. However, if an external magnetic field is applied all the magnets will be arranged along that field just like a compass needle is oriented along the magnetic field of the Earth. Then, when external magnetic waves of the radiofrequency band pass through the

---

[5] Magnetic fields are actually produced by ion currents in neurons. The currents of a single neuron can be thought of as a current dipoles. The current dipoles should not be mixed with electric charge dipoles that generate signals in EEG.

[6] MEG has been developed in the 1970s and has been greatly aided by recent advances in computing algorithms and hardware. Similar to EEG, MEG reveals relatively poor spatial and extremely high temporal resolution (around 1 ms). However, the high cost of the MEG machines and the low signal to noise ratio limit clinical applications of MEG. The clinical uses of MEG nowadays are mostly confined by localizing epileptiform spiking activity in patients with epilepsy.

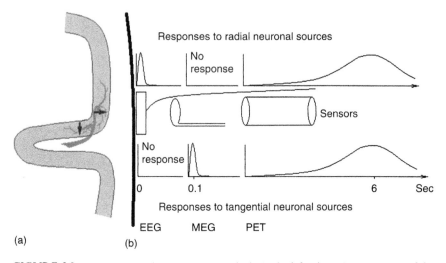

(a)   (b)

FIGURE I.2   EEG, MEG, and PET imaging methods. At the left: schematic presentation of the convoluted cortex with two electrical dipoles depicted by arrows. Blood vessels around neuronal generators are marked by a darker gray. Three types of sensors are schematically presented at the right middle. They are: metal electrode for EEG, SQUID (Superconducting Quantum Interference Device) for MEG and a photomultiplier tube for PET for detecting a burst of light emitted by a scintillator material when a gamma photon reaches the sensor. Changes in EEG, MEG, and PET in response to a short increase in neuronal activity for the tangential dipole (right, bottom) and for the radial dipole (right, top). EEG measures the radially oriented dipole while MEG measures the tangentially oriented dipole. There is almost no delay between the neuronal event and EEG or MEG signal. If radioactive water is used as a compound, the PET signal measures slow changes in local blood flow that follows neuronal events with a long (about 6 s) delay.

magnetized area they make the elementary magnets to rotate in a certain direction. When the radio waves are turned off, the atoms return to their original states and generate the waves that are registered by magnetic detectors of a tomography. These radio waves registered by magnetic detectors serve as source data for MRI. Density and magnetic features of elementary magnets define the power of the signal. To restore 3D density distribution pattern for these magnets, special mathematical image reconstruction methods are used[7].

---

[7] Many neurologists and neurosurgeons when examining MRI images do not even suspect that the source data look quite different from those shown on the MRIs. The source data are processed by complex mathematical algorithms requiring computational facilities of huge (even from today's point of view) capacity. Spatial resolution achieved by MRI is really astonishing. On MRI scans one can see separate convolutions, corpus callosum, caudate nucleus, and even smaller structures like mamillary bodies or thalamic nuclei.

F. PET

PET is based on physical properties of isotopes – radioactive forms of simple atoms (like hydrogen, oxygen, fluorine, etc.) – to emit positrons when they decay. The radioactive atoms are arranged into more complex molecules like molecules of oxygen, water, glucose, etc. During measurement in the PET scan, the radioactive substance is administered into the patient's blood and reaches the brain through circulation. The radioactive substance when it is accumulated in a certain area of the brain emits positrons. As positrons encounter with electrons they annihilate, emitting two gamma-quantums per one collision. Special detectors placed around the subject's head register the gamma-quantums, and number of collisions is directly proportional to metabolic activity of the brain area. In other words, the more active is the brain area, the more radioisotopes does it consume and the more gamma-emissions will be registered from that area[8]. To restore 3D pattern of radioactive substance distribution density, special mathematical reconstruction methods are applied similar to those used for MRI. However, spatial resolution of PET is significantly less than that of MRI. Due to a small resolution, it is impossible to detect brain structures like thalamic nuclei or mamillary bodies on PET images[9].

G. Functional MRI

An advanced modification of MRI, called functional MRI, was recently developed for studies of vascular/metabolic reactions of the brain tissue in response to different tasks. The physiology of the method is based on the fact that any local neuronal activity change leads to changes of oxygenation in the local blood supplying brain areas. The signal for the so-called blood oxygen level dependent (BOLD) fMRI comes from hydrogen atoms, which are abundant in the water molecules of the brain. The measured radiofrequency signal decays over time, owing to various factors including the presence of inhomogeneities in the magnetic field. The inhomogenity is associated in part with changes in blood oxygenation. Deoxy- and oxyhemoglobin have different magnetic properties with deoxyhemoglobin introducing the most of inhomogenity. Hence, an increase in the concentration of deoxyhemoglobin would cause a decrease in image intensity.

---

[8] The physiological parameter for PET is number of collisions – moments when two gamma-quantums are emitted. In a PET scanner there are quite many detectors registering gamma-quantums, and they surround the subject's head by sort of a ring – or rather by layers of rings, or cylinders.

[9] PET is rather expensive and invasive method. To apply it, a cyclotron and a special radiochemical laboratory are needed. To reduce the dose of radiation exposing the subject, relatively little quantities of isotopes are administered leading therefore to a poorer quality of PET images. However, for some scientific tasks (such as studying densities receptors of dopamine reuptake) PET seems to be the only method available at the moment.

H. Polarographic Recording of Brain Oxygen

The relationship between three processes (1) impulse activity of neurons, (2) oxygen and glucose consumption by neuronal cells, and (3) local blood flow is quite sophisticated and not fully understood. Any fast change in impulse activity of neurons results in slow (with delay of about 6–10s) changes in local blood flow and extracellular oxygen. In 1970s in our laboratory together with Valentine Grechin we used a polarographic method to study the level of extracellular oxygen in the brain of neurological patients[10]. Polarographic method of oxygen measurement is based on the fact that the voltage of $-0.63V$ applied to a polarizable electrode (such as a gold wire inserted into a brain tissue) creates a current that is proportional to the concentration of oxygen in the brain tissue. In our studies we showed that the level of oxygen in the local brain tissue does not remain constant but oscillates at very low frequencies about 6–10 cycles per minute (see Fig. I.3). These oscillations reflect complex metabolic processes in the brain associated with oxygen consumption of neuronal networks and local blood flow regulation in the local regions. The most thrilling feature of these oscillations was that at the cortical level they were associated with slow oscillations of electrical potentials measured from the skin of the head. The deco-second oscillations can be induced by tasks such as hand movements or arithmetical actions. An example of such reaction in the local concentration of pO_2 in the deep structure of the brain is shown in Fig. I.3. The sharp increase in multi-unit impulse activity induces slow changes in extracellular oxygen with a period of around 12s so that the first maximum of response has a delay period of 6s[11]. This example clearly shows that information processing in neuronal networks and metabolic activity take place at different time scales.

Almost 30 years later similar deco-second spontaneous fluctuations in the brain were observed in the BOLD signal by means of fMRI[12]. These oscillations reflect coherent performance of different spatially distributed regions belonging to a particular system such as the somatosensory, visual, or auditory systems. Functional meaning of these oscillations is unknown. In one of our studies (Kropotov and Gretchin, 1979) we showed that the phases of oxygen decreasing might be associated with memory consolidation when short lasting electrical signals of the neuronal networks are transferred to long lasing metabolic changes.

---

[10]Those were Parkinsonian patients who were unresponsive to all conventional forms of treatment and who agreed to undergo a stereotactic operation. Gold 100 micron wires were implanted to the globus pallidus, putamen of the basal ganglia and ventral nuclei of the thalamus. The results of these studies are summarized in our book published in 1979 by the Publishing House of Academy of Sciences of USSR (Grechin and Kropotov, 1979).

[11]In some areas the delayed increase in pO_2 was preceded by a short (about 1–3s) decrease in concentration of local extracellular oxygen.

[12]For a recent review see Fox and Raichel, 2007.

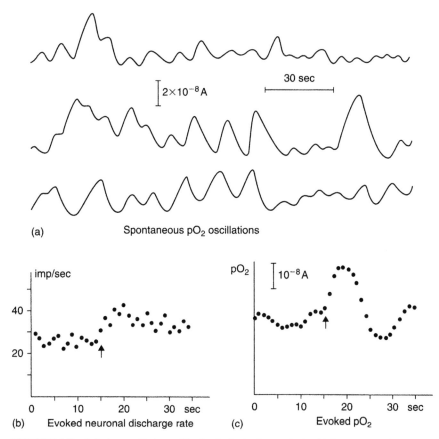

FIGURE I.3   Infraslow oscillations of local pO_2 in the human brain. (a) Spontaneous fluctuations of pO_2 in the caudate nucleus and two thalamic nuclei are recorded by the polarographic method in Parkinsonian patients to whom gold electrodes were implanted for diagnosis and therapy. Averaged over 10 trials simultaneously recorded multi unit impulse activity (b) and pO_2 (c) in the ventral thalamus of the human brain. Impulse activity of neurons and pO2 was measured by the same electrode. Each trial consisted of arithmetic operation (addition or subtraction) with two digits presented at the beginning of the trial.

III. FROM NEURONAL SPIKES THROUGH LOCAL FIELD POTENTIALS TO SCALP EEG

A. Impulse Activity of Neurons

We now are aware that the functions of the cortex are determined by collective behavior of neuronal ensembles, rather than by independent actions of single neurons. But, 40 years ago scientists were obsessed by an opposite view, suggesting that

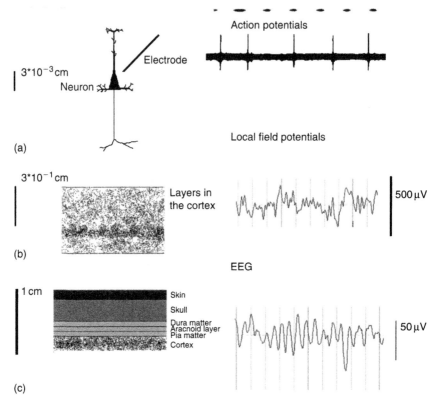

FIGURE I.4   Three levels of electrical events in the cortex. Single neuron level − corresponds to 30 microns of spatial scale and 1 ms of spike duration. Local field potentials − are measured with macroelectrodes within the cortex and are different at 3 mm scale. EEG recorded from the scalp has a spatial resolution of a few centimeters. Note 10 time difference in amplitude of potentials measures intracortically and from the scalp.

only behavior of single neurons would give a clue for understanding brain function. In those days a new method − the method for recording single unit activity − emerged[13] (Fig. I.4). Most electrophysiologists abandoned the field of classical EEG (the only electrophysiological method that was available in those days) and started recording activity of single neurons[14]. These were the years of euphoria.

[13]The technique implied the use of microelectrodes (with diameter of a few microns) and of special amplifies with the bandpass from 100 Hz to 10 kHz. The most exciting part of our work in those days was that in some (alas) rare cases spikes of single neurons could be recorded by macroelectrodes implanted into the brain of neurological patients.

[14]My scientific supervisor professor Natalia Bechtereva was the first who decided to record impulse activity of neurons in patients. These were patients to whom electrodes were implanted into deep brain structures for diagnosis and therapy. She used to tell me that EEG is very noisy and unspecific. She believed that impulse activity of neurons was the best way to study neuronal mechanisms of cognition.

To some extent the expectations were rewarded. Indeed, discovery of simple and complex cells properties in the visual cortex by Hubel and Wiesel (rewarded by the Nobel Prize in 1981) seemed to confirm the suggestion that reactions of single neurons could provide new insights regarding information processing in the animal brain[15]. It turned out that in some unique cases recording of impulse activity of single and multiple neurons during various cognitive tasks can be done in humans during stereotactic operations in epileptic and Parkinsonian patients.

B. Profiles of Neuronal Reactions

When in 1970s in our laboratory we studied reactions of single and multi-neurons in the human brain using tiny electrodes implanted into different parts of the brain of neurological and psychiatric patients we were struck by similarities of neuronal reactions in certain parts of the brain[16] (see Fig. I.5). These similarities were expressed in so-called profiles of neuronal reactions – a grand average representation of the responses of all neurons recorded in a particular anatomical structure. Comparing profiles of reactions with local field potentials recorded by the same electrodes showed that the collective behavior of neurons was quite accurately reflected in local field potentials recorded by the implanted electrodes (see Fig. I.6).

C. Local Field Potentials

Having in mind these data, in the beginning of 1990s in our laboratory we started using local field potentials as a method for analyzing stages of information processing in the human brain. The work was done in collaboration with Risto

---

[15]In the field of vision research, single neuron recordings had shown existence of several classes of neurons in the primary and secondary visual cortical area. Those types responded differently to specific visual patterns such as stationary and moving spatial gratings, colors, and other more complex visual stimuli. Moreover, some neurons kept their activity after stimulus offset revealing memory properties while others ceased the activity after extinction of stimulus.

[16]Invasive recordings in patients undergoing stereotactic operations are indispensable for defining the location where focal brain lesions or deep brain stimulations are appropriate. Such recordings involve measurement of local field potentials which reflect the coherent activity of small cell assemblies, or the use of microelectrodes to measure single-cell activity. As these studies require well-defined clinical indications, they never yielded data from normal brain circuits. Nonetheless, such data are valuable for understanding the pathophysiology of disorders and for linking animal models to the clinical situation. Beyond that, data from these studies can provide insight into the basic mechanisms of brain functions such as perception, movement control, memory formation, language processing, and even conscious awareness.

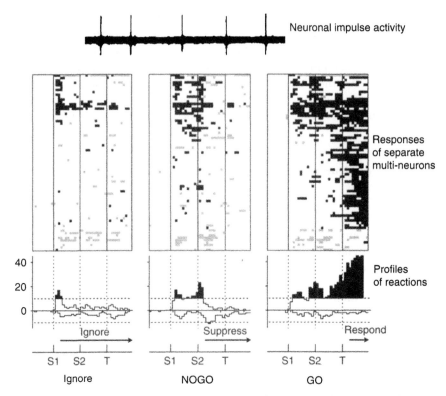

FIGURE I.5   Profiles of neuronal reactions in subcortical structures. Multi-unit activity (top) was measured from electrodes implanted into the basal ganglia and thalamus in patients performing the two stimulus GO/NOGO task. Each horizontal line (middle from the top) corresponds to a separate multi-unit. Black (gray) squares: significant ($p < 0.01$) increase (decrease) in the discharge rate above (below) background discharge rate. The binary post-stimulus histograms were averaged into profiles of reactions (bottom) with vertical axis: number of multiunits significantly activated (upward) or inhibited (downward) and dashed horizontal lines: confidence levels $p < 0.01$. Horizontal axis = time in 100 msec bins. Three types of trials are presented from left to right: Ignore trials, NOGO, and GO trials. S1, S2, T presentations of the first, second, and trigger stimulus in trials. Adapted from: Kropotov et al. (1997).

Näätänen and his colleagues from the Cerebral Brain Research Unit (CBRU) at the University of Helsinki[17]. In these studies we discovered that distinct cortical areas of the auditory cortex elicit quite different evoked potentials enabling us to study details on information processing the human auditory cortex[18].

---

[17]Long before that, in 1978 Risto Nataanen discovered an ERP component named mismatch negativity (MMN) that was attention independent and appeared in response to rare deviant stimuli when compared with ERPs to standard stimuli in the ODDBALL paradigm.

[18]Indeed, the primary auditory area 41 coded formant frequencies of acoustic stimuli in early (at 50 ms) intracranial evoked potentials but did not reveal any indication of memory effects, for example, did not habituate to repeated auditory stimuli. In contrast, responses in the secondary auditory area

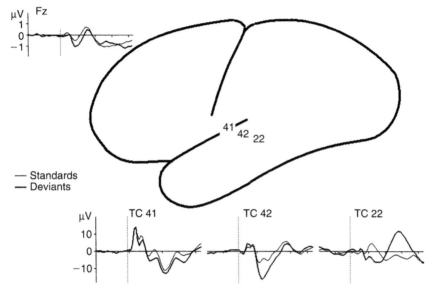

FIGURE I.6   Event-related potentials recorded from scalp and from intracranial electrodes. In the task standard acoustic stimuli (tone of 1000 Hz and 100 ms duration) were sequentially presented at 800 ms intervals and randomly mixed with rare (15 per cent of probability) deviant (tone of 1300 Hz) stimuli. Subjected were reading a book. Note 10 times difference in amplitude between scalp and intracranial recordings. Note also that patterns of responses are different for three auditory cortical areas: Brodmann area 41 – primary auditory area, Brodmann area 42 – secondary auditory area, Brodmann area 22 – association auditory area. Adapted from Kropotov et al. (2000).

D. Association of Local Field Potentials with Scalp EEG

The results of the study depicted in Fig. I.6 demonstrate two things: (1) local field potentials averaged over trials provide detailed knowledge both in time and spatial domains about local operations in cortical neuronal networks; (2) overall responses in local field potentials are reflected on the scalp in ERPs, although in significantly reduced amplitude. Similar inferences can be made regarding spontaneous scalp EEG and intracortical local field potentials. In our laboratory when we studied spontaneous local field potentials recorded with implanted electrodes we were struck by observation that different Brodman cortical areas reveal quit

42 habituated substantially indicating strong memory effects in this area. The most striking responses were produced in the association auditory area 21, which generated an additional potential when the stimulus did not match the repetitive sequence of the previous stimulation. The mixture of these three types of local field potentials seems to be expressed in scalp recorded negative fluctuation labeled as MMN.

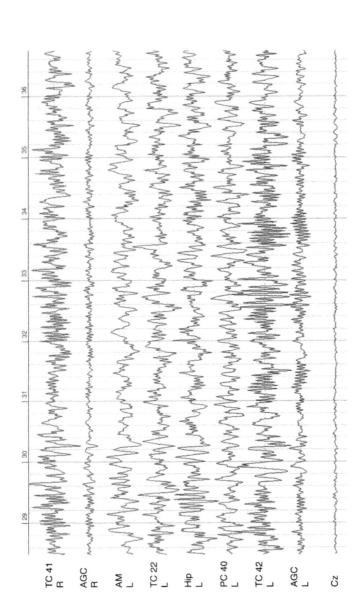

FIGURE I.7 Spontaneous local field potentials and EEG. Spontaneous local field field potentials recorded by means of intracranial electrodes in different brain areas (BA 41, 46, 42, 22, hippocampus, amygdala, anterior cingulate gyrus) in comparison to the scalp EEG recording at Cz. Note, that different areas generate quite different patterns of local field potentials. They are on average 10 times larger than scalp EEG, are quite independent and have different dominant frequencies.

different patterns of oscillations[19]. An example of such recordings in a patient with implanted electrodes is presented in Fig. I.7.

E. Modern Renaissance of EEG

Although EEG was discovered almost 80 years ago the fastest development of this filed was observed only recently. Nowadays we are facing a renaissance of EEG. There are at least four reasons for this: The first reason is related to a recent appearance of new methods of EEG analysis such as spatial filtration techniques in artifact correcting, independent component analysis of ERPs, wavelet analysis, electromagnetic tomography, and some others. The second reason lies in the relative cheapness of modern EEG devices. Indeed, nowadays EEG machines cost from few thousands US dollars to tens of thousands of dollars, which is very small in comparison to multi-million MRI and PET scans. The third reason is a dramatic increase of our knowledge regarding mechanisms of generation of spontaneous EEG waves and functional meaning of ERPs components. The fourth reason is a high temporal resolution of EEG and ERPs signals which principally can not be achieved by other neuroimaging techniques. EEG and ERP provide time resolution of few milliseconds, while PET and MRI are limited by few seconds (Fig. I.8).

IV. ENDOPHENOTYPES AND INDIVIDUAL DIFFERENCES

A. Biological Markers of Disease

The behavior itself can be considered as a set of all possible actions that the subject is able to perform – the repertoire of behavior. As we know from neuroscience, behavior is determined by multiple brain systems playing different roles in planning, execution, and memorization of human actions. These brain systems in turn are determined by genes and their complex interactions with each other and environment. So, in contrast to genotype the behavior can be considered as a phenotype of a subject. In psychiatry biological markers of disease have become known as endophenotypes. The term comes from the Greek word "endos" – interior, within. In another words endophenotype denotes a measurable component along the pathway between phenotype and genotype (Fig. I.9).

---

[19] It seems undisputable that invasive recordings provide detailed information that can not be obtained from scalp potentials. This is the reason why intracranial recordings are so important. They give us insights into pathophysiological mechanisms. For example, until now none of the available animal models of Parkinson's disease accurately reproduces all of the symptoms of the human disease, such as resting tremor, akinesia, and muscular rigidity. Intracranial recording in the human brain fills this missing gap.

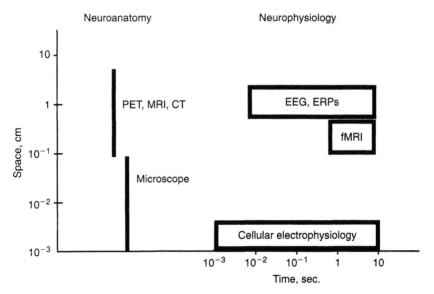

FIGURE I.8   Spatial and temporal resolutions of EEG and other methods. Spatial (Y-axis) and temporal (X-axis) resolutions are depicted as rectangles. Note the absence of time resolution in the techniques of neuroanatomy. Abbreviations: computer tomography (CT), positron emission tomography (PET), magnetic resonance imaging (MRI). Neuroanatomy is associated with different spatial scales. Microscope gives a space resolution lower than the size of the cell (around 30 microns – 3×10^{-3} cm). PET and MRI give much lower spatial resolution than microscope. Neurophysiological parameters include electric and electromagnetic properties of neurons and their networks and are studied by cellular electrophysiology, scalp EEG and ERPs.

Endophenotype is becoming an important concept in the study of complex psychiatric diseases[20].

B. Association with Functioning of Brain Systems

An endophenotype may be neurophysiological, biochemical, endocrinological, neuroanatomical, or neuropsychological in nature. Endophenotypes represent simpler clues to genetic mechanisms than the behavioral symptoms. The whole idea of introducing this concept is based on assumption that a more correct psychiatric diagnose can be made using the knowledge about brain systems (such as executive system) and brain operations (such as action selection, and action monitoring)

[20]The term was coined in 1966 and applied in psychiatry by Gottesman and Shileds in 1972 (for a review see Gottesman and Gould, 2003). Endophenotype is gradually substituting other semantically similar terms such "biological marker," "vulnerability marker" and "subclinical trait."

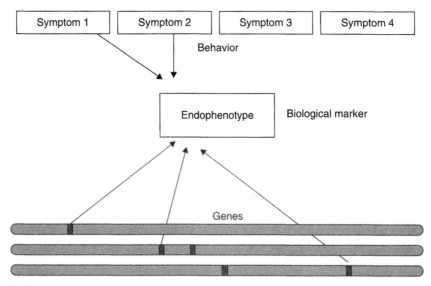

FIGURE I.9   Endophenotype as a biological marker of genetic expression in the behavioral pattern. Genes are responsible for production of specific peptides that define functioning of specific brain systems. The dysfunctioning of the brain system is associated with specific symptoms. The biological maker or endophenotype is a parameter that reflects functioning of the brain system.

associated with certain psychological processes. For example, impairment in action selection operation might be the core of some type of schizophrenia. Consequently, the aim of a modern biologically oriented psychiatry would be to find a biological marker of this operation and show that it is selectively impaired in schizophrenia. Functional MRI, EEG, and cognitive ERPs has been recently used for imaging neuronal circuits involved in brain diseases such as depression, schizophrenia, and ADHD.

C. Inverted U-Law

People are different. Behavioral responses of different people may be different in the same situation: some of us are almost always happy, some are prone to depressed moods; some of us are good in visual processing, some are much better in auditory processing; some of us never forget things, some of us do not remember what we ate yesterday[21] ... In this book we present a theory according to

---

[21]In chemistry the difference between chemical elements was recognized, and much of the effort in 19th century was spent in constructing Mendeleev's periodic table – a classification system of elements. In psychology the foundations of classification of personalities was laid down by Pavlov at the beginning of the 20 century and later in 1950 by Eysenk and his followers.

which the brain is divided into several functions systems, playing different roles in organization of behavior: sensory system, affective system, executive system, memory systems, and attentional networks. Each of the brain systems can be considered as a neuronal network with a complex structure. Neuronal elements in this structure receive multiple inputs and transfer them into action potentials (spikes). The transfer operation performed by a neuron (output versus input) represents a non-linear relationship described by a sigmoid function. Similarly, the transfer function of a neuronal net as a whole can be also described by the sigmoid function presented in Fig. I.10. The shape of this function actually means that (1) the neuronal network is poorly activated by a low input because the inputs in majority of neurons do not exceed thresholds, (2) the neuronal network changes activity almost linearly to a moderate input, and (3) the activation of the neuronal network reaches a plateau at higher levels of input – a so-called "ceiling" effect. We can further suggest that the performance of the system is defined by the ability of the system react to a small change in the input. Mathematically, the performance of the system is defined by the first derivative dO/dI (Fig. I.10). The first derivative is represented by a so-called inverted U shape. In psychophysiology it is known as Yerkes-Dodson Law[22].

As one can see in Fig. I.10 the neural network is characterized by two parameters: the level of activation, that is, input signal which drives the system, and the responsiveness of the system, that is, reaction of the system to a small change in the input. In neurophysiological studies these two parameters are usually named tonic and phasic activities. We speculate that for the brain tonic and phasic activities have two different functional meanings, the one associated with the state and the other with the response. For example, for attentional network the tonic activity can be associated with non-specific arousal, while the phasic activity can be associated with selective attention[23].

D. Pavlov's, Eysenk's and Current Theories of Personality Differentiation

Interindividual variation seems to be defined by differences in overall activation of the brain systems. As one can see from Fig. I.9 the "position" of the brain system on the input/output curve determines the tonic level of activation of the

---

[22] The Yerkes-Dodson law was formulated by psychologists Robert M. Yerkes and J.D. Dodson in 1908. The law describes an empirical relationship between arousal and performance. It says that the performance increases with the level of arousal only to a certain point: when the level of arousal becomes too high, the performance decreases.

[23] As will be shown below, the tonic overall input to the attention system is regulated by the level of noradrenalin, a peptide synthesized in the locus coeruleus of the brain stem, while the phasic activity is determined by a sensory stimulus attracting attention.

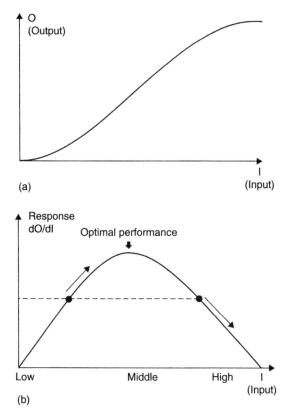

FIGURE I.10   The inverted U-law. (a) Schematic representation of the dependence of the overall activity of a hypothetical neuronal network on the input which drives the system. (b) Schematic representation of the dependence of the response of the system on its input. The response is defined as a reaction of the system to a small and elementary increase of the input.

system (such as arousal for attentional system) and a responsiveness of the system (such as attentional demand or load). For a particular brain system all subjects can be represented as dots on the inverted U-curve and can be also divided into three groups: Low, middle and high depending on the position on the curve. The subjects in these three groups react differently to a small unit increase in the corresponding input. The highest, and optimal, reactions are produced by the "middle" group. The low and high groups react similar with smaller (non-optimal) reactions but behave differently when the input level is increasing. The "low" group becomes better in response to agents elevating the level of the system input while the "high" group gets worse in performance. The agents that increase the input level may be associated with the stressful environmental factors, or with concentration of mediators in the brain stem ascending activation system of the brain.

During the times of Pavlov and Eysenk physiological foundation of individual differences was poorly understood. Pavlov used conditioned reflexes as a physiological parameter for discriminating types of nervous system, while Eysenk used reaction times as indicators of the speed of information processing. In 1960s, introduction of ERPs as indexes of stages of information flow opened new horizons. The first indication that subjects can be objectively divided into two groups came from research of relationship between the amplitude of N1/P2 complex in auditory evoked potentials and loudness of the auditory stimulus. Two groups, augmenters and reducers were separated: subjects from the first group increased amplitude of their ERPs with increase of intensity of the auditory signal, while subjects from the second group showed more shallow loudness dependence.

The most influential theory of personality differentiation is dividing people into extraverts and intraverts[24]. This theory (first suggested by Eysenk himself) associates the division with the level of arousal in the attentional system: extraverts having lower level of arousal[25]. The theory was recently tested in ERP experiments. The late positive component, named P300, served as indicator of reactivity of the cortex in response to attended stimuli. In agreement with the arousal theory of extraversion, introverts showed larger P300 to attended stimuli than extraverts (Beauducel et al., 2006).

Studies in EEG and ERPs have traditionally treated individual differences as unwanted statistical noise. Yet the individual differences exhibit a remarkable stability within individual subjects, suggesting that they are not just random fluctuations but rather reflect personality traits. To differentiate the interindividual differences from deviations from normality normative databases of QEEG and ERP are traditionally used.

---

[24] The notions of extraversion and introversion were used by C.G. Jung to explain different attitudes people use to direct their energy. If a subject likes to spend time in the outer world of people and things he belongs to extraversion type. He gets his energy from active involvement in events and having a lot of different activities. He's excited when he is around people and likes to energize other people. He often understands a problem better when he can talk out loud about it and hears what others have to say. If the subject prefers the inner world of ideas and images he belongs to introversion type. According to Hans Eysenk the ascending activation system determines how one reacts. If the activity of this system is low, the person needs more stimulation and belongs to extroversion type. If the activity is high, there is too much stimulation of the cortex and the person belongs to introversion type. Thus, introverts show stimulus aversion, and extroverts show stimulus hunger.

[25] The other idea of classifying different subjects is associated with the affective system. It presumes existence of three dimensions – three temperamental components such as negative affectivity (NA), positive affectivity (PA), and constraint (for a review see: Whittle et al., 2006). Inhibition, avoidance, and punishment sensitivity are heightened in individuals high on NA. These individuals have a propensity to experience a wide range of negative moods such as fear, anxiety, sadness, and guilt. Individuals high on PA have an active engagement in the world through high approach and reward sensitivity, and have a propensity to experience a wide range of positive moods such as joy, happiness, enthusiasm, and pride. Constraint refers to an individual's degree of control over impulses and emotions, their ability to direct attention and delay gratification. Individuals high on this dimension may be described as diligent, persistent, reliable, and responsible.

V. PHARMACO-QEEG

A. Goals

The idea that QEEG may be applied in pharmacology as an index of brain functioning in response to pharmaceutical agents was born in the early 1960s. At the beginning the goal was quite modest: to find a new functionally oriented method that would classify drug effects as alternative to structural methods based on chemical similarities between substances. During the last 50 years we faced a fast growth of studies in the field, foundation of the International Pharmaco-EEG society (IPEG) in 1980[26] followed by annual meetings of this society. It was shown that different classes of pharmaceutical agents affect spatial–temporal parameters (in a form of spectral maps) of background EEG differently[27]. However individual QEEG profiles for different classes of drugs often overlapped with each other due probably to three different reasons: (1) inappropriate extraction of parameters of QEEG with meaningful functional significance, (2) large interindividual differences that are probably exhibited in existence of several classes of QEEG patterns, (3) nature sharing of effects of distinct classes of drugs.

It was shown that some psychotropic drugs had EEG effects opposite to the EEG effects of the mental disorders treated with these drugs (key–lock principle). A parameter closely measuring the local metabolic activity and named concordance was invented[28] and was successfully used for predicting the response of patients to antidepressants. ERP components such as P300 were also used as parameters to monitor the efficacy of treatment of patients with schizophrenia and dementia.

B. Limitations

However in spite of this progress pharmaco-EEG until recently remained an empirical method with poor theoretical background and without any significant effect on drug industry and on clinical application. Hurdles that limit the use of pharmaco-EEG were associated with poor understanding of the mechanisms of EEG rhythms, components of ERPs, and poor methods of extracting the adequate information from the available data. One of the intentions of the present book is to lessen these

---

[26]The IPEG is an association of scientists involved in electrophysiological brain research in preclinical and clinical pharmacology, neurotoxicology, and related areas of interest. Goals of the IPEG are(1) t o act as a discussion platform for academic, and industrial research scientists as well as clinicians involved in pharmaco-EEG research, (2) to promote the use of electroencephalography for brain research in preclinical and clinical pharmacology and related fields, (3) to put forward guidelines on relevant aspects of pharmaco-EEG studies.

[27]The effect is measured as the change in QEEG parameters in contrast to placebo.

[28]The studies were made in UCLA.

hurdles: (1) to present new concepts regarding mechanisms of generation of different EEG rhythms; (2) to present recently developed methods of QEEG assessment such as s-LORETA, spatial filtration of artifacts, neurometrics… (3) to describe physiological meaning of ERPs independent components extracted by recently developed method of independent component analysis; (4) to present techniques that allow measuring reliable[29] parameters of brain electrophysiology.

C. New Horizons

In addition to maps of EEG spectra, ERP components have been also used in assessing the effects of pharmacological agents. The application was quite limited and confined mostly by N1/P2 and P3 components in auditory evoked potentials[30]. In this line of research, the serotoninergic system in depression was assessed the loudness dependence of auditory N1/P2 component, while for monitoring the cholinergic system P3b component was applied. The results are very promising. A new method of decomposition of raw ERPs into independent components makes this approach even more powerful and opens new horizons in pharmaco-EEG. The point is that the size effect of ERPs components in differentiation of psychiatric disorders seems to be bigger than the size effect of spectral amplitudes. The methodology implemented in the Human Brain Institute Database, described in the following chapters, provide a tool for the future research (Fig. I.11).

VI. PREREQUISITES FOR NEUROTHERAPY

A. Neurofeedback

Application of spectral analysis to EEG shows that in some brain dysfunctions the EEG amplitude in certain frequency bands significantly differs from the EEG amplitude computed for a group of healthy subjects[31]. Neurofeedback provides a tool for correcting such deviation from normality. Neurofeedback is based on three scientific facts. First, EEG parameters reflect brain dysfunction in a particular disease. Second, subject can voluntarily change the state of his/her brain so

---

[29]Reliability is a critical issue that limits application of EEG. The point is that the brain is a "noisy computer" which extracts the needed information from the background noise. The noisy processor produces noisy electrical currents. To achieve an appropriate signal to noise ratio several approaches in EEG and ERPs have been suggested.

[30]See a recent review on ERPs in neuropsychopharmacology by Pogarell et al. (2006).

[31]For example, a relatively large group of children with ADHD reveals an excess of the theta/beta ratio in central–frontal leads. This EEG abnormality is associated with hypo activation of frontal lobes.

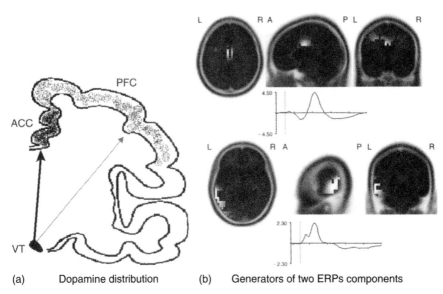

(a)   Dopamine distribution   (b)   Generators of two ERPs components

FIGURE I.11   Basis for pharmaco-ERPs (example). (a) Cortical distribution of dopamine arising from the ventral tegmentum of the brain stem. The densest distribution of dopamine is the anterior cingulate cortex. (b) Two of many components in ERPs in response to NOGO stimuli in the two stimulus GO/NOGO paradigm: top – monitoring P400 component generated by the anterior cingulate cortex (s-LORETA image and time dynamics), bottom – comparison P200 component generated by the occipital–temporal area. The P400 component can be used as an index of functioning of the anterior gyrus cingulus in the neuropsychopharmacology.

that changes can be associated with increasing or decreasing the parameter (see Fig. I.12 left). Third, the brain can memorize this new state and keep it for longer time not only in lab conditions but also in other environments, such as school, home. Historically neurofeedback was the first time applied in clinical practice for treatment epileptic patients. Its application was preceded by a solid research made in laboratories on cats. Later, neurofeedback was applied for correcting behavior of ADHD children. Nowadays this approach is used for a variety of brain dysfunctions.

It should be noted that spectral parameters of EEG are not the only physiological parameters that reflect functioning of the brain. A priory such parameters might be as follows: event-related de/synchronization (ERD/ERS) as measures of reactivity of the EEG rhythms, components of ERPs as measure of stages of information flow in neuronal networks of the brain, infra-slow potentials of the brain, fMRI signals and others measures of hemodynamic/metabolic activity of the brain. These parameters can be fed back to the subjects and, consequently, can be used for voluntary control of brain functions.

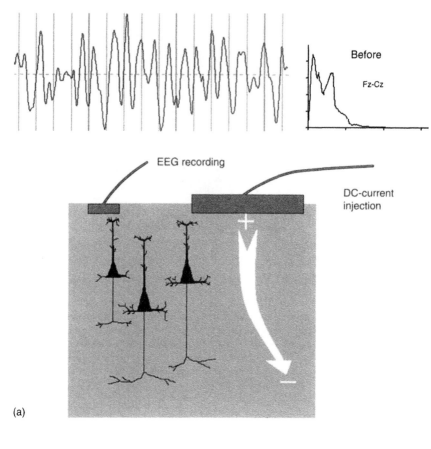

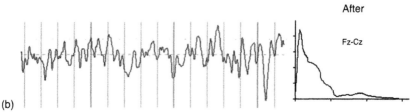

FIGURE I.12   Scheme of neurofeedback and DC stimulation. (a) An example of EEG in an ADHD children recorded from an electrode on the scalp. A power spectrum is computed and compared with the database (not shown). The neurofeedback parameter is computed and presented on the screen to the patient. The patient is able to suppress theta activity and to enhance beta activity in EEG (b). The same result can be achieved by depolarizing pyramidal neurons by injecting DC directly through a metal electrode placed on the skin of the head.

B. Brain–Computer interface

The feedback of electrophysiological parameters can be used not only for self-regulation of the brain but can be applied for communication with the external world as well as for manipulation of technical devices such prostheses and microprocessors. This type of biofeedback applications is named as Brain–Computer Interface (BCI). Usually the BCI requires the learning stage during which the subject learns to control his physiological parameters (such as EEG or ERPs) of the brain.

C. Transcranial Direct Current Stimulation

Our knowledge about brain functioning can be summarized in two postulates: information processing is expressed in fast action potentials of neurons[32] while modulation of this processing is expressed in more slow oscillations of potential. We also know that some psychological operations such as attention or motor preparations are associated with infra-slow shifts of scalp recorded electrical potentials. It is logically to suggest that direct injection of electric currents into the neuronal networks would modulate brain functioning. There are several methods of doing it. One simple way is to inject direct current with a goal to change polarization of cortical neurons. Application of anodal or cathodal electrical currents oriented along direction of apical dendrites of pyramidal cells of the cortex can change membrane potentials of pyramidal cells near their axon hillocks and, consequently, change the probability of neurons to fire in response to some external natural stimuli[33] (Fig. I.12 right). As shown in numerous studies the anodal transcranial direct current stimulation (tDCS) serves as activation procedure while the cathodal tDCS has an opposite effect[34]. The DC stimulation was introduced into laboratories in 1960s. In those days it was named micropolarization technique. The first positive results were challenged by success in psycho-pharmacology. Financial funding of DC-stimulation research in the west was dropped and for two decades the former USSR[35] remained the only place where the studies were continued. Nowadays we face a renaissance of the method. Recently, it was applied for rehabilitation of stroke patients. In our neurotherapy clinic of the Institute of the Human Brain of Russian Academy of Sciences we are using this method for children with ADHD and with speech delay.

---

[32]Recall, that duration of each action potential is just 1 ms.

[33]These changes are associated with increase or decrease of cortical excitability.

[34]In 1970s in our laboratory we were looking for a simple procedure that would temporally activate or suppress impulse activity of neurons near implanted electrodes. It was shown that application of direct current could provide such a procedure. Professor Bechtereva was the first to suggest this idea.

[35]One good side of the USSR science system in previous years was that a scientist got the salary irrespectively of what he or she was doing and most of the scientists did what they wanted to do.

D. TMS, DBS, and Other Stimulation Procedures

It should be stressed here that electrophysiologically based methods of brain modulation are not confined by direct current stimulation and neurofeedback. Neurotherapy as a set of methods also includes transmagnetic stimulation (TMS), AC electrical stimulation, electro convulsive therapy (ECT), deep brain stimulation (DBS) and some others. The basic idea of all these methods is to stimulate (or suppress) neurons in the corresponding cortical areas by means of using electromagnetic fields.

PART I

EEG Rhythms

*One of the most basic laws of the universe
is the law of periodicity*

György Buzsáki, Rhythms of the brain

I. INTRODUCTION

New insights in the field of electroencephalogram (EEG) discovered during the last few decades dramatically changed classical postulations which psychiatrists and neurologists used to learn in medical schools. These classical postulations presume that information processing in the human brain is carried out by impulse (spike) activity of single neurons. Oscillations of electrical events (such as EEG rhythms) were usually discarded and ignored, in the worst case, or considered as a background activity, in the best case. For example, in the fourth edition of "Principles of Neuroscience" edited by Eric Kandel, James Schwartz, and Thomas Jessel – the book that is considered as the bible for neuroscientists – electrical oscillations in EEG were missing and the chapter "The Collective Electrical Behavior of Neurons: the Electroencephalogram and the mechanisms of Epilepsy" by John Martin present in the third edition was discarded.

During the last few years the situation is slowly changing. Now we are facing the renascence of EEG. This renascence is associated with appearance of new methods in human EEG assessment and new experimental findings in animal research which allowed electrophysiologists to discover that alterations in oscillatory patterns of EEG play a critical role in maintenance of brain functions and consequently may be used as a powerful tool for diagnosis of brain dysfunctions.

From a general point of view, oscillations are present in all physical and biological systems trying to achieve the equilibrium. In almost all cases of oscillations emerge when the system is controlled by two opposite processes: the one that drives the system from the equilibrium and the one that returns it back. In this respect, EEG oscillations do not differ from oscillations in other biological systems. In the case of any observable EEG rhythm (such as alpha, beta, or theta) we always find a force that drives the neuron or the neuronal network from their equilibrium and a force that returns them back.

However, oscillations may be not only the reflection of two opposite forces in the neuronal networks but, hypothetically, can also serve as the source of combining factor in organization of neuronal networks. For example, changes in the overall local field potential created by the neurons – generators of this rhythm may entrain other neurons that do not participate directly in generation of the rhythm. This entraining synchronizes activity of all neurons of the neuronal network with the rhythm generators. In spite of several attempts to prove this suggestion, we still do not know whether it is correct or not.

This part of the book deals with EEG rhythms in frequency range from 0 to 70 Hz. The band covers several categories of electrical phenomena recorded from the scalp. These bio-electrical phenomena are conventionally divided into the following types: direct current (DC) shifts, decosecond oscillations, and slow waves, delta, theta, alpha, and beta EEG rhythms (Fig. PI.1). It should be stressed here that the notion of rhythm presumes that rhythm represents regular changes in electric potential measured by electrodes from the scalp. When Fourier or wavelet transforms are applied to EEG recordings containing rhythms these rhythms appear at the corresponding spectra in a form of peaks.

Recording of deco-second oscillations needs special amplifies. The deco-second oscillations are usually discarded in conventional EEG. Delta

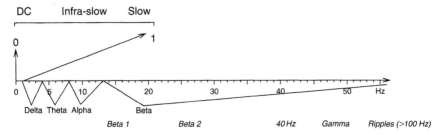

FIGURE PI.1   Frequency bands in EEG spectrum. The frequencies boundaries are not strictly determined. However usefulness of this classification was proved during the whole history of EEG.

rhythms cover the frequency range from 1 to 4 Hz, theta rhythms from 4–8 Hz, alpha rhythms from 8–13 Hz, and beta rhythms – frequency higher than 13 Hz. Theta, alpha, and beta rhythms are present in normal EEG recorded in resting (eyes closed or eyes open) state and in different task conditions. Delta rhythms in the normal brain are expressed on the spectrograms in a form of peaks only during the state of deep sleep. Although basic EEG rhythms are known since Berger's time in late 1920s their neurophysiological basis began to be elucidated only recently starting approximately at 1980s.

It should be stressed that EEG is a sensitive parameter of subject's state and EEG rhythms change dramatically when the subject falls asleep and transfers from one stage of sleep to another. For example, at stage II specific oscillations called sleep spindles emerge. Sleep spindles disappear while theta and delta rhythms develop at further stages of sleep. During wakefulness, rhythms can be a sensitive measure of brain responses to different psychological tasks. For example, occipital alpha rhythms are suppressed (desynchronized) while frontal beta rhythms are enhanced (synchronized) in response to behaviorally meaningful visual stimuli.

In the diseased brain normal mechanisms of EEG rhythms may be impaired and the rhythms may (1) become slower in frequency (so-called EEG slowing), (2) may appear in unusual places (e.g., alpha rhythms at temporal areas), (3) may become higher in amplitude (the phenomenon called hypersynchronization) and in more synchronicity with other areas (the phenomenon called hypercoherence), (4) in some severe cases (characterized e.g., by disconnection of cortical areas from subcortical structures due to stroke, trauma, or tumor) a separate slow rhythm in delta frequency (1–3 Hz) may appear. In some cases normal synchronization mechanisms may be enhanced and spike or spike/slow wave patterns appear indicating a so-called focus in the human brain which in some situations may cause a seizurer. Normative databases help an electroencephalographer to recognize those abnormal patterns and to assess the level of statistical significance of the abnormality. 3D location of generators of EEG rhythms can be assessed by different techniques such as dipole approximation and low resolution electromagnetic tomography (LORETA).

II. GLOSSARY

10–20 International system of electrode placement was accepted internationally in 1959. The name comes from the fact that any electrode is 10 or 20 percent of some distances from another.

Alpha rhythms are rhythmic activities in EEG recorded from the cortex of primary or secondary sensory areas during eyes open or eyes closed rest conditions and suppressed in response to activation of these areas. In EEG of healthy subjects alpha rhythms are found in posterior regions (occipital and parietal areas) and over the sensory motor strip (mu or sensory-motor rhythms) within the frequency range from 8 to 13 Hz. Alpha frequencies change with age: younger and older subjects have lower alpha frequencies.

Amplifier is a basic component of any EEG machine (or electroencephalograph). It amplifies a week (30–100 μV) EEG signal. 1 μV = 0.000001 V.

Barbiturates are pharmaceutical substances that bind to so-called "sedative–hypnotic" sites at $GABA_A$ receptors and promote opening of Cl^- ion channels. They belong to a class of GABA agonists. They are used as a sleeping medication, for example, to induce anesthesia before surgery as well as minor tranquilizers or antianxiety medication.

Beta band is a band beyond 13 Hz in EEG and MEG recordings. Sometimes, beta band is divided into smaller categories: low beta band (*beta 1*) from 13 to 21 Hz, high beta band (*beta 2*) from 21 to 30 Hz, and *gamma* frequency band for frequencies higher than 30 Hz.

Bispectral index (BIS) of the EEG is an empirical, statistically derived variable that provides information about the interaction of brain cortical and subcortical regions. BIS, which is expressed as a score between 0 and 100, is a consistent and reliable index of state of consciousness in normal subjects, with scores of 95 or greater typically indicating full consciousness.

Brodmann area is a region in the human cortex defined on the basis of its organization observed in microscope when a tissue is stained for nerve cells. Brodmann areas were originally defined in 1909 by a German neurologist Korbinian Brodmann and referred to by numbers from 1 to 52.

Burst of spikes is two or more discharges of a neuron followed by a period of quiescence. The burst mode of thalamic cells is generated in response to long hyperpolarization due to a rebound Ca^{++} spike. The bursts of cortical cells are induced in response to depolarizing injected currents.

Calcium spike is a rebound depolarization of the thalamo-cortical cells following strong hyperpolarization of the neurons. It is generated by a transient low threshold Ca^{++} current (I_t), ion current that is inactivated when the neuron is depolarized and becomes deinactivated during the hyperpolarization state.

Coherence is a measure of synchronization between EEG recorded in different scalp locations. It reflects a correlation between EEG powers computed for these two locations in the same frequency band.

Common average reference montage is a computational montage in which electrodes' potentials are measured in reference to "common average" potential, that is, a potential averaged over all electrodes.

Common Mode Rejection (CMR) defines the ability of a differential amplifier to be as close to the ideal (the output is zero when $V_1 = V_2$) as possible. It is expressed as ratio of the output signal when $V_1 = V_2$ (they are connected to the same source) to the output signal when only one input is non-zero. CMR is measured in dB.

Contingent negative variation (CNV) is a negative slow (with time constant of about seconds) shift in electrode potential associated with preparatory activity of the subject, such as preparation to receive a stimulus or to make a motor response.

DC potentials *are* potentials recorded from the scalp by non-polarizable electrodes (such as silver–silver chloride electrodes) in the frequency range from 0.04 to 0.16 Hz.

Delta rhythm (cortical) is EEG rhythm generated by intracortical thalamic mechanisms. It dominates in the EEG when the cortical area is disconnected from the corresponding thalamic nucleus.

Delta rhythm (thalamic) is EEG rhythm generated in the thalamus and recorded from the scalp by interplay of two ion currents in the thalamo-cortical neurons: a cation current that depolarizes the membrane potential, and a transient low threshold Ca^{++} current responsible for generation of so-called Ca^{++} spikes.

Depolarization is a decrease in neuronal membrane potential usually caused by cation (Na^+ and Ca^{++}) inward currents associated with opening of the corresponding ion channels in membrane. The potential changes caused by these currents are named excitatory postsynaptic potentials (EPSP).

Differential amplifier amplifies the difference between two input potentials V_1 and V_2.

ERD/ERS stands for event-related desynchronization/synchronization. It is a parameter that measures the percentage of decrease/increase of the EEG power in a given frequency band in a given time interval in response to a given event.

Excitatory neurons are neurons that when spiking generate a so-called excitatory postsynaptic potential which depolarizes (makes it less polarizable) the postsynaptic membrane and consequently, drives the membrane potential toward the threshold of action potential and increases the probability of action potential discharge. Glutamate serves as a fast excitatory mediator in many cortical neurons.

Forward problem is a problem of calculating the scalp potential of a single dipole or a set of dipoles located within the cortex. The forward solution can be expressed in a physical equation and numerically solved by computers.

Hebb's law is the law formulated by Donald Hebb in 1949 to identify a possible way for forming new memories. According to the law, if presynaptic neuron A is active (exhibits neuronal discharges) and a postsynaptic neuron B is active, then the synapse AB will be strengthen.

High frequency filter is analog or digital filter that suppresses lower frequencies in EEG signal and leave the higher frequencies intact. The filter is characterized by low cut in seconds.

Hippocampal theta rhythm is rhythmic activity from 3 to 10 Hz found in mammalian hippocampus and interconnected anatomical structures.

Human frontal midline theta rhythm is spontaneous or task related short bursts of rhythmic (from 5.5 to 8.5 Hz) activity over the frontal leads with maximum at Fz. This is the only normal theta rhythm in the human adult brain. This rhythm is synchronized in response to behaviorally important events and is associated with operations such as recalling from memory or encoding memory traces.

Hyperpolarization is an increase in neuronal membrane potential. The increase is usually caused by anion (such as Cl^-) inward currents associated with opening of the corresponding ion channels in membrane. The potential changes caused by this current are named inhibitory postsynaptic potentials (IPSP).

Independent Component Analysis (ICA) is a method of solving the blind source separation problem. In EEG the problem can be formulated as finding independent cortical generators of potentials recorded at the scalp.

Infra-slow activity is a type of EEG activity which can be recorded only by special (so-called DC) amplifiers and includes oscillations with periods from few seconds to few tens of seconds. The mechanism of their generation is unknown but the association with slow metabolic processes of the brain is hypothesized.

Inhibitory neurons are neurons that when spiking generate a so-called inhibitory postsynaptic potential which hyperpolarizes (makes it more polarizable) the postsynaptic membrane and consequently, drives the membrane potential away from the threshold of action potential and decreases the probability of action potential discharge. Gamma-aminobutyric acid (GABA) serves as a fast inhibitory mediator in many cortical neurons.

Inverse problem is a problem of finding multiple elemental dipoles in the cortex (sometimes named density of neuronal generators) that approximate potentials recorded by multiple scalp electrodes. Theoretically this problem does not have a unique solution, that is, a certain scalp distribution can be achieved by infinite number of cortical distributions.

Local average reference montage is a computational montage in *which a* local average potential is averaged over a small number of electrodes in the vicinity of a target electrode and is subtracted from the potential of the target electrode. There are several types of local average montages (Laplacian, Lemos, Hjorth).

Long-term potentiation (LTP) is the increase of synaptic strength between two neurons induced by high frequency stimulation of presynaptic terminals.

Low frequency filter is analog or digital filter that suppresses higher frequencies in EEG signal and leave the lower frequencies intact. The filter is characterized by high cut in Hz.

Montage is a rule according to which EEG potentials are computed. The simplest rule (linked ears montage) is measuring electrodes' potentials in reference to two linked electrodes located at left and right earlobes.

Non-polarizable electrode is an electrode that is not easily polarizable. It means that if you apply a current through an electrode, the potential of the electrode will not change significantly from its equilibrium potential. Silver–silver chloride electrode is an example of non-polarizable electrode.

Notch filter is a very sharp filter that attenuates a certain frequency in the signal. In EEG a notch filter at 50 (60) Hz is used to filter out the noise from the electrical system in the room.

Polarizable electrode is an electrode that is easily polarizable. It means that if you apply a current through an electrode, the potential of the electrode will change significantly from its equilibrium potential. Gold electrode is an example of polarizable electrode.

Polarographic method of measuring extracellular oxygen is a method of measuring oxygen in living tissues, in which an electric current induced by application of -0.63V is proportional to the concentration of extracellular oxygen.

Reaction of desynchronization corresponds to suppression of the corresponding rhythm.

Referential recording is a recording of EEG signal when the second (reference) electrode is usually located on the earlobes, mastoids, or the tip of the nose, that is, far away from the neuronal source. This is in contrast to sequential recording when two electrodes are located on the scalp near EEG generators in the cortex.

Sampling rate is the rate at which raw EEG signal is sampled (quantified). According to Naiquist theorem the sampling rate must be twice as much as the highest possible frequency of recorded EEG signal.

Slow waves of sleep is an EEG activity in a frequency range less than 1 Hz but higher than 0.3 Hz which dominates in EEG during deep sleep. This type of activity is generated by cooperative mechanisms in the recurrent cortical circuits and includes periodic fluctuations between UP and DOWN states.

Spectra are computed by means of fast Fourier transformation that decomposes EEG signals into series of sinusoidal functions with different frequencies, amplitudes, and phases. Spectra show how amplitude, power or phase of the sinusoidal harmonic depends on the sinusoid's frequency in the EEG signal.

Thalamus is a subcortical brain structure that controls the flow of sensory information to the posterior parts of the cortex through sensory-related nuclei and regulates activity in the prefrontal areas though a distinct set of nuclei.

Thalamo–cortical neurons are neurons of the thalamus that project to the corresponding cortical area and receive back the excitatory connections from this area.

Theta band in EEG is a band from 4 to 8 Hz.

Vertical organization of the cortex reflects the fact that pyramidal cells of the cortex with their long apical dendrites are oriented perpendicular to the cortical surface with distinct layers playing different roles in receiving inputs and sending outputs.

CHAPTER 1

Slow, Infra-Slow Potentials, and Delta Rhythms

I. ORIGIN OF SCALP POTENTIALS

A. Intracortical Organization

Electrodes placed on the scalp pick up potentials mostly from the cortical (locating near the surface of the head) areas. Here is the right place to describe in detail anatomy and physiology of cortical generators that produce potentials propagating to the surface of the head and measured by scalp electrodes in a form of electroencephalogram (EEG). Neurons with their axons, soma, and dendrites are primary candidates for such generators of potentials. One of the basic principles of the cortical organization is the existence of excitatory and inhibitory neurons in the cortex (Fig. 1.1). These types of neurons are designed by nature to shape up complex operations in the cortical neuronal networks, such as (1) coincidence detection[1], (2) spatial feature extraction[2],

---

[1]Coincidence detection is needed for enhancing signal to noise ratio of a signal processed by the neuronal network. When the inputs to the association cortex from the primary and secondary sensory areas extracting different features of the stimulus coincide in time, the coincidence detector signals that these inputs are not accidental but belong to the same stimulus.

[2]Spatial filtration serves the same function (enhancing signal to noise ratio) as coincidence detection but explores a different mechanism. This mechanism is based on spatial (not temporal as in the case of coincidence detection) integration of inputs coming to a particular neuron from a spatially distributed network. The excitatory and inhibitory inputs form a sophisticated spatial filter. For example, receptive fields of complex cells in the primary visual cortex could be considered as Gabor-like spatial filters while the corresponding operation in the visual system is considered as spatial filtration.

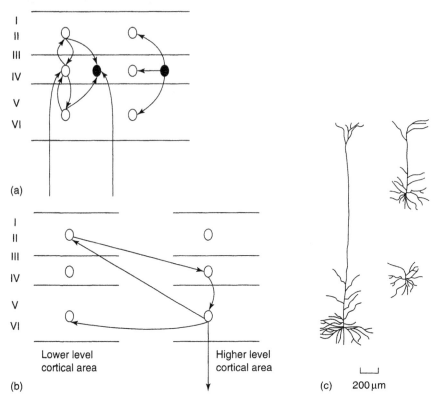

FIGURE 1.1   Organization of cortical connections. (a) Connections of excitatory neurons (depicted by empty circles) and inhibitory neurons (depicted by black circles) in superficial, middle, and deep layers of the cortex. (b) Connections between two cortical areas, the one located at the lower level (depicted at the left) and the one located at the higher level (depicted at the right) of cortical hierarchy. (c) Pyramidal and stellate sells in the cortex.

(3) reverberation of neuronal activity[3], (4) comparing inputs[4], and some other approved and hypothetical operations.

In general terms, excitation and inhibition are balanced within the cortex. In particular, the cortical organization is as follows. Both excitatory and inhibitory

---

[3]Reverberation of signals in the recurrent neuronal networks is needed for maintaining the signal in short-term memory. The theoretical concept of reverberation was known since 1940s but only recently direct neurophysiological evidence was obtained. The critical structural prerequisite for reverberation is the existence of recurrent pathways in neuronal networks of the brain.

[4]Comparing two inputs - the one generated by the expected model of behavior and the one generated by the current situation – plays a critical role in sensory and executive systems. In the sensory system it is needed for change detection, i.e. detection any change in a monotonous sensory stimulation. In the executive system the comparison operation is needed for detection mismatch between the planned action and the action that was actually performed by the subject. Detecting this change in its turn serves for monitoring behavior in general and for correcting errors in particular.

cortical cells receive excitatory inputs from the thalamus. The thalamus in its turn is considered as the gates to the cortex because all the pathways originating in the sensory organs (such as retina, cochlea, nucleus...) are passing through the so-called relay nuclei of the thalamus. The non-relay nuclei of the thalamus receive outputs from the basal ganglia as well as from the primary sensory cortical areas and project to the rest of the cortex. The input to the cortex from the thalamus is most heavily distributed within the middle cortical areas. In addition, inhibitory and excitatory neurons receive feedforward projections from the cortical areas located at a lower level of cortical hierarchy and feedback projections from the cortical areas located at a higher level of cortical hierarchy[5].

The *excitatory neurons* within the local module of the cortex are interconnected with each other forming a reverberation circuit, which is responsible for maintaining local activation for a time period longer than the duration of the stimulus. This process is named "reverberation" and functionally is based on the following local feedforward and feedback processes: when a group of neurons fire it sends the excitatory potentials to neighbor neurons, which fire with some delay and send the excitatory potentials back to the initial group of cells which activate them again (recurrently). This sequence of feedforward and feedback operations leads to avalanche-like behavior and is responsible for maintaining the activation within the local circuit.

The *inhibitory neurons* receive excitatory input directly from the thalamus and indirectly through the surrounding excitatory neurons. The inhibitory neurons are projected back on local excitatory neurons. The inhibitory neurons play at least three important functions. First, the recurrent inhibition does not allow over-excitation of the local cortical circuits. Second, a spatial pattern of distribution of inhibitory cells forms complex receptive fields of neurons in the cortex. Third, a combination of excitation and inhibition can form various types of comparison operations within the cortex.

The excitatory neurons in the cortex are divided into two types: pyramidal cells and stellate cells[6]. Examples of the two types of excitatory neurons are presented in Fig. 1.1. Short dendritic lengths enable the stellate neurons to process incoming signals fast and with high temporal precision. The pyramidal neuron

---

[5]These first-order and high-order thalamo-cortical interconnections, feedforward and feedback intercortical connections as well as local intracortical connections form complex neuronal circuits granting a basis for complex human behavior.

[6]The pyramidal cells have cell bodies that appear like pyramids with dendrites covered by spines. Spiny stellate cells are generally smaller and their cell bodies more resemble a star shape. They also have spiny dendrites which are covered by glutamate receptors. Interneurons (another type of cortical cells) have more rounded cell bodies and have little or no spines on their dendrites. Over the years anatomists have given descriptions to a number of unique subtypes of interneurons and neurons. Among them are chandelier cell (inhibitory cell with axons resembling candlesticks, neurogliaform cells (inhibitory; resembling glial cells), double bouquet cell – (inhibitory with axon collaterals and dendrites extend vertically in a tight bundle, basket cells (inhibitory with axonal branches terminating on pyramidal cells in a manner resembling a basket) and several other types.

differs from the stellate neuron by the presence of a very long, so-called apical, dendrite that is 6 times longer than the basal dendrites. The apical dendrite is oriented perpendicular to the cortical surface. This type of dendrite orientation is called a *vertical organization* in contrast to a horizontal (along the cortical surface) organization. Short dendrites of pyramidal cells extend outward from the soma in virtually all directions and are named the basal dendrites. There is a temptation to suggest that apical dendrites might play a specific function in information process-ing within cortical neuronal networks. This function still remains to be elucidated, but what we know for certain is that long apical dendrites of pyramidal cells of the cortex play a critical role in generation of scalp recorded EEG.

The variety of functions of the cortical inhibition is achieved by diverse classes of inhibitory interneurons, such as the basket, chandelier, double bouquet, neuro-gliaform cells. The axon of these interneurons reveal highly specific geometry and innervation patterns. The cellular mechanisms that specify inhibitory connections are only just beginning to be understood[7].

B. Membrane Potentials

To describe the mechanisms of generating EEG, let us start with description of membrane potentials. As we know from electrophysiology, membrane of neurons is the place where electric potentials are generated. In the resting state the mem-brane of neurons is electrically polarized. The membrane polarization is achieved by an active process, called the $Na^+–K^+$ pump (Fig. 1.2). Beside this pump, membrane potential is determined by functioning of so-called ion channels. The ion channels are pathways for ion movements across membrane. The ion fluxes across membrane form positively and negatively charged surfaces – a membrane potential[8].

In the resting state the membrane potential is negatively charged at the intra-cellular part in comparison to the extracellular part. So, membrane potential of neurons is defined as $V_m = V_{in} - V_{out}$, where $V_{in(out)}$ is the potential at the intra (extra) cellular part of the membrane. In majority of neurons V_m varies between −65 and −75 mV.

Ion channels consist of several different proteins, subunits, the α subunit of which contains the ion conducting pore as well as binding sites for endogenous

---

[7]For a recent review on this topic see paper by Huang, Di Cristo, and Ango (2007).

[8]The flux of ions through the opened ion channels is passive, requiring no waste of metabolic energy. Two forces determine the flux: chemical gradient and electrical potential across the membrane. The chemical gradient forces ions to diffuse from the places with higher concentrations to the places with lower concentrations of the corresponding ion. The positively charged surface of the membrane attracts negative ions called anions and keeps away positive ions called cations, and vice versa. Na^+, K^+, Ca^{++} ions are examples of cations. Cl^- is an example of anions.

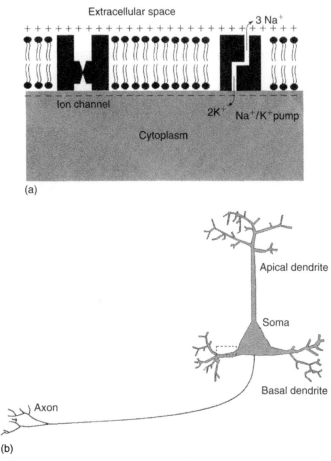

FIGURE 1.2   Main elements in the neuronal membrane. (a) Schematic representation of membrane with double layer of lipids forming membrane, with ion channel and K–Na pump and with external surface (upward) charged by positive ions (cations) and internal surface (downward) charged negatively. (b) Scheme of a pyramidal neuron with names of the basic parts.

ligands such as synaptic neurotransmitters (or artificial molecules such as some pharmaceutical agents). Ion channel, as a protein molecule, has several conformational states that are relatively stable. One of the states is closed state, another one is called inactivated state. In both states the channels do not conduct ions. There are several ways of opening ion channels and each channel has its own way of opening. According to this property ion channels are divided into several groups. The two of these groups are ligand-gated and voltage-gated channels (Fig. 1.3). Ligand-gated channels are opened in response to binding of the ligand (neuro-mediator or hormone) to its receptor on the ion channel. The energy from ligand

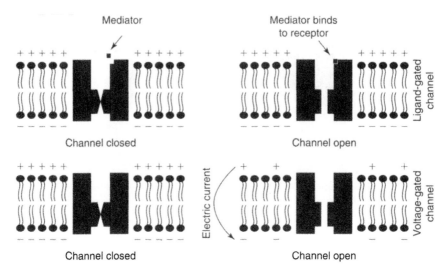

FIGURE 1.3   Ligand and voltage ion gated channels. Ligand-gated channel opens when a mediator molecule (depicted as a square) binds to the receptor part of the channel. Voltage-gated channel opens when the membrane becomes depolarized.

binding opens the channel. Voltage-gated channels open in response of changes in membrane potential and the energy for the opening the channel comes from electrical forces. Ligand-binding channels play a critical role in effects produced by pharmacological agents in treatment of different brain disorders. Voltage-gated channels play a critical role in effects of transcranial direct current stimulation and other electrophysiologically based therapeutic techniques.

More than a dozen basic channel types are known[9]. Each basic type has several subtypes (closely related isoforms) that differ in their rate of opening and closing and sensitivity to different regulation factors of gating. The rich variety of types of ion channel forms the basis for variety of functions of neuronal networks.

C. Synaptic Transmission

When a neuron fires it sends an action potential via the axon to another cell called a postsynaptic neuron. At the synapse, the contact between the two neurons, the action potential releases a mediator. The mediator diffuses into a synaptic

[9]In broad sense, all ligand-gated channels can be divided in two types: excitatory and inhibitory. Excitatory channels while opened ensure the influx of cations (such as N and Ca) inward the neuron and thus depolarize membrane, while inhibitory neurons while opened enable anions (such as Cl) to enter the cell thus hyperpolarizing membrane. Excitatory and inhibitory channels are divided into smaller categories, such as GABA-gated, glutamate-gated, dopamine-gated, and others.

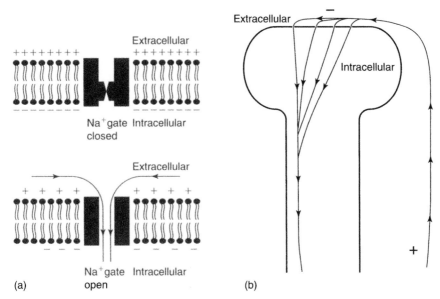

FIGURE 1.4   Ion currents through membrane. (a) Schematic presentation of closed and open Na channel at a dendrite. (b) Arrows indicate current flow in extracellular and intracellular space. Note that the current generates an electric dipole with positive pole at the base of the dendrite.

cleft and binds to a ligand-gated ion channel on the postsynaptic membrane. The channel opens and enables the flux of cations or anions (depending on the type of neurons – excitatory or inhibitory) inward the dendrite. Because the net charge of dendrite is zero, the outward current is generated in the opposite part of the dendrite thus compensating the inward current. This influx of ions inward and outward the dendrite produces a small electric current (Fig. 1.4).

D. Pyramidal Cells as Elemental Electrical Dipoles

The small currents of all dendrites of the same neuron sum up differently in different types of neurons. If a neuron is a stellate cell and excitatory synapses cover many dendrites oriented in different directions, the net current at the level of the cell as a whole will be close to zero and the net potential generated by the stellate cell will be negligible. But, if a neuron is a pyramidal cell and excitatory synapses are located on apical dendrites, the net current of the pyramidal cell will be directed along the apical dendrite and the neuron can be depicted as a small dipole with a negative part at the apical dendrites and with a positive part at the basal part of the neuron (Fig. 1.5). Similarly, if excitatory synapses are activated at

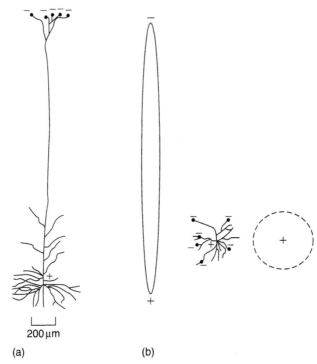

(a)   (b)

FIGURE 1.5   Schematic presentation of electric currents in pyramidal and stellate cells. (a) A pyramidal cell with a long apical dendrite. (b) A stellate cell. In this example the Na inward current is induced by binding molecules of the excitatory mediator glutamate to receptors on dendrites. Note that the currents in the pyramidal cell form a distinct dipole, while the currents in the stellate cell form a zero field outside the cell.

the soma and the basal dendrites of the neuron the neuron becomes a dipole that is charged negatively at the soma and positively at the apical dendrite.

EEG is a result of collective electrical behavior of pyramidal neurons, that is, a sum of hundreds of thousands small dipoles corresponding to those pyramidal cells. The dipoles are induced by local currents that are associated with excitatory and inhibitory postsynaptic potentials. Excitatory postsynaptic potentials depolarize the membrane driving its potential toward the threshold of spike generation and making probability of discharging higher. Inhibitory postsynaptic potentials hyperpolarize membrane, driving its potential from the threshold, and thus decreasing the probability of discharge. The duration of postsynaptic potentials is 10 times longer than duration of a single spike. The duration of postsynaptic potential depends on the type of receptor-mediator coupling, but at least lasts for 20–30 ms which corresponds to 30–50 Hz. The spike duration is about 1 ms which corresponds to 1000 Hz. In addition, the space occupied by synapses where postsynaptic potentials are generated is much larger than the space occupied by axonal hillocks where spike are generated. These two factors make postsynaptic potentials (not impulse activity of neurons) to play a critical role in generation of field potentials recorded at the scalp in 0–70 Hz frequency range.

When recorded by means of a grid of micro-electrodes inserted into the cortex, local field potentials measured at different cortical layers exhibit a clear reversal of potential that occur in the middle layers of the cortex, experimentally demonstrating dipole structure of intracortical potentials. These intracortical dipoles generate potentials at the scalp that can be computed according to the laws of physics. The problem of computing scalp potentials from the known intracortical dipoles is known as the direct problem.

Synchronization of neuronal elements is another factor that defines the electric potential on the scalp. Intuitively, to generate a significant potential at relatively remote distance from the cortical layers neurons must be not only properly oriented, but they must work together, in synchrony. For example, the source area of an epileptic spike, that pop out the background activity, was experimentally estimated of about 2000 mm², while for other elements of EEG a cluster of 40–200 mm² may be sufficient. Anyway the synchronization of neuronal elements over distances of tens of millimeters is a necessary factor for the EEG element to be recorded at the scalp.

II. INFRA-SLOW OSCILLATIONS

A. Spontaneous activity

Infra-slow potentials are measured by special amplifiers with time constant more than 10 s[10] and represent periodic fluctuations of scalp potential with periods from few seconds to few tens of seconds (Fig. 1.6). Although infra-slow potentials were discovered in early 1960 their physiological mechanisms and functional meanings remain unclear until now.

There exists strong empirical evidence indicating that the deco-second oscillations in the human brain might be associated with periodic fluctuations in the metabolic activity of the brain tissue characterized by slow oscillations in extracellular oxygen and local blood flow. In a study that was carried out in our laboratory in 1970s[11], concentration of extracellular oxygen was measured from polarizable (gold) electrodes by a so-called polarographic technique. In this technique

---

[10]Sometimes the amplifiers for measuring infra-slow potentials are called DC amplifiers.

[11]In those years I was working with Parkinsonian patients to whom electrodes were implanted for diagnosis and therapy. Those were patients who did not responds to all conventional forms of treatment and who underwent stereotactic operations. The patients bared electrodes inserted into the basal ganglia, thalamus and the premotor cortex.

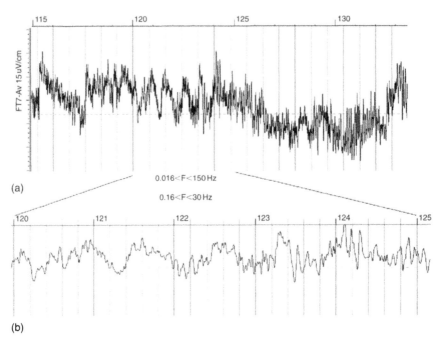

FIGURE 1.6   Infra-slow, slow, and faster EEG rhythms. Example of EEG recorded from FT7 electrode of a normal 19-year old subject in the eyes closed condition. (a) EEG in a wide band from 0.016 Hz (corresponding to 10 s time constant) to 150 Hz. (b) EEG recorded in a "conventional" EEG band from 0.16 to 30 Hz. Note different time scales – 7.5 mm/s for the top record and 30 mm/s for the bottom record.

a small negative voltage (−0.63 V) applied to the gold electrode induces an electrical current that is proportional to the concentration of extracellular oxygen. Examples of spontaneous oscillations of pO_2 are presented in Fig. I.3 from Introduction[12]. Similar oscillations were recorded from the non-polarizable electrodes located on the scalp of human subjects[13]. In a recent joint study from

[12]Recall that these oscillations are of relatively high amplitude with time periods of 30 s (0.03 Hz). They have different patterns in different brain regions and change in response to the tasks performed by subjects.

[13]Infra-slow oscillations became the subject of intensive research in 1970 and 1980 in the former Soviet Union. The pioneers in this field are Nina Aladjalova from Moscow and Valentina Ilukhina from Institute of experimental medicine in St. Petersburg. In Austria similar research was carried out by Herbert Bouer and Gezilher Guttmann from Vienna University. Research in these early years was mostly associated with empirical questions of how the infra-slow oscillations change in psychological tasks and of how they modulate quality of performance of the tasks. In particular, the Austrian group has shown that negative DC shifts were associated with improvement in performance (increase the number of correct responses) while positive shifts of cortical potentials were associated with decline of performance.

Universities of Helsinki (Finland) and Washington (USA) (Vanhatalo et al., 2004) the infra-slow oscillations were found to be strongly synchronized with faster activities in EEG. For example, negative phases of infra-slow oscillations were associated with increase in probability of occurrence of K-complexes and interictal spikes. These new findings support the early views on infra-slow oscillations as a slow, cyclic modulation of cortical gross excitability.

B. Preparatory Activities

Beside infra-slow spontaneous (i.e., not associated with observable behavioral changes) oscillations in cortical potentials there are specific slow brain activities associated with cognitive functions. A good example of "slow" cognitive function is given by a group of various preparatory operations. These operations emerge when in the absence of any behavioral event a subject is preparing to make a movement or to receive a stimulus. Such preparatory operations can last up to several seconds and more. Electrophysiological indexes of such preparatory operations are given by an EEG phenomenon called "contingent negative variation" and first discovered in 1950s by a famous English neurologist Grey Walter.

In 1970 and 1980 the preparatory activities in the human brain were studied by means of electrophysiological methods in Tubengen University in Germany (Brigitte Rockstroh, Niels Birbaumer). The Tubengen theory of preparatory activity can be briefly formulated as follows: when the brain is prepared to receive a stimulus or to make a motor action, apical (the most superficial) dendrites of pyramidal cells receive excitatory inputs from higher cortical areas. The pyramidal cells are thus preset so that information processing in the cortical networks is facilitated. This facilitation was demonstrated by showing improvement of the quality of performance (e.g., the ability to recognize a stimulus presented with near-threshold expositions) during negative shifts of deco-second oscillations.

If the theory is correct, negative shifts of DC potentials have to facilitate paroxysmal activity, such as spikes and spike/slow wave complexes, in the corresponding cortical areas, while the suppression of cortical negativity and increase of positivity might have an opposite effect – suppression of paroxysmal activity. In studies of the Tubengen group (Niels Birmbaum et al.) the attempt was made to use this regulatory function of DC potentials for treatment patients with epilepsy. Epilepsy patients were trained by means of neurofeedback technology to regulate their own slow cortical potentials. The most important finding was that patients with complex partial and secondarily generalized seizures were more likely to experience seizure reduction if they demonstrated good control of their infra-slow cortical potentials at the end of their training.

The other way of exploring regulatory function of DC potentials is expressed in a method of transcranial direct current (DC) stimulation. The method consists of injection of the constant electric current through scalp electrodes (anode and cathode) at very low intensities (below 1 mA). The systematic studies of the method started in 1960 but decayed because of extensive application of pharmacological approach for treatment of brain dysfunctions. We are now facing a renaissance of this method which can be used as an alternative method for activation (or inhibition) of the local cortical activity in treatment of conventional brain disorders (such as OCD, depression) or in rehabilitation of stroke or brain trauma.

III. SLOW WAVES OF DEEP SLEEP

A. Up and Down States

Slow oscillation is a dominant pattern during slow wave sleep and some forms of anesthesia. The frequency of slow oscillations is within 0.3–1 Hz band. Activity in this frequency band is also present during other states such as eyes open, eyes closed, and task conditions. However, the question whether the mechanism of these activities during wakefulness remains the same as during sleep remains to be answered.

The survival of slow oscillations after extensive thalamic lesions indicates that the slow waves are generated within the cortex. The slow wave represents a sequence of UP and DOWN states of a cortical neuronal network. The UP state is characterized by activation (increase of discharge rate) of cortical neurons associated with depolarization of these cells (Fig. 1.7). The activity in the UP state is maintained for about half a second due to a precise balance between excitation

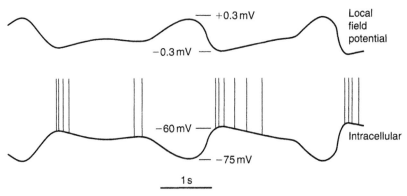

FIGURE 1.7   Local field and intracellular recordings of slow oscillations. Top – slow oscillations in local field potential. Bottom – intracellular recordings. Note that negative shifts in local field potential is associated with increase of spiking activity in neurons – UP state, while positive shifts in local field potential is associated with suppression of neuronal discharges – DOWN state. Note also, the slow oscillations of membrane potential of the neuron are inverse to the local field potentials. Adapted from Haider et al., 2006.

and inhibition within the recurrent neuronal network. The DOWN state is characterized by suppression of impulse activity of neurons associated with hyperpolarization of the cortical neurons. The neuronal mechanism of slow wave remains unknown. One of the hypothetical mechanisms (Bazhenov et al., 2002) suggests that occasional summation of the miniature excitatory postsynaptic potentials during the DOWN state may activate the persistent sodium current and depolarize the membrane above the threshold for spike generation.

Although the slow waves are generated by intracortical mechanisms, the periodic changes between UP and DOWN states group the thalamic electrical patterns (such as delta rhythms and sleep spindles) by means of the cortico-thalamic pathways. Owing to its synchronizing influence on neuronal activity within the neocortex and in a dialogue with thalamic and hippocampal circuitry, the slow oscillation has been suspected to underlie the consolidation of memory during sleep.

B. Transcranial Induction of Slow Waves

Whether slow cortical potentials and their extracellular equivalent have any physiological meaning per se is unclear. The attempt to test this hypothesis has been recently investigated by injecting the extracellular slow oscillating currents (Marshal et al., 2006). The currents were injected in young healthy humans through stimulation electrodes applied bilaterally at fronto–lateral locations and at the mastoids, with the fronto–lateral electrodes representing sites of anodal (positive) polarization (Fig. 1.8a)[14]. It was shown that inducing slow oscillation-like potential fields by transcranial stimulation during early nocturnal non-rapid eye movement sleep enhances the retention memories. The stimulation induced an immediate increase in duration of slow wave sleep and an increase of endogenous cortical slow oscillations and slow spindle activity in the cortex (Fig. 1.8b).

IV. DELTA OSCILLATIONS

Two types of delta oscillations have been separated in human EEG: the first one has a cortical origin while the second one is generated in the thalamus. The neuronal mechanisms of the cortically generated delta rhythm are unknown. The only

---

[14]The transcranially applied currents oscillated at a frequency of 0.75 Hz with maximum current density of 0.5 mA/cm². Stimulation started 4 min after subjects had entered non-REM sleep stage 2 for the first time, that is a time when sleep is expected to progress into the stage with slow waves. Subjects were tested twice, in a stimulation condition and a sham condition. In each condition, in the evening before sleep subjects learned different memory tasks. Recall of memories was tested the following morning. Declarative memory was assessed by a paired-associate learning task consisting of a list of 46 word-pairs to be learned before sleep to a criterion of 60 per cent correct responses in a test of immediate cued recall. At retrieval testing in the morning after sleep, cue words were again displayed and the subjects were required to recall the appropriate response word.

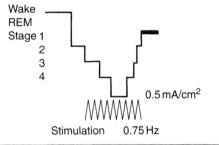

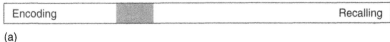

(a)

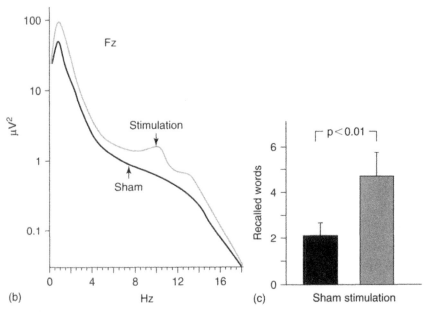

(b)   (c)

FIGURE 1.8   Slow oscillatory stimulation enhances declarative memory performance and increases slow wave activity. (a) Time-course of experiment. Indicated are time points of learning and recall of memory tasks, stimulation intervals, period of lights off (horizontal grey bar), and sleep represented by a hypnogram. W, wake; 1–4, sleep stages 1–4. (b) Performance on the declarative memory task across the retention period of nocturnal sleep for stimulation and sham stimulation. Performance is expressed as difference between the number of correct words reported at recall testing and learning. (c) EEG activity (average power spectra) during intervals between periods of electric stimulation (dark gray) and between corresponding periods of sham (black) at the midline frontal site. Adapted from Marshal et al., 2006.

thing we know is that both surgical removal of the thalamus and disconnection of the cortex from the thalamus result in significant enhancement of delta activity recorded from the scalp. These facts indicate that this type of delta rhythms is generated by intrinsically cortical mechanisms, probably associated with some slow lasting processes within the cortex[15].

A. Delta Rhythm of Sleep

In contrast to cortically generated delta activity, the neuronal mechanisms of thalamically generated delta rhythms are very well known. In intracellular recordings in animal preparations, it was shown that delta rhythm can be generated in a single thalamo-cortical cell, that is, in a thalamic cell projected to the corresponding cortical area. The scheme of thalamo-cortical circuit involved in delta rhythm generation is depicted in Fig. 1.9.

It should be stressed here that the same circuit is involved in generation of spindles (around 13 Hz periodic activity) during sleep and alpha rhythms (around 10 Hz periodic activity) during wakefulness. Those rhythmicities emerge at different levels

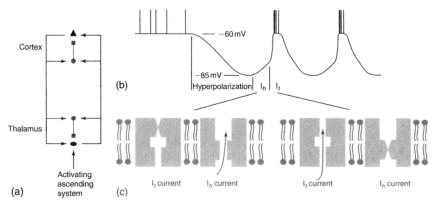

FIGURE 1.9   Generation of delta rhythm in thalamic neurons. (a) Thalamo-cortical neuronal network. Excitatory neurons and excitatory connections are depicted in black. Inhibitory neurons and inhibitory connections are depicted in grey. (b) A shift from depolarization to hyperpolarization is associated with the shift from single spike mode to burst mode. The burst mode is characterized by delta rhythmicity which in turn is a result of interplay of two currents: a cation current I_h that is activated when the neuron is hyperpolarized and a transient low threshold Ca^{++} current I_t that is responsible for generation of Ca^{++} spikes. (c) Opening membrane channels during the first two stages of Ca^{++} spikes.

[15]Delta oscillations might be related to slowly developing synaptic depression. We know that postsynaptic depression can last hundreds of millisecond that corresponds to the delta frequency range. Positive and negative phases of the cortically generated delta oscillation might be associated with synaptic depression that follows the recurrent activation.

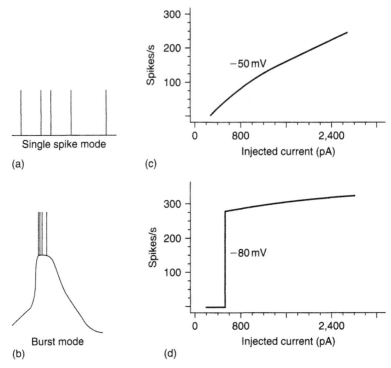

FIGURE 1.10   Tonic and burst modes of thalamo-cortical neurons. (a) Schematic representation of tonic and (b) burst modes of a thalamo-cortical cell. (c) Schematic representation of input–output relationships for a single cell in the two modes. The input variable is the amplitude of the depolarizing current pulse. The output variable is the firing frequency of the cell. The initial holding potentials are –50 mV for the tonic mode and –80 mV for the burst mode.

of polarization of the thalamo-cortical cells: alpha rhythms appear when thalamo-cortical neurons are relative depolarized, sleep spindles appear when these cells are relatively hyperpolarized. Delta rhythms emerge at the deepest level of hyperpolarization of thalamo-cortical neurons.

For generation of sleep spindles and alpha rhythms the networks properties, such as synchronized inhibition from reticular neurons, are needed. In contrast to sleep spindles and alpha rhythms delta waves are generated in single cells. The rhythm is generated by interplay between two intrinsic currents (and consequently two types of ion channels) in the thalamo-cortical neurons (Fig. 1.10).

---

[16]The I_t current is responsible for generation of so called Ca^{++} spikes. The Ca^{++} spike represents a transient inward flow of Ca^{++} ions that depolarizes the membrane of the thalamo-cortical neurons. The I_t is controlled by two gates: activation one and inactivation one. It is activated at –70 mV, so at relatively low threshold and in this association is called low threshold calcium spike. This is in contrast to conventional Na spike which has a higher threshold for activation which corresponds approximately to –50 mV. The other difference between conventional Na spikes and low threshold Ca spikes is the duration of spikes. Duration of Na spikes is 1 ms, while duration of Ca spikes is 50 ms.

The first current is called I_h. It is a cation current that is activated when the neuron is hyperpolarized and, as a consequence, it returns the membrane potential from hyperpolarized state back to a less polarized state. The second current is called I_t. It is a transient low threshold Ca^{++} current[16]. During a depolarization state of the neuron (that is usually found in the state of wakefulness) this current is inactivated. It becomes deinactivated only during the hyperpolarization state. This hyperpolarization state is produced during deep sleep due to the suppression of inputs from ascending activating system of the brainstem as well as due to suppression of inputs from the other brain systems. I_t current is responsible for generating Ca^{++} spikes. On the top of the depolarization phase of the Ca^{++} spike the neuron generates a burst of conventional K^+-Na^{++} spikes. These spikes through the thalamo-cortical pathways are transferred to the corresponding cortical area and generates postsynaptic potentials, which in turn are recorded from the scalp in a form of delta rhythm.

The generation of low threshold Ca^{++} spikes by the I_t current was first demonstrated in thalamic neurons by Rodolfo Llinas in 1984 and also recorded in vivo by Marcelo Steriade and colleagues. A big impact in our understanding cellular mechanisms of EEG was made by David McCormic and his collaborators.

B. Low Threshold Burst Mode of Thalamic Neurons

Delta oscillations are associated with a so-called burst mode of thalamo-cortical cells that emerges only when the thalamo-cortical cells are deeply hyperpolarized. In this mode the relationship between the input and output activity of a single cell represents a step-like function, reflecting the fact the output frequency of thalamo-cortical neuron in this mode does not depend on the injected current (Fig. 1.10b). This mode is quite different from a so-called tonic (or single spike) mode in which thalamo-cortical neurons respond to injecting depolarizing currents in a linear fashion − the larger is the input, the higher is the output spiking.

Rebound Ca spike is not the only way of generating burst mode of spiking. In the cortex a special set of neurons fire in burst mode. The mode may be defined by intrinsic properties of the neuron or by the properties of a neuronal network in which the neuron is embedded. The bursts of cortical cells that are induced by depolarizing currents are quite different from the bursts of the thalamic neurons (both reticular and relay cells) that are induced by hyperpolarizing currents.

C. Pathological Delta Rhythms

Phenomenology of appearance of delta activity in some severe brain abnormalities is quite complicated. In a Chapter of the famous book "Electroencephalography" edited by Ernst Niedermeyer and Fernando Lopes Da Silva titled "Nonspecific abnormal EEG patterns" Frank Sharbrough summarized all known phenomena associated with delta activities into several categories, such as intermittent rhythmic delta activity (IRDA), frontal intermittent rhythmic delta activity (FIRDA), persistent nonrhythmic delta activity (PNDA). For example, focal PNDA is considered as one of the most reliable indications of a local severe cerebral abnormality such as stroke or brain trauma. It should be stressed here that EEG reflects mostly cortical phenomena while the subcortical structures having little input to the scalp EEG. Consequently the cortical location of EEG abnormality and the 3D location of the corresponding brain damage on CT or MRI scans do not necessarily coincide. Moreover, sometimes focal EEG abnormalities are seen without any visible CT or MRI abnormalities and, vice versa, visible brain damage produces small changes in raw EEG. The brain damage related EEG abnormalities become more evident when visual analysis is supplemented by more sophisticated EEG spectral analysis and analysis of event related potentials.

V. SUMMARY

The frequency range below 0.1 Hz corresponds to so-called deco-second (with periods of tens of seconds) oscillations. Infra-slow potentials appear to be associated with slow metabolic processes. When these processes are measured by recording local blood flow and/or by recording concentration of local oxygen the most striking feature of dynamics of these two metabolic parameters is the appearance of infra-slow quasi-periodic fluctuations. Nowadays infra-slow oscillations are detected by fMRI studies and are associated with oscillations in local blood flow. Slow waves are in the range of 0.1–1 Hz. Slow waves are present in EEG during all states from the deep sleep to the state of focused attention. They dominate EEG recordings in deep sleep giving it the name "slow wave sleep." Slow oscillations are characterized by rhythmic cycles of cortical membrane depolarization (so-called UP states) following by hyperpolarization (so-called DOWN) states. UP states are associated with increase of discharge rate of a group of cortical neurons while DOWN states are associated with decrease of neuronal spiking. Delta oscillations of sleep (within the range 1–4 Hz) are generated by interplay of two ion currents (and consequently two types of ion channels) of the thalamic neurons projecting to the corresponding cortical areas. The interplay of the excitatory and inhibitory ion currents in the thalamic membrane is responsible for generation of so-called Ca^{++} spikes – rebound depolarization in response to prolong hyperpolarization.

CHAPTER 2

Alpha Rhythms

I. TYPES OF ALPHA RHYTHMS

A German psychologist Hans Berger was the first who observed alpha rhythms recorded from the human brain. He recorded this type of rhythms from the scalp of human subjects who were sitting quietly with eyes closed. He published his discovery in 1929 in the paper titled "Uber das Elektrenkephalogramm das Menschen" and named these electrical events "waves of the first order" or "α (alpha) waves."

Berger further showed that alpha waves were blocked upon eye opening or during certain types of mental effort, leading to the appearance of "waves of the second order" or "β waves." Berger's results were later confirmed by several investigators, in particular, by Adrian and Matthews, who introduced the brilliant concept (remains to be valid till now) stating that different cortical areas possessed their own alpha rhythm, which represented a "resting" or "idling" state of that brain region. In spite of the fact, that since Berger's time the science of electrophysiology accumulated a bulk of knowledge regarding phenomenology of alpha rhythms, the number of hypothesizes concerning mechanisms and functional meaning of these rhythms has not converged into a common theory. This ambiguity reflects, probably, the heterogeneity of alpha rhythms.

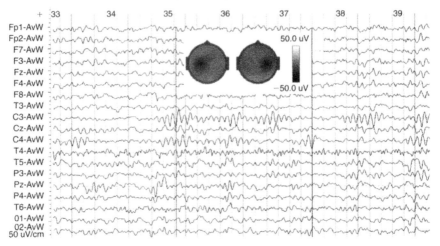

FIGURE 2.1   Mu-rhythms. A fragment of EEG recorded in a healthy adult subject during eyes open condition. Note distinct rhythms of about 10 cycles per second at C3 and C4. Insertion – two maps of potentials taken at two moments indicated bay black vertical lines.

A common view depicts alpha rhythms as rhythms in the human normal electroencephalogram (EEG) with frequencies that cover the range from 8 to 13 Hz. The definition of alpha rhythms as a single category of brain rhythmicity also presumes a distinct spatial distribution, a strong response to blocking the corresponding sensory input[1] and a distinct mechanism of generation. There are not one but several variants of "alpha rhythms." This fact was well known since 1950s (mentioned by the famous English electrophysiologist Grey Walter) but became well documented only recently when different mapping techniques became a routine procedure.

A. Mu-Rhythms

We start our description with sensory-motor alpha rhythms[2]. Figure 2.1 depicts a fragment of EEG of a healthy adult subject in the eyes open condition. One can clearly see two distinct EEG rhythmic patterns at C3 and C4 electrodes. These oscillations look quite independent of each other and have a peculiar form with sharp negative peaks that remind the Greek letter μ (mu). This specific form[3] gives one of the names of this EEG pattern – mu-rhythm. The other name – sensory-motor rhythm – is given because the rhythm is localized above the sensory-motor strip of the cortex (see also the maps of potentials measured at two

---

[1]For example, closing eyes, that is, decreasing sensory input to occipital-parietal areas, leads to increase of the power of posterior (occipital and parietal) alpha rhythms.

[2]Sensory-motor rhythms are of a slightly higher frequency than the posterior alpha rhythms.

[3]Mnemonically, mu-rhythm stands for motor.

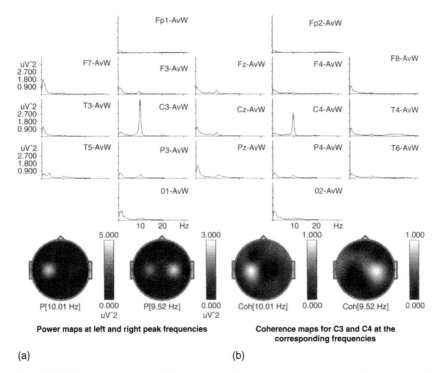

(a)   (b)

FIGURE 2.2   Independence of left- and right-side mu-rhythms. An example of power spectra for a healthy adult subject. (a) Maps of left and right mu-rhythms at the maximum of amplitude. Note, that they are at slightly different frequencies. (b) Coherence maps for C3 and C4 electrodes respectively. Note that a positive pick of coherency at one side is associated with negative pick of coherency in the opposite side indicating independency of the left and right mu-rhythms.

different time points). In some papers this rhythm is also called Rolandic because it is found above the Rolandic fissure. Sensory-motor rhythms can be blocked by the corresponding hand movement or by touching the hand. And vice versa, muscle relaxation will enhance the sensory-motor rhythms[4].

It should be stressed here that although mu–rhythms are found both at the left and right hemispheres (and in many cases look quite symmetrical at the EEG spectra) they are normally independent – that is, generated by independent generators. This is illustrated in Fig. 2.2 by means of coherence analysis.

Figure 2.2 represents the spectra computed for all 19 channels in eyes open condition for a normal subject. As manifested in EEG spectra, two distinct rhythms dominate EEG, the one with maximum of EEG power at C3 with peak

[4]The suppression of the sensory-motor rhythms to real or imagine movements seems to be caused by increase of the somato-sensory input from the body receptors to the sensory-motor strip. This kind of reactivity is similar to the reactivity of posterior alpha rhythms in response to opening eyes.

frequency of 10 Hz, and the other one with maximum of EEG power at C4 with peak frequency of 9.5 Hz. The maps of coherences computed separately for C3 and C4 are presented at the bottom at the right. As one can see the sensory-motor rhythm at C3 have the highest coherency at the left rhythm frequency (10 Hz) with the nearby electrodes from the left hemisphere and the lowest coherency with C4 electrode, and vice versa, the C4 rhythm does work in synchrony with the rhythm at C3 electrode at its peak frequency (9.5 Hz)[5].

In the neurofeedback-related literature there was some confusion in definition of this rhythm. In some papers one can find that this rhythm is defined in a frequency range from 12 to 15 Hz. This is a typical example of inappropriate extension of the results obtained in animal research to humans. The point is that the sensory-motor rhythm was intensively studied in 1960s by Barry Sterman from University of California in Los Angeles, USA. In experiments with cats he found that instrumentally rewarding the generation of the EEG rhythm recorded from the sensory-motor cortex of cats resulted in their resistance to developing seizures. He named this rhythm as sensory-motor rhythm. In cats it happened to be in the range of 12–15 Hz. In humans, as research unequivocally demonstrates the frequency of the sensory-motor rhythm varies in the range of 9 to 13 Hz. Barry Sterman at different conferences and workshops himself pointed out the cause of this confusion.

B. Occipital Alpha Rhythms

High amplitude rhythms recorded from occipital electrodes of the human cortex represent another example of alpha rhythms. Figure 2.3 depicts a fragment of EEG recorded in a healthy subject in the eye open condition. In the insertion of Fig. 2.3, power spectra for O1 and O2 electrode locations are presented. As one can see that the occipital rhythm in this subject is manifested in a form of a sharp peak at the spectra. The other thing that can be visually assessed is that in the rhythms at O1 and O2 electrodes of this subject are synchronous. Synchronicity is not a necessary feature: in some other healthy subjects, rhythms at O1 and O2 may be independent on each other.

The occipital rhythm is enhanced (synchronized) when a subject closes eyes. Grand averaged spectra in occipital leads for a group of healthy adults in eyes open and eyes closed conditions are presented in Fig. 2.4. As one can see closing eyes dramatically increase EEG power in alpha frequency band in occipital areas. This synchronization is caused by blocking the visual input to occipital areas. That is one of the reasons why the occipital alpha rhythm is considered as an idling rhythm of the occipital cortex. The occipital rhythm usually dominates in EEG

---

[5]We did not find in the literature any systematic research showing that the frequency of the sensory-motor rhythm significantly changes with age. This rhythm within the same frequency range can be found both in infants and elderly people, probably, reflecting an early maturation of the sensory-motor rhythm and mild aging.

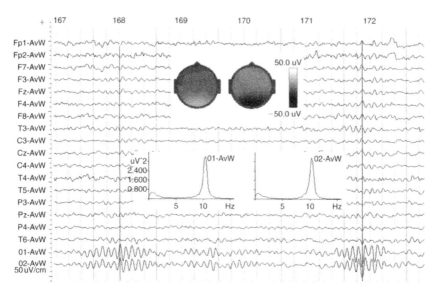

FIGURE 2.3   Occipital rhythm. A fragment of EEG recorded in a healthy adult subject during eyes open condition. Note a distinct rhythm of about 10 cycles per second at O1 and O2. Insertion (top) – two maps of potentials taken at two moments indicated bay black vertical lines. Insertion (bottom) – EEG power spectra at O1 and O2.

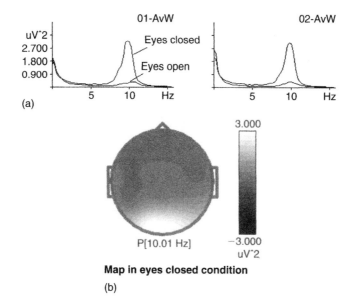

FIGURE 2.4   Synchronization of the occipital alpha rhythm during closing eyes. Grand average spectra for a group of healthy adults in eyes closed condition in comparison to eyes open condition. (b) Map in eye closed condition.

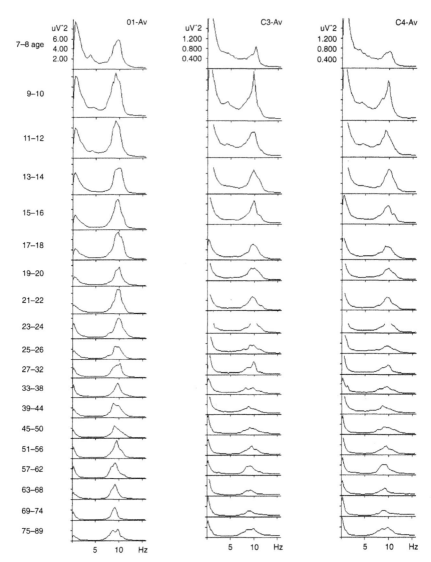

FIGURE 2.5   Age dependence of occipital alpha and mu-rhythms. Note that the averaged EEG power in the alpha range dramatically is decreasing with age while the frequency of the maximal power at the averaged spectra reveals much smaller changes.

recordings (as well in spectra) during eyes closed condition. In some rare cases, there exist not one, but two occipital rhythms. They may be generated in different areas of the occipital lobe and may reveal different peak frequencies.

According to the literature, the frequency of the occipital rhythms changes with age. Figure 2.5 depicts EEG spectra averaged over groups of healthy subjects of age from 7 to 89 years old. As one can see, there is a slight increase of the mean frequency from 7 to 20 years old and a slight decrease with later aging. However the variance of EEG spectra represented by the width of the peak is larger than changes with age. The frequency of the dominant alpha rhythm in healthy elderly people is around 10 Hz, so that an occipital alpha frequency less than 7.5 Hz is usually regarded as mild abnormality[6].

C. Parietal Alpha Rhythm

In some rare cases high amplitude rhythms in the alpha frequency band can be found at parietal areas with maximum at Pz. This is considered as a normal variant of alpha rhythm. This rhythm can be enhanced in the eyes closed condition in the same way as the occipital alpha rhythm, although in some subjects we saw a decrease of the parietal alpha rhythm in response to closing eyes[7]. The parietal rhythm may be present together with the occipital rhythm and seems to be independent from the occipital rhythm (Fig. 2.6). The frequency of the parietal rhythm is usually smaller than the frequency of the occipital rhythm when measured in the same subject. The overall power of parietal rhythms increases with the task load and is higher in the task conditions when compared with the eyes open condition. The functional meaning of the parietal rhythm is not fully understood. The functional analysis faces two difficulties: (1) the parietal alpha rhythm is present in few subjects and (2) it is masked by the neighboring occipital rhythm.

The recent success in developing electromagnetic tomography opens new possibilities in visualization of 3D generators of EEG rhythms. Low resolution electromagnetic tomography (LORETA) has been successfully used for these purposes. Nowadays LORETA is becoming a routine tool of brain imaging. Examples of 2D maps and the corresponding LORETA images of different types of alpha rhythms (occipital, sensory-motor, and parietal) in three healthy subjects of age 29, 19, and 18 years old are presented in Fig. 2.7.

---

[6] Because of the decline of alpha frequency with age, it has often been suggested that the frequency of alpha activity might reflect cognitive functions of the brain: smarter brain run at higher alpha frequencies. A group of researchers from Vrije (Free) University in Amsterdam, examined 271 twin families (Posthuma et al., 2001). IQ was assessed with the Dutch version of the Wechsler Adult Intelligence Scale (WAIS), from which four dimensions were calculated (verbal comprehension, working memory, perceptual organization, and processing speed). Individual peak frequencies were assessed according to the method described by Klimesch (1999). Structural equation modeling indicated that both peak frequency and the dimensions of IQ were highly heritable (range, 66–83 per cent) but there was no evidence of a correlation between alpha peak frequency and any of the four WAIS dimensions. However, our experience shows that slowing the dominant rhythm below the normative range for at least two standard deviations must be considered as an abnormality.

[7] This might indicate existence of at least two variants of parietal alpha rhythm.

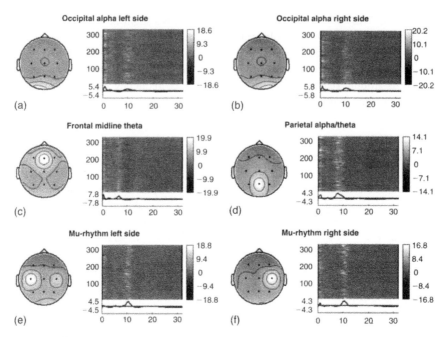

FIGURE 2.6   Independent component analysis (ICA) on amplitude spectra. ICA was applied to EEG amplitude spectra computed for more than 300 healthy subjects performing the visual two stimulus GO/NOGO task. Six independent components corresponding to different rhythms are presented. For each component, from left to right – topography of components, vertically stacking thin color-coded horizontal bars, each representing the corresponding component for a single subject, below – spectral characteristics of the components.

The three rhythms presented in Fig. 2.7 are found in three different subjects. However, in some cases all three rhythms can be found in a single normal subject. More over, even the alpha rhythm in a particular location (such as occipital) may exhibit two or more sub-rhythms with slightly different locations and different frequencies.

II. NEURONAL MECHANISMS

A. Association with Cortical Deactivation

Electrical stimulation of intralaminar nuclei of the thalamus suppresses alpha rhythms (reaction of desynchronization). The high frequency stimulation of the thalamic nuclei seems to increase overall activity of the cortex acting as reaction of arousal. In line with these observations, lesions in the thalamus lead to a pronounced disorganization or even complete suppression of EEG alpha activity.

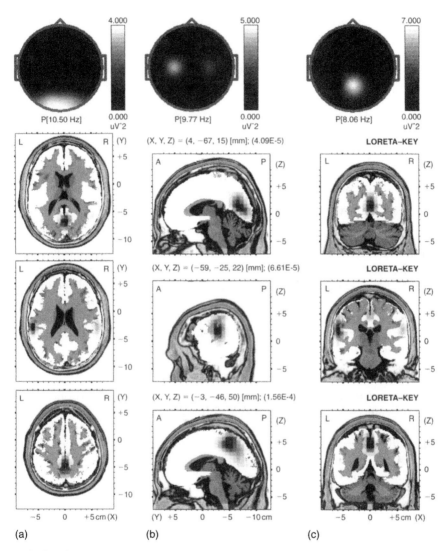

FIGURE 2.7   Maps and LORETA images of three types of alpha rhythms. Examples of maps and corresponding electromagnetic tomographies in three healthy adult subjects. All subjects were during eyes open condition. (a) An individual with occipital alpha rhythm. (b) An individual with mu-rhythms. (C) An individual with the parietal alpha rhythm. LORETA images depict generators in, correspondingly, occipital-parietal area, postcentral sensory-motor strip, and parietal middle area.

These data support the early suggestions that alpha rhythms are driven by regular thalamic activity.

Studies of correlation between EEG and positron emission tomography (PET) or functional magnetic resonance imaging (fMRI) signals support the hypothesis that alpha phenomena represent idling rhythms of the corresponding cortical areas. For occipital alpha rhythm it was shown in many independent papers. The behavioral paradigm used in these studies consists of sequential opening and closing eyes that produce corresponding suppression and enhancement of occipital alpha activity. The majority of current investigations show that during occipital alpha rhythm episodes, there is a decrease of activation in occipital areas as measured by blood oxygenation, blood flow, or glucose metabolism[8]. Subcortical (including thalamic) associations of metabolic parameters with EEG alpha amplitude are less well established and contradictive.

B. Thalamo-Cortical Circuits

One of the first ideas in 1960 was that the alpha rhythms have similar neuronal mechanisms as natural sleep[9] spindles. In those years Andersen and colleagues performed a series of elegant experiments showing that barbiturate spindles were generated at the level of the thalamus. The key role in generation of the barbiturate spindles was played by phasically firing inhibitory neurons, causing postinhibitory rebound bursts of action potentials in cortically projecting thalamic neurons. These inhibitory neurons were initially thought to be local circuit interneurons, but later it was shown that these cells were actually inhibitory GABAergic neurons located in the reticular nucleus of the thalamus.

Here is the right place to describe in more detail a scheme and principles of information flow in the thalamus. The thalamus is a paired nucleus located near the center of the brain and playing critical role in controlling information flow from receptors to sensory areas of the cortex. For this function the thalamus received its name "the gateway to the cortex." Indeed, almost every bit of sensory information enters the cortex through the thalamus. Besides this sensory-related function, the thalamus also plays important role in modulation information flow in cognitive, motor and affective cortical areas[10].

---

[8]For example, in a recent study by (Feige et al., 2005) alpha component was extracted by means of independent component analysis while metabolic activity was assessed by blood-oxygen-level-dependent (BOLD) parameter measured in the eyes open/closed paradigm. The thalamus was shown to be positively correlated with occipital alpha amplitude while widely distributed areas in occipital-parietal cortical areas were negatively correlated with the BOLD signal.

[9]In animal research sleep spindles in humans were modeled by barbiturate sleep.

[10]A different view to the thalamic function is presented in a book by S. Murray Sherman and R. W. Güllery "Exploring the thalamus and its role in cortical function." According to this view, for each nucleus the drivers and modulators are separated. The classical sensory afferents – visual, auditory, somatosensory, gustatory – are considered as drivers to so called first-order thalamic nuclei. The other types of drivers are the cerebellum and mamillary afferents for the ventro-lateral and anterior nuclei respectively. The third type of drivers are the layer 5 cortico-thalamic axons for the higher-order nuclei. The book includes a nice review of the current research regarding thalamo-cortical connections and their functional role.

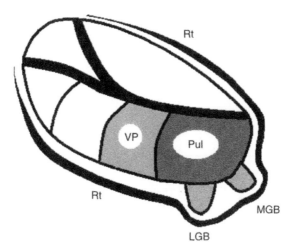

FIGURE 2.8   Main nuclei of the thalamus. Main sensory relay nuclei are LGB (lateral genicu-late body), MGB (medial geniculate body), and VP (ventral posterior nucleus). A large second-order nucleus is Pul (pulvinar). All nuclei (except the anterior nucleus) are shielded by the reticular nucleus of the thalamus.

There are two major components of the thalamus: the dorsal thalamus (for simplicity we will call it the thalamus) with roughly 15 nuclei and the ventral thalamus, the major part of which is the reticular nucleus. The reticular nucleus forms a kind of a shield against the dorsal thalamus (Fig. 2.8). It consists of inhibitory GABAergic neurons that project back to the thalamus. The reticular neurons receive feedforward excitatory projections from the thalamus, feedback excitatory projections from the cortex, and inhibitory projections from the ascending activating system of the brain stem (Fig. 2.9).

Sensory-related nuclei of the thalamus can be divided into first-order and high-order relay nuclei. The first-order relay nuclei receive sensory information directly from receptors, while the high-order relay nuclei receive highly processed sensory information (1) from the sensory cortical areas by means of cortico-thalamic projections and (2) from nuclei involved in motor actions such as orienting the body, head, or eyes. Examples of the first-order nuclei are the lateral geniculate body (LGB) in the visual modality, the medial geniculate nucleus in the auditory modality, and the ventral posterior nucleus in the somatosensory modality (Fig. 2.8). Examples of the high-order nuclei are the pulvinar in the visual modality, the posterior nucleus in the somatosensory modality (Fig. 2.8).

The simplest view to the thalamus emphasizes the relay function, that is, ability to relay sensory information to the cortex. However anatomical data indicate that even for the first-order thalamic nuclei primary sensory inputs constitute less than 20 per cent of all synaptic inputs. This fact favors another (and more realistic)

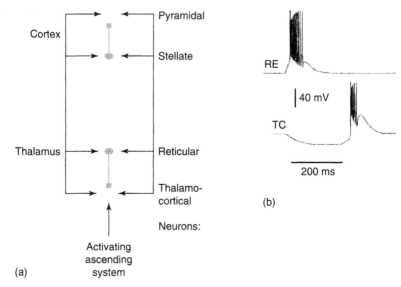

(a)

(b)

FIGURE 2.9   Thalamo-cortical circuit for generation sleep spindles. (a) The same as in Fig. 1.9. (b) Burst of a reticular neuron produces strong inhibition of a thalamo-cortical cell, this inhibition deinactivates Ca^{++} channels which leads to depolarization of the thalamo-cortical neuron. On the top of this depolarizaton the neurons produces burst of Na^+-K^+ spikes.

view to the thalamus emphasizing the significance of non-sensory inputs to the thalamus and, consequently, the modulatory function of the thalamus. The complex circuits involving thalamic, reticular, and cortical nodes play critical roles in modulating sensory information flow to the cortex. The mode of the sensory modulation seems to depend critically on the state of the brain and is different for different stages of sleep as well as for different stages of information flow during wakefulness.

C. Sleep Spindles

Description of the modulatory functions of the thalamus, we start with sleep spindles. Sleep spindles appear in EEG only during the light sleep (stage 2) or slow wave sleep (stages 3 and 4). They are rhythmic sinusoidal-like waves with frequencies between 10 and 14 Hz. The waves are grouped in sequences (bursts) of 0.5–3 s duration that may recur with intervals of 3–10 s. Sleep spindles appear quite early in life (at age of 6–8 weeks), are most prominent during childhood and adolescence and decline in voltage with age. Examples of sleep spindles in one healthy subject of 23 years old are presented in Fig. 2.10[11].

---

[11]There are actually two types of sleep spindles which are different both in topography and frequency. Fast frequency spindles show maximum of peak frequency at 14 Hz. The maximum amplitude

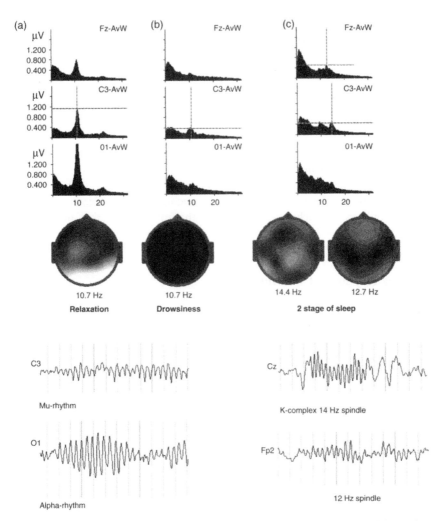

FIGURE 2.10   Sleep spindles. EEG was recorded in a healthy subject of 23 years old during three phases of falling asleep. (a) In the relaxation condition, two alpha rhythms are present in EEG: occipital alpha (O1 record) and mu-rhythm (C3 record). Spectra and maps are presented above. (b) The drowsiness phase is associated with suppression of the rhythms. (c) During the next stage of sleep, K complexes (vertex negativity followed by a sleep spindle of 14 Hz) appear with maximum of amplitude at central leads (see record at Cz). In addition, a 12 Hz rhythm with maximum of amplitude at frontal leads is also present.

of their topography is located near Cz. They are the first to occur in EEG during light sleep. Slower (with maximum around 12 Hz) spindles appear in sleep stage 2 as sleep deepens. During transition from stage 2 to stage 3 even slower (around 10 Hz) spindles appear. The maximum of the topography of lower type of sleep spindles is located near Fz.

A rough scheme of generation of sleep spindles is presented in Fig. 2.9. According to this scheme, the generation of spindles needs a network consisting of at least two elements – thalamic reticular neuron and thalamo-cortical neuron – and the interaction between them. According to this scheme burst firing of the inhibitory neurons of the reticular thalamic nucleus induces strong inhibitory postsynaptic potentials in the thalamo-cortical neurons. This hyperpolarization deinactivates the low threshold Ca^{++} current. This Ca^{++} inward current induces rebound depolarization of the thalamo-cortical cells (called Ca^{++} spike) and associated burst. The firing of the thalamo-cortical cell excites the reticular neurons by means of feedforward connections allowing the cycle to start again.

Spontaneous spindles are synchronized over large cortical areas. The cortico-thalamic pathway plays a critical role in this synchronization. Indeed, cutting this pathway induces desynchronization of the thalamic activity that dramatically changed into disorganized pattern with low spatio-temporal coherence.

D. Alpha Rhythms of Wakefulness

It should be stressed that the neuronal scheme described above is based on studies in anesthetized animals and explains the mechanism of a specific type of alpha-like oscillations – sleep spindles. Sleep spindles consist of waxing and waning potential oscillations at 10–14 Hz frequency band. In contrast to alpha bursts (that can last for long time intervals) sleep spindles are usually shorter in duration and last just only 0.5–3 s and recur every 3–10 s[12]. Although some authors attempted to transfer the mechanisms of sleep spindles generation for explanation of alpha rhythmicity in the state of wakefulness, recent studies brought doubt for this simple explanation. Indeed, a close consideration shows that sleep spindles and alpha rhythms are different phenomena.

First, alpha rhythms and sleep spindles occur in two very different behavioral states (relaxed wakefulness versus sleep or anesthesia). Second, alpha rhythms randomly wax and wane over episodes lasting several seconds, whereas barbiturate spindles are of a shorter duration. Third, alpha rhythms in humans show a restricted cortical distribution confined by primary sensory areas, whereas sleep spindles are more widespread having a maximum over central areas. And finally, alpha rhythms have a lower frequency than sleep spindles.

A new stage in search for neuronal mechanisms of alpha rhythms arrived on the scientific scene quite recently with the discovery that oscillations in alpha frequency band can be simulated in an in vitro slice preparation of the cat lateral geniculate nucleus – a part of the thalamus that conveys information to the visual cortex (Hughes et al., 2004). Recall that in this thalamic slice preparation the cortical part

---

[12]Although occipital alpha waves may show a better "spindle" shape (see Fig. 2.10) the term "sleep spindles" is widely used for the above mentioned EEG pattern to avoid confusion.

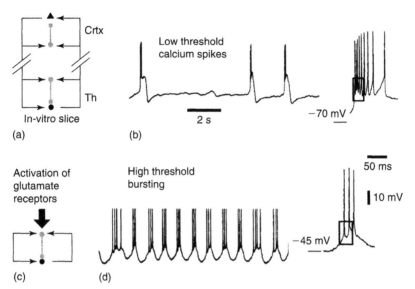

FIGURE 2.11   High threshold bursting in the thalamus. (a) A scheme of thalamic (LGB) slice preparation. (b) At the hyperpolarized membrane, a thalamic neuron displays low threshold Ca^{++} potentials and the corresponding bursting pattern. Individual bursts possess a characteristic interspike interval pattern consisting of short intervals between spikes at the start of the burst ($\sim$2–5 ms), which gradually increase as the burst progresses. (c) When cortico-thalamic feedback is mimicked in the thalamic slice by activating subtype of glutamate receptor, thalamic neurons are subject to a sustained depolarization. (d) In this depolarized state they exhibit high threshold (HT) bursting. Individual HT bursts exhibit a temporal pattern that is distinct to that of bursts on the top of low thresholds calcium spikes and that comprises relatively large intervals that do not alter significantly as the burst progresses. Adapted from Hughes et al. (2004).

is absent and consequently there is no direct way to mimic the thalamo-cortical interaction. The missed modulatory cortico-thalamic feedback interaction could be mimicked in the experimental condition by pharmacologically activating the glutamate receptors that are located postsynaptically to cortico-thalamic fibers.

E. High Threshold Burst Mode of Thalamic Neurons

Intracellular recordings of thalamo-cortical neurons in these slice preparations reveal a novel form of burst firing, which occurs at relatively depolarized (>-55 mV) membrane potentials and which has been termed high threshold bursting[13] (Hughes et al., 2002, 2004) (Fig. 2.11). The most salient property of

---

[13] With regard to ionic conductance, high threshold bursts appear to be critically reliant on the activation of dendritic I_t current, which is a transient Ca^{++} current. However, it should be stressed here that high threshold bursts are quite distinct from the low threshold bursts during sleep both in temporal pattern and in the level of hyperpolarization of thalamo-cortical neurons.

high threshold bursting is that it occurs repetitively in a wide frequency range, which encompasses the alpha and theta bands (i.e., 4–13 Hz), with the particular frequency at any one time being determined by the degree of neuronal depolarization. It has been found that a stronger activation of glutamate receptors leads to emergence of alpha frequency rhythms, whereas a reduction in the level of activation brings about theta waves. Thus, at the thalamic level, alpha and theta waves form a continuum of activity that is generated by the same intrinsic neuronal behavior. It might be also speculated that in vitro a decrease in the level of thalamic glutamatergic activation corresponds to a decrease of arousal state in vivo. Consequently, observation of slowing alpha (say below 7.5 Hz for occipital alpha rhythm in the wakefulness) in a particular subject may be associated with a decreased level of arousal in this subject.

A question arises: what makes the thalamo-cortical cells oscillate synchronously? In vitro experiments have demonstrated that the synchronization of high threshold bursts accompanying rhythmic alpha and theta activities are reliant on gap junction connectivity[14] between the thalamic neurons. Hughes et al. (2004) showed that alpha and theta rhythms in their slice preparations were susceptible to a large range of substances that target gap junction function but persist following a blockade of conventional chemical synaptic transmission.

Rhythmic bursts of spikes of the thalamo-cortical neurons in the alpha range are transferred to the cortical neurons via thalamo-cortical pathways. The arriving spikes generate postsynaptic potentials that are measured from the scalp in a form of alpha rhythms. The spatial distribution of cortical generators of different types of alpha rhythms (obtained by LORETA) indicates three different thalamic sources of alpha rhythms corresponding to three types of the alpha rhythms.

The first thalamic generator is located in the ventral posterior nucleus and corresponds to the sensory-motor rhythm (Fig. 2.12). This rhythm is generated at the postcentral strip of the parietal lobe which corresponds to the primary somatic sensory cortex. As we know from anatomy and physiology, this part of the human cortex receives projections for the ventral posterior nucleus of the thalamus – the first-order thalamic nucleus in the somato-sensory modality.

The two other thalamic generators correspond respectively to occipital and parietal alpha rhythms (Fig. 2.13). The occipital alpha rhythm is generated near the culcarine fissure that corresponds to the primary visual cortex. This area of the occipital cortex receives projections from the LGB – the first-order relay nucleus in the visual modality. The parietal alpha rhythm is generated in the Brodmann area 7. This area receives projections from the pulvinar nucleus of the thalamus – the second-order relay nucleus in the visual modality.

---

[14] A gap junction is a morphological structure of the electrical synapse – a quite rare type of connectivity between neurons in the brain. In contrast to conventional chemical synapses where transmission of the signals involves release and diffusion of a chemical substance – mediator – in the electrical synapse the conduction of electrical signal from one neuron to another takes place through the passive electric currents between pre- and postsynaptic membranes.

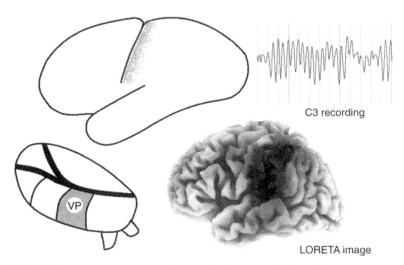

FIGURE 2.12   Generators of mu-rhythm. Mu-rhythm is recorded over the sensory-motor strip with maximum of amplitude at C3, C4 electrodes (see EEG record). Electromagnetic tomography (LORETA) indicates the somato-sensory cortex. The cortex receives inputs from the ventral posterior nucleus of the thalamus.

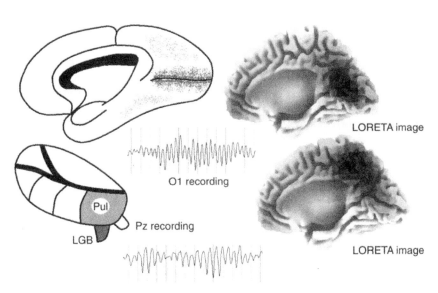

FIGURE 2.13   Generators of occipital and parietal alpha rhythms. Occipital alpha rhythm is recorded over occipital areas with maximum of amplitude at O1, O2 (see EEG record) while parietal alpha rhythm is recorded over the parietal area with maximum of amplitude at Pz (see EEG record). Electromagnetic tomography (LORETA) indicates the culcarine tissue for the occipital alpha rhythm and middle parietal cortex for the parietal alpha rhythm. The occipital and parietal areas receive inputs from the LGB and pulvinar respectively.

As one can see from Figs 2.12 and 2.13, only nuclei located in the posterior part of the thalamus (ventral posterior, pulvinar, lateral geniculate nucleus) are involved in generation of alpha oscillations in the healthy human brain. We do not know if this fact reflects the relatively lower level of depolarization of thalamo-cortical neurons in these nuclei or some other intrinsic cellular or network properties of the posterior nuclei[15].

III. RESPONSES TO TASKS

According to the theory of alpha wave generation presented above, any increase in the corresponding sensory input must suppress the associated alpha rhythm. This kind of suppressive reaction is named reaction of desynchronization, because high amplitude alpha rhythms can be considered as the result of synchronization in neuronal networks. The reaction of desynchronization of alpha rhythms to sensory stimulation has indeed been observed in many studies. These studies also provide some new insights regarding mechanisms of alpha rhythms generation and their functional meaning.

A. Event-Related Desynchronization of Mu-Rhythms to Motor Actions

The leading role in this field has been played by a group from Technical University in Graz, Switzerland headed by Gert Pfurtscheller. He was the first who in 1979 published the method for parametric assessing of the EEG desynchronization. The parameter was coined ERD – event-related desynchronization. In some specific cases instead of suppression of alpha activity, the enhancement of alpha wave power was observed – this reaction was named synchronization and the parameter corresponding to it – event-related synchronization-ERS[16].

---

[15] The first suggestion looks more realistic. If it is correct then the lower level of depolarization might be explained by fewer excitatory inputs to the thalamo-cortical neurons of first-order and second-order relay nuclei of the thalamus. In line with this suggestion, any behavior directed to decreasing the sensory input (such as closing eyes in the visual modality or muscle relaxation in somato-sensory modality) enhances the corresponding alpha rhythm. Another way of decreasing the depolarization in the thalamo-cortical cells might be associated with decrease of the overall excitation of cortical neurons projecting back to the thalamus.

[16] The classic method to compute ERD/ERS includes the following stages. Fist, bandpass filtering must be done on EEG recorded during trials in a given psychological task. This procedure enables the researcher to separate a distinct alpha rhythm. Nowadays, together with temporal filtration spatial filtration based on independent component analysis of raw EEG is sometimes applied. The second stage consists of squaring of the EEG signals. The procedure provides the power of EEG signal as the output. The third stage consists of averaging of power samples across all trials. The fourth stage is needed to smooth the data and to reduce variability and consists of averaging the obtained dynamics over time. And finally, relative values for ERD/ERS are obtained. The relative values may be calculated in percents (for more details see Methods of Part 1).

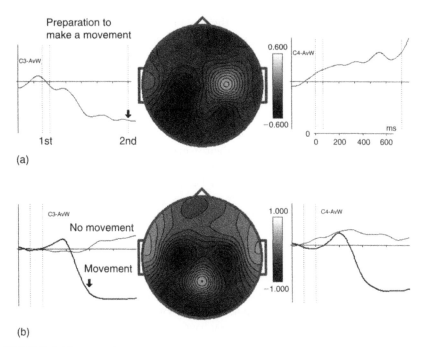

FIGURE 2.14   ERD during preparation to make a movement and during movement per se. (a) ERDs are computed for a healthy adult subject performing a two stimulus GO/NOGO task. Pairs of visual images of animals and plants in different combinations are presented with the task to press a button in response to two animals. Note a left-side mu-rhythm desynchronization accompanied by ERS at the right side during preparation to make a movement. (b) ERS are computed for the same subject performing an auditory oddball task. Strong ERD are observed to movements in response to targets. Note the desynchronization in one area is accompanied by an opponent reaction – synchronization – in the adjacent area.

For spatial mapping of ERD/ERS local average montages or Laplassian-like transformations are usually applied. An example of ERD computing and mapping is shown in Fig. 2.14. The data are taken from a healthy adult subject from the Human Brain Institute Database. In EEG spectra of this subject strong mu-rhythm has been observed both in eyes open and eyes closed conditions. The subject also performed the two stimulus GO/NOGO task and auditory oddball task. ERDs in response to stimuli required motor actions were computed according to the method designed by Pfurtscheller. In Fig. 2.14a ERD/ERS are presented between the first warning stimulus[17] and the second stimulus which can be either GO or NOGO stimuli. One can see that the preparatory period is accompanied

---

[17]Indicating that the subject has to wait for the second stimulus presentation while no movement – right finger pressing – is required.

by desynchronization of the mu-rhythm in the contra-lateral hemisphere and synchronization in the ipsi-lateral hemisphere. Figure 2.14b shows ERD/ERS in response to auditory stimuli: the target one (rare) that required right finger pressing and the non-target one to which no movement was needed. One can see that only the target stimulus induces strong desynchronization of mu-rhythm.

Using ERD/ERS methodology in behavioral paradigms associated with voluntary movements, the Graz group reported existence of several sub-types of Rolandic rhythms (Pfurtscheller et al., 1997). They showed that mu-rhythms may be differentiated on the basis of their spatial location. For example, face and foot areas in the sensory-motor strip produce different mu-rhythms. The Graz group also showed that mu-rhythms may be separated on the basis of frequency (Pfurtscheller et al., 2000). The lower frequency (8–10 Hz) mu-rhythm shows a widespread movement-type – unspecific ERD pattern similar for finger or foot movement, whereas the higher frequency (10–13 Hz) mu-rhythm shows a more focused, movement-type – specific ERD pattern, clearly different for finger and foot movement. Both are blocked before and during movement and should therefore be considered mu-rhythms[18].

According to the Graz group data the desynchronization of upper mu-rhythm is somatotopically specific and topographically restricted. The desynchronization of this rhythm starts over the contralateral hand area 2 s before unilateral voluntary hand movement onset. The desynchronization is often accompanied by synchronization in central-parietal areas and has been coined as "focal ERD/surround ERS" (Pfurtscheller, 2003). In general, this term describes the observation that desynchronization of rhythmic activity in the alpha band does not occur in isolation but can be accompanied by synchronization in neighboring cortical areas. The areas of lateral synchronization may correspond to the same sensory modality or to another modality.

To explain the focal ERD/surround ERS phenomenon Gert Pfurtscheller suggested a thalamic gating mechanism (Pfurtscheller, 2003). He argued that the same thalamic model that has been used for sleep spindles can be applied for mu-rhythm generation. The critical role in his scheme is played by interplay between thalamo-cortical cells and inhibitory neurons of the thalamic reticular nucleus.

---

[18] In contrast to the focal and somatotopically specific desynchronization in the upper frequency band the widespread non-specific desynchronization of lower mu-rhythm found over frontal, central, and parietal areas may indicate the existence of a distributed non-specific neural network in the sensorimotor cortex. This network is activated by different types of motor behavior, but it is not necessarily critical to support a specific movement. One hypothesis suggests that this system may act as a relatively non-specific mechanism that presents somatosensory and motor neurons before a specific motor act. Another interpretation of this non-specific, low-mu related system could be that this system serves as a neurophysiologic mechanism for general motor attention to all cortical areas involved in a motor task including premotor and parietal areas in addition to primary sensorimotor. Indeed, lower alpha desynchronization is also obtained in response to a variety of non-task-specific factors that may be best summed up under the term "attention." This ERD is topographically widespread over the scalp and probably reflects general task demands and attentional processes.

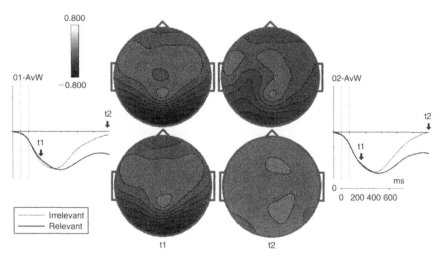

FIGURE 2.15   ERDs of the occipital alpha rhythms in response to visual stimulation. Grand average ERD calculated for 8–12 frequency band for relevant and irrelevant stimuli in the two stimulus GO/NOGO task. As an example, a group of healthy subjects of 12–13 years old was selected. Note that relevant stimulus elicits a longer response but with the same amplitude as irrelevant one at initial stages.

The latter forms a topographically organized inhibitory feedback mechanism that is capable of controlling the information flow through the thalamus. This controlling function of the reticular inhibitory neurons is named "gating." When the gate is closed, the thalamic neurons fire in the burst mode which is manifested in emergence of cortically recorded mu-rhythm. When the gate is open, the thalamic neurons fire in the tonic mode which is manifested in desynchronization of mu-rhythm. According to the proposed mechanism, the lateral inhibition that exists between the reticular neurons is responsible for the ERD-center/ERS surround phenomenon[19]. Summarizing the above mentioned results, we can conclude that Rolandic mu-rhythms are suppressed in response to real or imaginary movements.

B. ERD of Occipital Rhythms to Visual Stimuli

Similar results are shown for posterior alpha rhythms: they are suppressed in response to visual stimuli. Moreover, reactions in alpha band reflect the amount of mental effort associated with these stimuli. This is illustrated in Fig. 2.15 that presents the data taken from the Human Brain Institute database. ERD/ERS for the

[19]It should be stressed here the reticular thalamic nucleus is not the only place with lateral inhibition in the brain. A similar effect may be produced by the lateral inhibition in the striatum – a part of the basal ganglia – that is in position of controlling the information flow from the thalamus to the executive cortical areas – areas that are involved in action programming.

alpha (8–12 Hz) frequency band were computed for a group of healthy subjects of 12–13 years old. They performed a two stimulus visual task. ERDs in occipital areas in response to relevant and irrelevant stimuli are presented at the left. Presentation of the relevant stimulus in the pair indicated that the subjects had to wait for the second stimulus (after which GO or NOGO response were required) while presentation of the irrelevant stimulus indicated that the whole trial had to be ignored. As one can see, at the first stage of information processing (up to 240 ms poststimulus) both types of stimuli elicited the same occipital alpha desynchronization. However, the later stages of information processing are associated with more occipital alpha desynchronization for the relevant stimulus in comparison to the irrelevant one[20].

IV. FUNCTIONAL MEANING

A. Alpha Rhythms as Idling EEG Activity

As fMRI studies show that the amount of synchronization of alpha rhythms is negatively correlated with metabolic activity. Consequently alpha rhythms are considered as idling rhythms. According to this view we might expect that appearance of alpha rhythms in specific sensory areas would inhibit the sensory information processing in those areas[21]. As we learned from above, alpha rhythms are epiphenomena that reflect thalamic regular bursting transferred to the cortex. This bursting reflects the level of neuronal depolarization, which in turn reflects the dysbalance between excitatory and inhibitory postsynaptic potentials arriving to the thalamo-cortical cells (Fig. 2.16). If excitation is strong enough the thalamo-cortical neurons are depolarized, do not generate bursts, and the information from the receptive organs is transferred to the cortex without any constrain. We call such a sensory pathway as an active channel.

B. Lateral Inhibition in Activation of Alpha Rhythms

If the excess of inhibition or the lack of excitation drives the membrane potential toward the hyperpolarization state, the neurons start firing in bursts. The lack of

---

[20]Also note that preparation to the second stimuli that could be followed by the right finger pressing is associated with ERD of mu-rhythm in C3.

[21]This hypothesis was tested in a recent study by Ergenoglu et al. (2004). In this study visual stimuli were presented on a threshold so that approximately in 50 per cent of trials subjects could not detect stimuli. The intensity of stimuli was tailored to each subject according to his or her specific abilities. Trials were separated into two groups: trials with detected and undetected stimuli. Between the two conditions, a significant ($p < 0.01$) difference was observed in the relative power of the alpha band, which was significantly lower before detected stimuli in line with significantly ($p < 0.001$) higher amplitudes of the ERPs. These results show that short-lasting changes in brain's excitability state are reflected in alpha rhythms of the EEG.

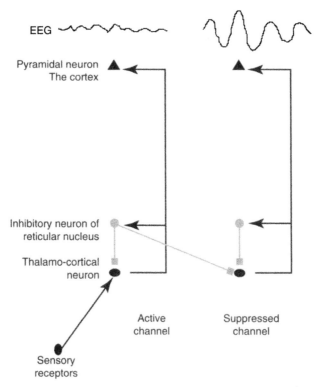

FIGURE 2.16   Lateral inhibition in the thalamo-cortical circuits. Two channels, the active one and the suppressed one, are schematically presented. Inhibitory neurons of the reticular nucleus in the active channel are activated and inhibit thalamo-cortical neurons in the adjacent channel. The neurons in the suppressed channel are hyperpolarized and generate alpha rhythms.

excitation can be achieved by suppressing the sensory input to the relay thalamic nuclei, for example, by closing eyes in visual modality. The excess of inhibition can be achieved by means of lateral inhibition that is produced by reticular neurons in the nearby (active) channel, which are excited through connections from neurons in the active channel both at the cortical and at the thalamic levels. The thalamo-cortical neurons in such a channel, that we call the suppressed channel, generate bursts at alpha frequencies. In order the alpha rhythms to be recorded from the scalp, neurons in the suppressed channel must be synchronized. In this synchronization mode the transfer of sensory information to the cortex is limited. It is not completely blocked as during early stages of sleep when the thalamic neurons generate sleep spindles, but it is limited to some extent, so that stimulus recognition in this mode is insufficient.

And finally, the frequency of bursts generated in the state of wakefulness in the suppressed channel networks is defined by the level of polarization of the thalamo-cortical neurons: the more they inhibited, the low is the frequency. In some pathological cases this frequency may become lower than 8 Hz in adults.

V. ABNORMALITY OF ALPHA RHYTHMS

A. Complete Absence of Alpha Rhythms

Moruzzi and Magoun in 1949 were the first to show that stimulation of the brain stem reticular formation activates the cortex and transfers the high voltage, low frequency EEG, that is, EEG with prominent alpha rhythms, into low voltage, high frequency EEG[22]. In the normal brain alpha rhythms of EEG appear to be the largest in amplitude. So, when alpha rhythms are absent, the EEG records look lower in voltage. Such EEGs are called low voltage records. If the higher frequency rhythms are not suppressed in comparison to norms, the records are called low voltage high frequency EEG. On power spectra such EEG records lack any significant peaks in the alpha frequency band both in eyes open and eyes closed conditions. Empirically, low voltage record is defined as a record during eyes open and eyes closed conditions with amplitude in the linked ears montage no greater than 20 μV over all cortical areas. As one can see this definition is quite subjective, very loosely defined.

Low voltage records are found in 4–10 per cent of normal adults depending on criteria and can be hardly considered as abnormality. Rather, low voltage records can be related to a certain personality trait. The low voltage records are found in families of alcoholics and drug addicts. Consumption of alcohol seems to work as a self-medication in this population with the objective to decrease the hyperactivation of the cortex.

B. Alpha Rhythms in Unusual Sites

In children and young adult EEGs alpha activities may be found in occipital areas (O1, O2), parietal area (Pz), and over the sensory-motor strip (C3, C4). However, the scalp distribution of alpha activities (especially in eyes open condition) changes with age and in elderly people temporal alpha rhythms become prominent. Ernst Niedermeyer (1997) considers the "temporal alphoid rhythm" found mainly over the anterior temporal and midtemporal region as of mildly abnormal character and suggests that it could be a sign of early cerebrovascular disorder.

---

[22] This effect is mediated, in part, by thalamic midline nuclei. Electrical stimulation of intralaminar nuclei of the thalamus alone also induces the same effect. Actually the reaction of activation consists of suppression of alpha rhythms (reaction of alpha desynchronization) and of increase of high frequency activity (reaction of beta synchronization).

He also mentioned that in early adulthood this pattern could be found over temporal lobe harboring an epileptogenic focus. The rhythmical alpha activity may camouflage a rhythmical paroxysmal discharge type without revealing any sharp/spiky component.

Our experience of working with normal subjects and patients enable us to propose the following rule: if in a particular patient: (1) the maximum of rhythmic activity within a range of 7–13 Hz is localized in leads different from mentioned above, and (2) the rhythm itself is a prominent one, so that there is a significant deviation from normality both in absolute and relative power, then this rhythm must be considered as an abnormal. In our practice maximums of distributions of abnormal alpha rhythms were found in posterior temporal areas (e.g., in connection with tinnitus or whiplash), in left parietal areas (in connection with dyslexia), in the middle temporal areas and in the anterior temporal areas (in connection with aging cerebrovascular disorder). Only in few cases, abnormal alpha rhythms were found in frontal areas.

An example of spectral characteristics of EEG of a patient[23] with abnormal alpha rhythms is presented in Fig. 2.17. As one can see, raw EEG recording of this patient exhibits two types of rhythms within alpha band: the first one with frequency of 9.5 Hz located in the left middle temporal area and the second one with frequency of 7.3 Hz located at Fz. The results of comparison with the normative database and s-LORETA images are presented in Fig. 2.17a.

In general, alterations in the normal functioning of the thalamo-cortical loop might result in neurological disorders: such as some types of epileptic seizures and the tremor of Parkinson disease both of which have rhythmic components. Stimulation or lesion of the appropriate portion of the thalamus (the ventral tier nuclei) is now a common method to alleviate movement tremor, presumably through a disruption of the oscillatory network activities. Abnormal rhythmic activity of thalamic cells (as revealed by recordings in patients with stereotactically implanted electrodes) is also present in some neurological disorders with behavioral symptoms that are not obviously rhythmic. For example, recordings of thalamic neurons in patients suffering from chronic pain as the result of sensory deafferentation (so-called phantom pain) show the presence of abnormal rhythmic bursts of action potentials. And again, stereotactic lesions of the thalamic nuclei lead to lessening phantom pain[24].

---

[23]This is a patient of 13 year old and IQ of 88. He visits a special school. He has Incontinentia Pigmenti – a rare disease from a group of gene-linked diseases known as neurocutaneous disorders. These disorders cause characteristic patterns of discolored skin and also involve the brain, eyes, nails, and hair. In most cases, IP is caused by mutations in a gene called NEMO. Discolored skin is caused by excessive deposits of melanin (normal skin pigment). Neurological problems include cerebral atrophy, the formation of small cavities in the central white matter of the brain. About 20 per cent of children with IP will have slow motor development, muscle weakness in one or both sides of the body, mental retardation, and seizures. They are also likely to have visual problems, including crossed eyes, cataracts, and severe visual loss.

[24]The condition in which thalamo-cortical loops generate inappropriate rhythmic activity (such as slow rhythmic burst firing in the awaked brain) has been coined as "thalamic dysrhythmia" by Llinás and

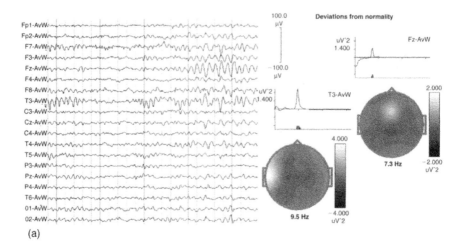

(a)

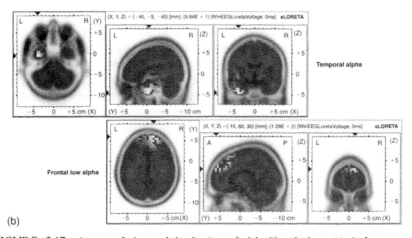

(b)

FIGURE 2.17 A case of abnormal localization of alpha-like rhythms. (a) A fragment of EEG in eyes open condition. Deviations from normality in EEG spectra and corresponding maps. (b) s-LORETA images of the abnormal rhythms.

---

colleagues (Llinás et al., 1999). "Dysrhythmia" in this sense is present in some forms of epilepsy and tremorgenic syndromes, both of which represent abnormal states of the thalamo-cortical network accompanied by stereotyped behaviors such as rhythmic hand movements in tremor or 3 Hz spike-and-wave oscillations in the electroencephalogram during generalized absence seizures. Could similar thalamo-cortical "dysrhythmias" underlie other disorders, including neuropsychiatric ones? At present, this interesting and provocative suggestion of Llinás and colleagues should be considered as strictly hypothetical and needs more research.

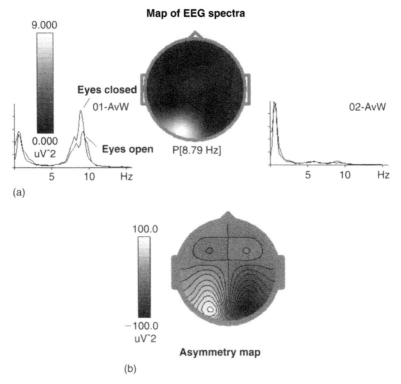

FIGURE 2.18   A case of abnormal asymmetry of the occipital alpha rhythm. (a) Spectra (for eyes open and eyes closed conditions) and spectra map (for eyes closed condition) of EEG recorded in a patient with the right parietal lobe stroke. (b) Asymmetry map for eyes closed condition.

C. Alpha Asymmetry

Another important characteristic of abnormality is alpha asymmetry. As was mentioned above, in spite of the fact that grand average spectra are quite symmetrical it is not uncommon for a healthy individual to reveal an asymmetry at the range of 10–50 per cent. However, if the asymmetry is larger than 50 per cent this might be an indication of pathology. In such cases the comparison with the database can show how much the observed asymmetry is deviant from normality. An example of abnormal alpha asymmetry is presented in Fig. 2.18 that depicts spectral characteristics of EEG of a patient with sensory neglect produced by a lesion in the right occipital-parietal area. Note a big (almost 100 per cent) asymmetry of occipital alpha rhythm both in eyes open and eyes closed conditions.

Grand average EEG power spectra in alpha band for different age groups look quite symmetrical (Fig. 2.19). In other words left and right hemispheres produce

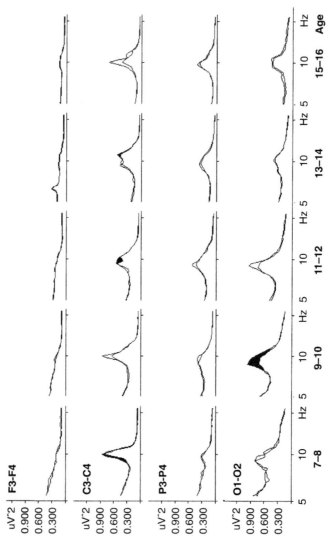

FIGURE 2.19   Alpha band asymmetry. Grand average spectra for five groups of healthy subjects of different age are super-imposed on each other in pairs F3–F4, C3–C4, P3–P4, O1–O2. The large negative (i.e., C3 < C4) difference are shown by black color. Note no asymmetry that would be consistent over all ages.

averaged EEG patterns of similar amplitude and frequencies. But, when measured in individuals the power asymmetry could be big enough. The question arises if this asymmetry might be a measure of some individual character, such introversion/ extraversion division, or prevalence of positive/negative affective states.

More than two decades ago, several researchers started to investigate EEG asymmetry during emotional states. The research was inspired by Richard Davidson's theory regarding asymmetrical involvement of the frontal cortex in the emotional reactions (for review see Davidson, 2004). Roughly, according to his theory the left hemisphere is biased to processing positive emotional stimuli, while the right hemisphere processes mostly negative emotional stimuli. This research led to the proposal that frontal EEG asymmetry in a resting state reflects a trait-like asymmetry of anterior cortical activity, which acts as a diathesis for emotion-elicitors and is a contributory factor for individual differences in affective/motivational behaviors[25].

Many findings supported the Davidson's theory, but several authors noted substantial inconsistencies in the evidence. Recently, this situation stimulated a search for methodological factors that may contribute to the divergence of findings. For review of methodological issues see (Hagemann, 2004). According to our experience, the inconsistency is due to two factors. First, the asymmetry index is a ratio of two random variables one of which is a difference between two variables. Consequently, a standard deviation of the alpha asymmetry as a ratio is proportional to the sum of two standard deviations of both parts of the ratio. The difference between EEG power at the left and right sides is quite small in many healthy subjects, consequently the error in computing the asymmetry index is quite big. Moreover, the recordings are made laterally, where a lot of muscle and eye movement artifacts are present. The second factor lies in the actual absence of prominent alpha activity at frontal areas. It is illustrated by Fig. 2.19. Note absence of any peak in alpha frequency band in EEG spectra at F3, F4 sites which unequivocally indicate absence of alpha rhythm generators at frontal areas.

VI. SUMMARY

During relaxed wakefulness in eyes closed condition, the human brain exhibits several types of distinct rhythmic electrical activity in the alpha frequency band

---

[25] In a typical study the steps of experimental procedure are as follows. The spontaneous EEG in a resting state is recorded in human subjects. The alpha power (P) asymmetry sites is computed as a ratio: $P(L)-P(R)/P(L) + P(R)$, where $P(L)$ and $P(R)$ are alpha power at the left (L) and right (R) homologous electrodes. This ratio serves as a measure of anterior asymmetry of cortical activity. Taking into account that alpha is an idling rhythm, the positive asymmetry $P(L) > P(R)$ serves as indicator of more cortical activation at the right side, and vice versa, the negative asymmetry $P(L) < P(R)$ serves as indicator of more cortical activation at the left hemisphere. Facets of affective style are measured with experimental procedures or questionnaires. The statistical analysis is focused on the associations between asymmetry and affect.

(8–13 Hz). At least three main types of alpha rhythmicity are separated. They are: (1) the posterior alpha rhythms, recorded at occipital or occipital-parietal areas, (2) the Rolandic or mu-rhythm, recorded over the sensory-motor strip, and (3) mid-temporal, the so-called third, rhythm which in normal conditions can be recorded only in magneto-encephalogram (MEG). These oscillations are driven by rhythmic activity from thalamic nuclei: each rhythm having an origin in a corresponding thalamic nucleus. The frequency of the occipital alpha rhythm slightly changes with age reaching its maximum at the age of 15–20. Posterior alpha rhythms are suppressed in response to visual stimulation while Rolandic rhythms respond by desynchronization (decrease of amplitude) to actual or imaginary actions. Alpha rhythms must be separated and distinguished from sleep spindles. These two distinct categories of rhythms are observed in different states (sleep versus wakefulness), have different spatial distribution (sleep spindles have broad central distribution while alpha rhythms are located near the primary sensory cortical areas), different frequencies (sleep spindles are about 13–14 Hz in contrast to alpha frequencies that vary between 8 and 13 Hz). The mechanisms of sleep spindles generation have been explored in detail in animal models. As far as alpha rhythms concerns, the mechanisms of their generation are still poorly understood. The power of alpha activity is inversely correlated to metabolic function of the corresponding cortical area giving rise to a functional explanation of alpha rhythms as idling rhythms of the cortex.

CHAPTER 3

Beta Rhythms

I. TYPES OF BETA RHYTHMS

Beta rhythms manifested in distinct peaks on the spectrograms may be found in various locations of the cortex in normal subjects. In the frequency between 13 and 30 Hz beta rhythms are more often found in frontal or central areas when compared to posterior regions of the cortex. At least two distinct beta rhythms can be separated: beta rhythms with maximums at electroencephalogram (EEG) spectra located over the sensory-motor strip – Rolandic beta rhythms and beta rhythms located more frontally – frontal beta rhythms. These rhythms are manifested in a form of peaks on individual spectra. However, quite few healthy subjects reveal a distinct peak on spectra and, as a consequence, grand average spectra both in eyes open and eyes closed conditions do not exhibit clear maximums in the beta frequency band. The amplitude of beta rhythms when measured in reference to linked ears is less than $20\,\mu V$[1].

---

[1]The asymmetry of beta rhythms usually does not exceed 35–40 per cent. Empirically, any asymmetry more than 50 per cent may be considered as abnormal and needs additional attention.

A. Rolandic Beta Rhythms

The Rolandic beta rhythms are observed as spontaneous activity during eyes open and eyes closed conditions in healthy subjects over the sensorimotor area (C3, Cz, C4). Although Rolandic beta rhythms quite often have a frequency of about 20 Hz (i.e., two fold frequency of mu-rhythm) they should not be considered as a sub-harmonic of this lower frequency oscillations. Indeed, as magneto-encephalogram (MEG) studies show, mu and beta rhythms have different sources in the primary somatosensory and the motor cortex, respectively (see Hari and Salmelin, 1997 for a review). In EEG beta Rolandic rhythms can be found in absence of Rolandic mu-rhythms as well together with Rolandic mu-rhythms but in different locations. The latter case is illustrated in Fig. 3.1. The frequency of Rolandic beta rhythm (the maximum of peak at spectra) may vary from subject to subject in a broad range from 14 to 30 Hz. It also depends on age.

B. Desynchronization/Synchronization Pattern to Motor Actions

The Rolandic beta rhythm is modulated during various motor and cognitive tasks. An example of dynamics of Rolandic beta rhythm during GO/NOGO task in a group of 15–16 years old adolescents is presented in Fig. 3.2. As one can see in Fig. 3.2, the Rolandic beta rhythm recorded at C3 is clearly suppressed during finger pressing after the second stimulus presentation in GO trials as well as during preparation periods when subjects were preparing to make a movement both in GO and NOGO trials, but not in Ignore trials when no preparation to make a movement was involved. Note also that the suppression of Rolandic beta rhythm (named desynchronization) is accompanied by a suppression of EEG power in alpha frequency range – mu-rhythm desynchronization. Note also that suppression of Rolandic beta rhythm associated with finger pressing is followed by rebound beta synchronization. This synchronization takes place during continuation of mu-rhythm desynchronization indicating that Rolandic beta and mu-rhythms exhibit different dynamics[2].

Because movement is associated with overall activation of neurons in the sensory-motor strip, we can speculate that the Rolandic beta appears when the corresponding neuronal system in the sensory-motor strip is relaxing after a strong

---

[2]It should be stressed that in the studies presented above stimuli presentations serve as synchronization events. However, because Rolandic beta rhythms are associated with movements, it is reasonable to use as synchronization events for computing ERDs movements themselves but not stimuli triggering movements. In experiments carried out in Graz by a group headed by Gert Pfurtscheller subjects with multiple electrodes located over the sensory-motor strip were asked to press a button voluntarily in a convenient pace. The studies showed that movement itself is accompanied by suppression of beta Rolandic beta activity. The suppression is followed by a strong rebound effect – beta synchronization.

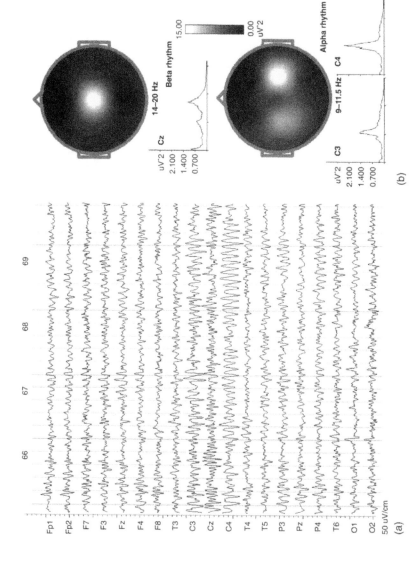

FIGURE 3.1 Midline central beta rhythm. (a) A fragment of 19-channel EEG in eyes open condition in a healthy subject of 48 years old. (b) Spectra in alpha and beta bands with the corresponding maps. Note that together with mu-rhythms recorded at C3, C4, EEG reveals a strong spindling beta rhythm recorded at Cz.

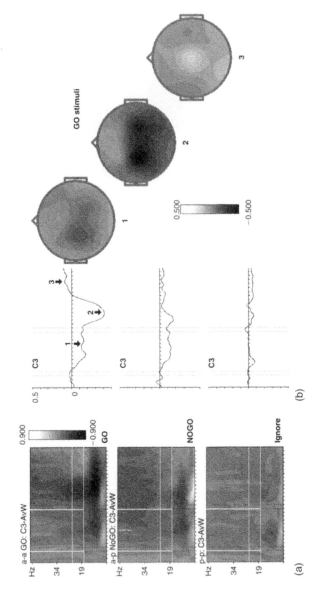

FIGURE 3.2 Suppression of Rolandic beta rhythms by motor actions. Grand average data for a group of 15–16 years old healthy children performing a two stimulus GO/NOGO task. (a) The power–time–frequency representations (wavelet transformation) of EEG responses in GO, NOGO, and Ignore conditions (in column from top to bottom) for C3 location. (b) Maps of responses in the frequency band of 18–24 Hz and time intervals shown by arrows.

activation phase. In other words, the Rolandic beta increase is a rebound phenomenon that can be considered as postactivation trace (for a recent review see Neuper et al., 2006).

C. Frontal Beta Rhythms

A second type of beta rhythms is associated with frontal beta rhythms. The frontal beta rhythms are usually expressed in spectrograms of frontal leads as wide picks with small amplitude. This appearance on spectrograms reflects low amplitude of these rhythmicities and their irregular pattern. Beta waves in the linked ears reference montage seldom – approximately at 2 per cent of normal population – exceed 20 μV. This is in contrast to alpha rhythms of central and posterior regions which usually have more regular patterns and expressed in narrow picks on spectrograms. An example of such activity is presented in Fig. 3.3. In F3, Fz, and F4 locations EEG spectra reveal distinct maximums at around 19 Hz.

D. Desynchronization/Synchronization Pattern to Cognitive Tasks

In contrast to Rolandic beta rhythms (that appear in motor-related tasks) frontal beta rhythms emerge in cognitive tasks related to stimulus assessment and decision making. In some subjects the frontal beta synchronization may be preceded by the beta desynchronization. But in all cases it needs several hundreds of milliseconds poststimulus for the frontal beta to develop. Frontal beta rhythm may be present in a subject together with the Rolandic beta rhythm. This is illustrated in Fig. 3.4. As one can see, the first stimulus presentation in GO and NOGO trials elicits a sequence of initial beta desynchronization and rebound beta synchronization in frontal areas (F3, F4). In contrast, beta in the sensory-motor strip (C3) desynchronizes during preparation for a movement with the beta rebound right after movement.

We have selected for the above example of rebound frontal beta synchronization a healthy adult subject with a prominent frontal beta rhythm. It is not a typical case. However similar data can be obtained for groups of healthy subjects. An example is given in Fig. 3.5 where grand average time–frequency representations of EEG responses in GO/NOGO task for a group of 15–16 years old adolescents are shown. Note that beta synchronization in response to the first stimuli in GO and NOGO pairs starts with considerable delay and reaches its maximum at around 800 ms. No frontal beta synchronization is observed in Ignored trials, that is, trials in which the presentation of the first stimulus indicated that the whole trial must be ignored.

Frontal beta synchronization induced by task can be also measured as a difference between overall EEG power in the beta frequency band in the task condition[3] and the corresponding parameter in eyes open condition. The difference

---

[3]Spectra are computed for the whole epoch of EEG recorded during the task.

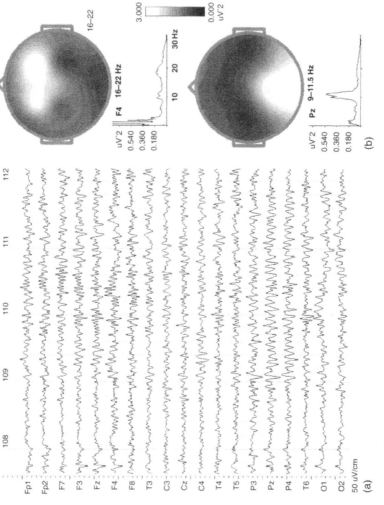

FIGURE 3.3 Frontal beta rhythm. (a) A fragment of 19-channel EEG in eyes open condition in a healthy subject of 53 years old. (b) Spectra in alpha and beta bands with the corresponding maps. Note that together with occipital alpha rhythm recorded at O1, O2, EEG reveals a strong spindling beta rhythm recorded at frontal areas with maximums at F3, F4. Note also that power of the beta rhythm is 3 times smaller than the power of the alpha rhythm.

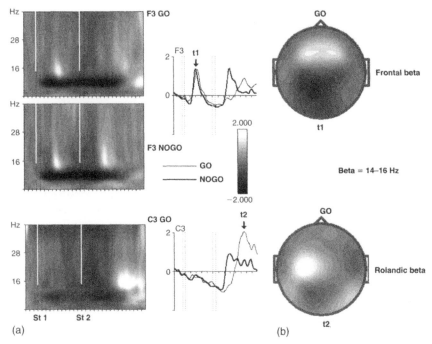

FIGURE 3.4   Rebound synchronization of frontal beta rhythm (single case). Data taken from a healthy 45 years old subject performing a two stimulus GO/NOGO task. (a) Power–time–frequency representations (wavelet transformations) of responses in GO and NOGO trials for F3 electrodes as well as responses in GO trials for C3 electrode. (b) Dynamics of relative EEG power in 18–24 Hz band and maps taken at the moments marked by arrows. Note that stimulus presentation (requiring decision making and not triggering movement) induced a small suppression of the frontal beta activity followed by rebound beta synchronization at 500 ms latency.

spectra in the beta frequency band might be a reliable measure of frontal lobe activation during task conditions. This is illustrated in Fig. 3.6 where EEG spectra for two different tasks (mathematical and GO/NOGO) are superimposed on spectra computed in eyes open condition. The map of the difference in the beta frequency band shows that the task-induced beta is distributed frontally. Moreover, the amount of frontal beta increase depends on the difficulty of the task[4].

---

[4]For comparison changes in beta activity associated with two psychological tests are depicted in Fig. 3.6. The first test is a quite difficult mathematical task that requires intense involving of working memory. The second test is an easier GO/NOGO task. In this test subjects are required to react only in 25 per cent of trials while performing a simple discriminating task. Difficulty of tasks is expressed in the number of errors which are much larger for the math task than for GO/NOGO task. One can see that the difficult task leads to increase of EEG activity in the frequency range from 14 to 20 Hz that is twice as much as the increase in beta activity generated by the simple task.

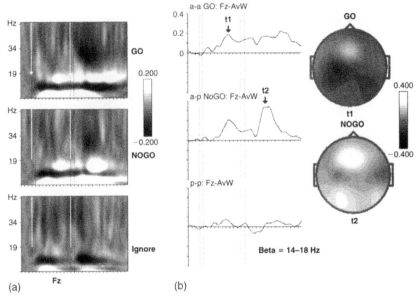

FIGURE 3.5   Rebound synchronization of frontal beta activity (group average). Averaged data from a group of 15–16 years old healthy subjects. Figure legends are the same as in Fig. 3.4.

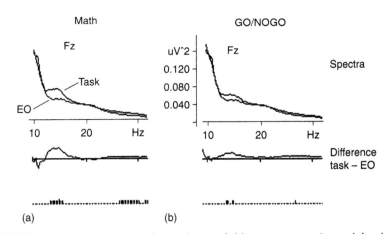

FIGURE 3.6   Task-related beta synchronization revealed by power spectra. Averaged data from a group of 13–14 years old healthy subjects. (a) Superimposed EEG power spectra computed in the mathematical (difficult) and two stimulus GO/NOGO (easy) tasks in comparison to the eyes open condition. (b) Difference spectra with vertical bars ($p < 0.05$) indicating the confidence level of difference.

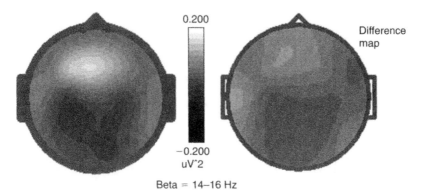

Beta = 14–16 Hz

FIGURE 3.6   (c) Maps of the difference for 14–16 frequency band.

II. NEURONAL MECHANISMS

A. Association with Cortical Activation

There is a close relationship between EEG power in beta band and metabolic activity in the corresponding cortical area of the human brain. It has been shown both for spontaneous EEG and evoked responses.

One of the most cited attempts in this respect was done by a group of scientists from UCLA (Cook et al., 1998). They performed simultaneous recording of multi-channel EEG and positron emission tomography (PET) scanning (by using radioactive water) in normal adult subjects, both at rest and during a simple motor task[5]. On the basis of their studies the authors concluded that (1) topographic EEG mapping can accurately reflect local brain function in a way that is comparable to other methods, and (2) the choice of EEG measure and montage have a significant influence on the degree with which EEG reflects the local metabolic activity. In relation to beta activity, the results show that EEG power in the beta frequency range of local average reference montage positively correlated with metabolic activity in a corresponding local cortical area (see Fig. 3.7)[6].

A strong relationship between EEG power and metabolic activity of the human brain suggests that absolute values of changes in all EEG bands may serve as an index of metabolic activation of the cortex in specific tasks. A comparison

---

[5]EEG data were processed using three different montages while two EEG power measures (absolute and relative power) were examined. The results of the studies showed that relative EEG power had much stronger associations with perfusion than the absolute power. In addition, calculating power for bipolar electrode pairs and averaging power over electrode pairs sharing a common electrode yielded stronger associations with perfusion than data from referential or single source montages.

[6]It should be noted that EEG power in other frequency bands is also correlated with metabolic activity but in different ways: alpha activity, for example, is negatively correlated with perfusion.

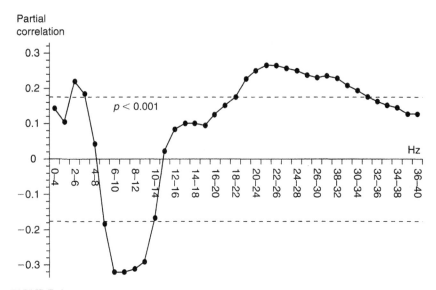

FIGURE 3.7 EEG-metabolism relationships. Relationship between local PET perfusion values and relative EEG power for relative source derivation montage. Statistical significance is indicated by horizontal dashed line representing the magnitude at which a correlation coefficient attains significance $p = 0.001$. Adapted from Cook et al. (1998).

between functional magnetic resonance imaging (fMRI) and evoked electromagnetic activity was made in a study of Singh et al. in 2002. They recorded MEG and fMRI data during a covert letter fluency task. The changes in MEG power were normalized and averaged across subjects. The results show that frequency-specific, task-related changes in cortical synchronization, detected in MEG, match those areas of the brain showing an evoked cortical hemodynamic response with fMRI. The majority of these changes were event-related desynchronizations (ERDs) in beta and alpha frequency ranges.

B. Sensitivity to GABA Agonists

The most striking feature of beta rhythms is their sensitivity to GABA agonists. Indeed, power of beta rhythmicity is enhanced after administration of barbiturates, some non-barbiturative sedatives, and minor tranquilizers[7]. Figure 3.8 schematically explains the action of the above mentioned drugs. It shows a Cl^- ligand-gated channel. When the channel is open it allows an influx of Cl^- ions inside the neuron. This influx hyperpolarizes the membrane and decreases the probability of

---

[7]Note that in contrast to increase of the power of the beta rhythm, the average frequency of the Rolandic beta rhythm decreases after administration of benzodiazepines (see Jensen et al., 2005).

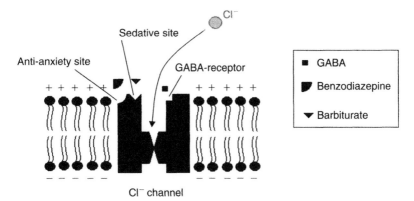

FIGURE 3.8   Scheme of GABA_A receptor. Shown a ligand-gated Cl⁻ channel that has three differ-ent sites (sedative site, anti-anxiety site, GABA receptor) with affinity to different substances depicted as different shapes.

neuronal discharge. The channel is a complex molecule that has several binding sites: the GABA binding site, the sedative, and anti-anxiety sites. The GABA site has affinity to GABA itself. The sedative site has affinity to alcohol or barbiturates such as phenobarbital. The anti-anxiety site binds benzodiazepines such as Valium, Librium, Halcion[8]. Inhibitory synapses differ in their position on the membrane from excitatory ones. Excitatory synapses usually occupy dendritic trees while inhibitory synapses are located on cell bodies.

The idea that oscillations may be generated as collective behavior of neuronal networks because of recurrent interaction between neurons appeared a long time ago. Many attempts were made to simulate such networks. Those attempts are in the frames of a separate, theoretical branch of neuroscience named neuronal networks.

C. Inhibition in Cortical Circuits

The research in neuronal networks simulation has shown that inhibitory neurons may play a critical role in generating oscillations. Networks generating oscillations consist of two types of reciprocally connected networks: inhibitory and excitatory. Imagine now that inhibition is blocked in such a net. Because of recurrent excita-tion the heavily interconnected network produces an avalanche behavior with a positive feedback. In such feedback the more neurons are active, the more they acti-vate other neurons through feedforward connections, and the more they get exci-tation via feedback connections. The positive feedback may lead to over-activation

---

[8]Because of their different actions on GABA receptors, sedative and anti-anxiety drugs should never be taken together. The combined doses of two types of drugs can produce coma or death.

Excitatory neuron

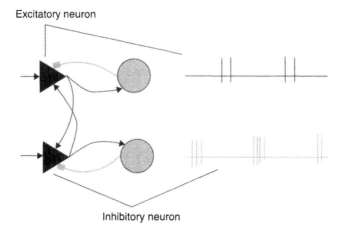

Inhibitory neuron

FIGURE 3.9   Neuronal model of beta oscillations. A simplified model of oscillations in a network with excitatory and inhibitory neurons. Note that activities in inhibitory and excitatory neurons are roughly reciprocal.

of the net. In reality, this over-activation is limited by inhibition. Inhibitory neurons impose breaking regulation on these avalanches: they periodically terminate over-activation of the network. The frequencies of these periodical terminations depend very much on duration of inhibitory postsynaptic potentials. The sequence of events in such neuronal network is schematically presented in Fig. 3.9. The network contains excitatory and inhibitory cells with interconnections between them and inputs from external sources. The external inputs serve as driving sources.

The above scheme of collective neuronal oscillations is a simplified and a hypothetical one[9]. Intuitively, such oscillations occur (1) if external inputs are quite strong to start an avalanche behavior, (2) if excitatory connections are strong enough to keep the excitation, (3) if the inhibitory connections are strong to stop the avalanche[10].

III. GAMMA ACTIVITY

Gamma rhythms (>30 Hz) have low energy and are difficult to record. Indeed 50 (60) Hz artifacts of electrical mains need special, so-called notch filters to eliminate those artifacts. The notch filters need to be very sharp to allow analysis in frequencies outside 50 (60) Hz. When special measures are taken to avoid the

[9]However, it reflects quite well internal connections of the canonical cortical circuit which is considered as good approximation of the real cortical networks.

[10]A new support for GABA receptor involvement in beta activity generation has recently come from combined electroencephalographic/molecular genetics studies. The strongest linkage with EEG power for the beta frequencies was observed on the short arm of chromosome 4. This region contains a cluster of $GABA_A$ receptor genes (Porjesz et al., 2005).

50 (60) Hz artifacts and to record EEG in the frequency range higher than 30 Hz, gamma oscillations can be analyzed.

A. Temporal Binding

In animal experiments the synchrony between neuronal elements at 40 Hz has been proposed as a special mechanism of neural cooperation, called temporal binding. This temporal coordination in spiking of spatially distributed neurons coded different features of the same image is needed to glue together representations of these different features of the image into a single percept. Much of the work in this field was done in Max-Planck-Institute for Brain Research in Frankfurt, Germany in a group headed by Wolf Singer. Recently, it was speculated that neuronal synchrony may be also critical for conscious processing (see, e.g., Engel and Singer, 2001).

In humans, scalp EEG recordings consistently reveal the existence of synchronized oscillatory activity in the gamma range when subjects experience a coherent visual percept. This was demonstrated by Tallon-Baudry and Bertrand in 1999. In this study the authors presented quasi-random dotted pictures to subjects. Naïve subjects perceived such stimuli as meaningless blobs. However, when the subjects were trained to detect the Dalmatian dog that was hidden in the pictures those now meaningful dotted pictures induced gamma activity at 280 ms after stimulus onset at occipital EEG recordings. A plausible interpretation of these findings is that objects giving rise to a coherent percept recruit visual areas that are synchronized in the gamma range.

Intracranial recording made by the same authors (Tallon-Baudry et al., 2005) showed that gamma induced synchronization can be found in the lateral occipital cortex and the fusiform gyrus. These areas consistently displayed large gamma oscillations during visual stimulus encoding, while other extrastriate areas remained systematically silent[11].

In our intracortical recordings of local field potentials in epileptic patients strong gamma synchronization was observed in Brobmann area 41 – the primary auditory cortex – in response to novel stimuli in the auditory odd-ball paradigm. This is illustrated by averaged wavelet transformations of responses in local field potentials in Fig. 3.10. As one can see only novel stimuli irrespectively whether condition of the task was passive (the patient just was watching a TV while the auditory stimuli were presented) or active (the patient had to press the bottom in response to deviant stimuli and to ignore both deviant and novel stimuli) elicit a strong (about 100 per cent) increase of the intracranial EEG power within the

---

[11]Simultaneously with wavelet analysis of induced EEG the authors also computed ERPs described in detail in Part III of the book. They showed that induced gamma activities and ERPs are different entities, because they could be present or absent in different intracranial areas independently of each other.

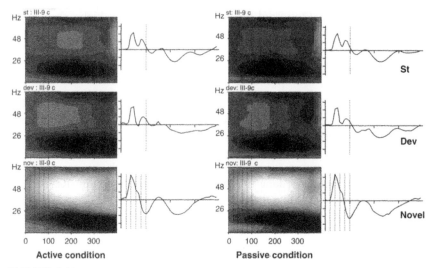

FIGURE 3.10   Synchronization of gamma activity in intracranial recording. Local field potentials were recorded in an epileptic patient to whom electrodes were implanted for diagnostic purposes into different areas of the left lateral (areas 41, 22) temporal cortex and the structures of the left medial temporal area (hippocampus, amygdala). The strongest synchronization of gamma activity was found in response to novel stimuli in the primary auditory cortex. Note that both local field potential ERPs and wavelet decomposition do not differ between the passive and active conditions indicating that information processing in the primary auditory cortex is attention independent. Stimuli of 100 ms duration start on 0 ms.

frequency range from 40 to 55 Hz and the latency of 120–250 ms. The functional significance of this response is not clear. Robert Knight who found similar responses in his intracranial studies associates this type of gamma synchronization with coding salient features of the auditory stimuli.

IV. FUNCTIONAL MEANING

Beta synchronization in tasks related to the visual modality can be observed not only in somato-sensory and frontal areas, but also in occipital areas (Fig. 3.11). In these areas beta synchronization occurs in response to Ignore or NOGO stimuli, that is, stimuli that were followed by subject's "relaxation," but not to stimuli (such as GO stimuli) that needed further processing or reactions. Figure 3.11 shows grand averages for wavelet transformations and ERD/ERS in beta frequency band for the left occipital area (O1 electrode). As one can see, beta synchronization in the occipital area is preceded by strong desynchronization both in alpha and beta frequency bands.

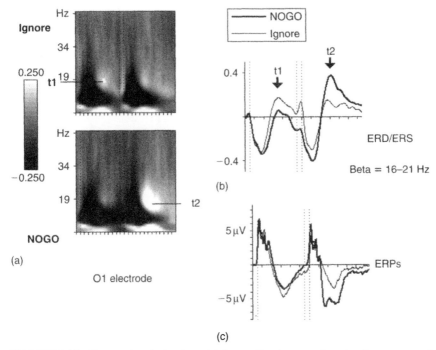

FIGURE 3.11   Beta synchronization in occipital areas. Grand average data taken from a group of healthy subjects of 14–15 years old. (a) Grand averaged power–time–frequency representations (wavelet transformations) of EEG responses at O1 electrode for NOGO and Ignore conditions. (b) ERD/ERS in beta band (16–21 Hz) in NOGO and Ignore conditions superimposed on each other. (c) ERPs computed for the same electrode and the same task conditions.

A. Beta Rhythms as Postactivation Traces

In Fig. 3.11 the most important fact, in regard to neuronal mechanisms, is the observation that beta synchronization was preceded by enhanced negative fluctuations in event-related potentials (ERPs) recorded simultaneously from the same electrode[12]. As will be shown in Part II of this book positive components of evoked potentials (at least in occipital areas in response to visual stimuli and for this particular age) are associated with excitatory postsynaptic potentials, while negative evoked potentials are, at least in part, associated with inhibitory postsynaptic potentials[13]. Taking this into account, we can conclude that beta synchronization

[12]The differences in negative components in response to the second stimuli between NOGO and Ignore conditions became evident 200 ms before any observed differences in beta synchronization. This observation indicates that beta synchronization follows changes in ERPs with significant delay.

[13]Note that this statement is a strong simplification and appears to be valid only for this particular case.

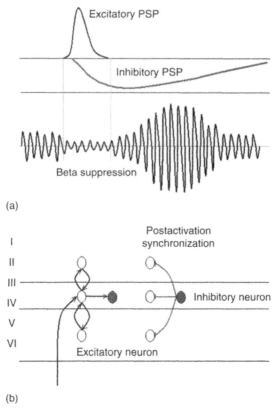

FIGURE 3.12   Beta synchronization as postactivation trace. A schematic representation of synaptic events in a cortical circuit in response to a sensory input. (a) Time course of postsynaptic excitatory and inhibitory potentials in response to a stimulus. (b) The main event during the two consecutive stages of information processing. The first stage is associated with activation of neurons via recurrent excitatory synaptic connections. During this stage beta rhythm is suppressed and information is processed actively. The second stage is associated with turning on inhibitory neurons and suppressing excitatory neurons. Increase of inhibition leads to strong synchronization of beta rhythm (middle). Functionally this postactivation trace resets the neuronal network for further processing new information.

is postactivation trace that follows a strong activation of occipital cortex. This postactivation trace is started by turning on inhibitory connections in the cortical network (Fig. 3.12).

This conclusion is in line with observations in regard to Rolandic and frontal beta synchronizations. Recall, that we associated beta event-related synchronization (ERS) with postactivation (rebound) effects in somato-sensory cortex and in frontal cortex. We speculate here that different types of beta synchronization (in a band from 14 to 30 Hz) observed in the tasks in response to stimuli and movements may be considered as a single phenomenon – postactivation trace.

B. Reset of Information Processing

The functional meaning of this trace is not clear. It could be a memory trace that the neuronal system keeps after its activation. However, under such assumption, the trace must be stronger for relevant stimuli. But we observe quite opposite, the trace is much stronger when stimulus is irrelevant and memory is needed no more. The most probable explanation of the observed phenomena is that beta synchronization, as a single entity, represents a reset operation. This operation is needed to erase the results of previous activation and corresponding computations and to prepare the system for new operations.

Anyway, beta activity must be considered as a delayed index of cortical activation. It occurs as a reaction to strong activation of cortical neuronal networks, when inhibitory neurons get enough excitation from the input and nearby excitatory neurons. During this phase of signal processing the inhibitory neurons start firing to suppress this strong activation. This inhibition occurs in cycles and each cycle is a wave of beta activity recorded at the scalp. In the normal brain, beta activity seems to act as a reset operation that clears all sequences of strong activation in neuronal networks and that enables the networks to process information again and again. In abnormal brain, when it occurs almost constantly and is reflected in too high level of beta activity it may be considered as an index of hyperactivation, irritation of the corresponding cortical area. Beta synchronization can be also enhanced if the inhibitory connections become potentiated such as after consumption of sedative and anti-anxiety drugs.

V. ABNORMAL BETA RHYTHMS

A. Need for Normative Databases

As we mentioned above beta rhythms are related to some specific states of the cortex. These states are characterized by a high level of external excitatory input and relatively strong intracortical inhibition. These states occur during a postactivation stage of information processing in response to a short stimulus presentation when inhibitory neurons switched on to suppress the neurons activated during the first stage of sensory processing. To define whether beta rhythm in a particular person is too large or too small one must rely on comparison with a normative database.

When the excess or lack of beta activity is found one have to interpret it with caution. First, the scalp distribution of beta excess is important. Uncommon locations, such as parietal or temporal must be paid more attention than sensory-motor or frontal locations. Second, asymmetry of beta activity itself (higher than 50 per cent) must be considered as additional indication of abnormality. Third, reactivity of the observed excessive beta rhythm is an important index of its functioning. If the excessive beta activity does not synchronize in response to task conditions in the way observed in the normative group, then this observation serves as additional indicator of abnormality. Fourth, patient's complains must be taken into account when a neurotherapy protocol or medication are to be recommended or prescribed.

B. Cortical Irritability

Increase of beta activity and a corresponding over-activation may be seen in areas associated with epileptic focus, for example, during pre-epileptic auras. Another example can be given by cortical hyperactivity associated with hallucinations. Auditory hallucinations are ones of the positive symptoms associated with schizophrenia. PET studies show that hallucinations are associated with hypermetabolism in the auditory cortical areas. In line with association beta activity with local brain metabolism, MEG studies show increase of beta activity (12.5–30 Hz) in the left auditory cortex that accompanies hallucinations (Ropohl et al., 2003).

Sometimes increase of beta activity can be visualized as spindling beta rhythms. This pattern has been reported to be associated with "cortical irritability," viral or toxic encephalopathies and epilepsy. This abnormal beta is seen in waxing and waning spindles over the effected cortex. Excess of beta activity has been found in less than 10 per cent of the ADHD population.

VI. SUMMARY

Beta band in EEG stands for the frequency above 13 Hz. Beta rhythm was first described by Hans Berger and was associated with focused attention. There are several types of rhythms in the beta band. To reflect this heterogeneity, the beta band is conventionally divided into the following sub-bands: low beta – from 13 to 20 Hz, high beta – from 21 to 30 Hz, gamma activity – from 31 Hz and higher. Sometimes, a special type "40 Hz activity" is separated in addition to the listed ones. This type of beta activity attracted a big interest of scientists in 1980s. The research was focused on a so-called binding problem in perception. Networks of inhibitory interneurons have shown both theoretically and experimentally to be crucially involved in generating beta rhythms. The involvement of inhibitory neurons is supported by the sensitivity of beta rhythms to GABAergic agonists – pharmaceuticals that mimic the action of GABA, the main inhibitory mediator in the central nervous system. GABA agonists such as barbiturates and benzodiazepines increase the power of high frequency bands. In the normal brain, beta activity was shown to be positively correlated with metabolic activity in the cortical area underlying the recording electrode.

CHAPTER 4

Frontal Midline
Theta Rhythm

I. CHARACTERISTICS

A. Spatial Distribution

According to the international nomenclature, the *theta band* is "the frequency band from 4 to under 8 Hz," and the *theta rhythm* is the "rhythm with a frequency of 4 to under 8 Hz". In 1950, Arellano and Schwab observed a 4–7 cycle/s rhythm in the midline just anterior to the vertex which occurred during problem solving. Ishihara and Yoshii in Japan induced the electroencephalogram (EEG) theta activity by administering a mental task consisting of continuous arithmetic addition. This theta activity was a train of rhythmic waves at a frequency of 6–7 Hz with a maximum amplitude around the frontal midline. The authors named this theta rhythm as the frontal midline theta.

An example of frontal midline theta activity recorded in one of the healthy subjects from our normative database is presented in Fig. 4.1. A 19 years old student participated in the task in which she has to make a simple arithmetic operation – to add two digits presented on the screen for 100 ms – and then to compare the result with a number presented 1 s later. As one can see, an effort associated with a mathematical operation evokes bursts of 2–3 cycles in the theta band.

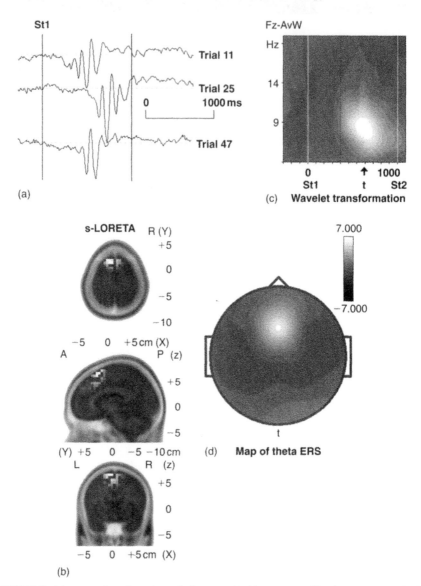

FIGURE 4.1   Frontal midline theta rhythm in a healthy 19 year-old subject. (a) Raw EEG recorded in three different trials at Fz during the math task. Visual stimuli were presented in pairs. The first stimulus (St1) in the pair was a brief presentation of two digits connected by a math operation (i.e., 2 + 2). The second stimulus whether corresponded to the result of the mathematical operation (i.e., digit 4) or did not (i.e., digit 5). The subject had to press button in response to the right stimulus. Note emergence of the not stimulus-locked bursts of the theta rhythm. (b) The s-LORETA images of the potential generators of those theta bursts are presented. (c) The averaged wavelet decomposition of EEG responses in the task. X-axis – time, Y-axis – frequency, color (see color scale) codes the averaged relative changes of EEG (event-related synchronization – ERS) in the theta frequency range. (d) The map of the ERS measured at $t = 700$ ms.

These bursts were not synchronized (time locked) with stimulus presentations and, consequently, could be revealed only by ERD/ERS method (see methods). The bursts of theta were observed not in every trial but randomly every 3 or 5 trials with a time period between separate bursts around 20 s. s-LORETA images indicate that those bursts are generated in the medial part of the prefrontal cortex (including anterior gyrus cingulate).

Frontal midline theta rhythm belongs to a separate category of brain rhythms and, consequently, is independent on alpha rhythms. This statement is illustrated in Fig. 4.2. Independent component analysis (ICA) was applied to raw EEG of a healthy subject performing the mathematical task. As one can see at the bottom the map of EEG spectra taken at 6.8 Hz (the mean frequency of theta rhythm recorded in the subject) overlaps with the maps of alpha rhythms (occipital and parieto-central) recorded in the subject. However application of the ICA method to the raw EEG clearly separate five different components with the first one belonging to the frontal midline theta rhythm.

In a study of Hiroshi Asada and colleagues (Asada et al., 1999), to clarify the source of rhythmic activity, magneto-encephalogram (MEG) and EEG were simultaneously measured in healthy volunteers during different mental tasks using whole head MEG system. MEG records were averaged every one cycle of frontal midline theta rhythms using individual positive peaks of frontal midline theta waves in Fz EEG as a trigger. Averaged theta components of MEG signals were analyzed with a multi-dipole model. Two sources were estimated to the regions both of the prefrontal medial superficial cortex and anterior cingulate cortex (ACC). These regions were alternatively activated in about 40–120 grades phase shift during one frontal midline theta cycle[1].

B. Personality Traits of People Generating the Rhythm

During the resting state with eyes open or eyes closed, the frontal midline theta as a prominent peak at EEG spectra is found only in minority of normal subjects. The rest of normal population does not reveal any signs of this rhythmicity. One explanation could be that because of deeply located generators the frontal midline theta becomes visible on the scalp only in rare cases. Indeed, for any cortical

---

[1]In a study of another Japanese group (Sasaki et al., 1996) medial location of FMT generator was questioned. This group demonstrated that current dipoles responsible for frontal theta 5-7 Hz burst activities scatter successively in wide cortical areas of the frontal lobes of both the cerebral hemispheres during mental calculation and mental tasks related to music. They gave an interpretation for this contradiction as follows: the theta activities generated in wide areas of both frontal cortices appeared to be seemingly maximal on the midline with EEG, because extracellular electrical currents generated in pyramidal neurons of wide frontal areas on both sides are summed, and flow densely along the midline through the volume conductor with several layers of different electrical impedances surrounding the hemispheres, mainly due to a shunting effect caused by the low impedance of the cerebrospinal fluid.

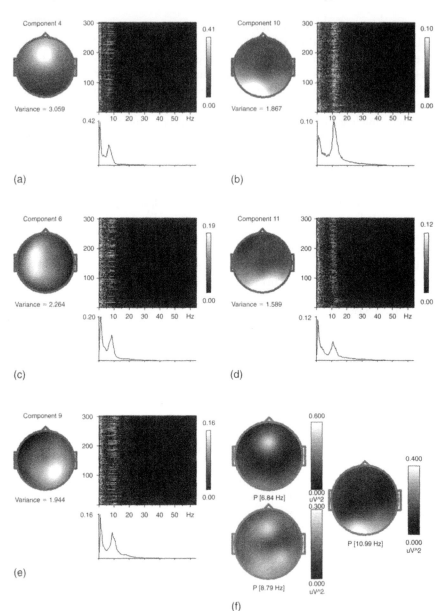

FIGURE 4.2   The frontal midline theta as a separate EEG rhythmic component. EEG was recorded in a healthy 20 year old subject performing the math task of the normative database. (f) Maps of EEG spectra computed at three different frequencies. The results of the ICA decomposition of raw EEG are presented in columns. For each component: left – topography, bottom – spectrum, right – color coded components for sequential 4s epochs of analysis with the first time intervals of the task is shown at the bottom.

rhythm to be recordable from the scalp the following requirements must be fulfilled. First, the sources have to be near the surface, but not too deep in the brain. Second, the sources must be synchronized over relatively large spatial scales. Third, the sources must be strong enough to be recorded on the skin of the head[2].

The incidence of frontal midline theta emitting subjects reported by the Japanese research groups is 43 per cent in young adults (18–28 years of age), and 11 per cent in older subjects. In their studies (for review see Inanaga, 1998) the normal subjects were divided into three groups according to the amount of the frontal midline theta generated in an arithmetic task at Fz: low, moderate, and high frontal midline theta groups[3]. The high frontal midline theta group showed the lowest anxiety score, the highest score in the extraversion scale, and the lowest score in the neurotic scale. The low frontal midline theta group, on the other hand, showed an opposite association; they showed the highest anxiety score, the lowest extraversion score, and the highest neurotic score. No differences were observed in these three groups in respect of the quality of the task. From these results, it is suggested that the appearance of the frontal midline theta showed a close relationship to personality trait and/or anxiety level of the subject.

II. NEURONAL MECHANISMS

A. Association with Cortical Activation

In contrast to alpha rhythms frontal midline theta was associated with activation and increase of metabolic activity in the medial frontal area and anterior cingulate cortex. In patients with intracranial recording for epilepsy assessment, electrical stimulation of the anterior cingulate cortex has been found to induce a 3–8 Hz rhythm in fronto-medial recordings as well as autonomic changes (Talairach et al., 1973). A research group from Harvard University and University of Wisconsin, USA (Pizzagalli et al., 2003) was the first that studied the link between frontal theta midline activity and metabolism in the human brain. Concurrent measurements of brain electrical activity (EEG) and glucose metabolism (PET) were performed in healthy subjects at baseline. EEG data were analyzed with a source localization technique that enabled voxel wise correlations of EEG and PET data. For theta, but not other bands, the rostral ACC (Brodmann areas 24/32) was the largest cluster with positive correlations between current density and glucose metabolism.

---

[2]The other possibility could be that frontal midline theta depends on genetic factors and is revealed only in a specific group of normal population.

[3]In order to evaluate the personality traits and the anxiety level of the subject, Maudsley Personality Inventory and Taylor's Manifest Anxiety Scale were adopted and completed by the subjects after the EEG measurements.

B. Association with Hippocampal Theta Rhythms

Frontal midline theta rhythm in human EEG is often associated with hippocampal theta in mammals. The reason for this association is straightforward: the most striking feature of the hippocampus in mammals is the ability to generate theta rhythm. This rhythmicity can be globally recorded by macro electrodes in all parts of the hippocampus and in majority of interconnected anatomical structures. This type of global, extracellular recorded phenomenon reflects cooperative behavior of large number of hippocampal pyramidal cells. The hippocampal pyramidal cells, all having similar orientations, fire in synchrony and periodically to produce theta oscillations. The frequency of these oscillations varies in a quite broad range from 4 to 10 Hz depending of species and functional state. These types of oscillations are usually combined under single name hippocampal theta rhythms or, in a broader sense, limbic theta rhythms.

C. Limbic System of Hippocampal Theta Rhythms

Brain structures in which theta rhythms can be observed are depicted in Fig. 4.3. These structures actually represent a loop[4]. The information flow in this loop

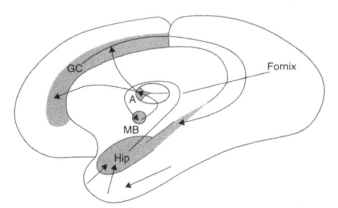

FIGURE 4.3   Anatomical structures where theta rhythms are observed. Hippocampus (Hip) receives multi-modal sensory inputs mixed with inputs from the gyrus cingulus, processes them and sends the results to mamillary bodies (MB) of hypothalamus through the pathway named Fornix, where they are integrated with other inputs to be sent to anterior nucleus (A) of the thalamus. The anterior nucleus serves as a relay nucleus to the gyrus cingulus (GC).

[4]This loop is also called Papez circle. In 1937 an American neuroanatomist John Papez described a brain circuit (or loop) beginning and ending in the hippocampal formation. He proposed that this circuit plays a critical role in emotional experience. Unlike its persistence as anatomical entity the function of the Papez circle has been less resilient. The early notion that Papez's circuit is associated with emotions has been abandoned and replaced by the proposal that it is primarily involved in mnemonic functions. This proposal was made on the results of studies showing that lesions of each of the major components of the circuit disrupt episodic memory but not affective functions.

could be simplified as follows: (1) the hippocampus receives polysensory signal through the rhinal cortex of the medial temporal lobe from various temporal and parietal sensory areas and a signal from the anterior part of the gyrus cingulus, (2) the hippocampus integrates this information and sends the results of processing to the mamillary bodies (MB) of the hypothalamus by means a bundle of axons called the fornix, (3) the MB send the information further to the anterior nucleus of the thalamus by means of so-called mamillo-thalamic bundle, (4) the anterior nucleus of the thalamus relays the information to the anterior gyrus cingulus, which through its connection to the hippocampus closes the loop.

D. Classic Model of Hippocampal Theta Rhythms Generation

As clinical evidence indicate, hippocampus is critical for consolidation of episodic memory. Despite intensive experimental research the link between memory-related phenomena at the cellular–molecular level, on one hand, and computations at the network level, on the other hand, remains unknown. One of the key issues of the current research is to understand how theta rhythm is generated by collective behavior of single neurons and what role this rhythmicity plays in memory formation. With this goal, hippocampal theta rhythms have been extensively studied in animal models, especially in rats. These studies revealed a classic model of theta generation in the hippocampus (see Fig. 4.4).

According to this model the theta rhythm originates in the brainstem as a non-rhythmic neuronal activation (indicated by arrow in Fig. 4.4). The neuronal elements of the brain stem include noradrenergic cells in the locus coeruleus, serotoninergic cells in the raphe nuclei, dopaminergic cells in the ventral tegmental area, and the substantia nigra pas compacta. Activation of these cells directly by sensory collaterals or indirectly through feedback projections from the cortex leads to activation of cells in septal nuclei – nuclei in the basal forebrain. The activation of septal neurons starts the burst of theta rhythm.

A critical role in theta rhythm generation is played by reciprocal connections of neurons in the septal region[5] with neurons in the hippocampus. In the resting state, a background activity of inhibitory neurons in the hippocampus suppresses the hippocampal pyramidal cells so that no sensory information is encoded into a memory trace. If a behaviorally meaningful stimulus (e.g., emotionally competent event) is presented, this stimulus through ascending activating system of the brain stem activates the septal excitatory and inhibitory neurons. The septal inhibitory neurons inhibit the inhibitory cells in the hippocampus. This inhibition of inhibitory cells (also named disinhibition) removes the background inhibition from the

[5]The area includes the medial septum and diagonal band of Broca.

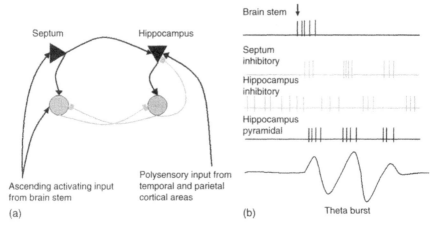

FIGURE 4.4   (a) Neuronal network for generating hippocampal theta rhythm. The network seems to be designed by nature to transform strong transient activation of the inputs from brain stem and multimodal cortical areas into a burst of theta rhythm. The network consists of excitatory and inhibitory neurons located in the septal region and hippocampus. The septal neurons through inhibition of inhibitory hippocampal neurons gate the sensory information flow through the hippocampus. Reciprocal inhibitory connections between the septum and the hippocampus generate a burst of theta rhythm. Excitatory neurons and excitatory connections are marked by black, while inhibitory connections – by gray. (b) Bursts of action potentials generated by different parts of the network.

pyramidal cells and eventually gates the pyramidal cells. This sequence of neuronal events starts a theta cycle.

Further on, the activation of pyramidal cells in the hippocampus inhibits the inhibitory cells in the septal nuclei, which in turn removes inhibition from hippocampal inhibitory neurons, and they in turn inhibit the pyramidal cells. This ends the cycle. In this scheme, the septal region is considered as the nodal point where ascending non-rhythmical inputs from the reticular system of the brain stem are converted into rhythmical signals of the septal neurons that are further transmitted to hippocampus. Hippocampal theta depends strongly on the strength of the input from the septal region: when a certain critical level of activation of septal neurons is reached, the hippocampal theta rhythm materializes[6].

E. Involvement in Memory Operations

Several lines of evidence support the concept that the theta rhythm plays an important role in specific memory operations. First, long-term potentiation (LTP)

---

[6]There seem to be not one but at least two types of theta rhythmicity in the animal hippocampus. Type 1 theta, associated with voluntary movements, is resistant to atropine or to cholinergic depletion. Type 2 theta, sometimes present during immobility, is abolished by atropine and occurs spontaneously during urethane anesthesia (Kramis et al., 1975).

as a mechanism of synaptic modification[7] is sensitive to the phase of the theta rhythm, with potentiation favored at the peak of the cycle and depotentiation favored at its trough (Huerta and Lisman, 1993). Second, a number of studies have reported that induction of LTP is optimal when the time interval between stimuli is approximately 200 ms, that is, in theta range. Third, septal lesions not only block theta in the hippocampus but also produce severe impairments in memory function. These finding suggests that the theta rhythm acts as a windowing mechanism for synaptic plasticity[8].

It should be stressed that the hippocampus is not the only area in the brain revealing theta rhythm. This rhythm was found in a large number of brain structures: parahippocampal cortex, anterior gyrus cingulus, MB of hypothalamus, medial dorsal nucleus of the thalamus (Fig. 4.3). All these structures belong to the limbic system. Although these structures cannot generate theta activity alone they are interconnected with each other and provide a complex network with several functions and, consequently, with several possible roles for theta rhythms. Gyorgy Buzsáki, the world expert in this field, suggested using the term "limbic theta oscillations" instead of hippocampal rhythm, reflecting the complexity and distributed nature of theta oscillations.

F. Theta Quantum

In line with this functional view on the limbic system is the discovery of LTP and its relation to the hippocampal theta rhythm. Indeed, as we mentioned above, induction of LTP is optimal when the stimulus is repeated with periodicity in theta range. To induce LTP a rhythmic stimulation at theta frequency is not needed: just two high frequency bursts with 200 ms interval are sufficient to induce long-term changes in synaptic strength. These data explicitly show that for memorizing the brain does not need sustained theta, only two incomplete cycles are sufficient. That is why a theta cycle may be considered as information quantum. This quantum seems to serve for functional linkage of different limbic structures allowing encoding of a certain episode of our daily life into a memory chunk.

[7]LTP was discovered in the mammalian hippocampus by Terje Lømo in 1966 (for review see Lømo, 2003). In vitro and in vivo experiments condition a series of short, high-frequency electric stimuli to a synapse strengthen, or potentiate, the synapse for minutes to hours and days. LTP is considered as one of the major mechanisms of memory formation.

[8]Theta appears to play a role in the neural coding of place (O'Keefe and Recce, 1993). As a rat traverses a place field, hippocampal "place cells" fire at a progressively earlier phase of the ongoing theta oscillation. This information may significantly improve accuracy in reconstructing the animal's position in space (beyond rate-coded information alone). Another view (Bland and Oddie, 2001) suggests that theta rhythm plays a role in sensory-motor integration. Consistent with this hypothesis, human theta oscillations occur during exploratory search and goal-seeking behaviors, as well as during virtual movement, when sensory information and motor planning are both in flux; compared with periods of self-initiated stillness.

G. Hippocampus as a Map of Episodes

The most popular view of the hippocampal function is that hippocampus encodes in compressed form and temporally stores the neocortical representation of an episode (McNaughton, 1989). There are actually two parts of any episodic event: sensory-related part (including neuronal elements encoding different properties of visual images, acoustic signals, body sensations…) and action-related part (including neuronal elements encoding executed action, emotional state, motivation…). These two parts of the episode are encoded in different cortical areas of parietal-temporal lobes for the sensory-related part and in different cortical areas of the frontal lobe for the action-related part. The anterior gyrus cingulus serves as intermediate integrating area in the prefrontal lobe. It integrates all information from various prefrontal areas and sends the results of processing to motor areas and to the hippocampus. Although the posterior and anterior parts are interconnected with each other they encode quite different representations of the episode. We suggest that the hippocampus is a place in the brain where all various and spatially distributed representations of the episode converge into a single activation pattern or segment[9] (Fig. 4.5).

H. Theta Rhythm and Memory Consolidation

Without hippocampus and related structures[10] the trace in these areas can be kept only in the working memory in a form of reverberation of neuronal impulses in recurrent neuronal networks. This working memory trace lasts few seconds and is very sensitive to interference – any new episode activates a distributed trace that overlaps with the trace of the previous episode destroys it.

We hypothesize that the hippocampal trace lasts for longer time intervals. The duration of the hippocampal trace might be determined by strong LTP induced by high frequency bursts of spikes that follow each other with an optimal (at theta period) time intervals. This process is proposed to allow the hippocampal system to rapidly learn new information without disrupting old memory stored in the neocortex, while at the same time allowing gradual integration of the new information into the older, structured information.

The above model actually suggests that the hippocampus serves as a temporally storage mechanism for the episode. An important episode induces a burst of theta activity which reflects synchronous activation of hippocampal cells associated with a compressed trace. If an episode is not important enough it does not evoke a theta burst and it will not be consolidated.

---

[9]Anatomically the hippocampus ideally fits a mapping mechanism. The hippocampus consists of a large number of segments aligned in long linear strip. Activation of a limited number of segments would successfully map the cortical representations of episode into a spatial pattern of hippocampal activity.

[10]Such as MB of the hypothalamus and anterior nucleus of the thalamus.

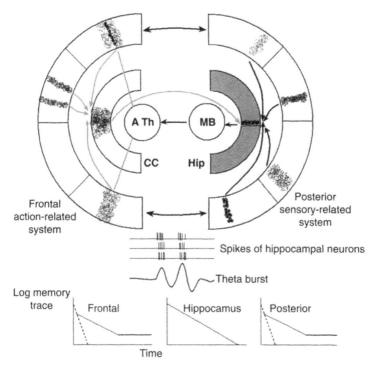

FIGURE 4.5   Hippocampus as a mapping memory device. The sensory part of the episode is mapped in the sensory-related posterior regions of the cortex, while the action part of the episode is mapped in the prefrontal areas. These two representations are in turn mapped into the hippocampus. The reverberation-based traces in the prefrontal-posterior regions are stored only for a short time (traces depicted in interrupted line) while the LTP-based traces in the hippocampus (because of strong LTP in hippocampal cells) are stored for a longer time (traces depicted in gray) before they become consolidated and kept in the permanent memory (traces in black).

The hippocampal representation later becomes active either in explicit recall, or in implicit processes such as sleep. This gives rise to reinstatement of the corresponding neocortical memory, resulting in incremental adjustment of neocortical connections, probably involving local, synaptic consolidation. So, the hippocampus uses its representation of the episode to recreate repeatedly the neocortical representation until it becomes consolidated, integrated, and independent of the hippocampus[11]. This temporal representation of the episode in the hippocampus

[11]Much evidence suggests that sleep plays a pivotal role in synaptic plasticity and memory. It has been shown that sleep is essential after visual training for the consolidation of some forms of procedural memory, such as visual discrimination skills. However, the facilitating effect of sleep is not limited to procedural memory, as sleep deprivation produces marked impairments of episodic memory. It was proposed that the facilitating effect of sleep on memory consolidation depends on the synchronized neuronal activity of slow wave sleep. For instance, an influential model of episodic memory

is relatively insensitive to interference because separate episodes are mapped into spatially separate parts of the hippocampus.

III. RESPONSES TO TASKS

A. Increasing with Memory Load

Inspired by animal research, human theta has been studied extensively in memory tasks during the last two decades. In one of the first studies performed by Alan Gevins from EEG systems Laboratory and SAM technology in San Francisco (Gevins et al., 1997), changes in cortical activity during working memory tasks were examined with EEGs sampled from 115 channels and spatially sharpened with magnetic resonance imaging (MRI)-based finite element deblurring technique. Subjects performed tasks requiring comparison of each stimulus to a preceding one on verbal or spatial attributes. A frontal midline theta rhythm increased in magnitude with increasing memory load. Theta signals increased, and overt performance improved, after practice on the tasks.

B. Two Types of Theta Responses

The leading role in studies of theta rhythms in humans belongs to a group of Wolfgang Klimesch from Saltzburg, Austria (for review see Klimesch, 1999). The group gained the evidence that there seem to be several theta activities with different associations to memory and attention. The first type of theta activity may be related to sustained attention or working memory. This type of attention-related theta activity is expressed in long lasting, tonic oscillations in the theta frequency band. As far as phasic bursts of theta activity concerns there seem to be two types of transient theta responses: the parietal theta activity that is associated with encoding of episodic memory and the frontal activity that is associated with retrieval operation. This conclusion is supported by numerous studies of the Klimesch's group who found that the extent of theta synchronization during encoding predicts later memory performance and that event-related theta synchronization during recognition for old words is larger than for new words.

(Buzsáki, G., 1989) postulates that during waking, information is initially stored in the CA3 region of the hippocampus, through changes in the strength of connections between pyramidal neurons. Later, during slow wave sleep, synchronized population discharges of CA3 neurons would "replay" the representations stored in the CA3 network and, via the rhinal cortices, reactivate associative cortical neurons representing features of the event of interest. Ultimately, this replay of stored representations would lead to long-term synaptic changes in associative cortical networks.

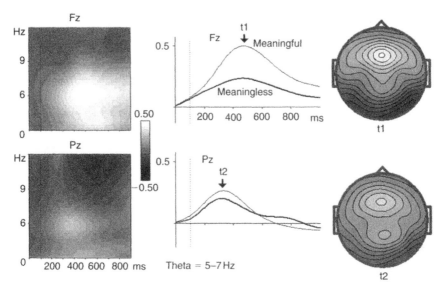

FIGURE 4.6   Two types of theta-like activity (wavelet analysis). Grand averaged wavelet transformations of EEG responses in the two stimulus GO/NOGO task. Meaningful (animal at the first place in the pair) and meaningless (plant at the first place) stimuli evoke theta-like activities in frontal and parietal areas: These induced rhythms have quite different temporal pattern: the parietal theta has a shorter latency: 350 ms versus 500 ms for the frontal rhythm. The frontal theta depends critically on the behavioral meaning of the stimulus, while the parietal theta does not depend on the stimulus meaning.

A support of existence of two phasic theta responses also comes from a study by Nobuaki Nishiyama and Yoko Yamaguchi from Brain Science Institute (BSI), RIKEN in Japan (Nishiyama and Yamaguchi, 2001). They recorded EEG from 64 channels during human virtual maze navigation. Theta oscillations were observed as bursts composed of several cycles. These burst were usually localized at two regions, the frontal region and the parietal-temporal region. The former is identified as the frontal midline theta. The activity in the parietal-temporal region was accompanied by bursts of the frontal midline theta while the phase difference between the two regions varied from time to time.

Two types of theta-like activity have been also observed in the data obtained from the Human Brain Institute Normative Database. Grand average power–time–frequency representations of EEG responses in the two stimulus GO/NOGO task are shown in Fig. 4.6. Stimuli are divided into two categories: meaningful and meaningless[12]. One can see that these stimuli induce synchronization of theta-like

[12]"Meaningful" stimuli are pictures of "animals" at the first place in pairs of stimuli. After presentation of these stimuli subjects had to prepare for the next stimulus presentation and to press a button if the second stimulus matched the first one. "Meaningless" – are pictures of plants at the first place. After presentation of these stimuli subject were able to relax and to ignore the whole trial.

activity in frontal and parietal areas. These theta-like activities are different not only in relation to spatial distribution (frontal versus parietal) but in relations to time dynamics, attention and mode of habituation to repeated trials. Indeed, first, the peak latencies of responses in the parietal areas are shorter than those in the frontal areas. Second, the frontal theta synchronization in contrast to the parietal theta synchronization is higher to Meaningful in Comparison to Meaningless stimuli. And third, frontal theta habituated to repeated trials while parietal theta did not habituate at all (not shown in Fig. 4.6).

Two types of theta-like activities may be revealed by simple subtraction of spectra in the eyes open condition from spectra in the task condition (the mathematical task is selected for example). The results of subtraction for a group of healthy 13–14 years old subjects are presented in Fig. 4.7. Note that the task is associated with larger EEG power in the theta (4–8 Hz) frequency range at the frontal area Fz and with larger EEG power in the frequency range from 5.5 to 9.5 Hz at the

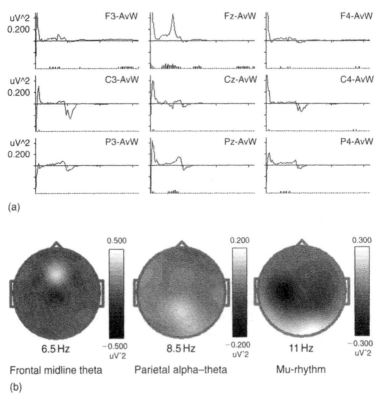

FIGURE 4.7   Two types of theta-like activity (spectral analysis). (a) The result of subtraction spectra computed for eyes open from spectra in the math task condition for a group of healthy 13–14 years old children. (b) Maps of difference spectra for different frequencies.

parietal area Pz[13]. Note also suppression of EEG power over the sensory-motor cortex due to constant button pressings which, as we know from above, induces suppression of mu-rhythm at the sensory-motor cortex.

The tasks in which frontal midline theta is most prevalent are those in which the subject is engaged in focused, but also relaxed, concentration. In examples presented above the tasks were the two stimulus GO/NOGO test and the mathematical task. Other examples of tasks associated with induction of the frontal midline theta rhythm are games such as Tetris, driving tasks ... In one study (Laukka et al., 1995), subjects were engaged in a simulated driving task in which they had to learn how to navigate through a series of streets represented as animation on a computer screen. It was found that the power of frontal midline theta activity increased as the subjects grew better at the task, making more correct decisions.

C. Appearance in Hypnosis

A condition that is also associated with appearance of the frontal midline theta is hypnosis. In order to be hypnotized, people have to focus their attention on themselves and the person that is hypnotizing them. If they are distracted, the trance is broken. Highly hypnotizable people exhibit significantly more theta before and during hypnosis than low hypnotizables (Crawford, 1994). Another unique human condition linking theta activity to attention is meditation. During zen meditation, EEG in experienced practitioners has been recorded (Takahashi et al., 2005). As the zen-practitioners reach deeper and deeper meditative states or trances, the typical patterns of EEG activity begin with alpha activity (8–10 Hz) and gradually move into the theta range as the trance progresses.

IV. FUNCTIONAL MEANING

A. Associating Two Types of Human Theta Responses with Two Types of Theta in Animals

A detailed analysis of wavelet transformation of neuronal responses in different tasks obtained in the Human Brain Institute Normative Database shows that there are at least two types of theta-like activities. The first one is frontal midline theta rhythm. It is expressed in short bursts of activity within the range of 5–8 Hz. This rhythm increases with task load, is higher to meaningful stimuli and habituates if the same stimulus is presented several times. The second, parietal alpha–theta rhythm can be hardly seen on spectra computed for eyes open or eyes closed

---

[13]This type of rhythmic activity occupies the range of alpha and theta activity. That is why we call it alpha–theta rhythm.

conditions and appears only with task load. The parietal alpha–theta rhythm seems to appear even in shorter bursts in comparison to the frontal midline theta. It is on average of lower amplitude than the frontal midline theta rhythm, it does not depend on behavioral meaning of the stimulus, and it does not habituate with repetition of the stimulus. This rhythm was quite recently observed and was not investigated in detail.

Mechanisms of generations of those rhythms are unknown. Their relationships to hippocampal theta rhythms have not been clearly proved. However there are some analogies between these human rhythms and two types of theta activity found in hippocampal system in animal studies which we can not avoid to mention in this context. In animal studies two types of hippocampal theta rhythms are distinguished on the basis of pharmacological sensitivity, frequency, and behavior. Type 1 is not blocked by acetylcholine antagonists, but is sensitive to anesthetic agents such as urethane, ethyl ether, and alcohol, has 6–10 Hz frequency, and occurs during voluntary (exploring) motor movements. Type 1 theta does not habituate. In human scalp recordings this high frequency theta may be associated with the parietal theta rhythm. It is evoked in short bursts, does not habituate and seems to be related to sensory encoding.

Type 2 theta in animals is eliminated by muscarinic (cholinergic) receptor antagonists such as atropine. Peak frequency of his rhythm is usually 4–6 Hz (lower than Type 1). This type occurs during locomotion, immobility, and urethane anesthesia. Type 2 theta, in contrast to Type 1 theta, habituates in the intact animal. Type 2 theta appears in response to sensory stimuli when an animal is in "aroused" state. Spontaneous production of Type 2 theta in the rat is exceptionally rare and of a very short duration. Type 2 theta is observed during conditioning and appears to be associated with learning. Type 2 theta generation is mediated by cholinergic inputs to the hippocampal formation from the medial septum[14]. In human scalp recordings the analog of this rhythm might be associated to the frontal midline theta rhythm which strongly habituates and seems to be related to episodic memory.

The frontal midline theta in the resting state can be found in the raw EEG only in a small group of normal population and seems to be related to a genetically determined behavioral trait, which is low in anxiety scale, low in neurotic scale, and high in extraversion scale. There are also studies suggesting that the frontal midline theta reflects feelings of relief from anxiety[15]. We are now aware of

---

[14]The most intriguing part of this story comes from the observation that the same pyramidal neurons can participate in generation of part 1 and part 2 theta oscillations indicating that the same anatomical structures can be involved in generating both rhythms.

[15]For example in a study of a Japanese group, EEG was recorded in patients with generalized anxiety disorder while the Hamilton Rating Scale for Anxiety and the State Anxiety Scale of Spielberger's State-Trait Anxiety Inventory were evaluated once a week. The data suggest that the appearance of frontal midline theta might be closely related to an improvement in the anxiety symptoms associated with generalized anxiety disorder (Suetsugi et al., 2000).

at least three different ways of inducing the frontal midline theta. They are meditation, neurofeedback, and binaural-beat technique[16].

V. ABNORMAL THETA RHYTHMS

Clinical significance of the normal frontal midline theta rhythm and the parietal alpha–theta rhythm is limited for several reasons. First, these rhythms are of short duration and appear only in task conditions, closely depending on the task difficulty. Second, even in task conditions they can be seen in EEG spectra in a form of peaks only in some part of healthy population. Third, the difficulty of recording these rhythms creates difficulty in systematic studies of their neuronal mechanisms.

A. Frontal Midline Theta Subtype of ADHD

At the current stage of research, we are now aware of one condition that is associated with abnormality in generating the frontal midline theta rhythm. This is a rare sub-type of attention deficit hyperactivity disorder (ADHD) population. In the symptoms that this group is exhibited the most important are poor social relationships and inability to correct behavior. From electrophysiological point of view this ADHD-subtype is characterized by very long runs of the frontal midline theta rhythm. The presence of the rhythm is expressed in extremely high and sharp peak on EEG spectra at Fz in frequency range from 5.5 to 8 Hz and extremely low theta synchronization in response to meaningful stimuli in the two-stimulus GO/NOGO and math tasks conditions.

B. Theta Rhythms in Non-frontal Areas

Appearance of theta rhythms in other than Fz (and to some extant at Pz) electrode positions must be considered as abnormal. In such cases comparison to the normative database is necessary to determine the confidence level of observed

---

[16]Binaural-beat stimulation is an important element of a patented auditory guidance system developed by Robert A. Monroe. In this method individuals are exposed to factors including breathing exercises, guided relaxation, visualizations, and binaural beats. The last factor is based on ability of the brain to detect differences in frequencies of auditory tones presented in the left and right ears. This perception of the binaural-beat is at a frequency that is the difference between the two auditory inputs. Binaural beats can easily be heard at the low frequencies (<30 Hz) that are characteristic of the EEG spectrum. The perception of the binaural-beat is associated with an EEG frequency following response. This phenomenon is described by Atwater (1997).

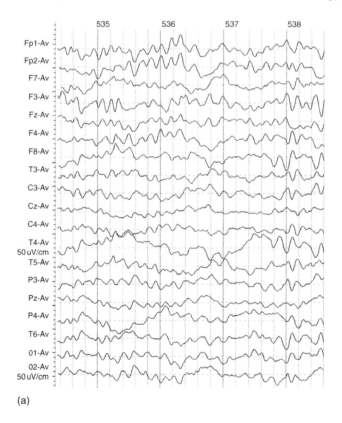

(a)

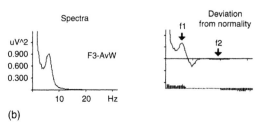

(b)

FIGURE 4.8   Abnormal theta rhythm. (a) A fragment of EEG recorded in a 32 years old patient after 5 days from the closed brain injury. (b) Spectrum at F3, deviation from normality at F3.

abnormality. An example of such case is given by EEG parameters presented in Fig. 4.8. The EEG was recorded in a patient after several days of closed brain injury. One can see a high amplitude theta rhythm at F3, F4 locations the power of which is significantly ($p < 0.001$) different from the normative data. Note also that deviations in the theta band are accompanied by extremely low power of beta activity widely distributed over the cortex.

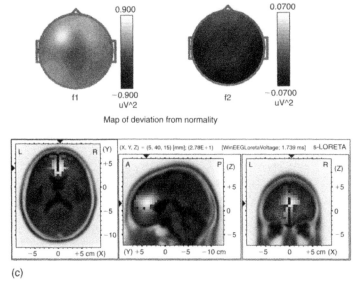

FIGURE 4.8   (c) Maps of deviations from normality at theta and beta frequencies and s-LORETA images of generators of theta rhythm.

VI. SUMMARY

Theta rhythm is the "rhythm with a frequency of 4 to under 8 Hz." Japanese scientists were the first who induced the EEG theta activity by administering a mental task consisting of continuous arithmetic addition. This theta activity was a train of rhythmic waves at a frequency of 6–7 Hz with maximum amplitude around the frontal midline and was labeled as the frontal midline theta rhythm. The frontal midline theta rhythm is often associated with the hippocampal theta rhythms. It was hypothesized that the hippocampal theta oscillations are involved in memory encoding and retrieval. Recordings in human hippocampus are available only in rare cases of stereotactic operations in epileptic patients with depth electrodes implanted for diagnostic purposes. The frontal midline theta shows individual differences and is related to certain personality traits: the amount of frontal midline theta negatively correlates with scores in the anxiety scale, while positively correlates with the scores in the neurotic and extraversion scales. The frontal midline theta correlates with changes in anxiety levels induced by anti-anxiety drugs.

CHAPTER 5

Paroxysmal Events

I. SPIKES

In visual inspection of electroencephalogram (EEG), abnormal patterns are basically divided into two groups: slower waves[1] and spikes. The spike is a paroxysmal (i.e., suddenly appearing) electrical "explosion" that pop out the background activity and looks like a large nail. Recall that in the normal brain excitation and inhibition within the cortex are well balanced. The balanced cortex during wakefulness produces normal regular electrical events such as alpha rhythms, beta rhythms, and the frontal midline theta rhythm. These rhythms are recorded on the scalp due to synchronous activations of millions of neurons. If the balance is disrupted so that excitation exceeds inhibition and neuronal networks become hypersynchronized the cortex starts producing abnormal patterns called paroxysms[2]. These abnormalities in majority of cases can be recorded from the scalp by conventional EEG in a form of specific electrographic patterns. There are several types of paroxysmal events, the most common of them are spikes, sharp

---

[1] Abnormal slow waves were described in the previous chapters portraining delta, theta, and alpha rhythms.

[2] Paroxysms in EEG stand for abnormal patterns of excessive synchronization.

waves, spike-slow wave complexes. In extreme cases the cortical hypersynchronization in the focus may produce seizures – stereotyped and involuntary paroxysmal alterations in behavior, such as jerking movements and convulsions accompanied by a transient loss of consciousness. The extent of seizures varies: some patients may shake and fall down, for others a seizures may be perceived only by most attentive family members.

A. Spatial-Temporal Characteristics

There are three characteristics that define a spike or a sharp wave in EEG. They are paroxysmal character, high degree of sharpness, and short duration. These parameters are presented in Fig. 5.1[3].

Paroxysmal character of spike is partly associated to its amplitude: the spike pops up from the background activity. The amplitude of spike in turn depends on several factors: (1) position of the focus within the brain with lower amplitudes generated by deeper sources; (2) the volume of the focus with lower amplitudes generated by smaller foci, (3) orientation of the electric dipole corresponding to spike with tangential dipoles generating smaller amplitudes in comparison to radially oriented dipoles. The amplitude parameters that we are using in the Human Brain Institute Database for automatic spike detection are presented in Fig. 5.1. The degree of spike sharpness can be estimated by the second derivative of EEG

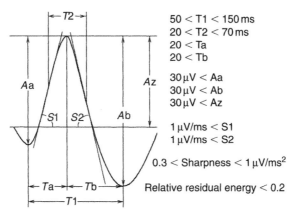

$$50 < T1 < 150 \, ms$$
$$20 < T2 < 70 \, ms$$
$$20 < Ta$$
$$20 < Tb$$

$$30 \, \mu V < Aa$$
$$30 \, \mu V < Ab$$
$$30 \, \mu V < Az$$

$$1 \, \mu V/ms < S1$$
$$1 \, \mu V/ms < S2$$

$$0.3 < Sharpness < 1 \, \mu V/ms^2$$

Relative residual energy < 0.2

FIGURE 5.1   Temporal and amplitude parameters of waveforms used for automated spike detection. See explanations in text.

[3] The parameters are taken from the paper of Ktonas, P.Y. (1987). Automated spike and sharp wave (SSW) detection. In Methods of Analysis of Brain Electrical and Magnetic signals. EEG Handbook (revised series, Vol. 1) Gevins A.S., and Remond A. (eds)., Elsevier Science Publishers, B.V. 211–241.

signal. The second derivative computed at the maximum (or minimum) of the spike was set larger than $0.3 \mu V/ms^2$. The other parameter of sharpness is slope, defined as the maximum magnitude of the first time-derivative during the leading (trailing) edge of an EEG wave. It was set larger than $1 \mu V/ms$. By definition, the duration of spike is less than 70 ms, while the duration of sharp wave is between 70 and 200 ms. The durations of certain time parameters of the spike are presented in Fig. 5.1. For example, duration between two successive maxima or minima is set less than 150 ms (but more than 50 ms).

Our experience shows that the selected parameters enable us to detect reliably most of the spikes that can be visually detected by an experienced electroencephalographer.

Another paroxysmal event is called spike and wave complex. It refers to a spike that is followed by a prominent wave. If the spike is associated with synchronous excitation of many neurons, the following wave is associated with the inhibitory postsynaptic potentials that follow excitation. It should be stressed here that the appearance of the wave after the spike does not place this paroxysmal event in a new category. Both belong to paroxysmal events and reflect synchronous activity in the focus.

The spatial position of an epileptogenic focus within the cortex strongly defines the character of a seizures. The locations of the focus differ from patient to patient. They can be frontal (i.e., premotor, mesial, or orbital), Sylvian, temporal (anterior, mediobasal, posterior), parietal, occipital. In some cases the epileptogenic focus is located in hippocampus and related structures. In such cases identification of spikes from the surface is difficult because of low amplitude of spikes recorded from the scalp.

B. Automated Spike Detection

An example of automated spike detection is presented in Fig. 5.2. EEG was recorded in an epileptic patient of 7 years old. Because the spikes are detected in a period between seizures they are called interictal spikes[4]. The advantage of automatic spike detection is that the procedure enables us to average the detected spikes and to get a reliable picture of potential distribution, spatial distribution of generators by means of s-LORETA and location of the equivalent dipole within the brain. The results of spike averaging are presented in Fig. 5.2[5]. As one can see

---

[4]The parameters of the detected spike fit all above listed parameters both in amplitude and temporal characteristics. For example, Aa = $130 \mu V$, T2 = 40 ms. The program automatically detects the spike that could be visually separated.

[5]According to the algorithm presented above the program automatically detects spikes by running separately through all channels. Further, the detected spikes in a channel are averaged. Potential distribution over the head at the time of the peak is approximated by a single dipole. The squired difference between the real potential and its approximation is averaged over all channels and divided by the total energy. The computed parameter is called a relative residual energy that defines how well the spike can be approximated by the dipole.

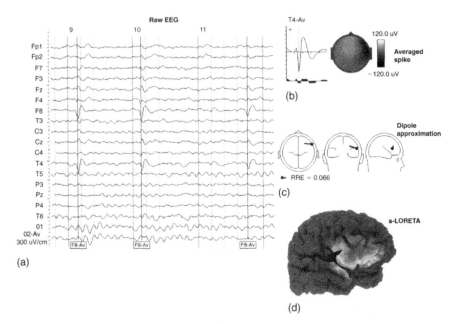

FIGURE 5.2   Automated spike detection. – (a) A fragment of EEG recorded in an epileptic 7 years old patient. Spikes (marked by a vertical line and a bottom box with the number of the channel of maximal amplitude) were detected by the computer algorithm realized in the Human Brain Institute software on the basis of temporal-amplitude parameters presented in Fig. 5.1. Bars in the bottom of the event-related potential (ERP) traces show confidence levels of deviation from the background. (b) Averaged spike and its 2D map. (c, d) Dipole approximation and s-LORETA image.

in Fig. 5.2 spikes at the electrode location with the maximum of amplitude at F8 are of negative value. This negativity is a scalp reflection of strong depolarization that takes place in the epileptic focus. However, because the dipole is oriented tangentially to the surface, a small positive peak can be simultaneously detected at Fz.

C. Intracranially Recorded Spikes

It should be stressed that there is no direct relationship between epilepsy and paroxysmal patterns. Sometimes, spikes can not be seen from the scalp and can be seen only with implanted electrodes (Fig. 5.3).

Sometimes, vice versa, raw spontaneous EEG shows spikes but they are not expressed in epileptic seizures and the subject might never have them. The last case is the situation when we have to be very cautious. The point is that having a focus in the cortex may not evoke visible seizures[6], but the hypersynchronization

---

[6] Or seizures are so subtle that can remain un-noticed by patients and others.

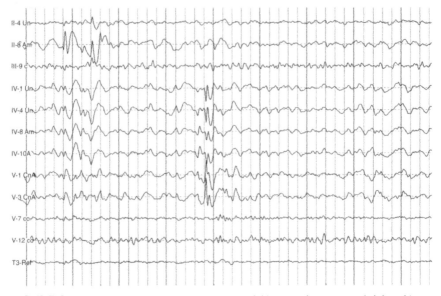

FIGURE 5.3   Spikes in intracranial recordings. Local field potentials were recorded from hippo-campus and adjacent structures in an epileptic patient to whom electrodes were implanted for diagnostic purposes. Note two distinct types of spikes generated in different structures. Also note that scalp electrodes (T3 is presented for comparison) do not reveal any noticeable spikes.

in the focus may disrupt the normal information flow in the cortex and may be associated with brain dysfunctions specific to a particular location. An example of such case is presented in Fig. 5.4.

II. NEURONAL MECHANISMS

A. A Lack of Inhibition

Most of our knowledge regarding mechanisms of epilepsy comes from experiments in animals. The interictal spikes reflect synchronous activity of many hundreds of thousands (or millions) of neurons. The excess of synchronization can be achieved by a shift of a balance between excitation and inhibition toward excitation. It could be due to increase of excitation or decrease of inhibition or both. Intracellular recordings in cortical neurons in the experimental epileptic focus show that the initial component of spike is accompanied by a so-called paroxysmal depolarization shift. The depolarization shift is generated by excitatory postsynaptic potentials that are enhanced and subsequently amplified by intrinsic voltage-dependent membrane responses. The enhancement may be due to a variety of mechanisms. One of them is reduction of intracortical inhibition. This was

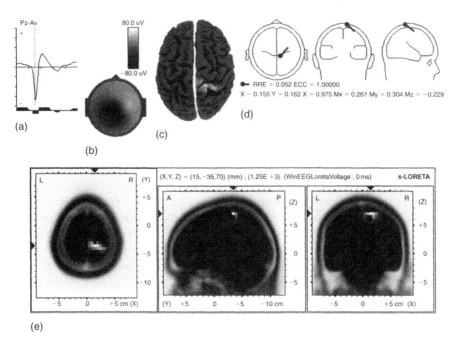

FIGURE 5.4   Spikes in EEG of a 6 year old patient without epileptic seizures. The girl was having speech difficulties. (a–d) Averaged spike, 2D topography, 3D s-LORETA image, dipole approximation. (e) Slice view of generators of the spike.

recently found in focal cortical dysplasia[7] which is a common cause of medically intractable epilepsy (Calcagnotto et al., 2005).

B. Neurofeedback

Having recurrent *unprovoked seizures* is a sign of epilepsy – a common chronic neurological condition[8]. Epilepsy is the first disorder for which neurotherapy has been applied. In certain types of epilepsy when medication either does not help or has undesired side effects training of the 12–14 Hz activity over the sensory-motor strip has reported to significantly decrease the number of seizures. Barry Sterman from University of California in Los Angeles was the first who introduced this methodology into clinical practice.

[7] This term refers to a condition where the cortex does not form properly in the developing fetus. Dysplasia means "bad form" in Greek.

[8] As one can see from this definition, simply having a seizure is not diagnostic of epilepsy, because seizure can be provoked by acute events, such as trauma, oxygen deprivation, tumor, expose to toxic chemicals, or high temperature. In the past, epilepsy was associated with religious experiences and even demonic possession. Nowadays seizures are associated with excessive synchronous neuronal activity in the brain. About 0.5–1 per cent of the population suffers from epilepsy. Epilepsy is usually controlled with medication, in difficult cases surgery may be considered as an alternative way of treatment.

C. Epileptology

There are many different types of epilepsy, each presenting with its own unique combination of seizure form, age of onset, EEG correlates, methods of treatment, and prognosis. Epilepsy as a subject of a separate branch of medicine – epileptology – is beyond the scope of this book. Here we just want to stress that EEG recordings in cases of suspicious epilepsy are accompanied by "activating" procedures such as hyperventilation (HV)[9], photic stimulation, and sleep deprivation while paroxysmal patterns are detected by visual inspections of qualified clinicians. In contrast quantitative electroencephalogram (QEEG) mostly focuses on quantitative parameters of EEG in eyes open, eyes closed, and task conditions, which are specifically designed to study sensory, affective, executive, and memory functions of the brain. So QEEG analysis is mostly used for other brain disorders, such as attention deficit hyperactivity disorder (ADHD), depression, schizophrenia… However, our experience working with QEEG shows that some behavioral problems (such as symptoms of ADHD) in rare cases might be consequences of having the focus in the cortex[10].

III. SUMMARY

In the normal brain excitation and inhibition within the cortex are well balanced. The balanced cortex during wakefulness produces normal regular electrical events such as alpha rhythms, beta rhythms, and the frontal midline theta rhythm. If the balance is disrupted so that excitation exceeds inhibition the cortex starts producing abnormal patterns called paroxysms. These abnormalities in majority of cases can be recorded from the scalp by conventional EEG in a form of specific electrographic patterns. There are several types of paroxysmal events, the most common of them are spikes, sharp waves, spike-slow wave complexes. Spikes are usually generated by a local area in the cortex – called focus. Using modern techniques of electromagnetic tomography, such as low resolution electromagnetic tomography (LORETA) or dipole approximations, focuses can be localized within the cortex with a good precision. Since 1950s detection of spikes by visual inspection remained the only method for many years. In the last 10–20 years, quite reliable methods for automatic spike detection were developed. Nowadays, most of the modern QEEG systems have additional tools for automatic spike detection that help practitioners for detecting and analyzing paroxysmal events in the brain.

---

[9] For example, in recent study with video-EEG monitoring of 97 eligible patients, in 24 patients clinical seizures associated with ictal EEG changes was found during HV, mostly in the first 4 min (Guaranha et al., 2005).

[10] If paroxysmal patterns are observed in EEG in any of conditions (EO, EC, or task) the patient is recommended to be referred to an epileptologist for more careful examination.

CHAPTER 6

QEEG *Endophenotypes*

In the introduction of the book we presented a concept of endophenotypes as biological markers of the brain disease. Endophenotype must obey the following requirements: (1) endophenotype must be stable and reproducible in time intervals during which behavioral patterns associated with the state of the brain remain unchanged; (2) endophenotype must reflect a function of a certain brain system that in a specific way determines the human behavior, (3) endophenotype must be inherited, that is, in the homozygotic twins it must be quite similar. In this chapter we are going to show that spectra, or better to say amplitude of the background electroencephalogram (EEG) in certain frequency bands, obey these requirements and, consequently, can be considered as endophenotypes.

I. TEST–RETEST RELIABILITY

EEG basic oscillations (such as alpha rhythms and the frontal midline theta rhythm) wane and wax in time. The degree of variability of the basic oscillation depends on the frequency band and the state (eyes open, eyes closed, task) of the subject. For example, alpha spindles in posterior regions vary with periods of few seconds, burst of the frontal midline theta appear with interburst periods of

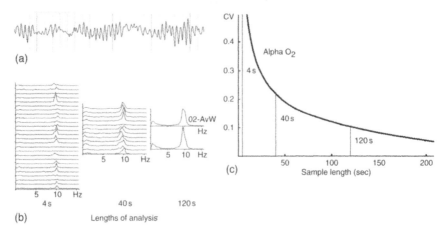

FIGURE 6.1   EEG variability. (a) Occipital alpha waves wane and wax over 1 s range. (b) Fourier spectra computed for 4 s sequential periods of analysis, for 40 and 120 s periods of analysis. Each period of analysis was divided into 4 s epochs. Fourier transform (left, bottom) was applied to each epoch separately and the resulted spectra were averaged. One can see that variability in spectra declines with the length of analysis. (c) Effect of sample length on EEG spectra variability. Y-values are the coefficients of variation (CV) for the power in the alpha frequency band when increasing the sample size (X-axis) from 4 to 400 s. For each sample size, values were obtained by calculating the CV of 100 randomly selected samples, resulting in a curve for each individual recording that was averaged across subjects. Adapted from Maltez et al. (2004).

few deco-seconds. However, if averaged over sufficiently long time intervals the resulting spectra become quite stable characteristics of the brain. The question arises, what is the minimal length of spectral analysis[1] that would give us a stable and reliable measure.

To give the reader a sense of EEG variability, in Fig. 6.1a we present raw EEG recorded in a healthy subject from O_2 electrode in eyes closed condition. The EEG spectra computed for sequential 4, 40, and 120 s intervals are presented below. One can see that at 4 s intervals spectra varied tremendously, however at 120 s interval of analysis they become almost identical. Several studies have been performed addressing the variability of different EEG spectral parameters using the variance, coefficient of variation (CV^2) and test–retest reliability measured as correlation coefficient between consecutive measurements. A recent study was performed by a group of scientists from Karolinska Hospital in Stockholm, Sweden (Maltez et al., 2004). EEG was recorded in healthy subjects during 15 min

---

[1]Do not mix the length of analysis with epoch for fast Fourier transformation. The epoch defines the frequency resolution of spectra with longer epochs corresponding higher resolution. The length of analysis defines the reliability of the spectra.

[2]Coefficient of variation is defined as standard deviation divided by the mean.

with the subjects instructed to open (5 s) and close the eyes every 60 s[3]. Epoch for fast Fourier transform (FFT) was selected of 4 s. CV varied proportionally to the inverse of square root of time (a schematic presentation of such dependence is presented in Fig. 6.1c. Alpha had the highest and theta the lowest CV.

On the basis of the graphics in Fig. 6.1 we can estimate that to get a coefficient of variability smaller than 0.05 we need to have recording length at least of 3 min. An example of the variability of spectra for 3 min recording is shown in Fig. 6.2. One can see that spectra obtained from EEG recordings made during 3 min eyes open condition with 7 days interval between recordings are very similar and could be considered as a reliable and stable estimation of the brain functional state.

II. REFLECTION OF FUNCTIONING BRAIN SYSTEMS

EEG is a complex combination of rhythms. For example spectra of EEG of a patient presented in Fig. 6.2 include frontal theta rhythm, posterior alpha rhythm, posterior temporal low beta activity, and central high beta activity. When compared with the normative database, frontal theta activity and posterior temporal low beta activity are out of the normal range.

Different oscillations reflect different mechanisms. Alpha rhythms reflect the state of thalamo–cortical pathways. Frontal midline theta rhythm reflects functioning of the limbic system. Beta rhythms are more local and reflect the state of local cortical areas. In the above chapters we tried to show the links between EEG rhythms and brain systems and correspondingly brain dysfunctions. So, defining abnormal rhythmic activities in EEG and associating these abnormalities with distinct brain systems fit the second requirement for endophenotypes as biological markers of disease.

III. HERITABILITY

There is strong experimental evidence indicating that spectral characteristics of EEG are inherited. The measures of heritability in EEG spectra are schematically presented in Fig. 6.3. The curves at the left are take from the Human Brain

---

[3] The test–retest reliability within the recording was evaluated when each recording was split into two sets of data. When splitting first half versus second half, the Pearson correlation coefficient was quite high ranging from 0.93 to 0.98 for alpha, beta, and theta power. When splitting the recordings in odd closed eyes periods versus even closed eyes periods the Pearson correlation coefficients were 0.97–0.99 for all power bands. The effect of the sample size on the variability was studied by calculating CV while varying the number of 4 s epochs chosen randomly from each recording with a minimum of 4 s (1 epoch) to a maximum of 400 s (100 epochs). For each sample size CV was calculated from an average of 100 selections and the obtained values were averaged across subjects.

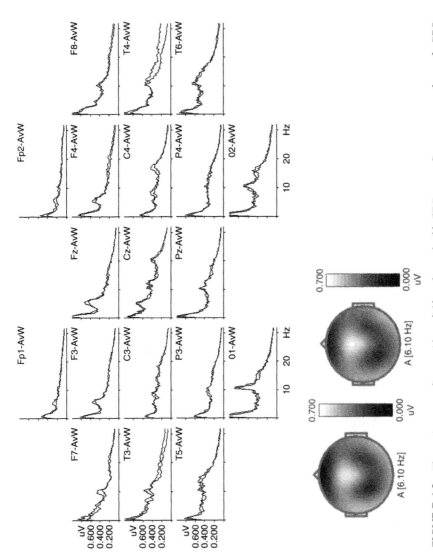

FIGURE 6.2 Three minute recording provide a reliable and reproducible EEG spectra. Power spectra and maps for EEG recorded in one patient for two 3 min periods of analysis made within 7 days.

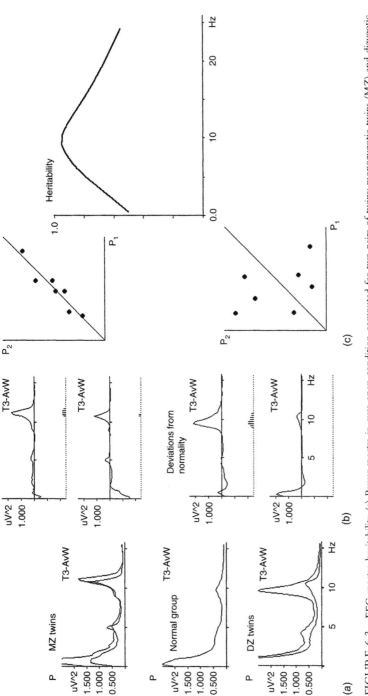

FIGURE 6.3   EEG spectra heritability. (a) Power spectra in eyes open condition computed for two pairs of twins: monozygotic twins (MZ) and dizygotic twins (DZ). (b) Difference spectra obtained by subtracting grand average spectra for a normative group from the individual spectra. Note that three of four twins exhibit deviation from normality in alpha band at T3 electrode. (c) Schematic presentation of scaterograms for two groups of twins, where P1 (P2) – power spectra for a given frequency band for the first (second) twin in a pair. Note that heritability computed according to the formula in the text is a function of frequency. Heritability graphic is adapted from Smit et al. (2005).

Institute Database while a schematic representation of heritability of EEG spectra are based on the results from a recent study by a group from Vrije Universiteit Amsterdam, in The Netherlands (Smit et al., 2005)[4]. The results show that across the scalp and most of the frequency spectrum, individual differences in adult EEG are largely determined by genetic factors.

Endophenotype is becoming an important concept in the study of complex psychiatric diseases. The term was coined in 1966 and applied in psychiatry by Gottesman and Shileds in 1972 (for a review see Gottesman and Gould, 2003). It is gradually substituting other semantically similar terms such as "biological marker," "vulnerability marker," "subclinical trait," and even "intermediate phenotype"[5]. For example, according to a MEDLINE search, the term was used in 16 papers in 30 year period before 2000, but in 116 papers in just 1 year in 2007. The notion of endophenotype is based on assumption that a more correct psychiatric diagnose can be made using the knowledge about the state of brain systems. Functional MRI has been recently used for imaging neuronal circuits involved in brain diseases such as depression, schizophrenia, and ADHD. In this chapter we have shown that spectral characteristics of background EEG might be also used as endophenotypes.

IV. SUMMARY

In psychiatry, endophenotype denotes a measurable index of brain functioning. Endophenotype obey the following requirements: (1) endophenotype must be stable and reproducible in time intervals during which behavioral patterns associated with the state of the brain remain unchanged; (2) endophenotype must reflect a function of a certain brain system that in a specific way determines the human behavior, (3) endophenotype must be inherited, that is, in the homozygotic twins it must be quite similar. In this chapter we showed that EEG spectra obey these requirements.

---

[4]It was a twin study that compared the intrapair resemblance between two types of sibling relationships, namely genetically identical (monozygotic twins, MZ) and non-identical twins (dizygotic twins, DZ). If MZ resemblance (r) for EEG power is higher than DZ resemblance, this constitutes evidence for genetic influences on the EEG. A simple formula computes the relative contribution of genetic influences to the total variance, also called heritability (h2), as: $h2 = 2(rMZ - rDZ)$, where rMZ and rDZ quantify the intrapair resemblance for MZ and DZ twins. Nineteen-lead EEG was recorded with eyes closed from 142 monozygotic and 167 dizygotic twin pairs and their siblings, totaling 760 subjects.

[5]An endophenotype may be neurophysiological, biochemical, endocrinological, neuroanatomical, or neuropsychological in nature. Endophenotypes represent simpler clues to genetic mechanisms than the behavioral symptoms.

CHAPTER 7

QEEG During Sleep

I. ANATOMICAL BASIS

A. Sleep and Wakefulness Promoting Nuclei

During the day the brain does not remain the same, it exhibits a super slow rhythm that roughly follows light–dark changes produced by the rotation of the earth around the sun. This rhythm is called circadian rhythm (from Latin "circa" – about, and "dies" – daily). Roughly the circadian rhythm can be divided into two phases: wakefulness and sleep. On average, we spend 30 per cent of our lives asleep. Sleep duration in humans shows a bell shaped distribution, with an average sleeping duration of 7.0–7.9 h. Behaviorally sleep is defined by four criteria: (1) reduced motor activity; (2) decreased response to external stimuli, (3) stereotypic postures; (4) and easy reversibility (distinguishing it from coma).

During World War I, the world was swept by a pandemic of encephalitis lethargica, a viral infection of the brain. The infection caused a profound and prolonged state of sleepiness in most individuals. A Viennese neurologist, Baron Constantin von Economo, reported that this state of prolonged sleepiness was due to injury to the posterior hypothalamus and rostral midbrain. He also reported that one group of patients had the opposite problem: a prolonged state of insomnia. It was

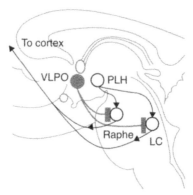

FIGURE 7.1   Brain nuclei involved in sleep-wakefulness regulation. VLPO – ventrolateral preoptic nucleus, PLH – posterior lateral hypothalamus, Raphe – Raphe nuclei of the brain stem, LC–locus coeruleus.

associated with lesions of the preoptic area and basal forebrain. Based on his observations, von Economo suggested that the region of the hypothalamus near the optic chiasm contains sleep-promoting neurons, whereas the posterior hypothalamus contains neurons that promote wakefulness with lesions in it causing narcolepsia[1].

In subsequent years, his observations on the sleep-producing effects of posterior lateral hypothalamic injuries were reproduced by lesions in the brains of monkeys, rats, and cats. However, the basic neuronal circuitry that causes wakefulness was clearly defined only in the 1980s and early 1990s, and the pathways responsible for the hypothalamic regulation of sleep began to emerge only in the past five years (Fig. 7.1). As neurophysiological data indicate, the ventrolateral preoptic nucleus (VLPO) contains GABAergic and galaninergic neurons that are active during sleep and that inhibit the monoaminergic cell groups in the ascending activating system (such as the raphe nuclei and locus coeruleus), and consequently, are necessary for normal sleep. The posterior lateral hypothalamus (PLH) contains orexin/hypocretin neurons that are crucial for maintaining normal wakefulness, while their damage leads to narcolepsy. A model is proposed in which wake- and sleep-promoting neurons inhibit each other (not shown in Fig. 7.1), which results in stable wakefulness and sleep.

II. EEG CORRELATES OF SLEEP

A. REM and NREM Sleep

For centuries, sleep has been regarded as a simple halt of behavioral activity. Today we know that sleep is a complex and highly organized global state that in turn can

[1]A disease in which individuals have a tendency to fall asleep at inappropriate times.

be divided into distinct stages. During sleep cortical neurons undergo slow oscillations in membrane potential, which appear in electroencephalograms (EEGs) as slow wave activity (SWA) of <4 Hz. The amount of SWA is homeostatically regulated, increasing after wakefulness and returning to baseline during sleep. It has been suggested that SWA homeostasis may reflect synaptic changes underlying a cellular need for sleep.

In mammals, there are two types of sleep – rapid eye movement (REM) and non-REM (NREM). They are defined in terms of electrophysiological signs that are detected with a combination of electroencephalography (EEG), electro-oculography (EOG), and electromyography (EMG), the measurement of which in humans is collectively termed polysomnography. REM sleep (also known as paradoxical, active or "desynchronized" sleep) is characterized by the following features: wake-like and "activated" (high frequency, low amplitude, or "desynchronized") activity in the EEG; singlets and clusters of REMs in the EOG; and very low muscle tone (atonia) in the EMG.

B. Stages of NREM Sleep

NREM sleep is divided into four stages, corresponding to increasing depth of sleep, as indicated by progressive dominance of the EEG by high voltage, low frequency ("synchronized") wave activity. Such low frequency waves dominate the deepest stages of NREM (stages III and IV, also termed slow wave sleep)[2]. The first steps of falling asleep represent a complex sequence of events. The state of relaxation is characterized by high incident of alpha rhythms in occipital or central areas. Periods of drowsiness (the first stage of sleep) are associated with suppression of those rhythms. In the second stage of sleep a new phenomenon called sleep spindles appear in EEG. Stage II NREM is also characterized by a slow (<1 Hz) oscillation, which influences the timing of K-complexes. NREM and REM sleep alternate in each of the four or five cycles that occur in each night of adult human sleep. Early in the night, NREM sleep is deeper and occupies a disproportionately large amount of time, especially in the first cycle, when the REM epoch might be short or aborted. Later in the night, NREM sleep is shallow, and more of each cycle is devoted to REM.

---

[2]The cyclic organization of sleep varies within and between species. The period of length of each REM–NREM epoch increases with brain size across species, and the depth and proportion of the NREM phase in each cycle increases with brain maturation within species. NREM sleep complexity is a function of brain systems, such as the thalamo-cortical circuitry, that reach their maximum development in mature humans. It can therefore be concluded that the differentiation of sleep is a function of brain differentiation, a rule that indicates both mechanistic and functional links between sleep and other brain functions.

III. FUNCTIONAL MEANING OF SLEEP

The functional meaning of sleep still remains unknown despite a number of facts and even larger number of theories. This ignorance is probably the main reason why our society has little respect for sleep presuming that sleep simply takes away precious moments of our life. Now we know that our immune system, cognitive ability[3], and mental health are all affected by sleep. Disruption of the sleep/wakefulness cycle results in a broad range of disorders, including poor attention and memory, depression, reduced motivation, metabolic abnormalities, immune impairment, and a greater risk of cancer.

A. Memory Consolidation

Evidence from both animal and human studies indicates that there is a strong association between sleep and so-called "sleep-dependent memory processing." In many animal studies, sleep deprivation after learning tasks has been shown to impair performance in subsequent tests. In humans, the learning of various tasks improves significantly following a night of sleep. Furthermore, the selective disruption of REM, but not NREM, sleep abolishes this performance gain. In more detailed studies individuals were selectively deprived of slow wave sleep (SWS), stages III and IV of NREM, and REM sleep. It was concluded that memory consolidation was initiated in SWS and then enhanced during REM sleep. If the sleep-dependent memory processing hypothesis is correct then one aspect of sleep disruption will be impairment of the mechanisms of brain plasticity.

B. Immune System

In humans the activity of natural killer cells can be lowered by as much as 30 per cent after only one night without sleep. Loss of sleep also impairs many other aspects of the immune system, including circulating immune complexes, secondary antibody responses, and antigen uptake. Sleep disruption and sustained psychological stress increase cortisol concentrations in the blood. One night of lost sleep can raise cortisol concentrations by almost 50 per cent by the following evening. High levels of cortisol suppress the immune system, so excessively tired people are more susceptible to illness.

---

[3]When people are sleep restricted to 3 or 5 h per day over 7 consecutive days, there is a dose-dependent decline in vigilance and performance. Similarly, when the length of sleep periods is gradually increased after cumulative sleep restriction, performance improves. Interestingly, the first few hours of sleep seem to be particularly important for recovery. This might explain why sleep naps of as little as 10 min have been shown to improve subjective alertness.

C. Psychiatric Disorders

Psychiatric dysfunctions are almost always associated with disturbances in sleep. Insomnia and early morning awakening are hallmarks of major depression. Furthermore, sleep disturbance is a strong predictor of a relapse into depression in medicated patients. Depression is often accompanied by anxiety disorders, which are also closely related to chronically disturbed sleep. When we experience excessive anxiety, our sleep, work, sense of pleasure, and relationships often suffer. Panic disorder, posttraumatic stress disorder, generalized anxiety disorder, and social phobia are all anxiety related disorders that are associated with sleep disruption. A population study involving several European countries indicated that anxiety is related to insomnia in 50 per cent of individuals who have a history of a psychiatric disorder.

IV. BISPECTRAL INDEX

A good measure of brain changes in a sleep-wakefulness cycle is provided by bispectra[4]. Bispectral analysis was first developed in the early 1960s to characterize the phase relationships and non-linear properties of wave motion during atmospheric pressure changes. Application to EEG analysis occurred with the onset of high speed, microcomputer technology. Bispectral analysis was adapted as an EEG processing tool in the late 1980s and early 1990s even though a theoretical link between neural network physiology in the cerebral cortex and frequency coupling had not been established. Current theories hypothesize that strong EEG phase relationships are inversely related to the number of independent EEG pacemakers in the brain.

A. Association with Anesthetic Depth

The bispectral index (BIS, Aspect Medical Systems, Natick, MA) is a complex parameter, composed of a combination of time domain, frequency domain, and high order spectral subparameters[5]. It is unique among the quantitative

---

[4]The bispectrum analysis is the next level beyond spectral analysis. Whereas the phase spectrum produced by Fourier analysis measures the phase of component frequencies relative to the start of the epoch, the bispectrum measures the correlation of phase between different frequency components (for more details see Methods).

[5]The particular mixture of subparameters in BIS was derived empirically from a prospectively collected database of EEG and behavioral scales, representing approximately 1500 anesthetic administrations (almost equal to 5000 h of recordings) that used a variety of anesthetic protocols. BIS was then tested in other populations. The weighting assigned to each EEG derivative varies with the approximate depth of anesthesia. Further, devices that implement BIS are the only ones currently approved

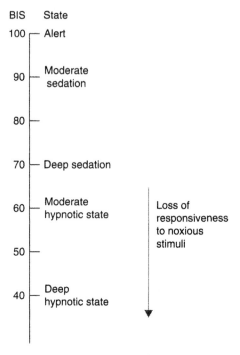

FIGURE 7.2   BIS values in association with various degrees of narcosis. Loss of responsiveness to noxious stimuli can occur over a range of BIS values from 0 to 65. Values larger than 65 are associated with increases in intraoperative responsiveness and postoperative recall of intraoperative experiences. For the various sedation scales used in these studies, the BIS value was inversely correlated with increasing depth of sedation. Values of 90–100 are associated with EEG pattern in focused attention and a value of 0 is associated with a completely suppressed EEG (isoelectric pattern).

electroencephalogram (QEEG) parameters because it integrates several independent descriptors of the EEG into a single variable. The BIS is a dimensionless EEG parameter ranging from 0 to 100. It is derived from Fourier and bispectral calculations performed on artifact-free EEG data. The BIS is calculated from an algorithm that relates three factors: (1) degree to which EEG waveforms are in phase (bicoherence); (2) amount of EEG power in the delta (1–4 Hz) versus beta (13–30 Hz) range (power spectrum); and (3) proportion of the EEG that is isoelectric. The degree of bicoherence of the EEG increases with increasing anesthetic depth (Fig. 7.2) and is inversely related to the derived BIS.

by the Food and Drug Administration for marketing as monitors of anesthetic effect on the brain. Although bispectral analysis involves complicated mathematics, modern computers are powerful enough for real-time computations. A BIS sensor is required for obtaining the EEG from a patient. The sensor is usually a 1-piece sensory strip that has location markers to facilitate placement.

V. SUMMARY

Sleep is a global state that is distinct from wakefulness both behaviorally and neurophysiologically. Sleep is defined by reduced motor activity; decreased response to external stimuli, stereotypic postures; and easy reversibility (distinguishing it from coma). Wakefulness and sleep can be further divided into separate periods with different behavioral patterns. Sleep consists of four stages (from drowsiness to deep sleep without eye movements and with eye movements). Each of these periods is characterized by distinct neurophysiological mechanisms generating different EEG patterns. As neurophysiological data indicate, the anterior part of the hypothalamus contains GABAergic that are active during sleep and inhibit the monoaminergic cell groups in the ascending activating system, and consequently, are necessary for normal sleep. The posterior hypothalamus contains orexin/hypocretin neurons that are crucial for maintaining normal wakefulness, while their damage leads to narcolepsy. A model of sleep suggests that wake- and sleep-promoting neurons inhibit each other which results in stable wakefulness and sleep. EEG may be considered as the best of known imaging method that enables us to index the states of sleep. The BIS is a complex parameter derived from Fourier and bispectral calculations performed on artifact-free EEG data. The BIS is calculated from an algorithm that relates three factors: (1) degree to which EEG waveforms are in phase; (2) amount of EEG power in the delta versus beta range; and (3) proportion of the EEG that is isoelectric. The degree of bicoherence of the EEG increases with increasing anesthetic depth and is inversely related to the derived BIS.

CHAPTER 8

Methods of Analysis of Background EEG

I. ANATOMICAL LOCATIONS

To describe locations of different anatomical brain structures a specific terminology is used (Fig. 8.1). The directions are named as: lateral – medial, anterior (rostral) – posterior (caudal), dorsal – ventral. Sections of the brain made with different planes are named as: coronal, horizontal, and sagital sections.

II. BRODMAN'S AREAS

The term cortex means "bark" because as in tree bark it contains many infoldings. The infoldings are sulci (the infolded regions) and gyri (the crowns of the folded tissue). About 2/3 of the cortex is confined within the depth of the sulci. When unfolded, the whole human cortex constitutes the area of about $2\,m^2$.

The whole cortex in each hemisphere is divided into four lobes: occipital, temporal, parietal, and frontal lobes. Cortex consists of 52 anatomically distinct areas described by a German anatomist Korbinian Brodmann in 1909 (Fig. 8.2). This classification is still in use. It should be noted that the numbering reflects just the order in which Brodmann sampled the brain and does not have any other systematic meaning. In addition to its Brodmann's number (such as Brodmann's area 17) a cortical area may be referred to by its cytoarchitectonic name (such as striate cortex due to its appearance at the microscope), anatomical position regarding sulci, and gyri (such as calcarine, i.e., surrounding calcarine fissure) and its functional name according to a suggested function of the region (such as primary visual cortex).

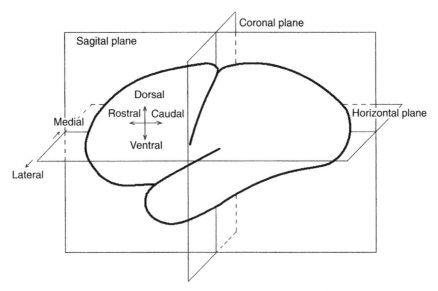

FIGURE 8.1   Anatomical terms used in neuroscience. A scheme of the brain is cut by horizontal, sagital, and coronal planes. Directions (medial – lateral, dorsal – ventral, rostral – caudal) are depicted by arrows.

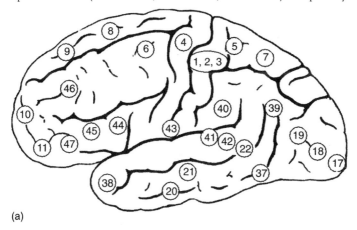

(a)

FIGURE 8.2   Brodmann's areas. A scheme of the human cortex with numbers corresponding to numbers of Brodmann areas defined by Brodmann in 1909 on the bases on the cytoarchitectonic organization of the cortex.

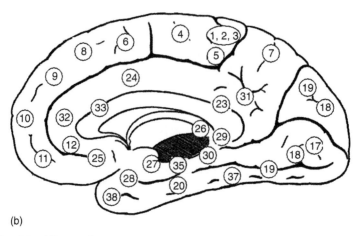

(b)

FIGURE 8.2   (*Continued*)

III. 10–20 INTERNATIONAL SYSTEM OF ELECTRODE PLACEMENT

In 1959 the first standards in electroencephalogram (EEG) recordings were laid down. Among them was the system of placement of electrodes. This system is called the 10–20 International System of Electrode Placement or simply 10–20 system (Fig. 8.3)[1].

The names of electrodes include the first letter associated with the area where the electrode is placed, and the number indicating the side and placement within this area. Fp1, Fp2 – prefrontal, F3, F4,– frontal, Fz – frontal midline, C3, C4 – central, Cz – central vertex, P3, P4 – parietal, Pz – parietal midline, F7, F8 – anterior temporal, T3, T4 – mid temporal, T5, T6 – posterior temporal, A1, A2 – earlobes. Odd numbers indicate left hemisphere. Even numbers indicates right hemisphere.

IV. ELECTRODES

In almost all commercially available electrodes' sets electrodes are made of metal. Theoretically the optimal electrodes for measuring slow shifts of potentials are non-polarizable electrodes such as silver–silver chloride electrodes, that is, electrodes made

---

[1]The name comes from the fact that any electrode is 10 or 20 per cent of some distances from another. In the direction from nose to back of the head this distance is defined by the circumference of the head measured from the nasion to the inion. In the direction from one ear to another the distance is defined by the circumference of the head measured from the small fossa just anterior to the one ear canal over the central vertex to the opposite ear. The distance between the peripheral electrodes is defined as 10 per cent of the circumference of the head measured just above the eyebrows and ears.

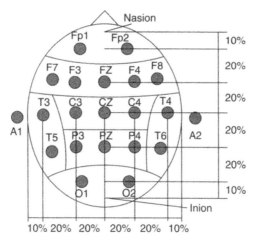

FIGURE 8.3   10–20 International system. Each electrode position (lead) has a letter (to identify the lobe) and a number or another letter to identify the location within the lobe. Any electrode is 10 or 20 per cent of some distances from another.

of silver (Ag) and covered with AgCl layer. Practically for recording conventional EEG (e.g., within the range from 0.1 to 70 Hz) other metals can be used[2].

Any metal electrode placed in a conducting solution forms a so-called double electric layer between the solution and the metal. This electric layer is formed due to the flow of ions from the metal surface to the solution and back. The double electric layer is the source of potential difference between the metal electrode and the solution. The value of this potential is a complex function of the electrode material, the electrolyte composition, and the temperature. In Ag/AgCl electrodes the exchange of ions in the double electric layer is very high so that any current applied to the electrode can not change the double layer potential, and such electrodes are called non-polarizable electrodes[3].

In the EEG machine the amplifiers magnify the potential between an EEG electrode and a reference one. Recall that each metal generates its own double layer potential between the electrode and gel. When the same metals are used for reference and recording electrodes these double layer potentials cancel each other, but using different metals for EEG and references electrodes can lead to a significant dysbalance between potentials and can alter the normal conditions of EEG recordings. That is the reason why all electrodes for EEG recordings must be made of the same metal.

[2]Such electrodes are made of gold (e.g.,, by Grass-Telefactor, USA), of tin (Electro-Cap International, USA), of silver (Technomed Europe, The Netherlands), of platinum (Ad-Tech Medical Instrument Corporation, USA), or stainless steel (Ad-Tech Medical Instrument Corporation, USA).

[3]"Non-polarizable" literally means that when applying electric current to the electrode, the potential of the electrode does not change significantly from its equilibrium.

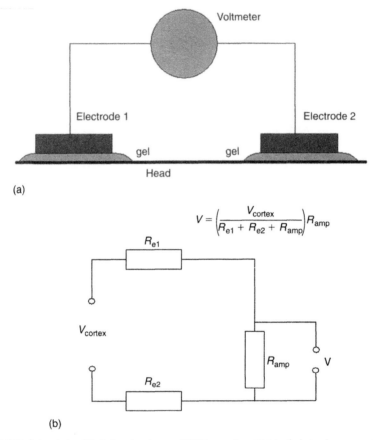

$$V = \left(\frac{V_{cortex}}{R_{e1} + R_{e2} + R_{amp}} \right) R_{amp}$$

(b)

FIGURE 8.4   A simplified electric scheme of EEG recording. (a) Metal electrodes are attached to the skin by means of electro-conducting gel, while the voltmeter is measuring the potential difference between two electrodes. (b) The potential V_{cortex} is amplified by the amps. V_{cortex} – is the potential generated by the cortex, R_1 and R_2 – are resistances of electrodes or better to say resistances of contacts of electrodes with the head mostly defined by the electro-conducting gel and by the quality of contact between the electrode and the skin. R_{amp} – is the resistance of the amps.

Electrical scheme for measuring the cortical potential by two electrodes is shown in Fig. 8.4. Note that a part of measured potential is falling on electrodes' resistors according to Ohm's law[4]. This is the reason why electrodes' resistance (some times referred to by a general name "impedance") is usually kept as low as possible. The requirements for scientific papers usually demand the electrode impedance for EEG recordings to be less than 5 Kohm.

[4]Ohm's law defines the relationship between voltage and current in a conductor. This relationship states that: The potential difference (voltage) across a conductor is proportional to the current through it. The constant of proportionality is called the "resistance," R.

V. AMPLIFIERS

The basic component of any EEG machine (or electroencephalograph) is an amplifier. It amplifies a week EEG signal. Recall that in adult EEG recording the signal is about 30–50 μV. Modern EEG machines comprise from 19 to 128 amplifiers or channels. The EEG machines use differential amplifiers (Fig. 8.5).

The differential amplifier simply magnifies the difference between two inputs. One goal of differential amplifiers is to get rid of common artifacts (affecting both V_1 and V_2) such as induced potentials from mains and other external sources of electrical signals. Ideally, when two inputs have the same common input the output signal is zero. In practice the output signal is small but different from zero. The ability of amps to be as close to the ideal as possible is reflected in a parameter called common mode rejection (CMR) expressed as ratio of the output signal when $V_1 = V_2$ (they are connected to the same source) to the output signal when only one input is non-zero. CMR is measured in dB. For example, CMR $= -100\,\text{dB}$ at $50\,\text{Hz}$.

VI. EEG DIGITIZING

Nowadays most of EEG machines are digital. They transfer continuous (so-called analog) EEG signals into a set of numbers. Numbers represent an electrode potential measured at discrete points. The amount of measuring points per second is called the sampling rate of the EEG machine. For example, sampling rate of 250 Hz means that the EEG signal from one electrode during 1 s is represented in computer as a set 250 numbers. At such sampling rate the interval between two sequential measurements is 4 ms. It is essential that the sampling rate is more than twice larger than the highest expected frequency in the incoming signal (Shannon's sampling theorem)[5]. Numbers are stored in computers in a binary form, that is, in set

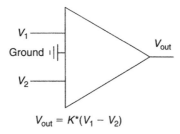

$$V_{out} = K^*(V_1 - V_2)$$

FIGURE 8.5   Differential amplifier. A simplified scheme of a differential amplifier. It amplifies the difference between two potentials V_1 and V_2. K is the coefficient of amplification.

[5]Conservative design actually calls for sampling at a rate 4–10 times higher than the highest frequency of expected signal.

of bits[6]. If the EEG machine uses 14 bit analog to digital (A/D) converter, its resolution is 1/8192 or approximately 0.0001 of the maximal output. So, if the machine is designed to measure a signal within the range of +1V and −1V, the step size in its 14 bit conversion is $0.1\,\mu V$.

VII. MONTAGES

A. Linked Ears Reference

In EEG machines with differential amplifiers we are measuring electrode potentials in reference to some other potential or potentials. However, traditionally one sort of measuring when a referential electrode is located on a part of the head presumably picking up a small amount of signals from the cortical neurons is called referential. In the referential recording a reference electrode is usually located on the earlobes, mastoids, or the tip of the nose. This type of recording is also named a monopolar recording. When two electrodes are located on the scalp near EEG generators in the cortex, this type of recording is named sequential or bipolar recording.

There are many schemes of EEG measurements. All of them are united under a common name – montages[7]. Montage – is a rule according to which EEG potentials are measured. The simplest rule (a so-called linked ears montage) is measuring electrodes' potentials in reference in two linked electrodes located at the left and right earlobes. Linked mastoids, chin or the tip of the nose can be also used as reference electrodes[8]. Ideally, the reference electrode must be electrically neutral, that is, its potential does not change throughout the recording. Unfortunately, due to the conductivity of the scalp, all locations on the head are in a sense electrically active and there is no place in which a reference electrode could be attached to meet the criteria of the ideal reference. This means that the electrical potential recorded from any single electrode will depend on the reference.

[6]A bit is a smallest chunk of information and can be 0 or 1. So, a number that includes 14 bits is a number between -10^{13} and $+10^{13}$ or − 8192 and +8192.

[7]The advantage of modern digital EEG systems (in comparison to old analog systems) is that the digital EEG system allows the montage and filter settings to be determined at the time the EEG is reviewed, rather than at the time it is recorded. The EEG is usually recorded with minimally restrictive analog filter settings and with potentials at all electrodes measured with respect to a single reference (such as nose or linked ears). A computer program can then process the data as they are displayed on a screen or printer, reformatting the original referential montage to any desired referential or bipolar montage and digitally filtering the data as needed. If necessary, the same segment of EEG can be displayed repeatedly, using different montages and filters. Historically, in electroencephalograpy many different montages have been used. The variety of these montages was defined by technical abilities that were available in the previous days.

[8]Note that in the book, if not mentioned otherwise, EEG was recorded in reference to linked ears.

B. Common Average Montage

One method, that tries to deal with this problem, is the common average reference montage. It was developed in the early 1950s. The procedure is straightforward: the potential is averaged over all electrodes (called common average potential) and is subtracted from any single potential. The procedure is expressed in the following formula:

$$V_i' = V_i - \sum V_j / n$$

where Σ is a sum over all electrodes (Fig. 8.6).

If the head were a sphere and electrodes could be placed in all places of this sphere, then the common average would be zero and the "*common average montage*" would be a perfect solution. However, in reality this is not the case: the head is not a sphere and electrodes are attached only to the upper and lateral surfaces of the head.

C. Local Average Montage

Another montage is a "*local average reference montage.*" The term local average reference refers to the construction of a unique reference for each electrode. In this case, a small number of electrodes in the vicinity of a target electrode are used to compute the synthetic reference.

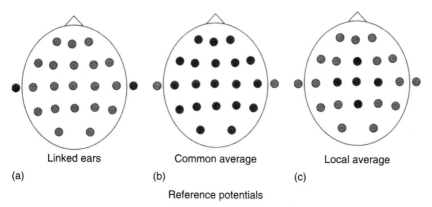

FIGURE 8.6   Three montages. (a) In the linked ears montage an electrode potential is measured in reference to the potential of two physically linked earlobe electrodes. (b) In the common average montage an electrode potential is measured in reference to the potential averaged over all electrodes. (c) In the local average montage the electrode potential (e.g., Cz) is measured to a potential averaged over adjacent (local) electrodes. Reference electrodes are depicted in black.

In the formula presented above Σ now is a sum over the electrodes surrounding the i-th electrode[9]. In general terms, any montage can be defined by the formula:

$$V_i = V_i - \sum w_{ij} \times V_j$$

where w_{ij} are the weights. Consequently, any montage is characterized by its weights w_{ij}. The values of the weights can be found in Setup of any modern software.

An example of a local average reference is the Laplacian montage. Constructing the Laplacian montage involves estimating the Laplacian operator for each electrode. Mathematically, the Laplacian operator is a second spatial derivative of the potential field. From the point of view of physics, the second spatial derivative is proportional to the current flow entering and leaving the skull at the corresponding point. In its turn, the current flowing toward or away from a point on the skull enables us to estimate the strength of the underlying neural generator.

Originally described by Pitts in 1952 the method required a 3D array of closely spaced electrodes, a situation that requires the use of intracranial depth electrodes. Modifications to allow applications to surface potentials were developed by Hjorth in 1975. Hjorth was able to show that calculations could be simplified by making a number of assumptions about the structure of the cortex. Hjorth assumed that within a particular layer of the cortex there exists homogeneity of conductivity. As a result, potential fields orientated parallel to the each layer are homogenous. A 1D derivation is therefore appropriate as the only fields perpendicular to the lamina are of interest. In this manner, the second spatial derivative of the potential field is confined to current flow perpendicular to the cortical surface[10]. The Horth method was later modified by Lemos.

Figure 8.7 represents maps of EEG spectra computed for two frequencies for the two montages: monopolar and local average (Lemos) montages. In this particular EEG recorded in a healthy subject taken from the Human Brain Institute (HBI) DataBase there are two distinct alpha rhythms with overlapping frequencies: mu-rhythm and parietal alpha rhythm. Note that a better spatial resolution and clear separation of the sensory-motor rhythm from the parietal rhythm is provided by the local average montage. In figures presented in the present book the local average montage is referred to as AvW while the linked ears montage is labeled as Ref.

---

[9]For example if we wish to determine the local reference for, say, Cz, we have to compute an average over the electrodes surrounding Cz, in this case: Fz, C3, C4, Pz. For our Cz electrode, we would have the following expression for a local average : $V_{Cz} = V_{Cz} 2 (V_{Fz} + V_{C3} + V_{C4} + V_{Pz})/4$.

[10]A number of limitations are associated with the Laplacian montage. First, the spatial accuracy is highly dependent on the number of electrodes and interelectrode distance. Second, potentials at the periphery of the measurement area cannot be reliably estimated since electrodes at these points are not encompassed by a complete array of surrounding electrodes. Third, the location of diffuse sources may be significantly distorted or even neglected. In view of these limitations it is clear the Laplacian is best suited for localization of relatively focal sources.

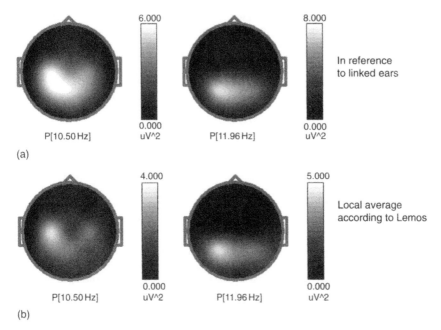

(a)

(b)

FIGURE 8.7 Comparison of two montages. Power spectra maps in a healthy subject in eyes closed condition in linked ears (a) and local average (b) montages. Note that the local average montage provides a more localized distribution of the potential sources.

VIII. FOURIER ANALYSIS

A. Spectra

One important element of EEG is its rhythmicity. As we learn in this part of the book there are several EEG rhythms that differ by their frequency, location, mechanisms of generation, and functional meaning. Rhythms are evolved in time, they wax and wane. As a representative EEG recording usually takes three or more minutes it is quite difficult to grasp the whole information about rhythms from viewing at each time only few seconds of EEG recording. Humans are limited! A powerful method of compressing the information about rhythmicity over time is given by Fourier analysis.

The Fourier theorem states that any signal $X(t)$ within the time limits from 0 to T[11] can be decomposed into a set of simple sinusoidal functions, called Fourier series (see e.g., Fig. 8.8), that is,

[11] T is the epoch for Fourier analysis or the sampling epoch. The larger is the epoch, the larger is the number of harmonics and the higher is the frequency resolution for spectra. For example, for the epoch of 4 s the frequency resolution is of $1/4 = 0.25$ Hz.

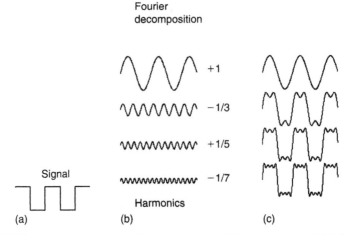

FIGURE 8.8   Decomposition of a step-like signal into sinusoidal harmonics. A signal (a) is decomposed into harmonics (b) with different frequencies and amplitudes (depicted as a number at the right). The more harmonics are added, the better the result of summating harmonics (c) corresponds to the signal.

$$X(t) = A_0 + \sum A_n \sin(nft + \varphi n)$$

where Σ is a sum over all frequencies (harmonics), f – is a fundamental frequency of the signal $f = 1/T$, ϕ – is a phase, $n = 1,2,3,\dots A_n$ – amplitude, ϕ_n – phase of a sinusoidal component (n – is a harmonic number).

The goal of Fourier analysis is to find these parameters. They can be represented in a form of amplitude spectra (A_n versus nf), power spectra (squared amplitude A^2_n) and phase spectra (ϕ_n versus nf). The direct integral-based approach in computing A_n and ϕ_n is computationally very laborious. In 1965, Cooly and Tukey published a more efficient algorithm for computation Fourier series, called the fast Fourier transform (FFT) algorithm.

The time interval of EEG recording, for example in eyes open condition, is usually about 3 min. It means that this interval can be sliced in 45 four-second epochs. The slicing of a continuous signal stream into finite epochs can introduce contamination of spectra by artifactual frequencies created by the abrupt transitions at the ends of the epoch. This type of distortion is minimized by multiplying each time domain amplitude point within the epoch against the corresponding value of a window function. A window function is a numerical series containing the same number of elements as the number of signal samples in the epoch. Window element values tend toward zero at both ends and toward unity in the middle. A variety of window functions have been described, including the rectangle, the triangle, the Hanning, and the Blackman functions.

Applying different time windows produce another problem: fragments near the beginning and the end of epochs of analysis give a smaller input to spectra in comparison to the middle fragments. To compensate for this distortion, epochs are selected with overlapping. The overlapping usually constitutes a half of the epoch[12].

B. Spectra Dynamics and Averaged Spectra

Spectra can be displayed in different ways. One of them represents a dynamics of spectra computed for each epoch (or a number of epochs) sequentially. An example is presented in Fig. 8.9a. As one can see peaks at spectra corresponding

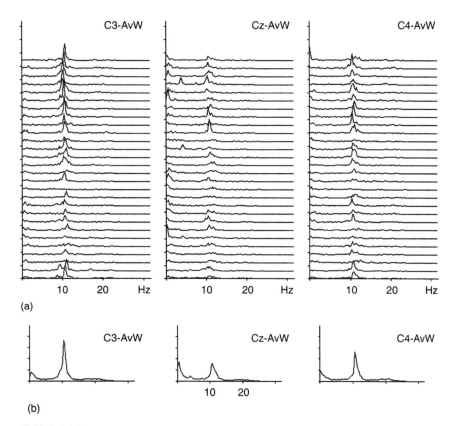

FIGURE 8.9   Two representations of EEG power spectra. (a) Dynamics of power spectra computed for three channels (C3, Cz, and C4) with time pointed from top to bottom. (b) EEG spectra averaged over all epochs. Montage – local average montage according to Lemos. Epoch = 4 s. In dynamics of spectra, each spectrum is an average over four sequential epochs.

[12]The parameters of Fourier analysis can be adjusted to the goals of a specific task. The parameters are: the length of epoch (usually from 1 to 8 s), type of overlapping between epochs (usually 50 per cent of overlapping is chosen), type of the time window (the best results are achieved by Hanning time window). In almost all commercially available software these parameters can be set up by the user.

to mu-rhythms at sequential time intervals wane and wax. The other way of pre-sentation of spectra is averaging spectra over the whole interval of recording (Fig. 8.9b)[13]. Averaged spectra are more stable and can reliably characterize the state of the subject. Three minutes is a minimal duration of EEG recording in order to get a relatively stable spectra.

C. Relative Spectra

Amplitude of EEG recorded in a particular subject depends on many factors including neurophysiological, anatomical, and physical properties of the brain and surrounding tissues (skin, bone, duramater, and piamater). These parameters vary from one subject to another and are basically unknown. These variations result in large variations in absolute EEG spectra (Fig. 8.10a). To compensate for this varia-tion, relative EEG power is sometimes computed (Fig. 8.10b). As one can see, the variability of the absolute power is higher than the variability of the relative power.

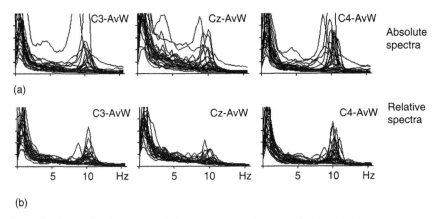

FIGURE 8.10   Absolute versus relative power spectra. Absolute (a) and relative (b) power spectra for a group of 28 healthy subjects of 15 years old are superimposed on each other. Note that variabil-ity is smaller for the relative power in comparison to the absolute power.

[13]Power spectra presented in Fig. 8.9 are calculated in following steps: (1) the epoch Length is set equal to 4 s, (2) the entire record interval (without intervals containing artifacts) is divided into the equal epochs, (3) the overlapping of the epochs is set equal to 50 per cent, beginning with the second epoch, the first 50 per cent of each epoch overlaps the final 50 per cent of the previous epoch, (4) Hanning time window is selected, (5) The power spectrum is computed by means of "fast Fourier transformation," (6) the average spectrum is calculated by averaging over all EEG epochs for each separate channel.

So, when Z-scores[14] are computed to assess the level of statistical significance of deviation of an individual spectrum from the mean averaged over a group of healthy subjects, large variations of the absolute EEG spectra in the normal group would lower the level of statistical significance of deviation from normality.

The formula for computing relative spectra is straightforward:

$$Pr(f) = Pa(f) / \left(\sum Pa(f_i) \right)$$

where $Pr(f)$ is a relative EEG power at frequency f, $Pa(f)$ is an absolute EEG power at the same frequency and Σ is a sum of EEG power over the whole spectrum or a part of it.

IX. EEG MAPPING

When EEG is recorded from many electrodes that cover the whole cortex it is possible to compute a 2D representation of a measured EEG characteristics. The characteristics could be either a current potential or an averaged power (amplitude, phase...) taken at a particular frequency[15]. Two types of maps are presented in Fig. 8.11.

X. FILTERING

A. Low and Highpass Filters

Digital filters play an important role in EEG analysis. Filters function by blocking (suppressing) given frequency components in a signal and passing the original signal minus these suppressed components to the output. In contrast to analog filters, digital filters work by performing mathematical operation on the signal.

In regards to function, there are many types of filters, such as lowpass, highpass, and bandpass... A *lowpass filter* allows only low frequency signals (below some specified cutoff) brought to its output. A *highpass filter* does just the opposite, by rejecting only frequency components below some specified cutoff. Filters are usually defined by their responses to the individual frequency components that constitute the input signal.

---

[14]Z-score for a statistical distribution is the ratio of deviation from the mean value divided by the standard deviation (variability).

[15]The idea of EEG brain topography was first suggested by Grey Walter in 1936. He used this technique for identification of abnormal electrical activity in the brain areas around a tumor. Nowdays mapping of EEG characteristics became a routine procedure.

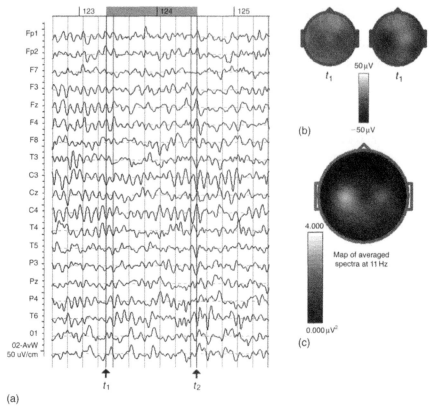

(a)

FIGURE 8.11   Two types of EEG mapping. (a) A fragment of EEG with two vertical lines marking two moments, t_1 and t_2. (b) Maps of potentials made for the first and second moments. (c) Map of power spectra at 11 Hz averaged over 3 min of recording.

B. FIR and IIR Filters

In regards to algorithm, there are *finite impulse response* (FIR) and infinite impulse response (IIR) or recursive filters[16]. For FIR filters the current output (y_n) is calculated solely from the current and previous *input* values (x_n, x_{n-1}, x_{n-2}, …). A *recursive* filter is one which in addition to input values also uses *previous output* values. The word *recursive* literally means "running back," and refers to the fact that previously calculated output values go back into the calculation of the latest output. The expression for a recursive filter therefore contains not only terms involving

---

[16]The impulse response of a digital filter is the output from the filter when a *unit impulse* (a single value of 1 at time $t = 0$) is applied at its input. The response of a FIR filter is of finite duration. The response of an IIR filter theoretically (but not practically) continues for ever, because of the recursive nature of the filter.

the input values $(x_n, x_{n-1}, x_{n-2}, \ldots)$ but also terms in $y_{n-1}, y_{n-2}, \ldots$ To achieve a given frequency response characteristic using a recursive filter generally requires a lower order filter, and therefore fewer terms to be evaluated by the processor, than the equivalent non-recursive filter. To filter out the 50 (60) Hz noise from the mains in the room, a so-called notch filter is applied.

XI. BISPECTRUM

Spectra represent second-order statistics of EEG signals. They do not provide information of how oscillations at different frequencies interact with each other. Higher order statistics include the bispectrum. Specifically, bispectral analysis examines the relationship between the sinusoids at two primary frequencies, f_1 and f_2, and a modulation component at the frequency $f_1 + f_2$. This set of three frequency components is known as a triplet $(f_1, f_2, \text{and } f_1 + f_2)$. For each triplet, the bispectrum, $B(f_1, f_2)$, a quantity incorporating both phase and power information, can be calculated. The bispectrum can be decomposed into (1) the phase information as the bicoherence, $BIC(f_1, f_2)$, and (2) the joint magnitude of the members of the triplet, as the real triple product, $RTP(f_1, f_2)$. A high bicoherence value at (f_1, f_2) indicates that there is a phase coupling within the triplet of frequencies f_1, f_2, and $f_1 + f_2$. Strong phase coupling may imply that the sinusoidal components at f_1 and f_2 have a common generator. So, functional meaning of bicoherence is straightforward: whereas the phase spectrum in the conventional Fourier analysis measures the phase of component frequencies relative to the start of the epoch, the bicoherence measures the correlation of phase between different frequency components. The bicoherence, $BIC(f_1, f_2)$, is a number that varies from 0 to 1 in proportion to the degree of phase coupling in the frequency triplet. We are still uncertain what exactly these phase relationships mean physiologically, but the simplest model suggests that strong phase relationships relate inversely to the number of independent EEG pacemaker elements.

XII. COHERENCE

A. Physiological Meaning

From structural (anatomical) point of view, the most striking feature of the brain is the abundant connectivity between neurons. From functional point of view, this connectivity is reflected in synchronous activities within the brain: neurons in anatomically connected structures tend to fire synchronously. Electrophysiological data show that this synchronicity is performed in bursts repeating at different frequencies. The frequency of the synchronization seems to define the functional meaning of connectivity. For example, alpha frequencies are idling rhythms of sensory systems and synchronization at 10 Hz frequency indicates the state of the sensory system when neurons do not relay sensory information but ready to commence when a relevant stimulus will appear. Oscillatory synchronization in gamma band has been proposed as a binding mechanism for combining different features of an object into a single percept. Synchronization at 40 Hz frequency indicates the synchronous activation of neurons responsible for detecting different features of the same stimulus. The disruption of "normal" synchronization may be a sign of neurological or psychiatric dysfunction. For example, an abnormal pattern of synchronizations between different parts of the basal ganglia seems to be responsible for tremor and dyskinesia in Parkinson's disease.

B. Representations of Deviations from Normality

In EEG the measure of synchronization between two different scalp locations is given by a parameter named coherence[17]. From functional point of view, coherence is a measure of correlation between EEG powers computed in the same frequency band but in different locations[18]. Mathematically EEG coherence is computed as follows:

$$\mathrm{Coh}_{xy} = |\, S_{xy}(f)\,|^2 / S_{xx}(f) S_{yy}(f)$$

where $S_{xy}(f)$ is the cross power spectral density at a given frequency f, $S_{xx}(f)$ and $S_{yy}(f)$ are power spectral densities of x and y at the same frequency.

Figure 8.12 shows the results of comparison of EEG coherences computed in a 45 year old subject with the normative data. This is a subject with a normal adaptive behavior, without any psychiatric and neurological complains but with a partial atrophia of the corpus collosum[19]. On the right, the results of subtraction of the normative coherences from the coherences computed for the subject are depicted. The coherences are computed for two electrodes' pairs: C3–C4 and F3–F4. EEG was recorded in three different conditions: eyes open, GO/NOGO, and mathematic task. In this picture only symmetrical interhemispheric connections are depicted. The EEG bandwidths were adjusted according to the individual characteristics of EEG spectra. This way of presenting the data clearly shows that

[17]Coherence is computed for two channels, so if one have 19 electrodes it gives a total number of pairs 19 $\times$ 18/2 $=$ 171. This number of values is impossible to map in one picture. Several ways of presenting coherence have been suggested. In Fig. 8.12 we present one of them.

[18]The correlation coefficient is defined by: $R = (\Sigma xy)/(\sqrt{x^2}\sqrt{y^2})$, where x and y are deviations from the means of two variables. In our particular case x and y correspond to EEG power measured in two electrode locations in a certain frequency band. R varies between -1 and $+1$. So, if two variables x and y change coherently and in the same direction in time, the correlation coefficient between these two variables is positive and close to 1. If two variables change in out of phase mode the correlation coefficient between these variables is negative 1.

[19]The axonal pathways connecting two hemispheres.

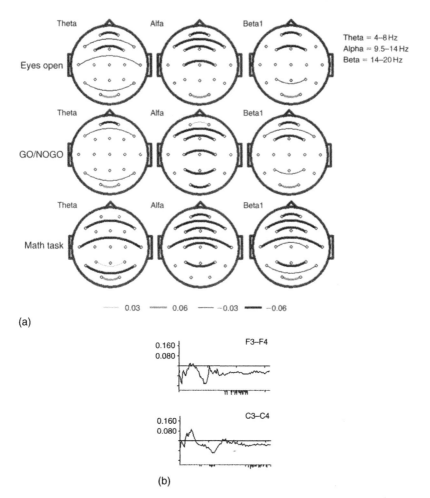

(a)

(b)

FIGURE 8.12   A lack of interhemispheric coherence in a subject with corpus collossum atrophy. (a) Connection diagrams for three frequency bands and three conditions of recording. Only interhemispheric connections in which the coherences are below thresholds (−0.03 and −0.06) are depicted. (b) Examples of deviations from normality in coherences for two pairs of electrodes.

the coherences between two hemispheres in this subject are persistently smaller than in the normal group.

XIII. EVENT-RELATED DESYNCHRONIZATION

The term desynchronization refers to a common observation that presentation of a relevant visual stimulus "desynchronizes" posterior alpha rhythm. This is

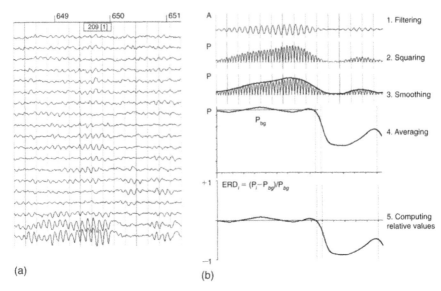

(a)   (b)

FIGURE 8.13   Computing event-related desynchronization/synchronization – ERD/ERS. (a) A fragment of EEG in GO/NOGO task filtered in alpha frequency band. (b) Stages of computing ERDs with description in the text.

exemplified in Fig. 8.13, which represents a fragment of EEG signal during a trial of GO/NOGO task. As one can see visual stimuli followed by the subject's response induce a decrease of alpha activity recorded at O1, O2.

To compute an index of "desynchronization" Gert Pfurtsheller in 1977 suggested the following method. It consists of several steps: first, EEG is filtered at a certain frequency band (in the case presented in Fig. 8.13 alpha band from 9 to 11 Hz was selected), then, the filtered EEG is squared to get EEG power and smoothed (actually in the variant suggested by Pfurtsheller smoothing is performed on the further stages), and finally power samples are averaged across all trials. To obtain relative values for the index of desynchronization, the mean EEG power in the background interval (i.e., the interval preceding the stimulus) – P_{bg} – is calculated and the relative decrease (or increase) of EEG after stimulus is calculated according to the following formula:

$$\text{ERD}_i = \left[\left(P_i - P_{bg}\right)/P_{bg}\right]$$

The parameter was named event-related desynchronization (ERD). However in other frequency bands and also for the alpha frequency band but in different time intervals increase of EEG power was observed instead of desynchronization. The increase was labeled as synchronization and the corresponding parameter was named – event-related synchronization.

XIV. WAVELET TRANSFORMATION

In Fourier analysis an EEG signal is decomposed into a set of sinusoidal functions of different frequencies, amplitudes, and phases. These functions are infinite in time domain. Consequently Fourier analysis lacks time dynamics. This transformation does not work when we want to study how different rhythms in EEG respond to brief presentations of stimuli or to brisk movements. In such cases, it is natural to decompose EEG not into continuous sinusoidal functions, but into discontinuous (finite length) oscillating waveforms (Fig. 8.14b). The discontinuous waveforms presented in Fig. 8.14 are named wavelets. In mathematics the wavelet transform refers to the representation of a signal in terms of a finite length oscillating waveform. This waveform is scaled and translated to match the input signal.

The mostly used functions are complex Morlet's wavelet, defined by equation:

$$w(t, f) = A \exp(-(t-t_0)^2/2s^2) \exp(2i\pi ft)$$

$w(t, f)$ have a Gaussian shape both in the time (around time t_0) and in the frequency domain (around frequency f): The wavelets have the same number of cycles for different frequency bands, resulting in different wavelet durations.

The signal to be analyzed $s(t)$ is convoluted by wavelets in similar way as it is convoluted with sinusoidal functions:

$$P(t, f) = |w(t, f) * s(t)|^2$$

The result is squared and gives the time-depending power of EEG around frequency f. Repeating this calculation for a family of wavelets, having different frequencies f, provides a time–frequency–power representation of the signal components (Fig. 8.14 continued).

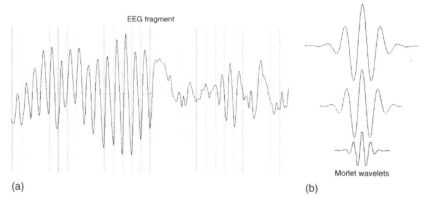

EEG fragment

Morlet wavelets

(a)   (b)

FIGURE 8.14   Computing power–time–frequency representation (wavelet analysis). (a) EEG signal − $s(t)$. (b) Morlet's functions, also called wavelets. (c) A schematic 3D presentation of the signal decomposition into Morlet's wavelets. (d) Time–frequency–power representation of the signal averaged over trials Y axis − frequency, X axis - time. Relative (in reference to the background) EEG power is color-coded at scale presented at Right.

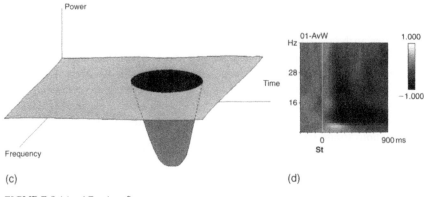

(c)   (d)

FIGURE 8.14   (*Continued*)

XV. BLIND SOURCE SEPARATION AND ICA

EEG is a sum of different rhythms produced at different frequencies by generators located in different cortical areas. For example, generators of 9–13 Hz mu-rhythm are located in the sensory-motor strip, while generators of the midline theta rhythm are located in the medial prefrontal cortex and anterior cingulate. Any electrode placed at the frontal–central area picks up a sum of these two rhythms. In a similar way, event-related potentials (ERPs) (see Part II of the book) represent the sum of different components generated by different cortical generators at different time intervals. For example, generators in the early (from 80 to 200 ms) stages of visual information processing are located in different areas of the posterior cortex such as the striate, pre-striate cortex, ventral visual stream (inferiotemporal cortex), and dorsal stream (parietal cortex). In these two examples, if we want to find independent generators that produce mixed potentials at the cortex we need to solve a so called blind separation problem.

A. Mathematical Formulation

Mathematically, this problem can be formulated as follows. Suppose, we have N source signals or variables (such as neuronal dipoles that reside in a particular cortical area and produce a particular rhythm) $s = \{s_1, s_2, \ldots, s_N\}$. Where s_i is a vector[20] and a function of time[21]. If we further consider time as a sequence of discrete time points t then the time dynamics of s_i can be considered as a matrix S with

---

[20]Vectors are a subject of linear algebra, a branch of mathematics concerned with the study of vectors, vector spaces, linear transformations, and systems of linear equations.

[21]In a special case, when the signal is transformed by Fourier or wavelet transformation into frequency domain, time can be replaced by frequency.

N rows (sources) and T columns (time intervals). Suppose further, that according to the laws of physics (such as volume conduction of electrical potentials) these signals almost instantly project to the surface of the head and are linearly mixed at a given electrode location. If a total number of electrodes is N then:

$P = MS$, where $P = \{P_1, P_2, ..., P_L\}$ is a matrix of time dynamics of potential (consisting of N rows and T columns), M is a so called mixing matrix that "mixes" independent sources into scalp potentials recorded by distinct electrodes:

$$M = \begin{vmatrix} M_{11} & M_{21}, ..., M_{N1} \\ M_{12} & M_{22}, ..., M_{N2} \\ M_{1N} & M_{2N}, ..., M_{NN} \end{vmatrix}$$

The goal of the blind source separation problem mathematically can be formulated as calculating an estimation of the vector S by finding a matrix W so that:

$$U = WP \text{ (note that U as an estimation of S)}$$

Note, that the matrix W is called "unmixing" matrix because it inverts the mixing potentials into their sources.

According to the linear algebra definitions:

$$P = W^{-1}U$$

where W^{-1} is the inverse matrix of W (recall that W^{-1} is called mixing matrix).

Further, according to linear algebra:

$$P = \sum P_i = \sum W_i^{-1} U_i$$

Where P_i is i-th component of the potential P and is the product of two vectors, the i-th column of matrix W^{-1} and the i-th row of U.

B. Spatial Filters for Decomposing Independent Components

Note that the i-th row of the matrix W^{-1} is called a spatial filter (or topography) of the corresponding component because it extracts (filters out) the independent component from the mixed combination of all of them. These filters can be considered as topographies of the corresponding components and visualized in a form of maps (see maps in Fig. 8.15c).

The source locations of independent components are assumed to be stationary, that is, not changing in space during time of recording. The activations of the corresponding sources (U_i) can be considered as the waveforms of independent

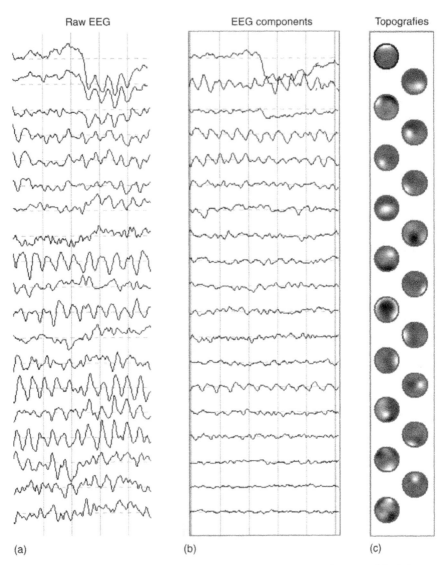

Raw EEG   EEG components   Topografies

(a)   (b)   (c)

FIGURE 8.15   Blind source separation in EEG. (a) Raw EEG, (b) Time dynamics of the independent components (U_i). Raw EEG is the sum of $W_i^{-1}U_i$, (c) Topographies of the extracted independent
components (W_i^{-1}).

components. Note that obtaining the actual amplitude of the independent source
on the scalp requires multiplication of the waveform and the corresponding topography. Because the only meaningful value is the actual amplitude of the source on
the scalp, we can multiply both topographies and waveforms by −1 without changing this value. This creates the ambiguity in defining polarities of waveforms and

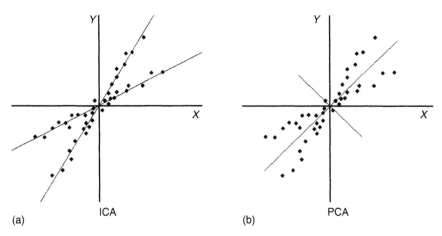

FIGURE 8.16   Comparison of ICA and PCA methods. ICA (a) reflects the nature of the distributions. A non-orthogonal mixture of two distributions at X–Y plane was separated by two methods. PCA (b) provides orthogonal axes ranked in terms of maximum variance.

topographies. So, neither the sign of the topography nor the sign of the waveform are meaningful in themselves.

Let us present the blind source separation problem in a graphical form. Here we have to stress that it is difficult to imagine a multi-dimensional space and even more difficult to imagine linear transformations in this space. So, for simplicity, we consider a 2D space (Fig. 8.16). Suppose, we have two independent sources (variables) that determine two parameters of a given system, such as X depicted at the horizontal axis, and Y depicted at the vertical axis. The X and Y parameters can be measured while the task is to find the independent sources. If the variables are independent and they vary in time, the set of the system states could look like that presented in Fig. 8.16 where each dot corresponds to a state of the system in sequential time intervals[22]. Note also that in Fig. 8.16 the variables are not Gaussian, that is, they are highly sparse. So, the blind source separation problem would be to separate vectors that correspond to the independent variables (or sources) knowing only the measured parameters of the system X and Y.

C. Independent Component Analysis Versus Principle Component Analysis

There exist several attempts to solve the blind source separation. The most powerful of them is independent component analysis (or briefly ICA). ICA was first

---

[22]Note, that in this example, information about time dynamics of the system is not taken into account.

introduced in early 1980s and for EEG was applied in 1995 for artifact correction. In general terms, ICA is a special field of mathematics and for its implementation uses numerical algorithms. These algorithms are based on optimization (finding minimum or maximum) of some objective functions. ICA is superficially related to classic methods such as principle component analysis (PCA) and factor analysis. But ICA is a much more powerful technique capable of finding the underlying variables or sources when these classic methods fail completely. The last statement is illustrated in Fig. 8.16. The figure represents a case of two independent, non-orthogonal and non-Gaussian variables that are mixed into two measured variables (X-axis and Y-axis).

The solutions given by PCA and ICA methods are schematically represented by thin line vectors. Clearly the ICA axes capture much more about the structure of these data than the PCA.

The key assumption used in ICA is that the sources are statistically *independent*. This assumption seems to fit EEG data quite well. Indeed all experimental evidence presented in this part of the book indicates that EEG is formed by potentials generated by different sources located in different cortical areas. The statistical independence means that measuring potential generated in a separate source (say, of the left sensory-motor strip that generates mu-rhythm) at a given moment does not allow any prediction regarding the source in an other brain region (say, in the right sensory-motor strip, or occipital area, or anterior gyrus cingulate) at the same moment. The assumption of statistical independence seems to be also true for components observed in ERPs (for more details see Part II of this book).

Most ICA methods are performed using information-theoretic unsupervised learning algorithms. Different laboratories are using different variants of the learning algorithms, such as JADE, infomax ICA, and FastICA. When these algorithms are compared, they generally perform near equally good. In the HBI Normative DataBase we are using the gradient-descent algorithm implemented for routine use by Makeig et al. (http://www.cnl.salk.edu/~scott/ica.html). It should be stressed that these ICA algorithms consider only statistics of the data maps recorded at different moments, without taking into consideration the time order of these maps[23].

An example of application of ICA to the raw EEG data is presented in Fig. 8.17 As one can see from EEG time dynamics (raw EEG traces) and from compressed frequency representations (spectra) the given EEG is generated by three distinct sources located correspondingly in vicinity of C3, C4, and O1, O2 channels. These sources correspond to the left mu-rhythm, the right mu-rhythm, and posterior alpha rhythm. The mean frequencies corresponding to these rhythms are quite close to each other, constituting 9.5, 9.3, and 10.2 Hz respectively. We applied the ICA method to 3 min of EEG recording. The topographies of three

---

[23]The so-called second-order blind identification (SOBI) approach has been designed in 1994.

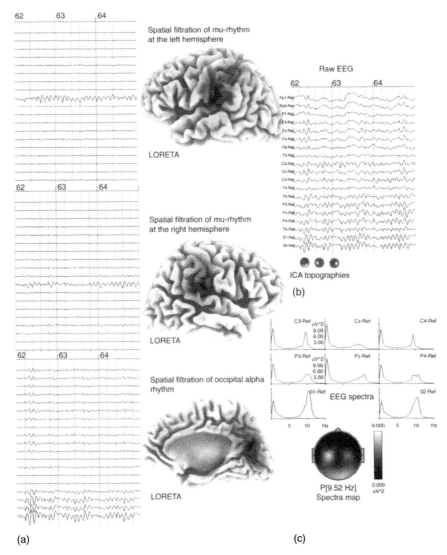

FIGURE 8.17   Decomposition of raw EEG into independent components. (a) Independent components with the corresponding electromagnetic tomograms. (b) A fragment of EEG signal of a healthy 19 years old subject during performing a GO/NOGO task with topographies of three independent components depicted below. (c) Power spectrum with a map at 9.5 Hz.

independent components are presented in Fig. 8.17(b). These topographies can be considered as spatial filters. Figure 8.17 at the left represents the results of application of such filters to the raw EEG. In the middle the low resolution electromagnetic tomography (LORETA) images of selected components are presented.

XVI. ARTIFACT CORRECTION BY SPATIAL FILTRATION

A. Eye Movements

EEG is contaminated by various artifacts. Eye movement artifacts are quite often the largest ones. They are generated by vertical and horizontal eye movements. The main source of the artifacts is the potential of the eyeball. The eyeball acts as an electric dipole with the positive pole oriented anteriorly. Eye blink results in reflexive upward vertical eye movement that produces positive deflection at frontal areas with maximum at Fp1, Fp2 electrodes. Eyes closing is associated with a similar artifact, while eyes opening results in downward vertical eye movement and negative deflection at Fp1, Fp2 electrodes. Horizontal eye movements (also called saccades) produce opposite changes of potentials at F7, F8 electrodes. Figure 8.18 represents a sequence of horizontal eye movement (saccade) and eye blink.

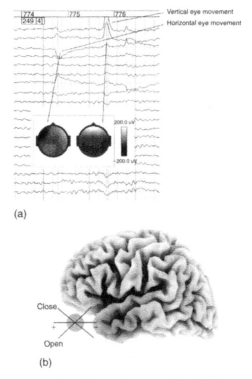

(a)

(b)

FIGURE 8.18   Horizontal and vertical eye movement artifacts.(a) Fragment of EEG recorded in the task condition in a healthy subject of 17 years old.Note: horizontal eye movement (at the left of recording) with a corresponding topography of potential (negativity at F7 and positivity at F8), and eye blink (at the right) with a corresponding topography (positivity at Fp1, Fp2). (b) The model of the eye as an electric dipole with the positive pole oriented anteriorly.

B. Correcting Eye Movement Artifacts

One way of correcting eye movements is to record the oculogram and to compute the proportion of ocular contamination in each EEG channel. Then the electrooculogram (EOG) signals are scaled by the estimated proportion and are subtracted from the original EEG signals.

Recently, a new method was suggested which is based on ICA approach. The basic idea is the decomposition of the EEG signal into two components: the one that corresponds to neuronal electric activity, the other one that corresponds to artifacts. Each component consists of a waveform, describing the time course of the modeled activity, and a topography vector, describing how the waveform contributes to each recorded signal. Artifact activity can be reconstructed as a product of artifact topographies and waveforms.

In Fig. 8.19 an example of application of ICA method for artifact correction is presented.

XVII. OTHER TYPES OF ARTIFACTS

EEG as a week signal may be contaminated by artifacts from various non-cortical sources. Beside slow shifts of potential associated with vertical and horizontal eye movements there are many other types of artifacts. We list here only the most common artifacts, such as muscle, ECG, and pulse artifacts.

A. Muscle Artifact

Muscle artifacts arise from electrical activity of muscles. In particular, frontalis and temporalis muscles are the most common source of myogenic activity respectively in frontal electrodes (mostly Fp1 and Fp2) and in temporal electrodes (mostly T3, T4). An example of temporal muscle activity is presented in Fig. 8.20. Usually, it is not difficult to separate muscle activity from beta cortical activity. Indeed, at the spectra the range of muscle artifact is usually broader than the range of beta activity. Because of that, at recordings muscle activity looks like a thicker line when compared with genuine EEG[24]. Single muscle discharges may look like epileptic spikes, but muscle "spikes" are shorter in duration and are limited to only one electrode.

B. ECG Artifact

In individuals with short necks and large hearts electrical fields of the heart may be detected by ears or other basal electrodes. It is difficult to confuse ECG

---

[24]One must remember that central electrodes such as Fz, Cz, and Pz are located over the places without strong muscle and avoid recording muscle activity.

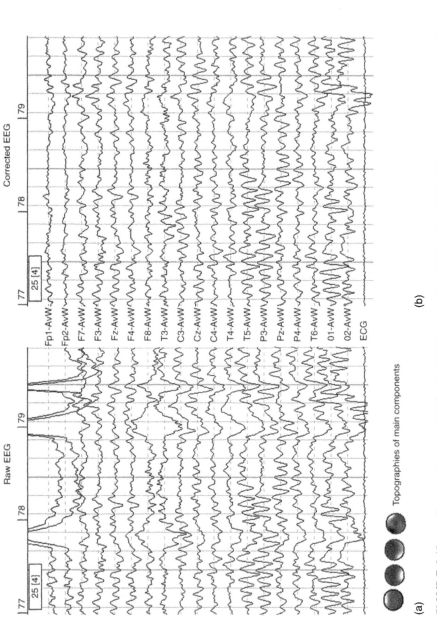

FIGURE 8.19 Artifact correction by spatial filtration. (a) A fragment of raw EEG with eye blinks, ICA topographies are presented below: the largest component corresponds to vertical eye movements and the smallest component – to horizontal eye movements. (b) The result of filtration of raw EEG by a spatial filter based on the topography of vertical eyes movements.

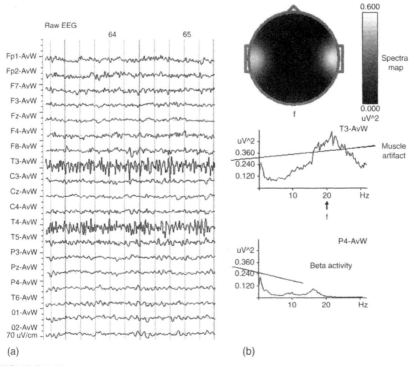

(a)   (b)

FIGURE 8.20   Muscle artifacts. (a) A fragment of EEG contaminated by myogenic artifacts at T3, T4 electrodes. (b) Power spectra of muscle activity (T3) in comparison to beta activity (P4).

artifacts with epileptic spikes because these artifacts are regular and usually seen with the same polarity in many electrodes (Fig. 8.21). Simultaneous ECG recording usually helps to differentiate these artifacts (labeled as *ECG artifacts*), but an experienced electroencephalographer can easily do it without such recording.

C. Cardio–Ballistic Artifact

Another common type of non–brain-related potential changes is called *cardio-ballistic artifact*. This type of artifact is caused by a periodic (with a period of heart beating) movement of electrode located just above a blood vessel of the head. Pulsation of the vessel moves the electrode which induces a periodic artifact. The cardio–ballistic artifact is usually observed under one electrode. This is the reason why it can be better seen when a local average montage is applied (compare EEG traces in Fig. 8.22 made for two montages: referential and local average montages). This artifact can be easily detected on the map of EEG spectra as a local peak in about 1 Hz frequency.

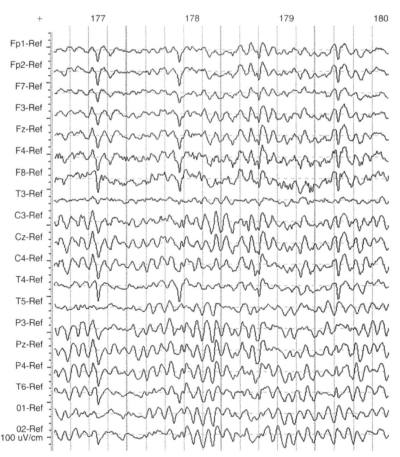

FIGURE 8.21   ECG artifact. A fragment of EEG with periodic (approximately one pulse per second) ECG artifact. Because of the low background EEG activity T3 record reveals the most distinguishable artifact.

XVIII. FORWARD SOLUTION AND DIPOLE APPROXIMATION

As we learnt from this part of the book, an element of EEG generator can be considered as a dipole located within the cortex and oriented perpendicular to the surface of the cortex. In some cases of EEG patterns, such as epileptiform spikes, a single dipole model may be a good approximation of the neuronal generator of the EEG pattern. For the cases, when the generator of the EEG patterns are localized and can be approximated by a single dipole, the scalp distribution of the potential can be expressed in a physical equation and mathematically computed.

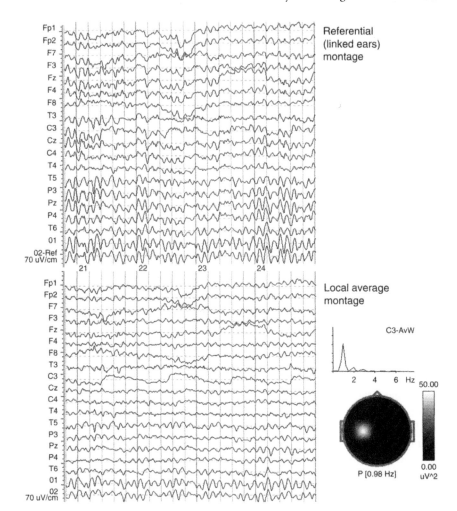

FIGURE 8.22   Cardio-ballistic artifact. A fragment of EEG with periodic cardio-ballistic artifact. This artifacts pops out when a local average montage is applied and when a spectra map is made at the pulse frequency.

In physics this is called the forward problem and its solution is called the forward solution. To solve the forward solution we need to know (1) location of the dipole on the cortical surface, (2) the orientation of the dipole, (3) the conductance of the shells (such as bone, skin …) that surround the dipole. A good solution can be given by the three or four concentric spheres models. Recently the realistic head models were introduced. They take into account parameters such as head shape and head anisotropy.

If the dipole model is correct, we can solve the inverse problem, that is, we can find the position, orientation, and strength of the dipole that fits the observed potential most of all. From mathematical point of view the procedure is finding a minimum of a functional that expresses the difference between the real and the simulated distributions. The procedure can be accomplished by several algorithms. Almost all of them are giving quite good and similar solutions.

In the Human Brain Institute software we are using the four-shell spherical volume conductor model of the head. This model seems to be the simplest approximation that considers the brain as consisting of four concentric spheres, which respectively represent (1) cortex, (2) cerebrospinal fluid, CSF, (3) skull, and (4) scalp. Least-square solution of inverse problem is performed by Nelder-Meade simplex method.

XIX. LORETA

A. Ambiguity of Inverse Problem

Spikes are quite rare patterns of EEG. In majority of cases EEG patterns are generated by distributed sources, that is, by cortical generators spread over wide areas of the cortex. In these cases the EEG potential recorded from a given electrode is a sum of numerous elemental dipoles located not only under the electrode but also in remote parts of the cortex. The problem of finding these multiple dipoles by knowing only potentials recorded by multiple scalp electrodes is called the inverse problem.

Theoretically the inverse solution is ambiguous, that is, there is infinitive number of different source configurations that would fit the measured electric field[25]. In 1984, Hämäläinen and Ilmoniemi were the first to introduce a tomographic solution to the EEG/MEG inverse problem: the well known minimum norm solution. However, the minimum norm solution misplaces actual deep sources onto the outermost cortex and thus produces excessively large errors in localizing cortical sources.

A better accuracy in localizing test sources is given by a methodological approach called low resolution tomography or briefly LORETA. LORETA was first introduced in 1994 by Roberto Pascual-Marqui and his colleagues. LORETA is based on certain electrophysiological and neuroanatomical constrains. It assumes that neighboring[26] cortical areas produce similar local field potentials, which electrophysiologically could be a result of synchronous activation of

---

[25]Non-uniqueness of the inverse problem was pointed out the first time by an outstanding German physician and physicist Hermann von Helmholtz almost 150 years ago.

[26]Neighboring in this context means those that have a spatial resolution of order of 7 mm. In our own studies with implanted electrodes we used bundles of electrodes with 3 mm interelectrode distance. Gold electrodes were stereotactically implanted into heads of patients for diagnostic purposes. In these studies, local field potentials recorded from neighboring electrodes in majority of cases looked quite similar.

neighboring neurons. From mathematical point of view these physiological constraints imply the smoothness of the spatially distributed generators. In essence, LORETA gives the smoothest of all possible inverse solutions. Its inverse solution corresponds to the 3D distribution of electric neuronal activity that has maximum similarity (i.e., maximum synchronization), in terms of orientation and strength, between neighboring neuronal populations (represented by adjacent voxels).

B. Matrix for Solution of the Inverse Problem

In LORETA approach, cortex is modeled as a dense grid of volume elements (voxels) in the digitized Talairach atlas (Brain Imaging Center, Montreal Neurological Institute). In the old version of LORETA, the number of voxels was 2394 that corresponded to a spatial resolution of 7 mm.

The current densities J in those voxels define the potential Φ[27] according to the Laplacian law of physics, that is, knowing the current densities in the cortex we can define potentials at any point in the scalp according to the formula[28]:

$$\Phi = K \times J + c$$

where K is a known operator[29].

C. Minimizing the Functional

Mathematically the inverse solution is to find J by knowing Φ. One way of finding the inverse solution can be obtained by minimizing the following functional:

$$F = \| \Phi - K \times J - c \|^2 + \alpha \| BW J \|^2$$

where α is a regularization parameter, B is the Laplacian operator. This functional is to be minimized with respect to J and c, for given K, Φ, and α. The explicit solution to this minimization problem is obtained:

$$J = T\Phi$$

where:

$$T = (WB^T BW)^{-1} K^T H \left[HK \ (WB^T BW)^{-1} \ K^T \ H + \alpha H \right]^+, H = I - 11^T / 1^T 1$$

---

[27]Note that Φ is a vector, that is, not one but many values corresponding to potentials recorded at different locations.

[28]This is a mathematical expression of the so-called "forward" solution.

[29]Matrix K is computed according to the formula of physics which analytically expresses the potential generated by an electric dipole.

As one can see T is a matrix that can be explicitly computed for a given position of electrodes and the regularization parameter. Knowing potentials Φ recorded from a given set of scalp electrodes in a given time interval we can compute the current density of sources generating these potentials simply by multiplication of the vector Φ by the matrix T. These are computations that are preformed by the LORETA software[30].

An example of application of LORETA for mapping N1 components of ERPs in response to visual and auditory stimuli is presented in Fig. 8.23. Note that generators are located in the occipital area for the visual stimulus and in the temporal cortex for the auditory stimulus. Those locations fit quite well our knowledge about information processing in the human brain.

We have to stress here that all currently available inverse tomographic representations are not precise solutions but rather approximations of the reality. The ability to correctly localize neuronal sources of potentials is the only criteria for

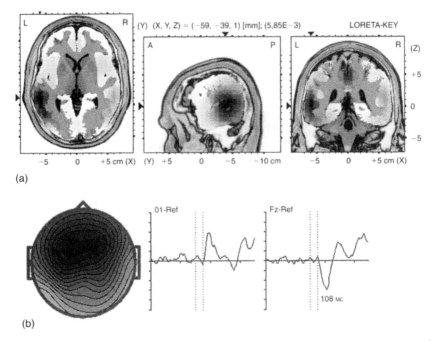

FIGURE 8.23 Low resolution electromagnetic tomography (LORETA). (a) LORETA images of visual and (c) auditory N1 components for a healthy subject. 1000 Hz tone of 100 ms duration served as an auditory stimulus, digit 9 presented for 100 ms served as visual stimulus. (b, d) ERPs and corresponding 2D maps.

[30]LORETA-KEY is free academic software unrelated to any form of profit-making undertakings. The software package that we are using in the Human Brain Institute Database is the same that Roberto Pacual-Marqui and his group use at the Key-Institute for Brain-Mind research in Zurich.

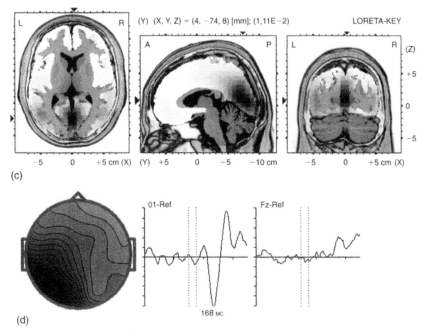

FIGURE 8.23   (*Continued*)

validation of any method in electromagnetic tomography. Practice is the criteria of truth. During the last decade many studies with EEG and ERP recordings showed a good correspondence between LORETA images and expectations that could be made on the basis on various neurophysiological studies[31].

D. s-LORETA – Zero Localization Error

Despite all previous efforts LORETA solutions produced images with systematic non-zero localization errors. One of the problems that pose the localization errors is variability of the "thickness" of cortical generators across the cortical mantle. One way to avoid the systematic localization error is to compute and depict a standardized current density. Roberto Pascual-Marqui in 2002 proposed a method in which localization inference is based on a standardization of the current density estimates. The free software can be found on his web-site. In the most of figures presented below in the book we are using s-LORETA images.

[31]The list of these publications can be found on the web-site of the Key Institute: www.unizh. ch/keyinst/NewLORETA

XX. BOLD fMRI

Although the book deals with electrophysiology we can not avoid discussing the method of functional magnetic resonance imaging (fMRI). This method has been widely used in numerous laboratories all over the world and during the last decade was the main source of our knowledge regarding brain functions. The parameter that is detected in fMRI studies is so-called "blood oxygen level dependent" or briefly BOLD. The signal for computing this parameter comes from hydrogen atoms, which are abundant in the water molecules of the brain[32].

After absorbing the radiofrequency waves, the hydrogen atoms emit energy at the same radiofrequency until they gradually return to their equilibrium state. The MRI scanner measures the total sum of the emitted radiofrequency energy. The radiofrequency signal decays over time, owing to various factors, including the presence of inhomogeneities in the magnetic field (Fig. 8.24).

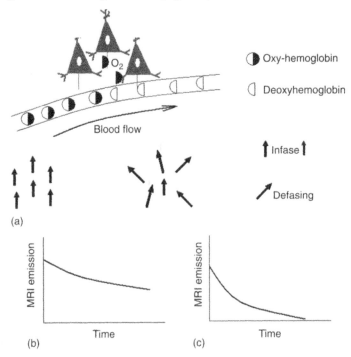

FIGURE 8.24   BOLD measure of metabolic activity. Blood flow in the vessel brings oxygen to neurons by means of oxyhemoglobin. After oxygen consuming by the neurons oxyhemoglobin turns into deoxyhemoglobin. Deoxyhemoglobin as a paramagnetic introduces inhomogenity which is measured by a sharper decay of MRI signal.

[32]As we already learnt in Introduction the MRI method is based on the fact that in the presence of magnetic field hydrogen atoms absorb energy that is applied at a characteristic radio frequency (~64 MHz for a standard, clinical 1.5–Tesla MRI scanner).

Greater inhomogeneity results in decreased image intensity, because each hydrogen atom experiences a slightly different magnetic field strength, and after a short time has passed (commonly called T2), their radiofrequency emissions cancel one another out. BOLD fMRI techniques are designed to measure primarily changes in the inhomogeneity of the magnetic field, within each small volume of tissue, that result from changes in blood oxygenation[33].

A. Transform Model of fMRI response

In EEG–fMRI correlation studies we need to take into account that changes in blood flow are quite slow and follow fast changes in electrical neuronal activity with a long (about several seconds) delay. A model of the hemodynamic response assumes that there are three phases of the BOLD fMRI response to a transient increase in electric neuronal activity (see Fig. 8.25): an initial, small decrease below baseline due to the initial period of oxygen consumption, followed by a large increase above baseline as a consequence of an oversupply of oxygenated blood, and then by a decrease back to baseline again.

Given the measured time course of neuronal activity, it is possible to compute the time course of the fMRI response. In EEG–fMRI correlation studies this is the way of finding association between EEG fast changing patterns and slow metabolic fluctuations measured by fMRI. It should be noted that most fMRI studies go the other way around: they infer the underlying neuronal activity from the fMRI response.

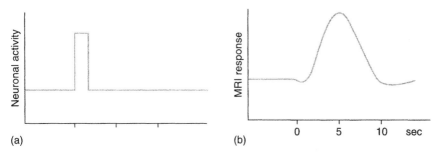

FIGURE 8.25   The transform model of fMRI responses. (a) Neuronal impulse response. (b) Hypothetical hemodynamic impulse response function (HIRF) measured as the response to a brief pulse of neuronal activity.

[33]Deoxy- and oxyhemoglobin have different magnetic properties; deoxyhemoglobin is paramagnetic and introduces an inhomogeneity into the nearby magnetic field, whereas oxyhemoglobin is weakly diamagnetic and has little effect. Hence, an increase in the concentration of deoxyhemoglobin (due to consumption of oxygen by nearby neurons) would cause a decrease in image intensity.

XXI. CORDANCE

Cordance as a complex EEG characteristic was first suggested by a group of scientists from University of California in Los Angeles (Cook et al., 1998). Cordance is computed by a normalization (deriving Z-scores) of absolute and relative EEG power values and adding these values. Cordance values are calculated in three steps: first, EEG power values are computed using a so-called re-attributional electrode montage in which power values from pairs of electrodes that share a common electrode are averaged together to yield the re-attributed power[34]. Relative power is calculated as the percentage of power in each band, relative to the total spectrum. Second, these absolute and relative power values for each individual EEG recording are normalized across electrode sites, using a Z-transformation statistic for each electrode site s in each frequency band f yielding $A_{norm}(s, f)$ and $R_{norm}(s, f)$ respectively. It should be noted that these Z-scores are based on the average power in each band for all electrodes within a given quantitative electroencephalogram (QEEG) recording, and are not Z-scores referenced to some normative population (as in the "neurometrics" approach, see below). The normalization process places absolute and relative power values into a common unit (standard deviation or Z-score units) which allows them to be combined. Third, the cordance values are formed by summing the Z-scores for normalized absolute and relative power for each electrode site and in each frequency band:

$$Z(s, f) = A_{norm}(s, f) + R_{norm}(s, f)$$

Cordance values have been shown to have higher correlations with regional cerebral blood flow than absolute or relative power alone (Leuchter et al., 1999). This measure was used for predicting response to antidepressants in a group of depressed patients.

XXII. NORMAL DISTRIBUTIONS AND DEVIATION FROM NORMALITY

A. Normative Database

Recording EEG and computing spectral characteristics such as power and coherence are only initial stages of QEEG analysis. The most important stage is comparing the computed parameters with the normative data[35]. The definition of a

---

[34]This is similar to a local average montage, but cordance recombines the power values whereas a local average method recombines voltage signals.

[35]It should be stressed here that we are talking about QEEG and not clinical (or medical) EEG assessment. The last one is based on visual inspection and search for meaningful EEG patterns such as spikes, slow waves, and different types of paroxysms. QEEG analysis does not exclude but actually implies clinical EEG assessment as one of necessary steps.

normative database as a representation of the range of "normal" within the whole population raises the issue of what is meant by normal. It is assumed that a normative database must be comprised of many individuals in a population who are rigorously screened for neuropsychiatric disorders, brain damage, for using drugs and medication, for history of neurological and psychiatric disorders. These are exclusive criteria for a normative database. The healthy (normal) individuals must be functioning well in family, school or work, and in society. The database must represent the mix of ages, gender, ethnicity, socioeconomic status, and other demographic factors present in the overall population. These are inclusive criteria for normative database. Special concerns apply to pediatric databases where dramatic developmental changes occur over relatively short time intervals. Such databases need quite many children for each year of age[36].

B. Normal and Log-Normal Distributions

It is a well known fact that any parameter of the normal population, if it depends on many factors, fits a normal (Gaussian)[37], or log-normal distributions[38]. In the case of log-normal distribution the so-called normalization procedure consists simply of taking a logarithm of the parameter.

The Gaussian (normal) distribution of a given random value x is characterized by only two parameters – mean (X) and standard deviation (σ). The mean reflects the averaged value of the parameter, while the standard deviation reflects how much an individual parameter differs from this average value – sometime this parameter is called "deviance."

C. Z-Scores

So, intuitively we feel that if, for an individual parameter x (e.g., the EEG power in 9–10 Hz frequency band computed for a single individual) we divide the fluctuation

---

[36]Practically no database fits these strict criteria. Consequently, the currently available databases are more appropriately considered "reference" rather than "normative" databases. However, for practical purposes the databases provide enormously significant information and they enable the practitioner to assess the patient's abnormality quite precise.

[37]In its simplest form, the Central Limit Theorem states that the sum of a large number of independent observations from the same distribution has, under certain general conditions, a normal distribution. It has been empirically observed that various natural phenomena, such as the heights of individuals, follow approximately a normal distribution. A suggested explanation is that these phenomena are sums of a large number of independent random effects and hence are approximately normally distributed by the central limit theorem.

[38]A variable might be modeled as log-normal if it can be thought of as the multiplicative product (not a sum as in the normal distribution) of many independent factors.

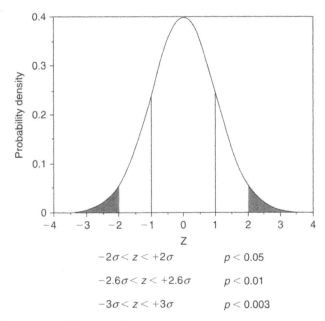

FIGURE 8.26   Normal distribution. See text.

from the mean by the standard deviation we get a measure of fluctuation from normality for this individual value x. In statistics this measure is called Z-score:

$$z = (x - X)/\sigma$$

The Z-score distribution is presented in Fig. 8.26 where Y-axis represents the probability density. So, the probability of Z-score to be smaller, for example, than 2 and larger than -2 is defined by the area under the corresponding curve. In contrast, for $|z| > 2$ this area is quite small and constitutes about 0.05. That defines the probability for which Z-score in a normal individual is larger than 2. In clinical practice the confidence level of 0.05 seems to be a reliable indicator of abnormality.

XXIII. CURRENTLY AVAILABLE DATABASES

A. NxLink

The first normative database was developed by group of researchers from the University of New York headed by Roy John. It became available in late 1980s. The term "neurometrics" was first used by this group to describe an analogy to psychometric assessment, commonly used in clinical psychology. The Neurometrics database is using the following EEG features: absolute power, relative power, coherence, mean frequency within band, and symmetry (left–right and front–back) extracted from approximately 2 min of EEG recorded in eyes closed condition and selected for being minimally contaminated by artifact. The analyzed EEG frequency range extends from 0.5 to 25 Hz. Extracted features were transformed to assure a Gaussian (normal) distribution. Two thousand and eighty-four (2084) variables are computed for each member of the database. The correlation of EEG features with age was noted and "best fit" age regression equations were developed to account for age effects. Univariate and multivariate Z-scores were computed for the purpose of characterizing an individual's deviations from the mean of the population. The NxLink database includes measures from some 782 "normal" individuals. Of this total 356 cases were between the ages of 6–16 and 426 cases were between the ages 16–90. Over 4000 clinical cases were used in the discriminant section of the software. The limitations of the database are as follows: (1) only recordings made with eyes closed at rest were analyzed and normed[39], (2) the comparisons are made only with banded EEG characteristics such as delta, theta, alpha, and low frequency beta bands[40].

B. Neuroguide

The database developed by Robert W. Thatcher (Thatcher Lifespan Normative EEG Database-Neuroguide) currently contains information from 625 individuals, covering the age range 2 months–82.6 years. Advanced methods are used including more extensive cross-validation and tests of Gaussian distributions for average reference, linked ears, Laplacian, eyes open and eyes closed. The NeuroGuide database has been tested and re-tested and the sensitivity of the statistical distributions has been calculated for each montage and condition. Nine hundred and forty-three (943) variables are computed for each subject including measures of absolute and relative power, coherence, phase, asymmetry, and power ratios. Z-score transforms are available in single Hz bins. Sliding averages are used to compute age-appropriate norms. Results are inspected for Gaussian distribution. The main limitation of the database is the absence of recordings in task conditions.

C. SKIL

The SKIL database developed by Barry Sterman and David Kaiser currently includes 135 adults ranging from 18 to 55 years old. The reference population is

[39]Recent studies show that the diagnostic power of EEG in eyes closed condition is inferior than EEG in eyes open and task conditions. Indeed, the dominant posterior alpha rhythm present in most of recordings in eyes closed condition masks other rhythms present in EEG.

[40]The analysis of a fine structure of EEG rhythms is impossible in such approach. However, as we saw above identification of several independent rhythms within a broad band may be of clinical importance.

comprised of students and laboratory personnel (50 per cent), volunteers recruited from the community (25 per cent), and US Air Force personnel (25 per cent). The SKIL database incorporates recordings at rest (eyes closed and open) and during task conditions including reading, math, and some others. A correction for the time of day of recording is available which is based on combined cross-sectional and longitudinal data rather than the preferred method of tracking within-subject changes over time. The SKIL database covers a restricted range of frequencies, from 2 Hz to 25 Hz. The database provides norms for each single Hz increment over this frequency range. The SKIL database relies exclusively on the linked ear reference. The limitations of the database are: (1) no normative information is currently available for children, (2) the tasks were not standardized in order to obtain ERPs.

D. Neurorep

Bill Hudspeth offers the "Neurorep AQR" (Adult QEEG Reference Database[41]). One of the most useful features of Hudspeth's work is the emphasis on *reliability* of measures obtained from individual patients, and the importance of EEG variability over time as a clinical index. EEG data are available for both eyes open and eyes closed conditions. The database includes measures of absolute and relative power for 19 scalp electrodes, and all combinations of pair wise electrode comparisons for coherence, phase, asymmetry, and correlation indices. The total number of individuals in the AQR is now rather small (<50) but additional data is being collected.

Frank H. Duffy, MD also has constructed an EEG database. This database includes both eyes closed and eyes open conditions, and spans a wide age range, including both children and adults. EEG data are available for 19 electrodes, and auditory and visual evoked potential measures also are included. This database was previously used in several commercial neurodiagnostic instruments (Nicolet, QSI) but to our knowledge, is not currently commercially available.

E. Novatech LORETA Database

First LORETA database was developed by Marco Congedo and Leslie Sherlin from the NovaTech. The database currently has 84 cases, and is actively adding new cases. This EEG imaging technology allows for a tomographic representation of EEG sources in 3D space. This database is useful in not only identifying deviations but in approximating the location of brain regions involved.

---

[41]Can be found at www.neurorep.com

F. BRC Database

One of the most exciting developments in this area during the last few years is the development of the first standardized International Brain Database. It overcomes the problems about the databases presented above. A consortium of leading neuroscientists was consulted to resolve an optimal choice of tests that tap the brain's major networks and processes in the shortest amount of time. Six sites have been set up with identical equipment and software (New York, Rhode Island, London, Holland, Adelaide, and Sydney) under the auspices of a publicly listed company (The Brain Resource Company[42]), with new sites to be added progressively. Hundreds of normative subjects have been acquired and the assessment of clinical patient groups has also recently begun.

The BRC Database involves data collection not only of EEG and ERP parameters in a battery of simple tasks (such as the auditory and visual oddball tasks), but also a comprehensive psychological test battery undertaken using a touch-screen monitor[43]. Structural and functional MRI data are also obtained for many selected individuals. Further, genetic information will be systematically collected for comparison to neuroanatomical, neurophysiological, and psychometric measures.

G. HBI Database

The Human Brain Institute (HBI) DataBase was recently developed as a joint venture of three people: programmer Valery Ponomarev, psychologist Andreas Mueller, and the author of this book. This database relies on the methodology developed in the laboratory for neurobiology of action programming of the Institute of the Human Brain of Russian Academy of Sciences (Director J.D. Kropotov)[44]. The methodology is presented in the present book and here there is no need to describe it even in a short form. But what is important to describe is the history of developing the database. It started in Cascais, a beautiful resort in Portugal, where the author of the book together with Jay Gunkelman was having a workshop on QEEG and neurotherapy. Andreas Mueller was among the attendees. He was impressed by the methodology of QEEG/ERP assessment and decided to collect the normative data. He invested quite a bit of his own money. With the help of his

---

[42]The information about this company can be found in www.brainresource.com

[43]Psychological test battery includes: choice reaction time (speed of motor performance), timing test (capacity to assess time), digit span (short-term memory), memory recall test, spot the word test, span of visual memory test, verbal fluency test, malingering test, verbal interference test, switching of attention.

[44]Note, that the name "HBI" is not the name of the Institute of the Human Brain (IHB) but rather reflects the fact that the database incorporates scientific knowledge obtained during fundamental research of the Human Brain obtained by one of the authors (Juri Kropotov) during the last thirty years at the Institute of Experimental Medicine of Russian Academy of Medical Sciences and at the Institute of the Human Brain of Russian Academy of Sciences in St. Petersburg.

co-workers at Institute of the Human Brain and Norwegian University of Science and Technology and students from St. Petersburg State University we were able to collect EEG data in 1000 healthy subjects of age from 7 to 89 years old. The database includes EEG recorded in eyes open, eyes closed resting conditions, and in five different tasks conditions (two stimulus GO/NOGO task, mathematic task, reading task, auditory recognition task, and auditory oddball tasks). It also includes recordings of more than 500 attention deficit hyperactivity disorder (ADHD) children and adolescents, as well as numerous recordings in other kind of patients (patients with epilepsy, obsessive-compulsive disorder – OCD, addiction, depression, whiplash, etc.)

To reduce the amount of time for preprocessing the data some procedures (such as artifact correction and spike detection) are automated. To assess both global and local features of EEG three montages (linked ears, global average, and local average) are used. Absolute and relative amplitude and power spectra, coherences, wavelet-transformations and ERPs are computed off-line and mapped into 2D representations or into 3D images using LORETA and s-LORETA technology. Dipole approximation methods are also provided. In addition, ERPs are subjected to ICA. Using this methodology, separate components associated with distinctive psychological operations are extracted. Each component is characterized by time dynamics and topography. Spatial filters are built up on the basis of these topographies and enable the users to extract the amplitude and latency of each component from the individual ERPs. Comparing these parameters with the normative data gives insights concerning different stages of information processing in the individual under assessment.

CHAPTER 9

Practice

I. INTRODUCTION

The book is equipped with an educational software. The software is a computer program (EdEEG.exe) that exploits basic algorithms of electroencephalogram (EEG) processing described in the book[1]. The software is stored in a zipped form and are provided via a web site created and hosted by Elsevier, and accessed through this one common URL: www.elsevierdirect.com/companions/9780123745125. There are two different pieces of software – EdEEG and Psytask. They are available separately in compressed zip files. After downloading, the user will need to extract the zip file and run 'Setup.exe' to install the software. Note that in this Part of the book you will need only EdEEG program. Besides the computational software, there are some EEG files recorded in normal subjects as well as in patients. For this part of the book we selected the EEG recordings in resting condition with eyes open and eyes closed (EO EC) conditions. It should

---

[1] The software was written by Valery Ponomarev – a senior research fellow from the author's laboratory at the Institute of the Human Brain of Russian Academy of Sciences in St. Petersburg. It is based on the methodological principles developed in the laboratory. The extended version of this software is commercially available.

be stressed that we are not going to present a complete atlas of the various EEG patterns[2]. Rather the goal of the educational software is to help the reader practice the basic methodological principles of background EEG analysis.

A. Categories of EEG Processing

The whole set of methods of background EEG analysis can be divided into the following categories: (1) EEG data format management, (2) EEG preprocessing including artifact correction, (3) representation of electric potentials on the head in a form of cortical generators by means of electromagnetic tomography or dipole approximation, (4) Fourier analysis that includes computing absolute and relative EEG spectra for separate channels, coherences for pairs of channels, (5) wavelet analysis including computing event-related de/synchronization (ERD/ ERS), (6) comparison of EEG parameters with a normative database including computation of z-scores as measures of statistical significance of deviation of the individual parameter from the normal distribution computed for healthy subjects of the corresponding age, (7) management of the files that store the results of EEG analysis, (8) compiling reports, that is presenting the results of processing in short and meaningful form with conclusions and recommendations for therapy.

These categories of EEG processing are schematically presented in Fig. 9.1. For the educational software we selected only few categories of EEG analysis. Those methods that are not included in the EdEEG software are briefly listed below to give the reader a flavor of what the methods might offer to the practitioner.

B. EEG Data Formats

As we learnt from this part of the book EEG is recorded by means of amplifiers. The amplifiers magnify low amplitude potentials of the human head into larger signals that are further converted into a digital form by means of analog-to-digit (AD) converters. To read the output of the AD converter the software, in its turn, needs a special routine called a driver[3]. The driver enables the software to "read" values of brain potentials from AD converters and to store them on the disc. There are several standard protocols (formats) of storing the EEG data on the

---

[2] For a modern atlas of EEG patterns and corresponding LORETA images see Zumsteg et al. (2004).

[3] In general terms a driver is a program that controls a device. Every device, such as a printer or an EEG amplifier, must have a driver program. Common drivers come with the operating system. For the EEG amplifier you need to load a new driver when you connect the amplifier to your computer. In Windows environments, drivers often have a DRV extension. A driver acts like a translator between the device and the program that uses the device by accepting generic commands from the program and translating them into specialized commands for the device.

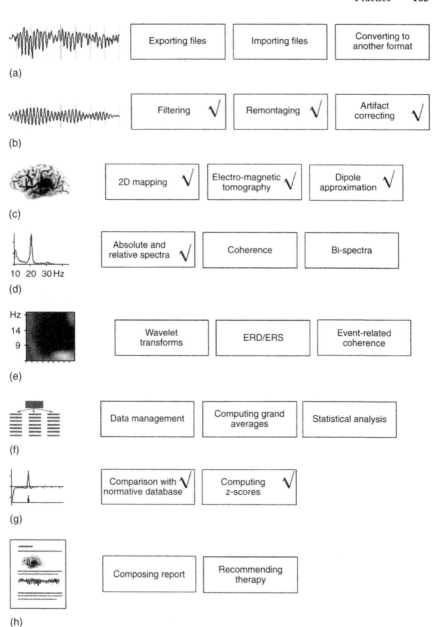

(a)

(b)

(c)

(d)

(e)

(f)

(g)

(h)

FIGURE 9.1   Methods of EEG processing. The methods are divided into categories (presented from top to bottom in rows). The items presented in EdEEG are marked. The categories are (from top to bottom): (a) EEG data format management, (b) EEG preprocessing, (c) 2D mapping and LORETA, (d) Fourier analysis, (e) wavelet decomposition, (f) management of the files, (g) comparison with a normative database, (h) compiling reports.

disc such as European Data Format (with extension .edf), Universal Data Format (with extension .udf), and EEG ASCII format (with extension .txt). The data files store numbers corresponding to potentials measured at sequential time intervals in each of the EEG channels in a form of tables (channels versus time). In addition, the data files store specific information, such as patient's name, date of birth, number of channels, sampling rate. In addition to standard data formats some companies make their own data formats specific to their EEG acquisition/processing systems[4].

C. Data Management

When the number of recordings that the user made in his/her practice exceeds a few hundreds it becomes difficult to manage the data[5]. Special tools enable the user to manipulate the data. One of them is an individual database[6]. The individual EEG Database is a structured collection of the EEG records obtained by the user. The records are stored in a computer in a special order so that a management program can consult it to answer queries. For example, raw EEGs and results of their processing (such as spectra, wavelet transformations, or event-related potentials) are usually stored in different folders. These different categories of files are described by a structural description known as a schema. For example, the schema describes the objects that are represented in the database by the patient's name, date of birth, date of recording, gender, diagnosis, computed parameter, etc. The schema becomes important when we want to make grand averages for a given age, gender, or diagnosis. It also helps to search for a particular patient or a particular date of recording. The computer program used to manage and query a database is known as a database management system. The first database management systems were developed in the 1960s. In the EEG field they became a standard tool.

D. Editing and Compiling QEEG Reports

Viewing and analyzing EEG data are usually accompanied by editing procedures for compiling a final report on a patient's EEG. These procedures enable the practitioner

---

[4] For Example, the Lexicor company has a specific data format with extension *.dat, while the Mitsar Ltd uses a specific format with extension *.EEG.

[5] For example, the user wants to test his impression that many from the recorded "whiplash" patients who visited his office during the last year has excess of alpha activity in the temporal areas. To test this hypothesis the user needs to select the data of all whiplash patients of a certain age (for example, from 20 to 30 years old), to average the data for a certain condition of recording (for example, to obtain grand average spectra in eyes open condition) and to compare the result with the normative data.

[6] Do not mix it with the normative database. The individual database comprises the data obtained by an individual practitioner.

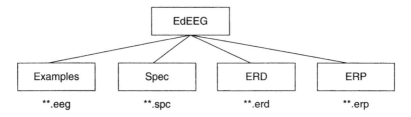

FIGURE 9.2   Organization of files in the EdEEG folder. Within boxes – names of folders, under boxes – extension of files that are stored in the corresponding folder.

to paste into the report all available information regarding the raw data (such as fragments of EEG in various conditions) and the results of processing (such as power, amplitude or relative EEG spectra, event-related desynchronization, etc.). Compiling also includes the interpretation of the observed results and recommendation for therapy, including recommendation for protocols of neurofeedback procedures and electrodes' placement in transcranial direct current stimulation.

II. EdEEG SOFTWARE

A. Installation

The procedure of installation of the program is a conventional one and consists of the following steps. After unzipping the downloaded file with EdEEG software run the SETUP.EXE program. Follow the instruction on the screen. Press "Finish" button to complete the setup. The program will be installed on the hard disc of your computer into the folder EdEEG.

B. Folders for Data Processing

In the subfolder *DATA* (Fig. 9.2) you will find files that store digital EEG recorded in normal subjects and in patients. The files have extension .eeg[7]. There are four EEG files: S1_EO EC, S2_EO EC, S3_VCPT, S4_VCPT recorded in healthy subjects and patients in correspondingly the EO EC resting conditions and during the two stimulus GO/NOGO task. Beside *DATA* subfolder, the EdEEG main folder includes three sub-folders named *SPEC, ERD*, and *ERP*. These sub-folders will store the results of EEG analysis that you are going to perform while practicing with the software. The sub-folders are supposed to include

[7] The files comprise 19-channel EEG + 1 channel of button press markers recorded by Mitsar amplifiers (Mitsar Ltd, St. Petersburg, Russia).

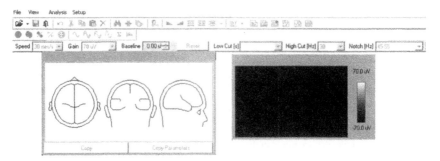

FIGURE 9.3   Main, dipole, and map windows of the EdEEG program. A view from the computer screen after starting EdEEG.exe. Big window – main (EEG) window which enables the user to view EEG records and make all types of EEG analysis. Small left window – dipole window that depicts length and orientation of electric dipole that fits the current distribution of the scalp potential. Small right window – map window that depicts 2D maps of the scalp potential at the left and right time markers.

the files with the corresponding extensions: ✶✶.spc for spectra, ✶✶.erd for event-related ERD/ERS and wavelet transformations, ✶✶.erp for event-related potentials.

To practice basic principles of background EEG analysis follow the steps described below. Note that in developing the software we pursued the main principles of Microsoft products. So, for those who are using the MS Windows platform the functional meaning and position of the main menus will appear familiar.

Step 1. Opening EEG file: Start EdEEG.exe program from the folder EdEEG. The following three windows will be opened up (Fig. 9.3). They are the Main, Dipole (left), and Map (right) windows.

In the main window you can see the following menus: *File, View, Analysis, Setup*. Each menu has its own *Commands* (see Fig. 9.4). Some of the most common commands are presented as *Toolbars*.

To view an EEG record stored in the subfolder *DATA* go to *File* menu and click *Open File* command. Select any file and open it. The *EEG window* similar to that presented in Fig. 9.5 will pop up.

Step 2. Viewing EEG record: The Main (EEG) window is used for viewing the recorded EEG. It has three bars: the *Channel Names bar* placed on the left side of the computer screen, the *Status bar* placed in the bottom, and the *Filters Bar* placed in the top. The *Channel Name bar* is used for indication and selection of channels.

Selection of the channel is performed simply by clicking a box on the *Channel Name Bar* with the corresponding name (for example, Fz). The box is highlighted. Selection of a time fragment needed for further analysis is made by two vertical markers. This is done within *the time bar* positioned just above the EEG record. The numbers in the *time bar* correspond to the time of recording measured in seconds. The left vertical time marker is set by clicking the left key of the mouse within the time bar. The right vertical marker is set by clicking the right key of the mouse. The selected interval is highlighted at the top.

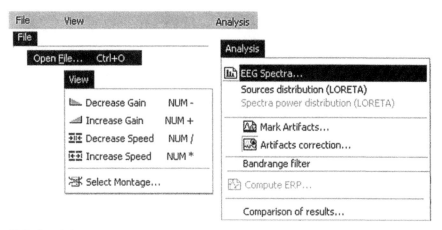

FIGURE 9.4   Commands of the File, View, and Analysis menus. Below File, View, and Analysis menus – main commands and corresponding tool bars.

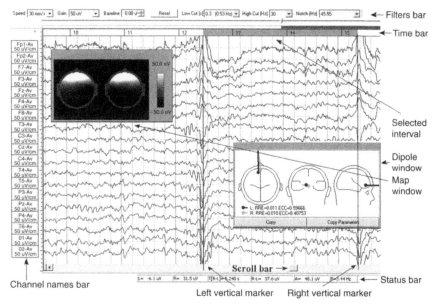

FIGURE 9.5   Viewing an EEG fragment. The main components needed for visualization and simple preprocessing are depicted. Filters bar – parameters of digital filtration for Low Cut, High Cut, and Notch filters. Time bar – current time of recording in seconds. Left and right vertical time markers are activated within this bar. Channel bar – names of channels ("active" electrode – Reference) and gain in μV/cm. Status bar – voltage at the left (L) and right (R) markers. T[R-L] – time interval between right and left markers, A – peak-to-peak EEG amplitude for the selected interval. F – "Average" frequency in the selected interval. Map window – 2D maps of the potentials at the left and right time marker. Dipole window – two equivalent dipoles that fit the distribution of cortical potentials at the left and right vertical time markers.

The 2D maps of the potentials at the left and right time markers are presented in the *Map Window* correspondingly on the left and right sides of the Window. In addition to 2D maps the software computes the parameters of two equivalent dipoles that fit the distribution of cortical potentials measured at the "left" and "right" time markers. These dipoles are presented in the *Dipole Window* in red color for the "left" marker and in blue color for the "right" marker. And finally, the software enables the user to perform the electromagnetic tomography (LORETA) either on instantaneous potentials at the left and right markers or on EEG cross-spectra computed for the interval between the markers[8]. To perform low resolution electromagnetic tomography (LORETA) on the EEG potentials defined by the two time markers, go to *Analysis/Source Distribution (LORETA)*. To perform LORTEA on the cross-spectra of EEG between the two markers, go to *Analysis/Spectra power distribution (LORETA)*. When doing it the first time the program will need to know the pathway to *Main* folder of LORETA software that must be already installed on the user's computer.

The *Status bar* of the EEG window presented on the bottom of an EEG record displays parameters for a selected channel, such as L, amplitude of potential in the selected channel at the left marker; R, amplitude of potential in the selected channel at the right marker; T[R-L], time interval between markers; R-L, potential difference between the markers; A, peak-to-peak EEG amplitude for the selected interval (difference between maximal and minimal values); F, "Average" frequency of the EEG fragment in the selected channel.

Step 3. Preprocessing EEG-record-filtering: The *Filter* bar is a multi-bar which enables the user to set up the *Low Cut* and *High Cut* parameters of the digital filters as well as to change time (*Speed*) and amplitude (*Gain*) scales. The *Speed bar* is used to choose horizontal (time) scale. The *Gain bar* is used to choose vertical (amplitude) scale. To change gain only for a selected channel, hold *Ctrl* pressed. The *High Cut (Hz) bar* is used to choose the EEG bandpass high frequency cutoff. To change the high cutoff only for a selected channel, press and hold *Ctrl*. The *Low Cut (Hz) bar* is used to choose the EEG bandpass low frequency cutoff. To change low frequency cutoff only for a selected channel, press and hold *Ctrl*. The *Notch (Hz) bar* is used to turn notch 50 or 60 Hz filter on or off. To change notch only for a selected channel, hold *Ctrl*. The *Baseline bar* is used to change the baseline of EEG recording. To change baseline only for a selected channel, hold *Ctrl* pressed.

In some cases[9] there is a need to filter EEG records in a narrow frequency range. This is made by bandpass filtering in the *Analysis* menu (see Fig. 9.6). But

[8] In order to be able to perform this option the user has to install LORETA-free software. The software is found on the site of The KEY Institute for Brain-Mind Research in Zurich, Switzerland http://www.uzh.ch/keyinst/NewLORETA/. The program was developed by Roberto D. Pascual-Marqui. To install the LORETA program follow the instructions on the site.

[9] These are, for examples, cases of computing ERD/ERS or cases of performing electromagnetic tomography (LORETA).

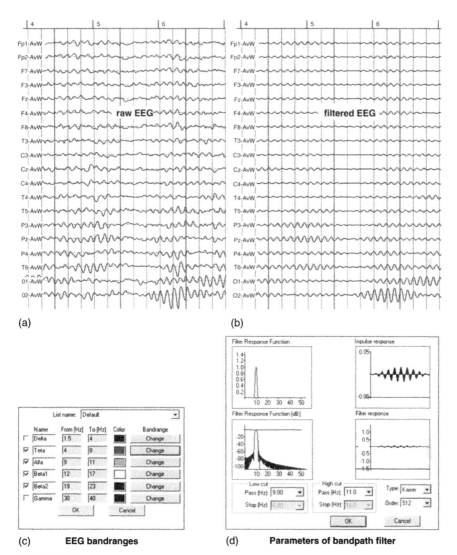

FIGURE 9.6   Electroencephalogram digital filtration. (a) Raw EEG, (b) filtered EEG, (c) EEG bands conventionally used for filtration, the bands can be changed by the user as well as new bands can be added, (d) parameters of an individual filter.

before doing it the user has to define the parameters of the filter. This is done by *SETUP menu* in *EEG bandranges*. In the example presented in Fig. 9.6 we selected the Kaiser digital filter of the order of 512 within 9.00–11.00 Hz frequency range. One can also use the default parameters, such as standard EEG bands or 1 Hz bands.

Step 4. Preprocessing EEG record – setting montage: The EEG is recorded and stored on the disc in the linked ears montage within the full bandwidth of EEG

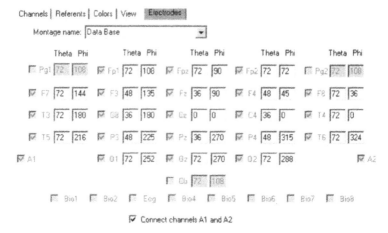

FIGURE 9.7   Coordinates of electrodes in 10–20 system. Each electrode position is defined by two spherical coordinates on the head – Theta and Phi values.

amplifiers. For viewing and analyzing the data other montages can be selected. This can be done by pressing *Select Montage* command in the *View Menu*. The *Montage Parameters window* will pop up.

In the *Montage Parameters* window there are five dialog boxes: *Channels, Referents, Colors, View, Electrodes*. Note the difference between electrodes and channels. *Electrodes* are physical places where the metal electrodes are applied. Each electrode position is defined by two spherical coordinates on the head[10]. They are presented in Fig. 9.7 as Theta and Phi values.

A *channel* by definition is a referential recording that measures potential difference between a physical *electrode* and a *reference*. Recording of the channel is depicted in the *Main (EEG)* window as an amplitude–time graphic. Several types of *References* are presented in the dialog box *View* (Fig. 9.8). They are from the left to the right: linked ears reference (*Ref*), common average (*Av*) and local average (*AvW*).

To define a channel one has to define the parameters of recording presented in Fig. 9.9. These parameters are *Electrode* (for the "active" site of recoding) and *Reference* (for the reference site of recording). Electrode and Reference are set to the defined channel simply by pressing the corresponding names at Electrode and Reference. Note that the user can design his/her own montage using this simple procedure. To add the channel use *Add* key, to delete the channel use *Delete* key. In default montages all these parameters are defined and the user does not need to worry about them. But in some cases the parameters have to be defined specifically by the user.

---

[10]The coordinate system is as follows: X-axis goes from the left ear to the right one, Y-axis – from the nape to the forehead, Z-axis – upwards.

Channels | Referents | Colors | View | Electrodes |

Montage name: [DataBase] ▾

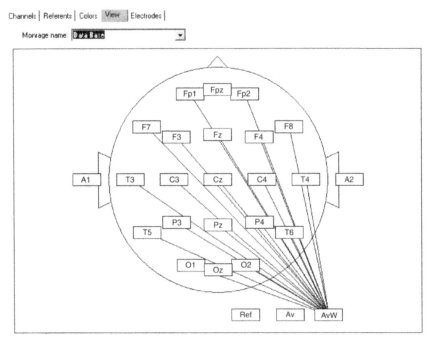

FIGURE 9.8   View of electrodes' montage. Electrodes are schematically presented in boxes. The boxes are connected with each other or with reference electrodes according the montage. In the example above the local average montage is presented.

We recommend starting with *DataBase* montage. For selecting it you just need to select DataBase in the list of montages from the Montage Parameters window (Fig. 9.10).

Step 5. Artifacting: Artifacting stands for methods of eliminating and correcting artifacts. We are presenting three methods: Manual Delete (or simply *Clear*), *Automatic Mark Artifacts*, and *Artifact Correction.* These methods represent different ways of dealing with artifacts.

There is a special toolbar (*Clear*) in the *Edit Menu* to implement the Delete function. Before pressing the toolbar, one has to find an artifact by visual inspection[11], select it by means of two vertical lines. After pressing the *Clear* bar you will see a gray bar instead of the deleted fragment.

The visual inspection mode of deleting artifacts is time consuming, subjective, and leads to different results depending on the experience and bias of the user. We offer a method that performs an automatic search for artifacts. The automatic

---

[11] Finding an artifact by visual inspection is an art. The methodology is described in the book "The art of artifacting" by D. Corydon Hammond and Jay Gunkelman, published by Society for Neuronal Regulation in 2001.

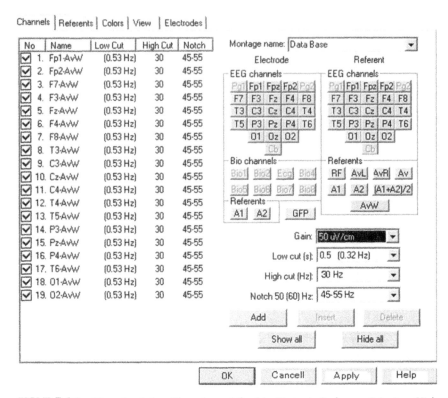

FIGURE 9.9 Channels window. Channels are defined by Electrode, Reference, Gain, Low, High Cut, and Notch frequencies. These parameters can be changed from the right part of the window and are depicted at the left part of the window. The montage name is shown at top right.

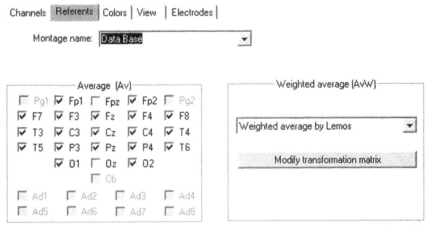

FIGURE 9.10 Reference window. The type of local (weighted) average montage is defined by clicking ▼ from the right. Electrodes to be averaged in common average montage are defined from the left.

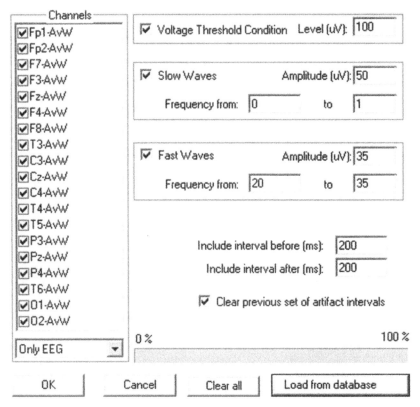

FIGURE 9.11   Parameters for automated artifact elimination. Left – channels that are going to be processed for artifacts. Right – amplitude threshold in μV, threshold parameters for slow and high frequency artifacts.

Marking artifacts is done by the corresponding command from the *Analysis* menu. The search for artifacts is made on the basis of preset parameters. An example of such a set of parameters is presented in Fig. 9.11. The parameters were defined experimentally. EEG fragments that fit the following criteria are considered as artifacts: (1) the amplitude of the raw signal exceeds 100 μV, (2) the amplitude of slow waves in the frequency range from 0 to 1 Hz is higher than 50 μV, (3) high-frequency activity in the frequency range from 20 to 35 Hz is higher than 35 μV. To run this procedure, press key *Mark artifacts* in *Analysis* Menu. The program will mark the artifacts with a blue mark and will not take the marked fragments into account for further analysis.

And finally, the third method of Artifacting is the method of spatial filtration (note that for actual EEG analysis one has to perform the spatial filtration of artifacts and then the marking artifacts). The best results of the spatial filtration method are obtained for eye movement artifacts. The procedure starts with defining

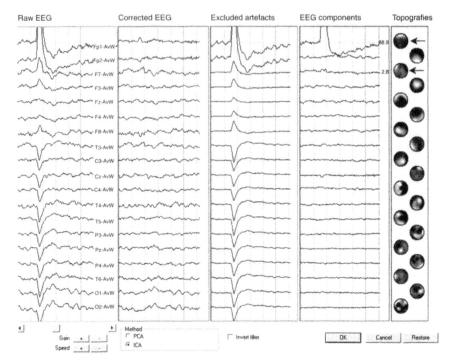

FIGURE 9.12   The window of artifact correction Bottom – scroll bar, Gain, Speed buttons, and Method of spatial filtration (PCA or ICA). Right – topographies of components extracted by PCA or ICA. Top (from left to right) – Raw EEG, Corrected EEG, Excluded artifacts, and time dynamics of extracted PCA or ICA EEG components.

an EEG epoch. This epoch will be used as a template for constructing the filters for artifacts. After defining the EEG epoch the procedure is initiated by pressing the command *Artifact Correction* from *Analysis* menu. The software decomposes the selected EEG fragment into components using principle component analysis (*PCA*) or independent component analysis (*ICA*). Time dynamics and topographies of the PCA components are presented at the right of the window which pops up after pressing the *Artifact Correction* command (Fig. 9.12). Some of the components correspond to EEG signal while others correspond to artifacts such as vertical or horizontal eye movements as marked in Fig. 9.12.

We recommend the reader to use the ICA method for artifact correction. To perform this function, click the corresponding icon (*ICA*) in *Method* of the *Artifact correction* window. Note that the ICA method needs quite long-time interval for analysis. We recommend selecting the whole EEG fragment by pressing the left button of the mouse within the time window at the beginning of the record and the right button at the end of the record. After clicking the *ICA* icon the program will decompose the raw EEG into independent components. Note that the computations might take

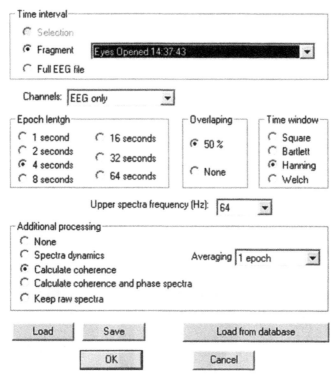

FIGURE 9.13   The window of parameters for spectral analysis. From top to bottom – interval of analysis, parameters of Fast Fourier Transformation, additional processing with the number of averaged epochs used for spectra dynamics.

a few minutes! Time dynamics and topographies of the ICA components will appear at the right side of the window.

The user has to select the topography of the artifact that needs to be corrected. Topographies of vertical and horizontal eye movements are marked in Fig. 9.12 by arrows. The selection of the needed component is made by simply clicking on the corresponding topography on the right of the Window and the corresponding topography is highlighted by red. On the basis of the selected topographies a spatial filter is computed. This spatial filter is further on applied to the EEG record after pressing the *OK* key on the *Artifact Correction Window.*

Step 6. Fourier analysis: After eliminating and correcting artifacts we can perform Fourier analysis of the EEG signal. This is done by clicking command *EEG spectra* from *Analysis* menu. The Window *Parameters of spectra computation* will appear (see Fig. 9.13). The parameters describe (1) the part of the EEG record we are going to analyze: *Selection* (a time interval defined by the left and right vertical time markers), *Fragment* (a fragment that was defined during recording such as EO, EC), or *full EEG record*; (2) parameters of Fast Fourier Transformation such as

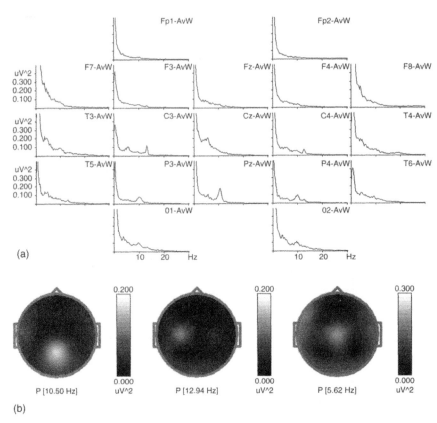

FIGURE 9.14   An example of results of spectral analysis. (a) Spectra of 19 electrodes positioned similar to electrodes' location on the scalp. Y-axis, EEG power in μV², X-axis, EEG frequency in Hz. (b) Maps of EEG power at three different frequencies (10.5), (12.9), (5.6). Scales are presented at right of each map.

Epoch length, mode of *Overlapping*, and type of *Time window*; (3) types of additional processing such as computing spectral dynamics, calculating coherence, and phase spectra; and (4) number of averaging epochs for computing dynamics of spectra.

We recommend downloading the parameters of spectral analysis from the database by clicking the corresponding dialog box (*Load from database*). After pressing *OK* button the spectra will appear in a way depicted in Fig. 9.14. In this figure each electrode is presented as a single graph with EEG power (squired amplitude) along the Y-axis and EEG frequency along X-axis. The EEG power at a selected frequency can be mapped into a 2D topography. To make a map, one has to select a certain frequency by activating a cursor in any of the graphs. This is done by holding the right button of the mouse pressed within any graph. When this button is released a pop-up menu appears on the screen. Use the *Add Map* command to add

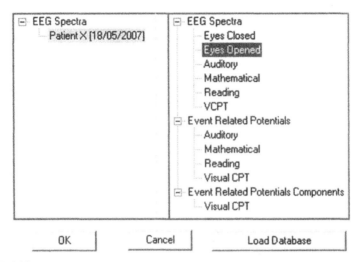

FIGURE 9.15   Window of comparison with the database. Left – name of the patient and date of recording. Right – EEG spectra, Event Related Potentials, and Independent Components of Event-Related potentials. Right categories are downloaded from the normative database by clicking button from Right Bottom – Load DataBase.

the map for the selected frequency. Spectra can be also presented in absolute amplitude, relative power, and logarithmic values. Use the corresponding *Value* to choose the parameter you want to depict in graphs and topograms: In Fig. 9.14 we present the power spectra of 19 channels of EEG. Each spectrum is averaged over 3 minute of the EO condition. Three maps made for three different frequencies are shown at the bottom of Fig. 9.14. The frequencies are defined by peaks of EEG spectra and correspond to the mu-rhythm (with peaks at C3, C4), parietal alpha rhythm (with peak at Pz), and central theta rhythm (Cz).

Step 7. Comparison with normative database: After finding peaks on the spectra and mapping them, we need to know whether the EEG power of the individual spectra significantly differs from the normative data or not. In this context "significantly" is defined by a confidence level of deviation of a particular feature of the individual spectra (absolute power or amplitude, relative power, coherence) from the mean value computed for a group of healthy subjects of the same age. To perform this operation in the *Analysis* menu click tool bar *Comparison of results.* In the following dialog press *Load Database* and you will get the window presented in Fig. 9.15. At the left of this window you can see the name of the patient you are analyzing and the date of recording. At the right of the window you can see different options for comparison. If you are analyzing EEG spectra in EO condition click *EEG spectra Eyes Open* and then press *OK*.

The program will compute differences between the individual spectra and the mean values of the normative group. The difference spectra (patient-norm) will be

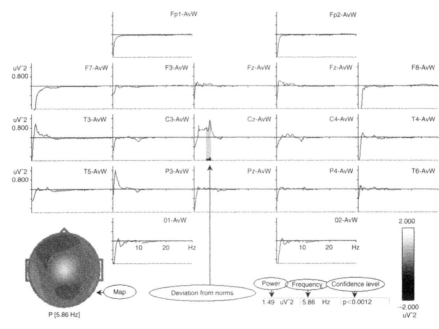

FIGURE 9.16   The results of comparison of the EEG spectra with the HBI normative database. Graphs – differences between the individual spectra and the normative database for 19 electrodes. Below each graph – vertical bars corresponding to the confidence level of deviation from normality. Small bars – $p < 0.05$, middle bars – $p < 0.01$. Bottom Right – difference value, frequency, and confidence level at the selected frequency. Bottom Left – map of the difference spectra at 5.9 Hz.

displayed for each channel. Below the difference spectra you can find vertical bars that correspond to the confidence level of deviation from normality. Depending on the length the following confidence levels are depicted: small bars – $p < 0.05$, middle bars – $p < 0.01$, long bars – $p < 0.001$. In addition, the exact value of the confidence level is displayed at the right side of the window when you position the cursor (by pressing the right button of the mouse) at a particular frequency on a spectra corresponding to the channel of your interest (for example, Cz in the case at Fig. 9.16). Together with the confidence level the program displays the frequency and the amplitude of the parameter under analysis (Fig. 9.16 right, bottom).

III. EXERCISES

The EdEEG software is provided with two EEG files, S1_EO_EC.EEG and S2_ EO_EC.EEG: one for a healthy subject and the other one for a patient. Both subjects belong to the same age group of 13–14 years old. EEG was recorded in two resting conditions with eyes open (EO) and eyes closed (EC). The corresponding fragments are labeled as *Eyes open* and *Eyes closed*.

We suggest the reader to exercise with the two files and to answer the following questions:

1. *Which file corresponds to a healthy subject and which one corresponds to a patient?*
2. *What normal rhythms can be found in the EEG records?*
3. *What type of brain dysfunction is found in the EEG record of the patient?*
4. *What brain disorder (ADHD, OCD, or Dyslexia) can be associated with the observed brain dysfunction?*

To answer these questions perform the steps of EEG analysis described above. Briefly the actions are as follow:

1. Start *EdEEG.exe* program.
2. From *File menu* click *Open File* command.
3. Open file from *EdEEG* folder *Data* subfolder (which if installed Typical is located on Disk C). There are two files, S1_EO EC and S2_EOEC. Analyze each of the files separately.
4. Use buttons from the Input Control toolbar (■ ◀◀ ◀ ▶ ▶▶) to view the record. These buttons correspond to Stop, Fast rewind back, Slow rewind back, Slow play back, Fast play back. You can also view the EEG at different time intervals by moving the scroll bar located just below the EEG record.
5. From *View menu* click *Select Montage* and in the window *Montage Name* select *DataBase Version 1 montage*. This montage name is the last in the list of montages. By clicking *References* dialog box in the *Montage parameters* window make sure that it is the *Weighted average by Lemos* montage. Then press *OK*. The EEG record will appear in the selected montage.
6. By visual inspection find artifacts of vertical and horizontal eye movements.
7. Select the whole record. This is done by clicking the *left button* of the mouse at the beginning of the record and the *right button* at the end of the record. Clicking must be done within the *time bar* located above the record. After clicking the *right button* the time bar will become yellow.
8. From *Analysis menu* click *Artifact correction* command. The program will automatically decompose the EEG fragment into 19 components by means of the Principle Component Analysis (PCA). From *Method* menu (presented at the bottom) select ICA (Independent Component Analysis) and click OK. The program will start iteration procedure of extracting independent components from the EEG fragment. The procedure usually takes more than 20 seconds and consists of 100 iterations or more. In topographies presented on the right of the appeared window the first (from the top) topography is highlighted by a red circle. This component is

the most strong and corresponds usually to Eye blink artifacts. Make sure that this is the case and click *OK*. The software will filter out this type of artifacts from the whole EEG record. By visual inspection of the record make sure that the corresponding artifact is corrected.

9. From *Analysis menu* click *Mark Artifacts* command. Load the parameters of artifact rejection from the database by clicking command *Load from database*. After pressing *OK* the software will mark the artifacts that fit the criteria.

10. From *Analysis menu* click *EEG spectra* command. Load the parameters of EEG spectra calculation from the database by clicking command *Load from database*. Select the time interval of by clicking *Fragment* and further *Eyes Open*. The software will compute spectra for *Eyes open* condition for each electrode separately and present them in a form 19 graphs located in a way similar to which the electrodes are located on the scalp.

11. From *Analysis menu* click *Comparison of results* command. The window named *Processing Results comparison* will appear. To load EEG spectra from the normative database click *Load Database* bar. At the left of the window the name of subject's EEG spectra is present while at the right the names of EEG spectra from the normative database are present. Click the spectra of the subject from the left and the *EEG spectra Eyes Open* condition from the right. Press *OK*.

12. The difference spectra (subject-database) will appear in *Comparison Window* (an example is presented in Fig. 9.16). Note that the confidence level of deviation from normality is presented in a form of small vertical bars below the spectra graphs.

Do the same analysis with the second file and try to answer the questions presented above.

PART II

Event-Related
Potentials

I. INTRODUCTION

As was presented in Part I different electroencephalogram
(EEG) rhythms are characterized by different neuronal
mechanisms. These rhythms are observed in resting states
with eyes open and eyes closed and are considered to represent background or spontaneous activities. In response to
stimuli or movements alpha and beta rhythms are suppressed
(desynchronized) during the first 200 ms. These dynamic
characteristics of alpha and low beta rhythms in healthy brain
indicate that the beta and alpha rhythms themselves do not
participate in signal processing per se but rather modulate the
information flow in the brain. Here is the right time to stress
the difference between two distinct functions in information
processing in the brain: (1) the function associated with flow

of sensory-related and action-related information in neuronal networks of the brain, and (2) the function associated with modulation of the information flow. As was shown in Part I of the book, modulation of information flow is manifested in synchronization and desynchronization of EEG rhythms.

The stages of information flow are measured by event-related potentials (ERPs). In contrast to EEG rhythms the necessary condition for eliciting ERPs is time locking to a certain event, either a stimulus or a movement. The tasks that are used to elicit ERPs cover a big variety of human sensory, motor, and cognitive functions. They include various types of detection and recognition tests in different sensory modalities, delayed response tests for measuring working memory, GO/NOGO tests for assessing executive functions and many, many others. Each task is associated with a group of distinct psychological operations such as detection and recognition of stimuli, updating working memory, initiation of action and action suppression, monitoring the results of actions and so on. Each psychological operation in turn involves temporal activation/inhibition pattern of neurons in a certain brain area. The sum of synchronously generated and event-locked postsynaptic potentials is recorded at the scalp in a form of an ERP component – a potential deflection that is spatially localized and temporally confined.

At the early years of ERP studies the components were associated with peaks and troughs on ERPs themselves or on ERPs difference waves. The difference waves were obtained by subtraction of ERPs in a task condition that presumably did not involve a studied psychological operation from ERPs in another task condition that presumably included this operation[1]. Potential deflections at difference waves could be divided into classes on the basis of their latency and direction of deviation (positive or negative)

---

[1]A simple example of such task could be a threshold recognition task used in one of our studies (Bechtereva and Kropotov, 1984). In this task visual stimuli (digits) were briefly presented to subjects. The exposition of stimuli was individually tailored so short that approximately in 50 per cent of trials the subjects could not recognize the stimuli, while in other 50 per cent of trial they recognized digits. The subjects had to name the digit or to say NO one second later the digit presentation when a trigger stimulus appeared. It was logical to assume that two categories of stimuli ("recognized," "non-recognized") differ from each other by one psychological operation – object recognition and the difference wave between responses to these categories of stimuli would give us a spatial–temporal correlates of this psychological operation.

such as P100, N100, N200, P200, P300, N400, where P stands for positivity, N – for negativity, and the number stands for the peak latency in milliseconds. However, latency of peaks and troughs does not really capture the essence of a component. For example, the peak latency of a so-called P3b component may vary by hundreds of milliseconds depending on the difficulty of the target–non-target discrimination. Even polarity of a certain components may depend on conditions of recording. For example, the C1 wave, which is generated in area V1 of visual cortex, is negative for upper-field stimuli and positive for lower field stimuli due to the folding pattern of area 17 in the human brain.

Another type of classification of components presumes their functional meaning. There are several ERP components that are elicited in certain type of behavioral paradigms and that have specific names according to their presumed function[2].

ERPs method was introduced in cognitive neuroscience more than 40 years ago – in 1960s. The first attempts to decompose ERPs into separate components were made in 1970 by means of factor analysis and principle component analysis. However these techniques provided only orthogonal (in a strict mathematical sense) components, while it was clear that the ERP components had not necessarily to be orthogonal. Recently emerged methods of objective separation of components (such as independent component analysis) lack this disadvantage of old methods and open a new horizon in this field. Accumulating knowledge shows a diagnostic power of independent ERP components as endophenotypes of brain dysfunctions.

This part of the book is devoted to ERP components, their generation, functional meaning, and diagnostic value[3]. We classify components on the basis of their functional meaning. We presume that the ERP components reflect distinct psychological operations carrying out in distinct systems of the brain.

---

[2]The most studied of them are the mismatch negativity (MMN) as indicator of change detection in repetitive sound, the processing positivity (PN) as indicator of focused attention to a certain sensory channel, error related negativity (ERN) as indicator of errors in continuous performance task, N2 NOGO component as indicator of motor suppression, P3b components as an index of updating the working memory, P3a components as indicator of involuntary switch of attention.

[3]For introduction to the ERP technique I recommend to read a clear written and detailed description of ERPs methods presented in the recently published book by Steven Luck (2005).

II. GLOSSARY

Affective state is a state of the brain characterized by drives, emotions, and motivations.

Agnosia is a condition of a patient who, when faced with a visual object, is unable to name it, show its use, or sort it into a group of morphologically dissimilar objects with identical functions. Shape, color, and movement agnosias are separated.

Amygdala is a nucleus that receives sensory information from polimodal areas of the temporal and parietal cortex through the hippocampus and sends the results of processing to the prefrontal cortex via the thalamus. Its main function is to express fear and initiate associated with fear behavioral reactions.

Anticipating schemata are cognitive structures that prepare the perceiver to accept certain kinds of information rather than others.

Attention, from psychological point of view, is a cognitive mechanism that enables one to process a selected source of sensory information in more detail in comparison to unselected sources by means of limited resources of the brain processor. Attention could be also defined as a state of readiness to receive a certain stimulus – that is, a state for looking forward for a sensory event. In this definition, attention must be separated from motor preparatory set as a state of readiness to make a movement.

Bottom–up processing is the flow of information from lower to higher centers transferring sensory information in a hierarchical manner. These bottom–up processes are usually accompanied by top–down processes in recurrent neuronal networks of the brain, so that separation of bottom–up processing from top–down processing is only of theoretical significance.

Canonical cortical circuit is a hypothetical neuronal network that enables the cortex to perform complex computations of its input. The circuit was first described by Rodney Douglas and Kevan Martin in 1989. The basic idea of the model is that cortical circuits are organized in recurrent excitatory and inhibitory local pathways and that this organization leads to a number of important emergent properties.

Comparison operations are hypothetical operations performed in sensory cortical areas with the goal of detecting any deviation from the anticipatory schemata and adjusting human behavior for those deviations.

An example of such operation in auditory modality is given by the so-called mismatch negativity – a component of ERPs elicited in response to a deviant acoustic stimulus presented at background of repetitive standard stimulus.

Disengagement operation – a process opposite to the engagement operation, which involves inhibition of prepared resources needed for action execution.

Dorsal and ventral streams in the visual system originate in segregated areas of the primary visual cortex of the occipital lobe and target correspondingly temporal and parietal cortical areas. The ventral stream is involved in recognition of separate objects (mostly defined by shape and color) while the dorsal stream is involved in encoding spatial relationships between objects and in controlling actions with those objects such as manipulating with them and orienting toward them.

Emotion is a behavioral response (change in heart rate, facial expression, speech) to a reward (positive emotion), punishment (negative emotion), or images of those behavioral events. Emotion as a psychological entity can be divided into two parts: emotional response and feeling.

Emotional response is defined by somato-sensory (facial and body) responses as well as endocrine responses to emotion-triggered stimuli-rewards and punishers.

Engagement operation is an operation performed by the executive system and involved activation of cortical–subcortical resources needed for action execution. The engagement operation implies the existence of an active process within the brain that exerts disinhibition of cortical neurons that are preset in a recent past to perform a certain action: either motor or cognitive.

Episodic memory is memory for specific events that are temporally dated. It also includes memory for relationships between different events.

ERPs (event-related potentials) brain potentials associated with information flow in the cortical areas evoked by some event (e.g., a repetitive stimulus presenting sequentially during a sensory discrimination task or repetitive flexing a finger during a simple motor task). ERPs are usually obtained by averaging technique that enhances the signal to noise ratio.

Executive functions refer to operations of control and monitoring of motor, sensory, and cognitive actions in goal-directed behavior. These functions are mostly attributed to frontal lobes however the basal ganglia and some other subcortical structures are necessarily involved.

Explicit memory (that is, conscious memory) is a memory which is stored and retrieved consciously. This type of memory can be acquired during an episode and declared by the subject afterward. It is often is called declarative memory.

Feeling (or emotional feeling) is a subjective experience of the state produced by emotion-triggered stimuli. Examples of emotions are joy and sadness, courage and fear, anger and happiness, love and hate... The cortical center for mapping emotions into separate activation patterns is the orbito–frontal cortex.

Implicit memory is an acquired skill or knowledge that a subject can demonstrate without explicit awareness of it. It is often is called non-declarative memory or procedural memory.

Information processing in the brain is a broad class of transformations of impulse activity of output neurons of the receptive organs (such as retina) to impulse activity and to slower membrane potentials of neurons within different neuronal networks of the brain. In its turn information processing can be divided into two functions: *information flow* and *information modulation*. These two operations are maintained by two different classes of neuromediators: *fast acting mediators* (such as glutamate and GABA) and *slow acting mediators* (such as dopamine, norepinephrine, serotonin, and acetylcholine).

Lateral inhibition is a type of connectivity in neuronal networks in which neurons inhibit the surrounding neurons and thus unable the spreading of activation in the lateral direction. Lateral inhibition was first described in retina of the eye in 1950s. The function of the lateral inhibition in the visual system is to emphasize the highest gradients of luminosity in visual images (such as Mach bands).

Leukotomy is a procedure of psychosurgery by which a leukotome (a special knife) is inserted through the eye socket and the inferior/ventral part of the prefrontal cortex is disconnected from the rest of the brain. This operation was started by a Portuguese neurologist Egas Moniz and was very popular in 1950 until the discovery of anti-psychotic drugs.

Limbic system – the term was coined by Paul Broca to define under the same name a group of structures that form a border around the brain stem. Limbic system plays an important part in emotional reactions.

Long-term potentiation (LTP) is an enduring increase in the amplitude of excitatory postsynaptic potentials as a result of high frequency (tetanic) stimulation of afferent pathways. LTP is considered to be a cellular model of learning and memory.

Memory consolidation at neuronal level is a process of developing irreversible changes in synaptic transmission. At psychological level, memory consolidation is associated with forming of long-term memory which decays very slowly (comparable with a life span).

Monitoring as a new concept defines a hypothetical psychological operation that enables the brain to evaluate the quality of action execution and alerts the executive control mechanisms to allocate resources for compensating the conflict between intended and executed actions.

Motivation is desire or drive that steer the behavior by determining goals.

Motor preparatory set is a cognitive mechanism that enables one to focus on performing a certain motor action while suppressing all other irrelevant actions. It is expressed in preparation to make a movement. Attention and motor preparatory set are elements of working memory.

Negative reinforcer (or punisher) is a stimulus that increases behavior pattern directed to avoid the punisher.

Neglect is a neurological syndrome in which patients with brain lesions show a marked deficit in the ability to attend to sensory information presented in the contralesional field. Neglect is often associated with lesions in the right parietal lobe, however lesions in subcortical structures (such a thalamus, basal ganglia, and superior colliculus) can be also responsible for neglect.

Neuromodulator is a slow acting neuromediator that modulates (slowly changes) the information processing.

Neuronal network is a net of neurons in the brain that maintains a distinct function. In this book we distinguish this concept from the notion of *neural net* that stands for a model of the real neuronal network.

Neurotransmitter is a fast acting neuromediator that provides the flow of information within neuronal networks.

Orbitofrontal cortex is a part of the prefrontal cortex that receives strong inputs from all sensory systems and maps rewards and punishers into separate spatially temporal patterns. Patients with damage of the orbitofrontal cortex (such as famous Phineas Cage) lost the ability to map effectively rewards and punishers and consequently lost their ability to make appropriate decisions between selecting appropriate rewards and avoiding punishers.

Positive reinforcer (or reward) is a stimulus that increases the frequency of a behavior pattern leading to acquisition of reward.

Priming is the facilitation of recognition, reproduction, or biases in the selection of stimuli that have recently been perceived.

Receptive field of a cell in the sensory system is a discrete area in the extrapersonal space (for vision and audition) and in the intrapersonal space (in somato-sensory modality) where the presentation of a corresponding stimulus causes activation or inhibition of the cell. Stimuli presented outside of this receptive field do not affect activity of the neuron.

Representation is a localized or distributed neuronal network which stores particular information (memory) and when activated, enables access to this information. Representations can be genetically determined or formed during learning.

Scotomas is a loss of visual perception in a local part of the visual field due to a localized damage in the primary visual areas.

Selection operation is a process of activation of a representation. In temporal domain the selection operation seems to be accompanied by synchronous oscillations in theta (4–8 Hz) and gamma (around 40 Hz) frequency bands. These synchronous oscillations form an optimal mode of recall from memory.

Semantic memory is a memory for factual information about the world, concepts, and word meaning.

Sensory modality refers to a sensory system that processes a certain type of receptor information. The most well-studied sensory systems are: visual system (seeing form, color, depth, motion, spatial relationships of visual objects), auditory system (hearing and localizing sounds), somatic sensory or somato-sensory system (feeling touch, pain, thermal sensations, mechanical displacement of muscles and joints).

Sensory systems include receptor organs and subcortical and cortical neuronal networks that specifically respond to activation of the corresponding receptors.

Top–down processing is a flow of information from "higher" to "lower" centers within hierarchy of sensory systems, controlling (modulating) sensory information processing in lower levels by extracting memories from the higher levels.

Working memory implies an active manipulation with the temporary stored information in order to perform sensory-motor and cognitive actions such as language, planning, decision making, etc.

CHAPTER 10

Sensory Systems

Knowledge comes to man through the door of senses

Heraclitus, 6th century, B.C.

We assess changes inside and outside us by means of different types of receptors[1]. They can be divided into two types – extra- and inter-receptors. Extrareceptors tell us about the external interactions with environment, while intra-receptors tell us what happens inside the body. The activity of some of the intra-receptors never reaches our consciousness. The sensory elements for perception of the external world are highly specialized from species to species[2]. There are different *sensory modalities* that give us sensations of images, sounds, body movements and produce pain, taste, touch, smell.

It is important to stress that we are aware not of objects themselves but of impulse discharges of output neurons in receptor organs. This neuronal activity in turn is induced by interaction of the objects with receptors. The brain regions

---

[1]The specific receptor cells transfer stimuli in specific modality into discharges (impulse activity) of output cells in receptor organs. For example, cones in the retina are sensitive to light and not sensitive to sound and transfer their reactions to the light toward ganglion cells of the eye.

[2]Mammals, for example, can not see in infrared light or perceive a magnetic field. The architecture and function of vision of hunting animals is different from those that eat the grass. Moreover the ability of perception depends very much upon experience. Eskimos people that spend their life among snow can distinguish many hues of snow. A good musician can distinguish absolute note of the sound.

where neurons respond to stimulation of a certain type of receptors are usually referred to as a corresponding *sensory system* (visual, auditory, system). Visual system is the most studied of them. In this chapter we confine the analysis by considering only visual, somato-sensory and auditory modalities, which are the most studied and carrying to the brain the most of sensory information.

I. ANATOMY

A. Brodmann Areas and Thalamic Nuclei

Sensory signals from receptive organs enter the cortex at the primary sensory areas through relay nuclei of the thalamus. The basic modalities are mapped into the following cortical areas: Brodmann's area (BA) 17-primary visual cortex or area V1, BA 41-primary auditory or area A1, and BA 1-primary somato-sensory cortex or area S1. The relay thalamic nuclei are lateral geniculate body (LGB) for visual modality, medial geniculate body (MGB) for auditory modality, and lateral posterior nucleus (LP) for somato-sensory modality.

B. Topographical Organization

Each primary sensory area is characterized by topographical order of projections[3]. The primary sensory areas and corresponding thalamic relay nuclei form heavily interconnected neuronal networks. A striking feature of these thalamo-cortical networks is ability to generate rhythms in alpha frequency band (for more details see Chapter 2). As was shown in Part I the function of such rhythms is to keep the sensory areas in an idling state – the state in which the cortex does not actively process the sensory information but can be switched to the active processing mode in a fraction of a second.

C. Parallel Pathways

Let us describe information flow in the visual modality[4]. If we look at the world around us from mechanical point of view, we can say that there are nothing in the world but different objects located in different parts of the space and moving

---

[3]Topographic representation literally means that adjacent cells in the receptive organ project to adjacent cortical neurons thus forming a map of the receptor organ within the cortex.

[4]In the visual modality the information from the retina of the eye is carried to the cortex by a bundle of approximately 1,000,000 axons while in the auditory modality we have only 30,000 axons carrying information from the cochlea of the ear.

with different speeds. Vision provides us with a tool to know (1) *what* is located in the space, (2) *where* in this space "the what" is located, and (3) *how* the subject can manipulate "the what" and make directional movements toward it.

To answer these different questions nature has developed different brain pathways (or streams) of information flow dealing with different kind of visual information. These pathways originate as early as at the LGB of the thalamus. This thalamic relay nucleus comprises two types of cells locating in different layers of the nucleus: smaller (parvocellular) and larger (magnocellular)[5]. These two systems (parvocellular and magnocellular) remain segregated at the level of the primary visual area (BA 17) and give rise to the two streams.

One of the streams is named the ventral or "What" stream (see Fig. 10.1). The stream includes the ventro-lateral prestriate cortex (parts of BA 18, 19) and the inferiotemporal cortex. The striate, prestriate, and inferiortemporal cortical areas compose a hierarchical structure in which signals are transferred from the first to the second level, from the second to the third and so on: The main goal of the hierarchical structure of this visual pathway is to decompose the initial image[6] into different sub-images characterized by different features such as orientation, spatial frequency, and color.

Speed and position of the visual image are decomposed in the hierarchical structure of the so-called dorsal visual stream. The dorsal stream includes areas of the parietal cortex. It should be stressed that the parietal cortex (as well as the dorsal stream in general) is involved not only in mapping spatial relationships in the visual scene ("Where" function), but also in organizing visually guided motor procedures ("How" function). Posterior parietal areas are interconnected with premotor regions of the frontal lobe and provide pathways that enable the human being to execute a class of orienting and manipulating motor actions, such as positioning eyes in direction of the selected object, grasping the object, and manipulating with it. In this respect the dorsal stream is closely related to procedural memory (see Chapter 14).

The ventral and dorsal streams can not be considered as pure parallel: they interact with each other at different levels of hierarchy. In addition, in both pathways there are recurrent connections by which the higher levels send back the information to the lower levels. The recurrent connections provide top–down processing necessary for attention and working memory while connections between parallel pathways coordinate information processing and seem to participate in binding different sensory features into a single percept.

---

[5]Smaller cells are located in the upper four layers of the lateral geniculate nucleus and constitute about 80 per cent of all relay cells in the LGB. Larger cells are located in the lower two layers and constitute respectively 20 per cent of the neurons.

[6]Talking about the initial image I mean the activities of ganglion cells of the eye that encode the light projecting to a distinct spot on the retina into bursts of action potentials.

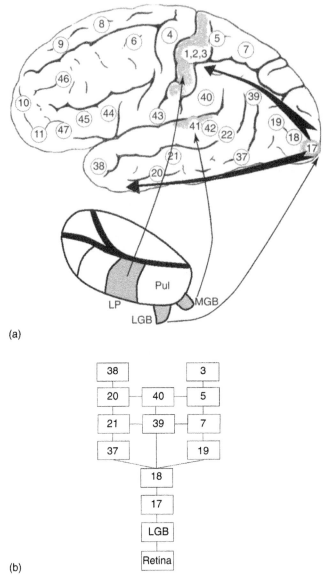

(a)

(b)

FIGURE 10.1 Ordered cortical projections in sensory systems. (a) Sensory-related thalamic nuclei (bottom) serve as gates to the primary sensory areas (top) in the cortex. Three modalities (visual, auditory, and somato-sensory) are depicted. (b) Schematic representation of ventral and dorsal streams in the visual modality. LGB – lateral geniculate body, MGB – medial geniculate body, LP – lateral posterior nucleus.

D. Pulvinar Nucleus as Coordinator of Information Flow

The information processing in ventral and dorsal pathways of the prestriate, temporal, and parietal cortical areas is not confined by mere cortical interconnections. An important role in coordination and modulation of information flow in these cortical areas is played by a thalamic nucleus – the pulvinar (see Fig. 10.1). Recent studies show that neurons in the pulvinar enhance their responses to attended (behaviorally relevant) events while suppress their activities to irrelevant stimuli[7] thus indicating the involvement of the pulvinar in control of information flow within the cortex, particular in attention operations. Some pulvinar neurons, for example, respond to moving stimuli during periods of fixation, while do not respond during saccadic movements, thus discriminating movements of the stimuli from eye movements. Control of the cortical information flow by the pulvinar is not confined by the visual modality: there is some evidence of pulvinar responses to somatic and auditory stimuli.

The sensory information after processing (1) transfers to the prefrontal cortex through the ordered (posterior–frontal) pathways and (2) funnels to the hippocampus through the rhinal cortex. Additionally, there exist "feedback" projections to ventral and dorsal streams areas from the prefrontal cortex and hippocampus.

II. VISUAL INFORMATION FLOW

A. ON and OFF Receptive Fields

Most of our knowledge regarding neuronal mechanisms of visual information processing comes from single neuron studies in animals. In a typical experiment, impulse activity of a single neuron is recorded while various visual stimuli are presented to the animal. For example, in the visual modality light spots, oriented bars, spatial gratings have served as stimuli. Such experiments enable researchers to define the properties of receptive fields of neurons. Two classes of cells labeled as ON and OFF neurons were separated on the basis of their responses to lightness and darkness. These cells are mostly found at the lower levels of visual information flow[8]. The receptive fields of these types of cells can be approximated by difference of two Gaussian functions (a so-called DOG function – see Fig. 10.2) characterized by respectively small and large spatial distributions: the one corresponding to excitatory inputs and the other one corresponding to inhibitory inputs to the neuron. This finding clearly indicates that the lateral inhibition plays a critical role in forming such receptive fields (see also Fig. 10.3).

---

[7]For review see (Robinson and Petersen, 1992).

[8]The lower levels include ganglion cells in the retina and neurons in the LGB of the thalamus.

B. Spatial Filtration at Thalamic and Cortical Levels

At the level of the primary visual cortex, neurons exhibit quite different receptive fields when compared with those of the thalamic neurons (compare the two filters

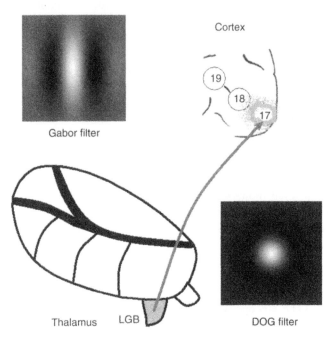

FIGURE 10.2   Receptive fields of neurons in the thalamus and visual cortex. DOG filter corresponds to the difference of two Gaussians and approximates the receptive fields of neurons in the LGB. Gabor filter is a product of a harmonic and Gaussian functions and approximates the receptive fields of the simple cells of neurons in the primary visual cortex.

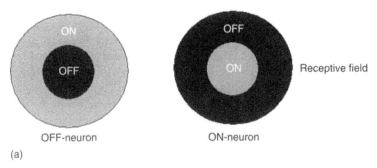

FIGURE 10.3   ON- and OFF-neurons in the visual system. (a) Receptive fields of ON- (right) and OFF-(left) cells. Gray (black) color indicates the part of the receptive field in which the neurons responds by activation (inhibition) to a small dot of light. (b) Responses of the two types of neurons to stimuli representing "light" and "dark" stimuli shown at the right.

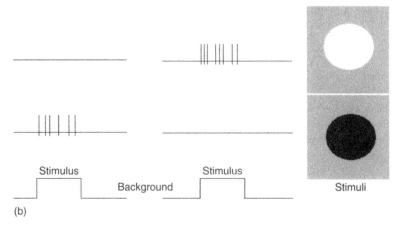

Stimulus   Stimulus

Background   Stimuli

(b)

FIGURE 10.3 (*Continued*)

corresponding to the receptive fields of neurons in the LGB and the visual cortex in Fig. 10.2). The cortical receptive fields in the visual cortex can be approximated by Gabor functions[9] while the thalamic and retinal receptive fields can be approximated by DOG functions.

In 1990s in our laboratory we developed a so-called canonical cortical module that simulated the structure and function of the visual cortex (see Methods of Part II of the present book for more details). This model was based on spatial segregation of ON and OFF cells in the inhibitory layer of the visual cortex. We also presumed that ON and OFF cells are distributed in segments forming the pinwheel structure. As a consequence of this spatial distribution and inhibitory nature of these input neurons shaping responses of the output cells, receptive fields of the simple cells of the module were approximated by Gabor functions.

The involvement of inhibitory neurons is a necessary condition for extracting specific features from the sensory input at all levels of the visual information flow in the brain. Indeed DOG and Gabor functions describing receptive fields of neurons in the visual system include both positive (excitatory) and negative (inhibitory) parts. In scalp recordings activation of excitatory and inhibitory neurons may be expressed in opposite fluctuations of the potential. For example, if the arrival of sensory information to the layer IV of the striate cortex is associated with scalp recorded positivity over the occipital areas, while the activation of the inhibitory neurons is associated with an opposite (negative) component.

---

[9]A Gabor function is a linear filter whose impulse response is defined by a harmonic function multiplied by a Gaussian function. The filter is convolved with the signal, resulting in a so-called Gabor space that is very useful in technical vision.

C. Ventral and Dorsal Streams

Visual cortex in the macaque comprises about 60 per cent of neocortex. The experimental findings show that the retinal images are mapped into multiple cortical areas. The number of these representations (the number of visual areas) in monkeys is more than 20[10]. Anatomically and functionally visual cortical areas can be separated into two streams: the dorsal and ventral pathways first described by Ungerleider and Mishkin as early as in 1980 (for a recent review see Creem and Proffitt, 2001). They suggested that these streams are associated with different capabilities: (1) the parietal stream is involved in visual assessment of spatial relationships; (2) the temporal stream is concerned with visual recognition of objects. Further studies showed that the functional streams in the visual system may be divided into finer pathways. These pathways originate within distinct *subdivisions* called blobs and interblobs of the primary visual cortex[11]. Neurons in the blobs are involved in color perception, while neurons in the interblobs participate in processing form and motion. In the secondary visual cortex (BA 18) neuronal representations of color, form, and movement remain segregated, but in a way different from the one in the primary visual cortex[12].

Within the dorsal and ventral streams of information flow distinct representations of visual world (such as shape, color, motion, and spatial relationships) are separated from each other by means of segregated streams associated correspondingly with different functions such as recognition of separate objects, differentiation of spatial relations between objects, and defining how these objects can be approached and manipulated. For example, neurons in the ventral stream show response selectivity for stimulus attributes as shape, color, and texture. By contrast, neurons in the dorsal stream are not tuned for these attributes; rather, they show response selectivity for the speed and direction of stimulus motion, or to stimuli presented in the attended spatial location.

Recall that neurons in the dorsal stream are mainly associated with the magnocellular (M) system originated in the larger cells of the LGB. In recent studies it

[10]In theory, a visual area should be identified by combination of several criteria, including separate representation of visual world (topographical representation is one of them), specific anatomical connections, and specific (different from others) neuronal response properties, architectonics and behavioral deficits resulting from ablation. In practice, application of all these techniques is very difficult and as a result identification and localization of specific areas is not yet complete.

[11]These subdivisions may be visualized when the cortex is stained for the enzyme cytochrome oxidase. This enzyme plays an important role in cell metabolism. When stained, the images of the tangential sections of the primary visual cortex under microscope appeared like random blobs (Wong-Riley et al., 1993).

[12]When stained for the cytochrome oxidase BA 18 appears as a pattern of thick and thin stripes intermixed with pale zones.

[13]This study was done by Mathew Schmolesky et al. in 1998 using the same experimental and analytical techniques for all brain areas.

was shown that neurons in the dorsal stream respond with faster latencies[13] when compared with the ventral (associated with the parvocellular) stream. For example, in monkey latencies of responses in M-system at the thalamus constitute 30 ms on average, while latencies of the P-system are at least 20 ms longer. At the cortical level the differences between the corresponding areas in the dorsal and ventral streams become even larger reaching 40 ms.

D. Hierarchical Organization

Within the visual streams the processing of information is hierarchical (Fig. 10.1). For example, processing of the shape of the image begins with Gabor filtering in BA 17 while the cells the inferior temporal cortex respond selectively to global object features, such as specific shapes of hand, face ... Likewise, the average receptive field size increases along the pathway from the occipital lobe toward the temporal one[14]. Consequently, neurons in the primary visual cortex process local features of visual images, while regions in the inferior temporal cortex appear to deal with visual objects as a whole – a term known as Gestalt. Indeed, patients with right anterior temporal lobotomy are markedly impaired in recognition of complex visual patterns (such as faces and irregular abstract designs). To describe this syndrome the term psychic blindness was initially used. Later, Freud introduced the term agnosia. Visual agnosia denote the conditions of patients who, when faced with a visual object, were unable to name it, show its use, or sort it into a group of morphologically dissimilar objects with identical functions, but at the same time shows evidence of preserved vision in the usual test of central visual acuity and peripheral visual fields[15].

E. Computational Maps

Each hierarchical level of cortical organization represents an ordered map of a distinct feature of visual images. For example, single cortical cells in the primary visual cortex selectively respond to light bars at certain orientations[16]. Cells with these features were named line detectors. The line detectors are organized in an

[14]At parafoveal eccentricities, RFs of neurons are about 1.58 grades in BA 17, and about 48 in the area 37, whereas neurons in area 38 have a median receptive size of 26 × 268. It thus appears that large receptive fields in the higher levels of cortical hierarchy are built up from smaller receptive fields at the lower levels.

[15]The impairment is specific to the visual modality, and performances are normal when the patient touches the objects or hears its characteristic sound. Visual agnosia is divided in smaller categories such as motion and color agnosia depending on the location of lesion within the ventral stream.

[16]For these studies carried out in 1960s David Hubel and Torsten Wiesel from Johns Hopkins University were awarded the Nobel Prize.

ordered fashion: the parameter of orientation changes slowly along the cortex and has a regular pattern. This regularity has lead to the notion of repeated computational maps in the visual cortex. The computational map now is viewed as a key building block in the infrastructure of information processing in the brain. Further, maps of neurons tuned to movement direction and spatial frequencies were experimentally found in higher levels of visual information processing[17].

F. Schemata

Imagine a person having a cataract disease of the eye manifested in a clouding of the lens of the eye or of its surrounding transparent membrane that obstructs the passage of light into retina. Further, suppose that this patient has undergone an operation – the lens has been removed and a new artificial one has been installed. The signals from retina are now coming to the brain!!! But could he or she see the world as we do? The psychological observation shows that if the person has had this disease from early childhood the patient can not deal with the visual world properly and considers the operation as unsuccessful. This simple observation shows that perception needs some kind of a guide that directs the sensory information in a proper way. This "guide" seems to develop during maturation on the basis of genetically determined neuronal structure. We are actively learning to deal with objects in the external world step by step from early childhood. We explore the world by shifting our heads and eyes, manipulating with objects by our hands and fingers.

This idea of schemata as an organizing factor in visual perception was first expressed by Neisser. According to his view the schemata are anticipatory cognitive structures that prepare the perceiver to accept certain kinds of information rather than others. The schemata not only direct perceptual activity, but are modified during perception (Neisser, 1978). In recent literature the Neisser scheme is modified into notions of bottom–up and top–down processing while the concept of schemata is replaced by concepts of representations (memories) for objects and their spatial relationships.

G. Face Recognition

One of the most striking human abilities is processing face images. With a brief look at the face we can recognize whether a person is familiar or unknown to us, we can judge his/her emotional state, and in some cases we even can read the subject's mind from the face expression. In several laboratories attempts were made

---

[17]It was shown that a local cortical area of approximately $500\,mcm \times 500\,mcm$ includes all possible types of orientations and spatial frequencies. This structure was labeled "cortical module." In our study in order to describe the modular organization of the visual cortex mathematically we suggested a model of the canonical cortical module (see Methods of Part II).

to find so-called "grandmother" neurons, that is, neurons which are selectively responded to a certain face. Although, such cells were indeed found in the inferior temporal areas it is difficult to prove conclusively that the neurons encode information that is specifically related to a certain face. It is possible that these neurons are signaling information about either a broader class of complex objects or some simple pattern such as topography that is common to faces.

H. Multiple ERPs Components

In a recent study of John Foxe and Gregory Simpson from Department of Neuroscience at Albert Einstein College of Medicine high density event-related potentials (ERPs) were acquired from 128 scalp electrodes. Visual stimuli were bilateral red discs. They were presented on a computer monitor with duration of 280 ms. The surface Laplacian transformation was applied to the ERPs. This local transformation enabled the scientists to reveal an elaborated structure of a so-called C1 component, presumably originated within the striate cortex. The data obtained in the above mentioned study indicate that multiple visual generators are active in the latency range of the traditional C1 component of the ERP with the dorsal generators associated with shorter latencies than the ventral generators. The other striking result was an observation that the dorso-lateral frontal cortex is involved in visual processing as fast as 80 ms after stimulus onset. Given that the occipital cortex was activated at 56 ms it means that the widespread system of sensory, parietal, and prefrontal areas is activated in less than 30 ms, which is considerably shorter than typically assumed in the human ERP literature.

I. Cortical Topography

Cortical topography is one of the fundamental organizing principles of the brain[18]. Topographical representations are present not only at lower hierarchical levels of information flow but can be also found at higher levels. Within the high levels of the visual cortex different object categories activate areas with specific eccentricity biases. In particular, faces, letters, and words appear to be associated with central visual-fields, whereas images of buildings are associated with peripheral ones. For

---

[18]Clinical evidence supports the topographical organization of striate and prestriate cortex. Patients with small lesions (caused by small strokes or tumors) are not able to see objects located in the corresponding part of the visual scene. This kind of brain dysfunction is called visual cortical (to emphasize the involvement the cortex in conscious visual perception) blindness and visual deficits are named *scotoma*. It is amazing that all of us have this kind of defect. It is induced by a so-called blind spot of the normal retina – a small (about 2 mm) area in the retina without retinal receptors where the optic nerve leaves the eye. Since the disc is medial to the fovea in both eyes, light coming from a single point in the binocular zone never enters both optic discs, so we are normally unaware of this blind spot.

example, in a recent functional magnetic resonance imaging (fMRI) study it was explicitly shown that faces activate cortical areas superimposed on areas associated with fovea topographical representations while objects such as buildings whose recognition entails large-scale integration activate representations of peripheral fields (for review see Malach et al., 2002).

J. Enhancement of N170 ERPs Component in Response to Faces

In line with the fMRI experiments are ERPs recordings. Roxane Itier from The Rotman Research Institute in Toronto and Margot Taylor from Paul Sabatier University in Toulouse, France recorded ERPs in response to brief presentation of different categories of pictures such as faces, houses, textures, etc. Their data show that the N170 component of ERPs was significantly higher in amplitude for human faces, both upright and inverted (Fig. 10.4).

Although the authors did not perform low resolution electromagnetic tomography (LORETA) analysis of the obtained data, the dynamics of 2D maps of ERPs show that the distribution of the N170 component is spatially different from the distribution of ERPs to other stimulus categories. Their data also indicate one of advantages of ERPs in comparison to other imaging methods. The advantage is expressed in superior temporal resolution of ERPs. Indeed, ERPs can index brain operations with a time resolution of few milliseconds while positron emission tomography (PET) and functional magnetic resonance imaging (fMRI) are limited by a few seconds time scale. This distinctive feature of ERPs enables scientists to study stages of information processing in the human brain.

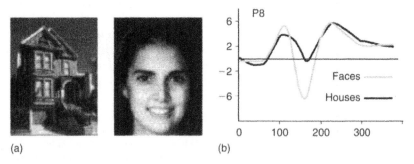

FIGURE 10.4   ERPs to different categories of visual stimuli. (a) Examples of stimuli from the nine categories used in the experiment. (b) Grand-average ERPs displayed between 0 and 400 ms for the two categories of stimuli at a parietal (P8) site. Note larger P1 and N170 components for faces compared to all other categories. Adapted from Itier and Taylor (2004).

III. DECOMPOSITION OF SINGLE TRIAL EVOKED POTENTIALS INTO INDEPENDENT COMPONENTS

In the same way as the background electroencephalogram (EEG) is composed of several rhythmic components, evoked potentials represent sums of several components generated by different cortical areas at different time intervals. This statement is illustrated in Fig. 10.5. ERPs have been computed in a single healthy subject of 26 year old in response to visual stimuli of the same category and to combinations of visual stimuli of the other category with auditory stimulation. The visual stimuli are short (100 ms) presentations of images of different plants or people while auditory stimuli are random temporal sequences of 20 ms tones of different frequencies. Because the tones in different trials are sequentially presented in different combinations, the auditory stimuli sound quite new every time they are presented. The subject is supposed just to view and hear stimuli without any particular response to them.

As one can see from the evoked potentials averaged over trials in Fig. 10.5a, the visual stimuli presented alone elicit a widely distributed fluctuation of potential which at 160 ms after stimulus has a negative value at the occipital regions. The visual stimuli presented simultaneously with "novel" auditory stimuli in addition to the occipital negative fluctuation elicit a positive fluctuation at 120 ms at the left temporal area and a widely centrally–frontally distributed fluctuation with maximum of positivity at Cz at latency of 200 ms. Consequently, one can hypothesize that ERPs to the visual + auditory stimuli consist of at least three different components differently distributed over the frontal–temporal–occipital areas and reaching extremes at different time intervals.

Say in order to prove this hypothesis we need to use the information regarding raw EEG from each trial. To be able to do it we need to know how potentials at different electrodes correlate with each other. Indeed, we presume that the potentials of electrodes that peak up activity from generators of the one component correlate with each other much stronger than electrodes potentials belonging to two different generators. This information is reflected in a so-called covariance matrix. During many years scientists tried to solve the problem of separation components from the covariance matrix. One way of solving the problem, a so-called principle component analysis (PCA), was suggested as early as in 1960s. From a mathematical point of view the method is a technique used to reduce multidimensional data sets (in our case 19-channel EEG) to lower dimensions (in our case three or more components). Unfortunately, the PCA produces orthogonal components while the physiologically meaningfull components are not necessarily orthogonal[19]. For this reason, the PCA obtained a limited application for analysis of biological data in general and EEG/ERP data in particular.

[19]In 1980s in our laboratory we developed the PCA method for analysis of neuronal reactions in the brain of patients with implanted multiple electrodes. The discharge rate of single- and multi-units

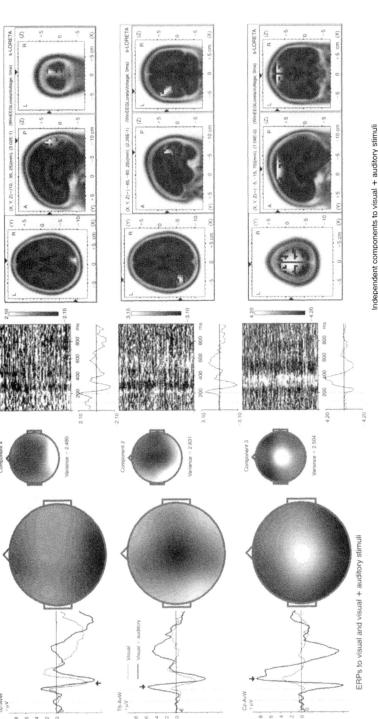

(a)

(b)

Independent components to visual + auditory stimuli

FIGURE 10.5 Decomposition of single trial EEG responses into independent components. 19-channel EEG was recorded in a healthy 26 year old subject performing the two stimulus GO/NOGO task. 50 per cent of trials were irrelevant (requiring no response of the subject) and composed of sequential presentation of two stimuli "plant–plant" and "plant–human + acoustic novel stimulus." ERPs in response to the second stimulus averaged over the "plant–human + acoustic stimulus" trials together with the maps of averaged potential taken at different times are presented at (a). The results of application of the ICA to single trials EEG in response to simultaneous presentation of visual and acoustic stimuli are presented at (b). Topographies, single trial dynamics, and s-LORETA images are presented at (b). Note that components are generated in different cortical locations and reveal different dynamics.

A few years ago a new method called the independent component analysis (ICA) appeared. The method was based on assumption that the sources of components are statistically independent (not necessarily orthogonal as in the PCA analysis). This assumption seems to fit the nature of generators producing different components in ERPs. Indeed, the information flow in the brain induced by stimulus presentation sequentially activates different cortical hierarchically organized areas so that the generators of different components are activated in different time intervals and at different cortical locations.

The results of application of the ICA to single trial multi-channel evoked responses are presented in Fig. 10.5b. Note that single trial responses are decomposed into three components with different localization of generators and different latencies.

Note that single trial ERPs components look quite noisy. Indeed the maximal amplitudes of averaged evoked potentials varied from 6 to 8 μV while the maximal amplitudes of raw EEG varied around 10 μV. These parameters are associated with the signal to noise ratio about 1. At the same time, averaging EEG over 100 trials increases the signal to noise ratio 10 times. So, it looks like that working with averaged ERPs we might get better results. However in this case we need to have not a single subject but quite many subjects (more than 100–200 depending on conditions).

IV. DECOMPOSITION OF AVERAGED ERPS INTO SINGLE COMPONENTS

ICA can be applied to a set of individual averaged ERPs. In this case the extracted components will reflect generators that are common for the selected group of subjects. Below we are going to illustrate this particular approach. Individual ERPs are taken from almost 1000 healthy subjects of the Human Brain Normative Database[20].

In the case of ERPs data the goal of ICA is to utilize the differences in scalp distribution between generators of ERPs common for the whole population of healthy subjects to separate their activation time courses. We suggest that different stages of information flow are associated with activities in distinct cortical areas and

---

recorded from different electrodes in response to repeated trails was computed, the covariance matrix and eigen-vectors were assessed. Strong changes in component weights in response to stimuli were observed, but interpretation of these changes was so ambiguous that after few years of trying to find any physiological sense in these reactions we stop using the PCA method.

[20]In Part I we presented basics of ICA analysis. It was described in association with finding independent generators of background EEG rhythms in raw EEG. The method was applied to the individual raw data and to a set of individual spectra. In the first approach we were able to separate individual sources while in the second approach we separated general sources common for all healthy subjects. Theoretically, the same procedures can be made with ERPs recorded in response to stimuli or movements.

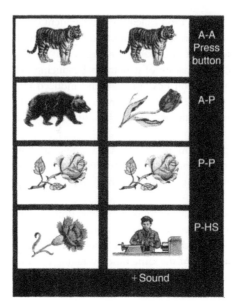

FIGURE 10.6   Stimuli for the two stimulus GO/NOGO task. See text for description.

with different (and to some extent independent) time patterns. Recall, that components are constructed by optimizing the mutual independence of all activation time curves. In more detail, ICA decomposition for ERP analysis is based on the three general assumptions: (1) generators located in different cortical areas produce potentials that are linearly summed at the recorded scalp electrodes, (2) ERPs represent the sum of activations in a specific set of spatially stable brain networks, and, (3) the time courses of activation in different subjects are temporally independent[21] (see Methods of Part II for details).

As an example, we are going to use the two stimulus GO/NOGO task developed specifically for the Human Brain Institute Database. The task consisted of 400 trials presenting to a subject every 3s (Fig. 10.6). In the task we selected four categories of stimuli: (1) 20 different images of animals – referred to later as A, (2) 20 different images of plants – P, (3) 20 different images of humans presented together with an artificial novel sound – HS[22]. Trials consisted of presentation of a par of stimuli with interstimulus interval of 1.1 s. Four categories of trials were selected: A-A, A-P, P-P, and P-HS. The trials were grouped into four sessions with

[21]The assumptions 2 and 3 are based on numerous experimental finding in animals indicating the activations of neurons in different brain areas are associated with different stages of information flow. These stages are characterized by stimulus properties encoded and by temporal pattern of activation.

[22]The randomly varying novel sounds consisted of five 20 ms fragments filled with tones of different frequencies (500, 1000, 1500, 2000, and 2500 Hz). Stimulus intensity was about 75 dB SPL at the patient's head.

100 trials each. In each session a unique set of five A stimuli, five P, and five HS stimuli was selected. Each session consisted of a pseudo-random presentation of 100 pairs of stimuli with equal probability for each category and each stimulus.

ICA decomposition was performed as described in (Makage et al., 1997) after re-referencing to common average reference. In Fig. 10.7 we present the results of ICA analysis of the whole set of ERPs computed for a group of healthy subjects from 7 to 89 years old. Only ERPs to the second stimulus in P-P pairs have been subjected for analysis. We will refer to this condition as "Irrelevant" condition. As you can see, in response to irrelevant visual stimuli (i.e., stimuli not changing behavior) the following main independent components are separated (Fig. 10.7).

The first component is generated in occipital–parietal areas. The time dynamic of this component dramatically depends on age. At age from 7 to 13 years the first fluctuation in this component is of positive value with latency of 116 ms. After age of 13 the positive initial fluctuation turns into a negative fluctuation[23].

The second component has a peak latency of 132 ms. It is amazing that in contrast to the early part of the first component, the early positive fluctuation of the second component is not changed significantly with age. The component is independently generated at the occipital–temporal areas of the left and right hemispheres.

The third component starts later than the previous components. The early part of this component represents a positive fluctuation with a peak latency of 148 ms. The first positive fluctuation is followed by a sequence of negative/positive waves.

We can speculate that the first and third components represent sequential stages of information flow in the dorsal (Where) stream, while the second component is associated with information flow in the ventral (What) stream.

A. ERP Component as a Sequence of Excitatory–Inhibitory Events (Model)

The time dynamics of the components presented in Fig. 10.8 explicitly shows that neuronal responses in a distinct cortical area are reflected in several phases of

[23]We do not know why electrophysiological correlates of visual processing differ between children and adults so dramatically. However we know from MRI studies that the brain anatomy undergoes quite large changes during adolescence (Lenroot and Giedd, 2006). This issue needs a further correlational research.

[24]The first component is generated in the occipital cortex. The component exhibits three temporal phases: (1) a very small and short positive phase with peak latency at 116 ms, (2) a strong negativity at about 150 ms for adults and a strong positivity for children (age 7–12 years old) at the same latency, and (3) a strong positive phase at 260 ms. The second two components are generated in areas of the ventral pathway (near the middle temporal gyrus) at the left and right hemisphere correspondingly. The components exhibit three phases: (1) a positive fluctuation with peak latency of 130 ms, (2) a negative fluctuation at 184 ms, and (3) a small positivity at 260 ms for adults and at about 360 ms for children (age 7–12 years old). The fourth component is generated in the parietal areas of the dorsal visual pathway. It consists of two positive fluctuations with peak latencies at 148 and 330 m, separated by a negative phase with peak latency of 220 ms.

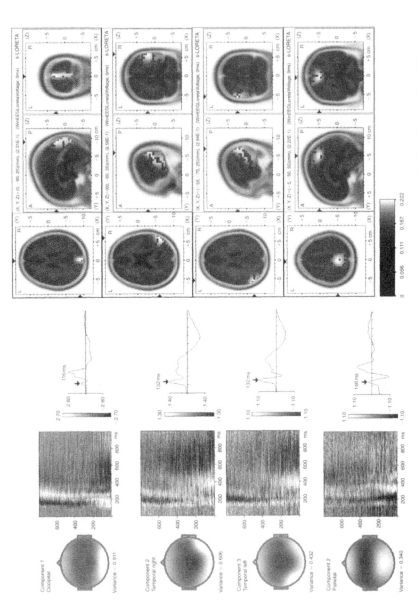

FIGURE 10.7 Independent components for "Irrelevant" visual stimuli in the two stimulus GO/NOGO task. From left to right – (1) topography of components with numbers below corresponding to the variance of the component, (2) vertically stacking thin color-coded horizontal bars, each representing the corresponding component for a single subject, almost 800 healthy subjects of age from 7 (bottom) to 89 (top) are depicted, (3) time courses of components with arrows and numbers corresponding to latency of the first positive peak, (4) s–LORETA images of cortical generators of components. Scales are presented near corresponding pictures.

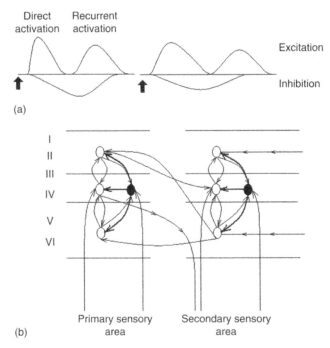

Direct   Recurrent
activation   activation

Excitation

Inhibition

(a)

I

II

III

IV

V

VI

Primary sensory   Secondary sensory
(b)   area   area

FIGURE 10.8   Sequence of events in primary and secondary cortical areas (scheme). (a) Positive and negative potentials associated with excitatory and inhibitory postsynaptic potentials. (b) Neuronal networks of primary (left) and secondary (right) cortical areas. Empty circles – excitatory neurons, black circles – inhibitory neurons. See explanation in text.

positive and negative fluctuations of the scalp recorded potential[24]. With a certain caution, these positive and negative fluctuations may be associated with periods of excitation and inhibition of neurons in the corresponding neuronal networks. This inference regarding phases of excitation and inhibition fits quite well observations in animals with recordings of impulse activity of neurons. In animal studies the first phase of activation of single neurons was often followed by a phase of inhibition exhibited in the absence of spiking. These excitation and inhibition phases were usually followed by a second activation.

In more detail, mechanisms behind successive phases of excitation/activation phases might be as follows. Let us first consider activity in the primary cortical area 17. The excitatory neurons in the primary visual cortex receive excitation from the relay nucleus (LGB) of the thalamus. Via local excitatory interconnections this initial activation spreads over the local neuronal network. The spread of activation excite the local short axon intracortical neurons. Because of short time constants of excitatory postsynaptic potentials the phase of excitation is very fast. When inhibitory neurons become activated they inhibit nearby neurons and because of the slower time constants of inhibition, the phase of inhibition lasts longer that the one of excitation[25]. The phase of the second activation might be associated with either a local rebound effects following inhibitory phase[26] or with a recurrent activation coming back via feedback connections in cortical networks. Figure 10.8 illustrates the second option. In any case, the consecutive stages of information flow in a distinct cortical area as revealed in scalp recorded ERPs indicate that information is processed twice (or may be more) in order to extract the needed content of the sensory input.

V. AUDITORY INFORMATION FLOW

A. "What" and "Where" Streams

The cortical part of primate auditory system is organized into a "core" of primary auditory cortical areas[27] that project to a surrounding "belt," with the belt projecting to "parabelt" areas. Each of these regions – core, belt, and parabelt – has a distinctive histological composition, specific thalamo-cortical and cortico-cortical connections, and unique physiological and functional characteristics.

The concept of multiple, parallel processing streams similar to those in the visual modality has been recently established for the auditory modality (Fig. 10.9). Electrophysiological studies in primates and fMRI studies in humans indicate a functional dissociation between anterior and posterior streams. A "What" stream associated with vocalizations (presumably subserving auditory object identification) involves the anterior belt and parabelt, that are further projected to anterior temporal and ventro-lateral frontal (not shown) regions. A "Where" stream for sound localization involves the posterior belt and parabelt, and posterior temporal and dorso-lateral frontal (not shown) regions. Posterior auditory regions have been shown to respond to spatial auditory cues in similar way as parietal neurons respond to visual spatial cues supporting the existence of posterior temporal–parietal stream in the processing of auditory spatial information. Zatorre and coauthors (Zatorre et al., 2002) suggest that this "dorsal" route of processing might subserve perception of spectral dynamics of sound reflecting its fast changes in time[28].

---

[25]It looks like that in case of young (below age of 13 small) healthy children, the excitation exceeds inhibition and we do not see a negative phase in ERP components. With maturation the first excitation is gradually decreased and inhibition starts exhibiting in the negative fluctuation of the scalp potential.

[26]The mechanism of such rebound effect may be similar to those discovered for cortico-thalamic neurons, that is, associated with calcium spikes.

[27]In humans, the "core" or primary auditory cortex is located in the first transverse gyrus of Heschl (BA 41). It receives thalamic input for the MGB of the thalamus.

[28]The property to respond to fast changes in spectral power is important for localizing and orienting to the sound.

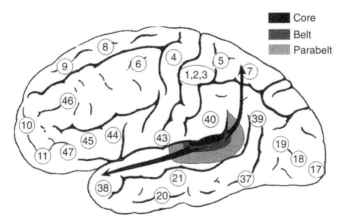

FIGURE 10.9   "What" and "Where" streams in auditory cortical system. Core, belt, and parabelt auditory areas are depicted in different colors. Arrows indicate "What" (anterior) and "Where" posterior streams of auditory information.

B. Cortical Tonotopy

Tonotopy (ordered maps of sound frequency selectiveness) is present at all stages of auditory processing. It is noticeably found in the core regions that respond to pure tones. Further, projections of belt and parabelt areas beyond the auditory region are also topographically organized. And finally, belt and/or parabelt (but not core) areas project to the caudate and putamen (part of the basal ganglia) in a topographic fashion.

C. Speech Processing

Activation specific to intelligible speech is observed in the left anterior superior temporal sulcus. This region is multimodal, receiving projections from auditory, visual, and somato-sensory cortex in primates, and may be important in representing the meaning content of utterances. In humans, support for the role of this part of the cortex in extracting semantic information[29] comes from patients with semantic dementia, who having grey matter loss in the left anterior temporal lobe exhibit a progressive deterioration in the comprehension of single words. In its turn, the temporoparietal junction, which forms the interface between auditory cortex and parietal and frontal systems, is anatomically heterogenous. A recent

[29]In this context semantic means accessing word meanings.

study in humans indicates at least four distinguishable areas on the anterior planum temporal alone.

Early babbling and word production require neuronal activity in cortical areas controlling face and articulator movements and actions. These areas are located in the inferior motor cortex and adjacent inferior prefrontal areas. The articulations cause sounds that activate neurons in the auditory system, including areas in the superior temporal lobe. Strong fiber bundles between inferior frontal and superior temporal areas provide the substrate for associative learning between neurons controlling specific speech motor programs and neurons in the auditory cortical system stimulated by the self-produced language sounds.

D. ICA of ERPs (HBI Database)

The method of decomposition of a set of many individual ERPs into independent components described for visual processing above enables us to separate different stages of auditory information flow. As an example, we are going to use the Auditory task developed specifically for the Human Brain Institute Database. The task consisted of random presentation of tones with different frequencies but with the same duration of 100 ms. Occasionally the duration of a stimulus became longer (400 ms instead of 100 ms). The subject's task was to press a button to longer stimuli. ERPs to short auditory stimuli were computed for each subject and were further analyzed by means of ICA. In Fig. 10.10 we present the results of ICA of the whole set of ERPs computed for short (Irrelevant) auditory stimuli for a group of healthy adult subjects of age from 7 to 89 years.

As one can see, two symmetrical components are generated in the temporal areas correspondingly at the left and right hemispheres in vicinity of the primary auditory areas. The peak latency of the right temporal component is 84 ms[30]. These temporal components are multi-phasic in a way similar to that found in the visual-related occipital component. The third component was generated in the posterior gyrus cingulus, while the fourth component – in the parietal area. Note that the third and the fourth components exhibit just opposite changes with age: the posterior cingulate component is getting stronger with age while the parietal component decreases in amplitude with age.

One can speculate that the two components generated in the temporal lobes in auditory ERPs correspond to the ventral (What) stream in auditory modality, while two other components are associated with the dorsal (Where) stream of auditory information flow.

---

[30]Note that the first early component in the visual modality peaks at 116 ms almost 30 ms later the early auditory component. This fact reflect difference in reactivity of thalamic nuclei in visual and auditory modality as well as difference in complexity of information processing in the two modalities.

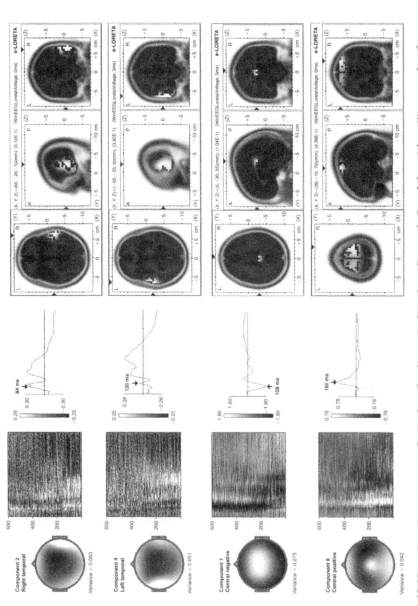

FIGURE 10.10 Independent components for "irrelevant" auditory stimuli in the auditory task. From left to right – (1) topography of components with numbers below corresponding to the variance of the component, (2) vertically stacking thin color-coded horizontal bars, each representing the corresponding component for a single subject, around 600 healthy subjects of age from 7 (bottom) to 89 (top) are depicted, (3) time courses of components with arrows and numbers corresponding to latency of the first positive peak, (4) s-LORETA images of cortical generators of components. Scales are presented near corresponding pictures.

VI. SOMATO-SENSORY MODALITY

Our bodies are covered with sensory receptors that give us feelings of pain, visceral function, and touch. These receptors are located on the surface and deeper layers of the skin as well as they are embedded within muscles, tendons, and joints. Somato-sensory receptors can be classified into three groups: nocio receptors, carrying information about pain and temperature, hapsis receptors, carrying information about fine touch and pressure, and proprio receptors carrying information about position of the body and its parts. In addition to the receptors telling us about external surfaces of our bodies there are receptors conveying information about the internal (visceral) parts of our organisms[31].

A. Somato-Sensory and Insular Cortical Areas

External somato-sensory receptors are projected to the somato-sensory cortex (Brodmann's areas 1, 2, and 3) through the ventro-posterior nucleus of the thalamus, while internal visceral receptors are projected to the insular cortex through the ventro-medial nucleus. The insular cortex is located deep within the brain and we know little about oscillations that are generated in this cortical area. The somato-sensory cortex lies at the outer surface of the cortex just under the central electrodes C3, C4, Cz. This cortex is known to generate mu-rhythms (see Chapter 2).

VII. CHANGE DETECTION

A. Functions of Change Detection

In real life, the sensory world is reflected in continuous activity of neurons of the sensory systems. Some part of the world remains constant for a relatively long time and we often are not aware of this unchanging world[32]. But if a change occurs, such as somebody touches the sleeve of our dress, or the engine of the car changes its regularity, or a mushroom appears within our gaze, this change might enter our consciousness. It seems the brain is constantly monitoring the sensory

---

[31]In somato-sensory modality there is a sub-modality called the sense of flutter. Flutter is felt when we touch a vibrating object. The frequencies of mechanical vibration we can feel vary from 5 to 50 Hz. The flutter is mediated by rapidly adapting cutaneous mechanoreceptors. The modality is similarly organized in monkeys and humans.

[32]Recall, that we do not feel the pressure of the clothing on our body, we are not aware of a gentle noise of the car we are driving in, and we do not see minor changes in the visual scene when we are in the forest and occupied by our thoughts.

world and is comparing incoming stimuli with a sensory model formed by a previous stimulation. In a similar way the brain is monitoring actions in order to correct behavior if a real action does not fit a planned action. In this book, these basic operations will be referred to as comparison operations. Historically, in sensory systems comparison operations are named change detection.

Two types of comparison operations are associated with two models of the world that are built up in our brain: a sensory model and a model of actions. These models are stored in different parts of the brain, named sensory systems and executive system. Although the systems are heavily interconnected, each of them has a distinct neuronal circuitry, distinct mechanisms of information processing and serves different functions. Consequently, in the human behavior detecting changes in the world serves two different purposes.

First, a change in the sensory world shifts attention either voluntarily (attention dependent) or involuntarily (automatic). For example, a sudden change in the humming of the car engine can be assessed by the driver when he pays attention to a road or when he attentively listens to the engine. In this case a *sensory* model is constructed in the sensory system and a change in the current stimulus not matching the model activates the corresponding part of the sensory system. The sensory model is formed on the basis of previous experience with the sensory world. So, the purpose of this type of change detection is confined by the sensory system itself – selecting the source of a change in sensory information with a purpose of more detail processing[33].

Second, a change can indicate that the actions which are prepared in a given situation are not valid any more and, consequently, have to be suppressed or changed. Imagine a subject who is ready to cross a street to a green light but is stopped by a sudden change of the light into red. In this case, an *action* model – to cross the street – is constructed within the executive system. A change in the current behavioral situation means that a prepared action is not appropriate and must be suppressed. So, the purpose of this type of change detection is to inhibit the executive system in order to suppress the prepared action.

B. Mechanisms of Change Detection (Model)

The mechanisms of sensory-related change detection have been most extensively studied in auditory modality. So, we start with this modality. The leading role in this research belongs to the Cognitive Brain Research Unit at University of Helsinki founded by Professor Risto Näätänen in 1980s. Näätänen was one of the

---

[33]The change can be further detected by executive system and navigate the body or the eyes (overtly or covertly) toward the selected source of sensory information, but the change can be also remained without any notice from the executive system.

first who suggested existence of two mechanisms of change detection in the auditory modality[34].

The first mechanism is reflected in the early component of ERPs and is associated with the information flow in the primary and probably secondary auditory cortical areas (Fig. 10.11a). Risto Näätänen associated the first mechanism with N1 component of auditory ERPs. The existence of two types of neurons (stable and refractory neurons) in these areas is hypothesized. The stable neurons do not change the response to the stimulus with repetition. The refractory neurons decrease their response while the same stimulus is repeated several times. The phenomenon of decreasing responses to repeated stimulus is called refractoriness. Although synaptic depression[35] seems to be the main cellular mechanism of decrease of neuronal response to repetitive stimulus, complex interactions between neurons also play some (albeit still undetermined) role in this phenomenon.

In addition to these two types of neurons the existence of a separate mechanism, called change detection, is hypothesized. The hypothetical neurons associated with this mechanism respond only to the change of the stimulus. Having

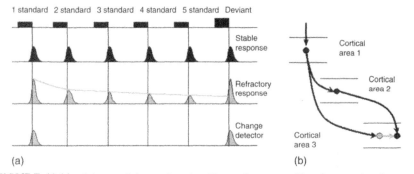

FIGURE 10.11   Scheme of change detection. Neuronal responses (a) and connections between neurons (b) in three hypothetical cortical areas. At the right, black color – excitatory neurons and excitatory connections, gray color – inhibitory neurons and inhibitory connections. The model postulates that comparison operations are preformed in neuronal networks consisting of three cortical areas. The first (rigid) area receives inputs directly from the thalamus. The responses of this area to the repeated stimulus are stable. This area is projected to excitatory neurons of the second (plastic) area and to inhibitory neurons of the third (change detectors) area. The second area in its turn is projected to neurons in the third area that receive inhibitory inputs for the local inhibitory neurons. Thus error detectors compare (that is, compute the difference) two inputs – a rigid one and a plastic one. If the stimulus is new, excitation exceeds inhibition and the neuron fires. If the stimulus is a repeated one, inhibition exceeds excitation the neurons remains silent.

[34]This hypothesis is presented in his book "Attention and Brain function" published by Lawrence Erlbaum Associates in 1992. This is clear written review of all available in that time literature and deserves reading even now after 15 years.

[35]At synaptic level depression is associated with decrease of postsynaptic potential in response to repeated stimulus.

in mind the non-linearity of neurons[36] it is easy to suggest a neuronal network for change detectors (see Fig. 10.11b). The model suggests that the association cortical area (cortical area 3 in Fig. 10.11) receives two inputs: the one from the primary cortical area that depends only on physical characteristics of the input and does not habituate with repetition of the stimulus and the other one from the secondary cortical area that decreases with the stimulus repetition. Neurons in the association area compare these two inputs by means of lateral inhibition so that some neurons in this area fire only when a new stimulus is presented.[37]

Auditory stimuli possess not only physical properties (such as frequency and intensity) but also an integrated property which could be named regularity. For example, in the auditory modality regularity is present in many auditory signals of our daily life, such as hammering of the engine in the car, steady noise of computer ventilator, monotonous speech of a lecturer … As we know from neuroscience, distinct properties of stimuli are assessed by neuronal elements located in distinct areas of the sensory systems. Regularity as a separate feature seems to be assessed in a separate location in the auditory cortex. Moreover, this feature is probably extracted by a specific mechanism. Indeed, in contrast to physical features of the stimuli regularity is formed on the basis of integration over quite long (for tens of second) periods of time. Mechanisms of such integration are still unknown. However electrophysiological correlates of brain response to regularity change are very well studied during the last 30 years. In auditory modality such electrophysiological index is coined as mismatch negativity (MMN).

C. MMN in Oddball Paradigm

The MMN is an electric response to a discriminable change in regularity of auditory stimulation. This response usually peaks at 150–200 ms from change onset and is elicited even in the absence of attention. The MMN has been first observed in the auditory modality and its presence in the visual modality is still debated[38].

---

[36]In this case the non-linearity means that the excitatory neurons at the cortical area 3 fire only if the excitatory inputs to these neurons exceed the inhibitory inputs by a threshold of firing.

[37]It should be noted here that the scheme we presented here is only one of the many possible. The real neuronal networks for change detection are not fully understood.

[38]The reason for that lies in the nature of the comparison operation. It is based on comparison with a memory trace. This trace is formed by reverberation processes and synaptic depression/ potentiation processes in the sensory short-term memory. In the auditory modality the duration of echoic memory is quite long – up to 10s, while the duration of iconic memory is very short – less than few hundreds of milliseconds. So, the property of regulatory is formed during the conventional auditory oddball paradigm but can not be formed in a visual variant of the oddball paradigm. It should be stressed here that the MMN disappears when interstimulus interval becomes longer than 10s which is in agreement with the estimated duration of the auditory sensory memory.

The behavioral paradigm for studying the MMN in auditory modality is an odd-ball paradigm. In its simple form, the oddball task consists of repetitive sequence of an auditory stimulus – standard (e.g., 1000 Hz tones of 100 ms duration) which is rarely interrupted by a deviant auditory stimulus (e.g., 1100 Hz tones of 100 ms duration)[39]. For more details see Methods of the Part II.

The MMN was discovered in 1978 in a classic work by Näätänen, Gaillard, and Mantysalo. A commonly accepted interpretation of the MMN is that it is generated by an automatic change-detection process in which a disconcordance (a mismatch) is found between the deviant stimulus and the memory representation (the trace) of the preceding repetitive auditory standard stimuli[40]. Grand-average ERPs in the oddball paradigm for a group of healthy subjects of age from 15 to 89 years are presented in Fig. 10.12a. Note that the deviant stimuli in comparison to the standard tones generate an enhanced negative potential distributed over frontal–central areas.

Using the ICA method, the ERPs are decomposed into three independent components presented at Fig. 10.12b. The first of the components is generated near the primary auditory cortical area with peak latency of 116 ms. The component is practically the same for standard and deviant stimuli. The second component generated over the association auditory cortical areas, has a latency of 132 ms and twice larger for deviant stimuli in comparison to the component generated by the standard stimuli. And finally, the third component is generated near the anterior cingulate cortex. At latency of 236 ms the component for deviant stimuli is associated with an additional positive fluctuation that is absent in response to standard stimuli.

D. Intracranial Correlates of MMN

In a joint study of our laboratory with a Finnish group headed by Risto Näätänen (Kropotov et al., 2000) we showed the existence of at least three separate neuronal mechanisms that form the basis of MMN generation. They are presented in Fig. 10.13 as local field potentials recorded from intracranial electrodes implanted in Brodmann areas 41, 42, and 22 of the temporal cortex. As one can see, responses in the primary auditory area (BA 41) are stable. They do not habituate with repetition and appear to encode physical properties (such as a tone frequency) of the auditory stimulus. Responses in the secondary auditory area (BA 42) strongly habituate,

---

[39]To avoid the effect of refractoriness in the generation of the MMN the difference between the standard and deviant stimuli are usually chosen as small as possible.

[40]For a review see a book of Risto Näätänen (1992). Attention and brain function, Erlbaum, Hillsdale, NJ.

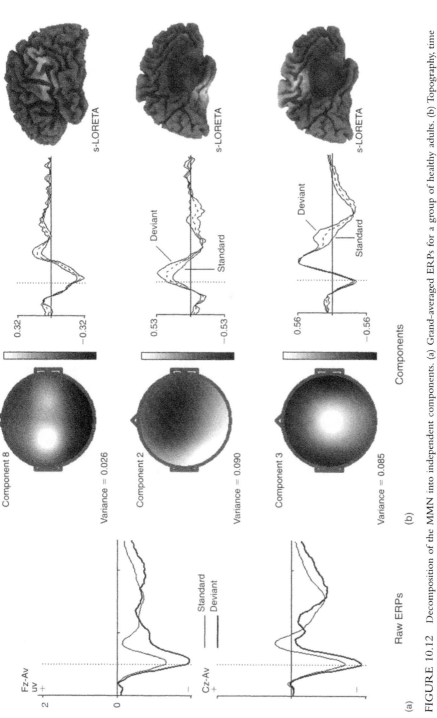

FIGURE 10.12 Decomposition of the MMN into independent components. (a) Grand-averaged ERPs for a group of healthy adults. (b) Topography, time course, and s-LORETA image of three independent components that compose ERPs. At (b) dotted line – the ICA component for both stimuli while continuous lines correspond to deviant and standard stimuli separately.

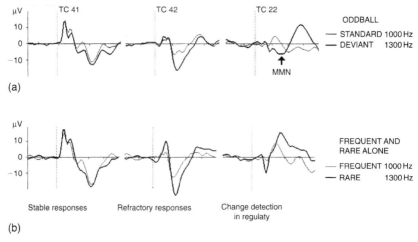

FIGURE 10.13   Three mechanisms of comparison operation (intracranial recordings in auditory modality). Intracranial local field potentials were recorded in epileptic patients with electrodes implanted for diagnosis and therapy into different areas of the temporal lobe (Brodmann's areas 41, 42, and 22 labeled as TC 41, TC 42 and TC 22). During recordings patients read a book while were presented with sequences of tones. In the oddball paradigm (a) standard tones of 1000 Hz were interspersed with deviant tones of 1300 Hz. In two other recordings (frequent and rare alone – a) standard and deviant stimuli were presented alone corresponding to short and long interstimulus intervals. Thin lines – ERPs to standard (a) and frequent (b) stimuli. Thick lines – ERPs to deviant (a) and rare (b) stimuli. Adapted from Kropotov et al. (2000).

that is, decrease with consecutive repetition of the same stimulus. We suggest that synaptic depression in this area might be responsible for the habituation. Operation of comparison of the input stimulus with the memory trace of repetitive signal appears to be carried in the association area 22. If the stimulus does not match the memory trace developed by the previous repetitive stimulation, this area generates a strong negative component followed by a positive component[41]. It should be noted here that the temporal lobe seems to be not the only place that contributes to generation of scalp recorded MMN. Besides the temporal lobe, a different source located in the prefrontal cortex has been identified[42].

[41]Note that this component is present in the oddball paradigm but is absent when rare and frequent auditory tones are presented alone.

[42]The activation of the prefrontal generator follows the activation of the temporal generator with a short time delay. The prefrontal generator appears to play a critical role in the initiation of an involuntary attention switch to sound change detected in the temporal lobe. It was further proposed that change-detection process occurs pre-perceptually in the auditory cortices (generating the temporal subcomponent of the MMN), which in turn triggers frontal-cortex processes (generating the frontal MMN subcomponent and the subsequent P3a component) underlying the possible attention switch to and conscious perception of stimulus change.

E. Change Detection in Two Stimulus Discrimination Tasks

It should be noted that the MMN represents a special case of a more general operation. This special case is associated with change in "regularity" of the auditory stimulation. However, regularity as a characteristic of sensory stimulation is the most prominent only in the auditory modality[43].

A more general operation is associated with comparison of any characteristic of the sensory stimulus with the previous memory trace. We call this operation as "change detection." If our task is not to study detection of a sudden change in the regularity of stimulation, we do not need to repeat the previous stimulus many times. Consequently, in general terms the change detection can be experimentally studied in different than the oddball tasks. For example, we designed a two stimulus discrimination task in order to measure change detection in different features of visual stimuli. In this task stimuli are presented in pairs in which the second stimulus match or mismatch the first one with the task to respond differently for two categories of trails.

In monkey studies (for review see Romo and Salinas, 2003), the research was focused on flatter discrimination task and included recording of impulse activity of neurons located in somato-sensory areas S1 and S2, ventral prefrontal, and medial premotor cortical areas. In these experiments a mechanical stimulator was placed on the fingertip of one digit of the monkey hand and produced short lasting mechanical oscillations. Each trial consisted of presentation of two vibrations with different frequencies f1 and f2 separated by a time delay. The monkey's task was to press one or another button depending on whether f2 was higher or lower than f1. The sequence of psychological operations in this task is as follows: (1) encoding the first stimulus frequency f1, (2) maintaining it in the sensory memory, (3) encoding the second stimulus frequency f2, (4) comparing it with the trace in the memory, (5) transferring the results of the comparison operation to motor neurons.

The results of the study show that neurons in the secondary (but not in primary) somato-sensory area perform a comparison operation. They "compute" the difference between of two vibrations (f1–f2). This difference is reflected in the discharge rate of these neurons in response to second stimulus in the pair of stimuli[44]. It takes about 200 ms for the comparison operation to develop. No evidence of such computation is observed in the primary sensory area S1, where neurons simply respond as a function of the vibration frequency of the stimulus.

---

[43]This seems to be the reason why the existence of the MMN in the visual modality is hotly debated.

[44]In the case of flatter sense the frequency of mechanical vibration is encoded by the spike rate of neurons in S1 area: the higher the frequency of mechanical vibration, the higher is neuronal activity. This type of encoding seems to be a simple frequency representation.

F. Modality Specificity

In our laboratory we studied comparison operations since early 1990s. We developed a so-called two stimulus paradigm in which stimuli were presented in pairs and the subject's task was to compare two stimuli and to make different response depending on whether the second stimulus matched the first one in the pair. The tasks we were using in the auditory and visual modalities were as follows. Stimuli were high (H) and low (L) frequency tones presented in pairs HH, HL, LH and LL pairs in auditory modality and digits 6 and 9 presented in pairs 99, 96, 69, 66 in visual modality. The patient's task was to identify pairs of stimuli, to compare the second stimulus in each pair with the first one and to press a button when the second stimulus (high tone or digit 9) corresponded to the first high stimulus. We presume that after the instruction and several probing trials the subject develops a behavioral model that associates a presentation of a pair of two stimuli of the same designated category (e.g., two images of digit 9) with a certain action (pressing a button). We also presume that a model consists of two parts: (1) a sensory model – a template of a category of the relevant stimuli (e.g., of the digit 9); (2) an action model – a template of an action (pressing a button) that must be done as fast and precise as possible.

A priori, several psychological operations are involved in the task. The psychological operations induced by the first stimulus are: (1) encoding relevant features of the stimulus; (2) comparing the features with those of the sensory template; (3) in the case of match, updating the sensory preparatory set and initiating the motor preparatory set; (4) in the case of mismatch, suppressing the preparatory set. The psychological operations induced by the second stimulus (GO or NOGO) are: (1) encoding relevant features of the stimulus, (2) comparing these features with those of the previous one[45]; (3) in case of match, selecting the action and updating the preparatory set; (4) in the case of mismatch, suppressing the automatically selected action and updating the preparatory set; (5) comparing the results of the NOGO trial (no action performed) with the action template (the button is to be pressed) and to correct the further behavior.

For simplicity reasons, here we are going to present only responses to the second stimuli in trails and, for the purposes of this chapter we will consider only first stages of sensory information processing. We are going to show that the early differences between ERPs for GO (match) and NOGO (mismatch) conditions are (1) modality specific, (2) consist of two (spatially overlapping but separating in time) components reflecting correspondingly physical and semantic changes in the stimulus, and (3) are distinct from components associated with motor actions.

Figure 10.14 illustrates the fact that the early ERPs difference waves between NOGO (mismatch) and GO (match) conditions are modality specific. Note that for the visual modality maximum of positivity is located near T5 electrode, while for the auditory modality the positive part of the difference wave reaches it maximum

---

[45]These two operations are similar to the corresponding operations induced by the first stimulus.

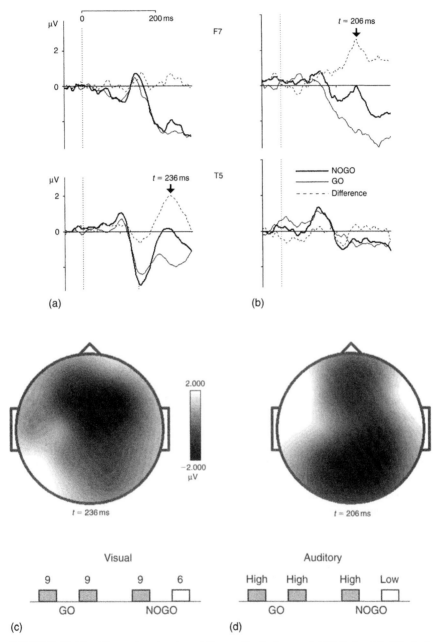

(a)

(b)

(c)

(d)

FIGURE 10.14   Change detection is modality specific. Scalp recorded ERPs for GO (thin line), NOGO (thick line) conditions superimposed on the difference waves (NOGO–GO) (dotted line) for F7 and T5 electrodes in (a) visual modality and (b) auditory modality. (c) Map of the difference waves in the visual modality. (d) Map of the difference waves in the auditory modality.

at F7. Note also that information processing in the auditory modality is faster than in the visual modality: peak latencies of the difference waves are 200 ms for the auditory modality and 240 ms for the visual modality.

G. Physical and Semantic Change Detection

Figure 10.15 illustrates the fact that the difference wave at the early stages consist actually of two components. Recording were made in an epileptic patient to whom electrodes were implanted for diagnosis and therapy. The patient participated in the two stimulus auditory task twice: one day he responded by button pressing to HH pair (GO condition) while the other day he responded by button pressing to HL pair (GO condition). NOGO condition in both tasks was associated with positive component elicited at latency of about 200 ms. However, the early negative component with latency of about 100 ms was elicited only in response to the physical change of expected stimulus. Note that the early negative component also appeared for the first stimulus when the stimulus did not match the expectation (L stimulus at the first place in the pair instead of expected H stimulus).

H. Change Detection and Motor Suppression

To illustrate the fact that change detection takes place in the area distinct from the place where the signal for action suppression is generated, we are presenting the results of ICA that has been made on ERP differences in the two stimulus – visual GO/NOGO task[46] (Fig. 10.16). The two strongest components are presented. One can see that the first component is generated in the left temporal lobe and seems to reflect both physical and semantic change detection[47]. The second component is generated over the left premotor cortex[48] and seems to reflect operation of suppression of the prepared movement.

Recently a group of researchers from Hokkaido University in Japan (Kimura et al., 2006) observed ERPs correlates of change detection in a visual S1–S2 matching task. Similar to our results, they showed that change of stimuli elicit a posterior positive component with a latency of 100–200 ms. They varied the properties of stimuli that were changed (such as color and motion change detection) and showed that components associated with those changes were localized in different cortical areas and revealed different temporal patterns.

---

[46]This task was specifically designed for the Human Brain Institute Database. Instead of simple digits, images of plants and animals were presented. Those ecologically valid stimuli elicited larger responses and were less boring than digits 6 and 9 in the first version of the task.

[47]Similar component was generated at the right temporal lobe. This component is not shown in the figure.

[48]Recall that the subjects were instructed to press a bottom with the right (contralateral) finger.

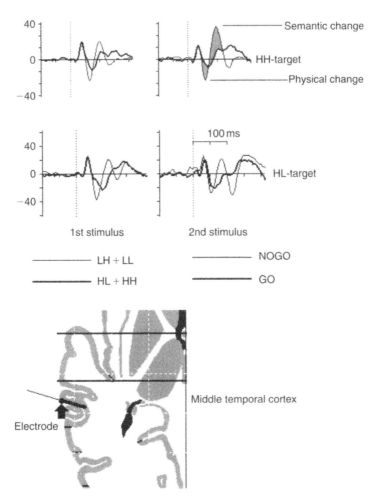

FIGURE 10.15   Change detection evolves in two stages: physical and semantic stages. Intracranial recording made in the middle temporal gyrus from an implanted electrode (bottom) of an epileptic patient. Recording were made in two different days presented at top and middle. Patient participated in the two stimulus auditory task in which four different pairs of high (H) and low (L) tones were randomly presented with equal probabilities. During the task in the first day the patient had to press the button in response to HH pair, while during in the second day he had to press the button in response to HL pair.

VIII. TYPES OF SENSORY SYSTEMS

A. U-Shape Curve of the System Reactivity

As for any neuronal network, overall activity in the sensory systems depends on the sensory input according to sigmoidal function (Fig. 10.17) while reactions of

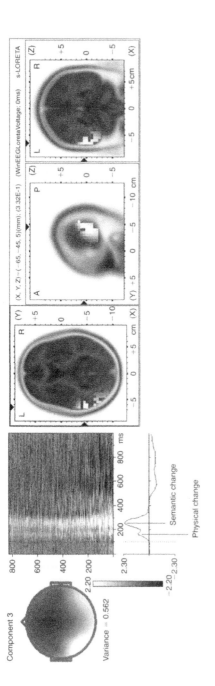

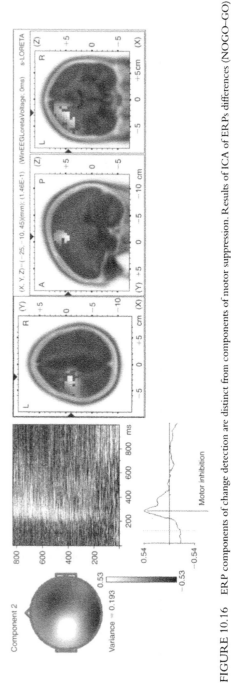

FIGURE 10.16 ERP components of change detection are distinct from components of motor suppression. Results of ICA of ERPs differences (NOGO–GO) for more than 800 healthy subjects of age from 7 to 89. From left to right – (1) topography of components with numbers below corresponding to the variance of the component, (2) vertically stacking thin color-coded horizontal bars, each representing the corresponding component for a single subject, almost 800 healthy subjects of age from 7 (bottom) to 89 (top) are depicted, (3) time courses of components with arrows, (4) s-LORETA images of cortical generators of components. Scales are presented near corresponding pictures.

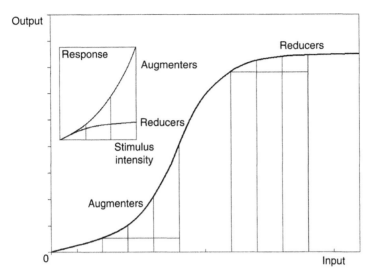

FIGURE 10.17   Two types of sensory systems. The sensory system output activity in relation to the input represents a sigmoidal function. If the sensory input is increased in intensity the output of the system is also increased but in different way depending on the initial state of the system. The system in which activity increases slower (faster) than the input is called the reducing (augmenting) system.

the system to the same stimulus obey to the inverted U-law (see Introduction). In short, the law declares that the system reacts poorly to the stimulus when the overall activity of the system is too low (threshold effect) or too high (ceiling effect).

B. Augmenting and Reducing Sensory Systems

Suppose that for a given system we study how the system reacts to stimuli with increasing intensities (Fig. 10.17). As one judge from Fig. 10.17 the response of the system will increase. However, the way of this increasing will depend on the state of the system. If the system is characterized by the initial low input and low overall activity (the point at the bottom of the curve), relative changes in the response will be higher than relative changes in the sensory input. These systems can be labeled as augmenting sensory systems (see insertion of Fig. 10.17). If the system has much higher overall activity, then relative changes in response will be lower than the relative increase in stimulus intensity. These systems can be labeled as reducing sensory systems.

In animal research the serotoninergic neurons of the brain stem were found to innervate the auditory cortex. The serotoninergic innervation in its turn leads to a strong dependence of overall activity of the auditory cortex with the level of serotonin. Auditory N1/P2 component serve as a good indicator of functioning of the auditory system. So, if the level of serotonin and correspondingly the input activity is increased the loudness dependence of auditory evoked potential reduces (i.e., the system shifts from the left point on the curve of Fig. 10.17 to the right point). In the studies of Gallinat et al. (2000) this property of the auditory system and N1/P2 component was used as a predictor of the acute response to serotonin reuptake inhibitors in depression.

C. Auditory P2 in Augmenters and Reducers

One practical way of assessing the type of the sensory system is presenting to a subject auditory stimuli with increasingly changing intensities. ERP over the primary cortical areas are recorded, the P200 amplitude is measured and is plotted against stimulus intensity. As predicted from Fig. 10.17, on the basis of the slope of the P200 amplitude, normal subjects can be classified into two groups: augmenters and reducers.

IX. DIAGNOSTIC VALUES OF SENSORY-RELATED ERPS COMPONENTS

A. MMN

The most known of the sensory-related ERP components is the MMN. It was intensively studied during the last 30 years both from theoretical and practical points of view. The MMN has recently been used to study phonological and auditory dysfunctions in dyslexia. For example, in one of the studies (Schulte-Körne et al., 1998) the MMN was used to compare the discrimination of speech and non-speech stimuli were in dyslexic and control adolescents. The speech stimuli were syllables ("da" as the standard stimulus and "ba" as the deviant stimulus) and the non-speech stimuli were sine-wave tones. It was found that the MMNs for the tone stimuli did not differ between the two groups, whereas the syllables elicited a smaller MMN in dyslexics than in controls. This result was interpreted as reflecting a deficit specific to the phonological system rather than a general failure in processing auditory information in dyslexia. When dyslexic children were trained by means of an auditory visual training their MMN increased and became more similar to those of norms.

One of the most interesting clinical research lines using the MMN involves schizophrenia. The effect of this psychiatric condition on two types of the MMN generators (temporal and frontal) was studied. In the light of the results obtained so far, it appears that the frontal generators are more affected than the auditory cortex ones.

Studies of the aging effects on the MMN amplitude suggested that this amplitude is reduced with aging. Consequently, aging appears to reduce the duration of auditory sensory memory without affecting auditory. In Alzheimer's disease the MMN (especially with long – about 3 s – ISI) is dramatically decreased.

In coma output prognosis the MMN seems to be an objective measure. The appearance of a MMN kind of fronto-central negativity to a wide frequency change in serial MMN recordings seemed to herald the recovery of consciousness.

B. Comparison Component

Even a brief summary of practical applications of the MMN shows that this parameter can discriminate different psychiatric and neurological conditions from healthy norms. However the size effect of these discriminations is quite small which confines the practical application of the MMN in clinical use. The small size effect can be partly explained as a small value of the component itself. Recall that the mean value of the MMN constitutes just only 1 μV which is 10–50 times smaller than the average amplitude of the background EEG.

In this respect the comparison component in the two stimulus visual GO/ NOGO task represents a more powerful tool. At least the amplitude of the comparison component is 4 times larger than that of the MMN (Fig. 10.18). Moreover using

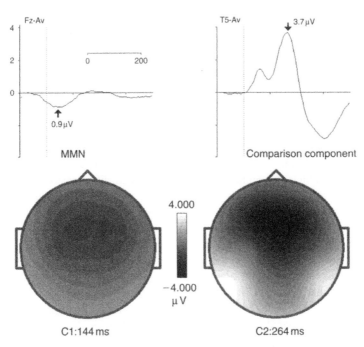

FIGURE 10.18   MMN versus comparison component. MMN was computed as a difference wave between ERPs for deviant and standard tones in the auditory oddball task. Comparison component was computed as a difference wave between ERPs for NOGO and GO conditions in the two stimulus GO/NOGO task. Grand averages were computed from the same group of healthy subjects (age 14–80) from the Human Brain Institute Database.

spatial filtration based on ICA enables us to increase signal to noise ratio of this component and to reliably assess it in individuals. Further studies are certainly needed but even the current data show the higher power of this approach in comparison to old methods for defining biological markers (endophenotypes) of some psychiatric and neurological disorders (such as ADHD, see Part III).

X. SUMMARY

We assess changes inside and outside us by means of different types of receptors. There are different *sensory modalities* that give us sensations of images, sounds, body movements and produce pain, taste, touch, smell. We are aware not of external and internal objects themselves but of impulse discharges of output neurons in the receptor organs. The brain regions where neurons respond to stimulation of a certain type of receptors are usually referred to as a corresponding *sensory system* (visual, auditory … system). In any modality at least three hierarchical cortical areas (primary, secondary, and association) can be separated with higher level areas extracting more complex features of sensory stimuli. The neurons that extract a certain feature of the sensory world form topographically organized computational maps. For example, face recognition, as a specific human feature is associated with activation of certain neurons in the temporal cortex expressed in a specific component of scalp recorded sensory-related potentials. Each class of objects in the external world and each class of spatial relationships appears to have a separate memory. These categorical memories actually perform the role of anticipating schemata. The sensory-related potentials generated by activation of the schemata can be decomposed into several components. A recently developed ICA represents a powerful tool for such decomposition. The sensory-related components extracted by means of the ICA have different time dynamics with peak latencies ranging from 110 ms in the visual modality and from 80 ms in the auditory modality. Different components are generated in different cortical locations varying from the primary sensory areas to the association areas including the anterior cingulate cortex. Different components appear to be associated with different psychological operations such as primary visual (auditory) processing, comparison operation (that can be in turn decomposed in physical and semantic change detection), and engagement operation. In the visual modality, the comparison and engagement components are generated correspondingly in the areas of ventral and dorsal visual pathways. In the auditory modality the comparison operation at the lower hierarchical level is expressed in the mismatch negativity (MMN). The MMN is generated by an automatic change-detection process in which a mismatch is found between the deviant stimulus and the memory representation (trace) of the preceding repetitive auditory stimulation. The MMN is found in the auditory oddball paradigm and has been used for diagnostic purposes in different neurological and psychiatric conditions.

CHAPTER 11

Attention Networks

My experience is what I agree to attend to
William James, 1890

I. PSYCHOLOGY

A. Attention as Selection Operation

Imagine you have closed your eyes in a room with a mechanical clock in it. At first you do not hear the clock, but then you start attending to it. Attending to the sound looks like "turning on" the loudness of the loudspeaker: the ticking is getting louder. Attending to another source of sound such as a whisper of your friend sitting in a corner "turns off" the sound of the clock in your mind. This is how our attention works! As this example shows, attention is associated with enhancement of relevant sensory information and suppression of irrelevant sensory information. These enhancement/inhibition operations can be named by a single term – selection operations. In the same way, attention as a psychological process can be determined as selection operations in sensory modalities with a goal to process relevant sensory information more accurately.

During the first part of 20th century the theory of conditioned reflexes by Ivan Pavlov as well as the theory of operant conditioning[1] of Burrhus Skinner

[1] These two approaches laid down the foundation of behaviorism as a methodological approach in psychology. Behaviorism is based on the proposition that all things which organisms perform can be regarded as behaviors, which in turn can be described objectively without referring to internal subjective physiological events or to hypothetical constructs such as the mind, consiousness....The behaviorist school opposed the psychoanalytic and Gestalt approaches in psychology.

dominated in scientific approach. In late 1940s and early 1960s the emphasis in psychology was made on distinction global states of behavior such as arousal and sleep. Giuseppi Moruzzi and Horace Magoun showed that stimulation of reticular system in the brain stem resulted in awaking a sleeping cat, while stimulation of other brain stem areas induced sleep[2]. The term "arousal", as a state of physiological reactivity of the subject, was introduced and electroencephalogram (EEG) correlates of arousal were discovered. In late 1960s a new scientific paradigm named information processing based on computer metaphor replaced behaviorism[3]. Attention had become a hot topic of this approach.

B. Sensory Selection Versus Motor Selection

Selection operations in a broader sense take place not only in sensory processing but also in the motor domain. The repertoire of human motor actions is tremendous. We can dance, play musical instruments, talk, read and write (some of us in several languages)... In each of these big categories of actions the number of possible elemental actions could be tremendous. Just consider only the number of words that we know[4]. So, at any time interval many potential actions are available. The aim of our behavior is to choose among those actions and to select only one action that is the most appropriate in a given moment. Selection operations are not restricted by motor actions. The selection operations are also performed with cognitive actions – thoughts. Recall words of William James "To think is to select"[5].

C. Preparatory Sets

An attempt to combine these separate psychological entities under a single concept was made by Edvard Evarts, Yoshikazu Shinoda, and Steven Wise in their classical book "Neurophysiological approaches to higher brain functions" published in 1984. The notion of preparatory set as a state of readiness to receive a stimulus or to make a movement was introduced. Using modern concepts we can say that the

---

[2] G. Moruzzi and H. W. Magoun published their book "Brain Stem Reticular Formation and Activation of the EEG" in 1949.

[3] Information processing is an approach in psychology that considers cognition as computational in nature, with mind being the software and the brain being the hardware. Information processing may be sequential or parallel, centralized or distributed. In mid 1980s the parallel distributed processing in neuronal networks became an explanational paradigm in cognitive psychology.

[4] The vocabulary of William Shakespeare constituted around 30,000 words!

[5] In his book "The Principles of Psychology" published in 1890 William James, a pioneering American psychologist, devoted chapters to habit, attention, perception, association, memory, reasoning, instinct, emotion, and imagination.

preparatory set in sensory domain is associated with attention, while the preparatory set in motor or cognitive domain is associated with executive functions[6].

In any time interval a behavioral pattern can be divided into two parts: execution of a cognitive-motor action and sensory perception associated with this action[7]. Sensory and action elements of behavior are interconnected. Indeed, almost any voluntary movement is associated with perceiving of how the movement is performed (perception of tension of muscles, position of limbs...) and how the subject interacts with the outside world during this movement (perception of changes of light flow, of acoustic waves in the air....). Vice versa, almost any perceptual act (assessment of color, or position, or velocity...of a certain object) is associated with movement of a subject or his head and eyes in the external world (gaze positioning to the corresponding point of visual space, following the flying object by eyes, making saccadic eye movements while viewing the complex figure[8].

Although from psychological point of view attention, motor preparatory set, and selection of thoughts can be considered as similar entities associated with preparatory activities in neuronal networks, in experimental work they have been usually studied separately. These studies showed that neuronal circuits responsible for executive and perception functions are different. In action selection an important role is played by the basal ganglia thalamo-cortical system while in selecting the source of sensory information from a mixture of many different sources an important role is played by feedforward and feedback connections between distinctive cortical representations in sensory systems. These cortical representations have reciprocal connections with subcortical structures (thalamus and superior colliculus) playing an important role in shifting operations of attention[9].

D. Processing Multiple Objects

In everyday life, the visual scenes typically consist of many objects different in shape, color, motion, etc. and located in different space positions and cluttered with each other. Our experience tells us that we do not process all objects simultaneously.

---

[6]Executive functions in detail will be described in the following chapter.

[7]For example, the action part of speech production is manifested by complex synergic movements of tongue, lips, and throat, while the sensory part is manifested in perception of sounds produced by the subject and in perception of somato-sensory signals accompanied the movements. From lesions studies we know that the representations of the action part of the speech are located in Broca's area, while the representations of the sensory part are located in Wernike's area. Although these two areas are reciprocally interconnected, the damage to only one of them produces a specific dysfunction called either Broca's or Wernike's aphasia depending on location.

[8]Walking in the forest (movement), we need to see where to put a foot (perception). Watching the TV (perception) we need to follow the action by shifting the gaze (head and eye movements).

[9]Shift of attention can occur covertly, without noticeable movements, but even in this case the shifting operation involves the same brain structures that are associated with overt actions.

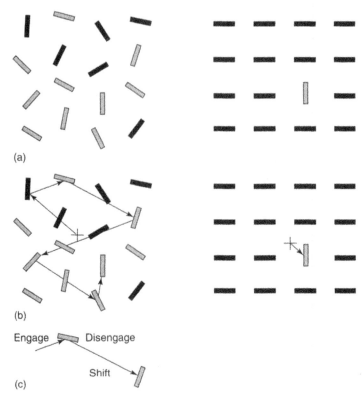

(a)

(b)

Engage / Disengage

Shift

(c)

FIGURE 11.1 Attention operations. (a) Two ways of attracting attention. According to the instruction attention has to be attracted to a gray vertical bar. Because of the limited processing capacity of the visual system, simultaneously presented multiple stimuli compete for a selected neural representation. This competition is difficult at the left fig (a sequential search for the target) and easy at the right fig (a parallel search for the target). One can speculate that in the first case the top–bottom controlled search finds a target, while in the second case, the bottom–up process pops up the target. (b) Shifts of attention are marked by lines with arrows. The shifts can be overt and measured by recording eye movements, namely position of the fovea of the eyes on the scene while a subject is viewing a picture in a search of the target. The technique of measuring eye movements during observation of pictures was first applied by a Russian scientist Alexander Yarbus. Shifts of attention may be also covered, that is, occur without any visible movements of eyes. (c) Three operations of attention after Michael Posner (Posner et al, 1988) – engagement, disengagement and shift operations.

Just look at Fig. 11.1a, left and try to locate a vertical gray bar. It takes time to do it. Your focus of attention seems to sequentially search for different locations until the appropriate object is found (Fig. 11.1b, left). A metaphor of a "search light" comes to mind when we consider how we search for the target. It looks like that the ability of our visual system to process information regarding multiple objects at any given moment in time is limited. In Fig. 11.1a left bars with different orientations and colors compete for the selected representation.

E. Engagement, Disengagement and Shift Operations

As one can see from the above example, attention is a dynamic process. According to Michael Posner, a world expert in psychology of attention, three different operations can be separated in this dynamic process (Fig. 11.1c). The first one is engagement operation – facilitation of neuronal representation of attended source of information[10]. The second element of attention is disengagement operation – inhibition of unattended source of information[11]. The third operation is shift or move operation – intermediate state between processing two different sources of information. These three operations can be easily distinguished in the examples depicted in Fig. 11.1b left representing a superposition of a scene and trajectories of eye movement during its viewing. As one can see, sequential fixation points of eyes are located at different (not repeated) bars during the search of the target.

F. Bottom–Up and Top–Down Factors

A critical prerequisite of attention is existence of several sources of information – several visual images in the visual modality, for example. They compete with each other for representation[12]. The competition between different stimuli can be resolved by two different ways: top–down and bottom–up factors. The top–down factor is exemplified in Fig. 11.1a, left. Giving to the subject instruction to look for a vertical gray bar defines the higher order process that in turn governs the saccadic actions that shift attention from one location to another until the required stimulus is found. The bottom–up factor is exemplified in Fig. 11.1a, right by attributing a salience feature to a selected object, such as its specific orientation and color that is quite different from orientations and colors of the other stimuli. In this case a single vertical gray bar among the multiple distracter lines is effortlessly and quickly detected because of its salience in the display, which biases the competition in favor of the vertical gray bar. Such "deviant" stimulus is pop up in Fig. 11.1a, right. Processing of visual scenes combines bottom–up sensory aspects with top–down influences. This combination constitutes the essence of attention.

---

[10]One important features of attention is that the engagement operation can last quite long thus allowing us to sustain a perception for extended periods of time. A good example of such sustained attention could be listening to music or solving a mathematical problem or playing a chess game. We need time (and some times quite long) to solve a certain problem!

[11]A special case of disengagement operation is inhibition of return. This phenomenon is manifested in a lower probability to return to the previously attended object, for example, in Fig. 11.1 middle a shift attention rarely returns to a spot that was already attended.

[12]It looks like the world is too complex for us – the environment contains far too much information to perceive it at once.

II. ANATOMY

A. Sensory Systems

Attention works on sensory information and, consequently, involves circuits within the sensory systems (Fig. 11.2). Besides bottom–up and top–down operations in the hierarchical cortical areas of sensory systems, the sensory information is controlled by subcortical structures such as thalamus and superior colliculus. The pulvinar nucleus of the thalamus have reciprocal connections with secondary and association sensory cortical areas and together with the corresponding part of the reticular nucleus controls the information flow in these areas. The other subcortical structure, the superior colliculus, is involved in covert and overt shifts of gaze. Through its connections to sensory areas the pulvinar is involved in selecting local parts of 3D environment for detailed analysis.

B. Executive System

Attention implies selection operations in sensory domain. However, any sensory event including attention modulation can not be separated from its action

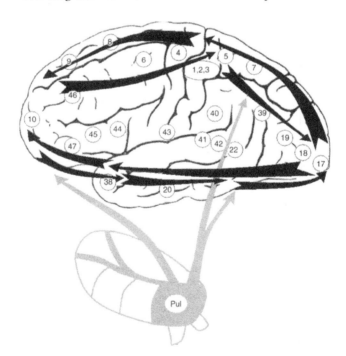

FIGURE 11.2   Attentional pathways of the brain. Arrows indicate bottom–up and top–down interactions between posterior and anterior cortical areas. These interactions are supported by projections from the pulvinar nucleus to the corresponding cortical areas.

counterpart. For example, to switch attention from one part of the visual scene to another an orienting action including eye movement and pupil dilation must be performed. The cortical areas of sensory systems located in posterior parts of the cortex have reciprocal intercortical connections with the anterior cortical areas of the executive system involved in selection of actions that we need to perform in order to process sensory information in detail. As we mentioned above, selection of actions takes place in the frontal executive system and involves distinct mechanisms reviewed in Chapter 12.

III. MODULATION OF SENSORY INFORMATION FLOW

A. Mutual Inhibition in Animal Experiments

Most of our understanding of neuronal correlates of attention comes from monkey research[13]. In this research, vision is the modality that was mostly studied[14]. Schematic results of a typical experiment in monkey are presented in Fig. 11.3 (for more details see Reynolds et al., 1999). Impulse activity of a neuron located in the ventral stream is recorded while visual stimuli (e.g., oriented bars) are presented within the receptive field of the neuron. When only one stimulus is presented and attention is directed outside the receptive field, the stimulus evokes a response consisting of two parts: the early response and the late response. When in this condition the second stimulus is presented within the receptive field of the neuron the late response of the neuron is suppressed. When the monkey attends to the first stimulus while ignoring the second one, the response to the joint stimulation is enhanced. These findings clearly indicate that two stimuli presented at the same time within a neuron's receptive filed are not processed independently, but interact with each other in a mutually inhibitory way. Attention appears to be a process that inhibits the suppressive effect of the unattended stimulus, thus enhancing the response of attended stimulus. In short, these findings imply that attention resolves

---

[13]Vernon Mountcastle in 1970s pioneered experimental research of attention in monkeys by recording reactions of neurons in the dorsal stream (Mountcastle, 1978). He showed that neurons in both parietal area 7a and the pulvinar were enhanced while monkeys attended to stimuli.

[14]As we know from Chapter 1, Part II monkey's cortex contains more than 20 separate visual areas, which are organized into two functionally specialized processing pathways: ventral and dorsal streams. The ventral stream is critical for the identification of objects, whereas dorsal stream is designed by nature for assessing spatial relations between objects as well as for directing movements toward the objects. Neurons in the ventral stream show response selectivity for stimulus attributes that are important for object vision, such as shape, color, and, texture. Neurons in the dorsal stream show response selectivity for the spatial location of an attended object and for the speed and direction of stimulus motion. Taking these facts into account, we would expect that modulatory effects of attention to spatial cues have to be found in the dorsal stream while attention to visual features (such as shape or color) has to modulate responses of neurons in the areas of the ventral stream.

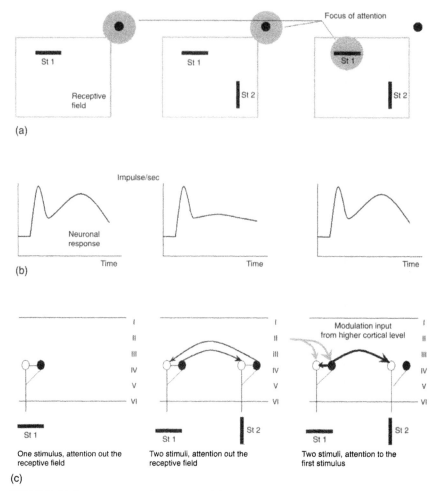

FIGURE 11.3   Attention resolves mutual inhibition between competing stimuli. (a) Receptive field of the neuron in the visual system (depicted by square) at three situations: left – only one visual stimulus (horizontal bar) is presented inside the receptive field with attention outside the field (depicted by gray color), middle – an additional visual stimulus (vertical bar) is presented within the visual field with attention outside the receptive field, right – attention is directed to the horizontal bar. (b) Reactions of the neurons to the brief presentation of stimuli in three different conditions. Note that the competing stimulus reduces the late component of neuronal reaction while attention restores the late component. (c) Schematic representation of neuronal networks responsible for these effects. Open circle – excitatory neuron, black circle – inhibitory neurons. Note that attention activates the inhibitory neuron corresponding to the first stimulus thus enhancing the detecting properties of the neurons and inhibiting adjacent irrelevant neurons.

the competition among multiple stimuli by counteracting the mutual inhibition between different sources of information, thereby enhancing (facilitating) information processing at the attended source and suppressing the unattended source[15].

B. Involvement of Subcortical Structures

Two main subcortical structures are involved in sensory processing and in attentional modulation of information flow. They are the superior colliculus and the pulvinar nucleus of the thalamus. The superior colliculus is involved in generating saccadic movements needed for overt search of relevant sources of sensory information. Its activity is controlled by the ocular-motor pathway in the basal ganglia. Some of recent studies suggest that superior colliculus participates not only in goal directed and saccadic eye movements but also in covert attention that takes place without any observable eye movements. The pulvinar nucleus of the thalamus is another subcortical structure involved in attention. This nucleus has reciprocal connections with cortical areas of ventral and dorsal visual pathways as well as with pathways in other sensory modalities. In addition, the pulvinar establishes connections with prefrontal areas, thus coordinating the joint functioning of executive and sensory systems. Neurons in this nucleus exhibit attention-related effects such as enhancement of responses to attended stimuli.

C. Attention-Related Negativities in Human ERPs

One of the first paradigms for studying event-related potentials (ERPs) correlates of attention in humans was a dichotic listening task introduced by Broadbent in 1954[16]. When EEG is recorded in the oddball task in which standard and deviant tones are presented to the left and the right ear with the subject's job to attend to either the left or right ear, ERPs difference waves between attended and unattended irrelevant stimuli reveal a negative wave, called processing negativity. A schematic result of such an experiment is presented in Fig. 11.4a (a review of processing negativity see in the book "Brain and attention" by Risto Näätänen).

[15]Mechanism of lateral inhibition could account for competition between stimuli. A neuronal model that might explain the above mentioned results is presented in Fig 11.3 bottom. Note, that lateral inhibition in the cortical layers plays a critical role not only in attention but also in extracting features from the stimulus by shaping the weight function of the neuron (see "Information processing in neuronal networks" in Chapter 8 of this part of the book).

[16]In the dichotic listening task, subjects listen through a set of headphones to two different streams of auditory stimuli presented to each ear independently. The subjects are asked to focus on the information that is being played to one ear. An experiment, done by Cherry in 1953, showed that the subjects can recall a little regarding the information that was going into their unattended ear aside from base characteristics such as the sex of the speaker.

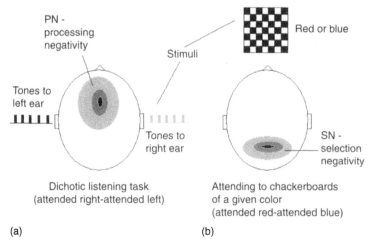

FIGURE 11.4   Attention-related negativities (schematic representation). (a) Processing negativity (PN) in auditory modality; the map of a difference wave between ERP to attended versus unattended ear in a dichotic listening task. (b) Selection negativity (SN) in color vision; the map of a difference wave between ERPs to attended color versus unattended one. In the task red and blue flashed checkerboards were presented in a rapid, randomized sequence at the center of the screen. Either the red or blue checks were attended on separate runs. Difference waves were formed by subtracting ERPs to the unattended color from those to the attended color, collapsed over red and blue stimuli. Adapted from Hillyard and Anllo-Vento, 1988.

A result of another paradigm to study ERPs correlates of attention is presented in Fig. 11.4b. Stimuli are presented in the visual modality. Checkerboard patterns of different colors (red and blue) are randomly presented in the middle of the screen with the subject's task to attend either to red or blue stimuli. The difference wave (attended–unattended) reveals a negative component called selection negativity (SN). Selection negativity is an example of ERPs index of attention in the ventral visual stream[17].

D. Parietal-Frontal Network in PET and MRI Studies

Although this chapter deals with control of sensory processing in posterior regions of the cortex, we could not avoid mentioning interaction of these areas with the frontal parts of the cortex which are traditionally associated with working memory. Indeed attention and working memory are interconnected operations: to keep the item in working memory one must attend to it, and vice versa to attend to some

[17]Negativities in difference waves are not the only components. Positive components can be also found in ERPs difference waves depending on the specific design of the task. There is a temptation to associate negative components in the visual modality with inhibitory postsynaptic potentials in the middle cortical layers, while to associate positive components with excitatory postsynaptic potentials.

expected stimulus one must keep it in memory. PET and fMRI studies in humans indicates that neuronal networks for these operations are similar. A network consisting of areas in the parietal and frontal cortex has been found to be activated in a variety of visuospatial tasks that require attention and working memory.

IV. NEUROPSYCHOLOGY

A. Sensory Neglect and Right Parietal Lesions

As we learnt from the previous chapter, neurons in the parietal cortical areas of the dorsal visual pathway ("where" pathway) are responsible for coding spatial locations of objects and are modulated during spatial attention tasks, that is, during tasks that require focusing attention on a distinct spatial location. On the basis of this knowledge we can suggest that damage to parietal areas would impair spatial attention. This is indeed the case, and unilateral parietal damage often leads to a so-called neglect syndrome, where in the patients fail to attend to objects in the hemispace, contralateral (opposite) to the side of lesion. In severe cases, patients suffering from neglect will completely disregard the visual hemifield contralateral to the side of the lesion. For example, they will read from only one side of a book, apply make-up to only one half of their face, or eat from only one side of a plate[18]. In less severe cases, the deficit is more subtle and becomes apparent only if the patient is confronted with competing stimuli, as in the case of visual extinction[19]. It must be stressed that visuospatial neglect may be induced not only by unilateral parietal lesions, but also by lesions in the frontal lobe, the anterior cingulate cortex, the basal ganglia, and the thalamus, in particular the pulvinar (for a review see Kastner and Ungerleider, 2000).

B. Balint's Syndrome

A complete loss of feeling of space and relations between objects is seen in bilateral damage in parietal lobes. Behavioral impairment induced by such damage

---

[18]Neglect occurs more often with right-sided parietal lesions than with left-sided parietal lesions, which suggests a specialized role for the right hemisphere in directed attention. Based on this hemispheric asymmetry, it has been proposed that the right hemisphere mediates directed attention to both sides of visual space, whereas the left hemisphere mediates directed attention only to the contralateral, right side of visual space (Mesulam, 1981). According to this view, in the case of a left-hemisphere lesion, the intact right hemisphere would take over the attentional function of the damaged left-hemisphere, whereas a right-hemisphere lesion would result in a left sided hemispatial neglect because of the bias of the intact left-hemisphere for the right hemifield

[19]In visual extinction, patients are able to orient attention to a single visual object presented to their impaired visual hemifield; however, if two stimuli are presented simultaneously, one in the impaired and the other in the intact hemifield, the patients will only detect the one presented to the intact side, denying that any other object had been presented.

is known under the name of Balint's syndrome. Patients with Balint's syndrome lose spatial information outside their own bodies and are functionally blind except for the perception of one object in the visual scene at a time. They cannot locate the item they can perceive, nor can they tell when an item is moved toward or away from them. They lose explicit spatial awareness. It is as if "there is no there, there"[20].

V. NEURONAL NETWORKS

A. Recurrent Depolarization of Apical Dendrites

Activation of recurrent circuits (both intercortical and thalamo-cortical) appears to be crucial for sustaining attention to a certain location (spatial attention) or a certain object (non-spatial attention). Several models simulating the mechanisms of attention have been suggested. Empirical evidence is still not enough to choose the most adequate one. However, one neuronal element of attentional networks is supported by numerous experimental finding and is accepted by the majority of models. This element is associated with sustained depolarization of apical dendrites of pyramidal cortical cells during various preparatory sets. A critical role in generating this depolarization is played by recurrent pathways from the deeper layers of higher order cortical areas to the upper layers of lower order cortical areas. In Fig. 11.5 this type of pathways is marked by a gray thick arrow. The recurrent pathways are excitatory in nature and depolarize apical layers of the cortex. This apical activity seems to be manifested in slow negative fluctuation recorded from the scalp during preparatory sets[21]. The apical depolarization modulates activity of pyramidal cells and decreases the threshold of their activation. Pyramidal cells in the middle layers of the cortex might work as coincidence detectors that fire only if both apical and basal dendrites are depolarized[22].

---

[20]It has been argued that Balint's syndrome is a type of double neglect. For instance, a patient with neglect might overlook the left side of a room but also the left side of a flower. However, Balint's patients neglect both sides of the room but they can see a single object. In fact, they see nothing but objects. So the relationship between double neglect and Balint's syndrome might not be as straightforward as it first seems.

[21]These types of activities are usually combined under the common term – contingent negative variation (CNV). CNV depends on modality of the preparatory set and localized near the corresponding sensory areas.

[22]However, another possibility of attentional modulation can not be ruled out. It is associated with activation of inhibitory neurons via the same recurrent pathways. The inhibitory neurons are located in the middle layers of the cortex and exhibit intracortical inhibition within the cortical area thus shaping receptive fields of pyramidal cells and tuning them to the expected stimuli. The inhibitory cells by lateral inhibition inhibit the competing cortical areas thus suppressing information flow in the irrelevant channels. The inhibitory postsynaptic potentials at the middle cortical layers produce negative potentials at the cortical surface similar to those generated by apical depolarization.

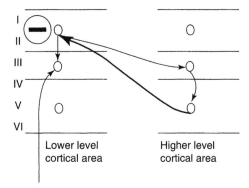

FIGURE 11.5   Schematic representation of attentional neuronal network. From left to right – networks of first order and second order sensory areas. Attentional control is provided by a recurrent pathway (depicted in thick black arrow). The recurrent pathways depolarize (denoted by thick minus sign) apical dendrites of pyramidal cells. The depolarization of apical dendrites is manifested in scalp recorded negativity.

B. Attention and Arousal

From our experience we know that sensory perception and object recognition depends on the level of arousal. In the waking state, the lowest end of arousal is drowsiness. The opposite extreme end is hypervigilance. We can hardly notice anything in the state of drowsiness because the threshold of activation of sensory neurons is very high, so that even relevant stimuli are not able to activate these sensory neurons. Consequently, performance of the attentional system is very poor. In the state of hypervigilance we are distracted by many irrelevant stimuli, because the threshold of activation of sensory neurons is so low that even irrelevant stimuli are able to activate them. Consequently, the performance of the system is also poor. So, if we define the ability of a sensory system to discriminate a certain stimulus from a noisy background as P (performance) and a general level of activation of this system as A (arousal level) we get a so called inverted U-shaped relationship.

Arousal reflects a fundamental property of behavior and, partly, is associated with the ability of sensory systems to process information. The effective thresholds of activation of sensory neurons appear to reflect the ability of the brain to process sensory stimuli (Fig. 11.6). The way how these thresholds are set by a general level of arousal is different from the way how these thresholds are set in specific preparatory sets. While setting the thresholds in attention is quite specific and is confined to a small set of relevant neurons, arousal reflects general or "non-specific" changes in thresholds. These changes are induced by a separate "non-specific" system.

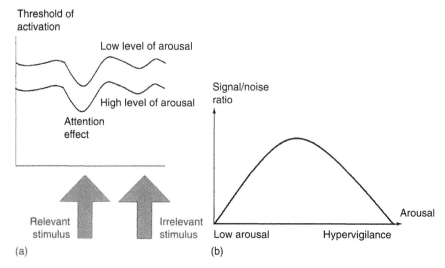

FIGURE 11.6   Global effect of arousal and local effect of attention. (a) Threshold of activation of sensory neurons: high level of arousal decreases the threshold non-specifically both for relevant and irrelevant stimuli, attention decreases the threshold specifically for the relevant stimulus. (b) Too much of and too low of arousal decreases the signal to noise ratio in the sensory system.

C. Tonic and Phasic Reactions of Locus Coeruleus

The origins of the non-specific arousal system reside in the brain stem in general and in a nucleus called the locus coeruleus (LC) in particular[23]. The overall level of activity of neurons in the LC strongly correlates with changes of arousal from deep sleep to hyperarousal. The neurons in the LC are silent during rapid eye movement (REM) sleep and exhibit progressive activation while the state of the human subject shifts from non-REP sleep to arousal. In fact, silence of LC neurons is one of few physiological parameters that discriminates REM sleep from wakefulness[24].

Neurons in the LC are characterized by two types of activity: the tonic or background activity that slowly changes with slow alterations in the state of the brain and the phasic component that reflects a fast response of the system to a brief sensory stimulation. The phasic part is thought to play a role of temporal enhancer (or filter) that intensifies processing of the most important stimuli.

---

[23]Locus coeruleus means blue spot in Latin. The name reflects the pigmented color of neurons in this nucleus. The locus coeruleus in humans comprises a small number (about 16.000 per hemisphere) of neurons.

[24]Recall that REM or paradoxical stage of sleep is characterized by cortical activation and corresponding changes in EEG patterns including appearance of frontal midline theta oscillations.

The following properties of neurons in the LC support this thought. First, the latency of neuronal reactions in response to stimuli in the LC is quite small – about 100 ms. Second, only targets, that is, behaviorally meaningful stimuli activate neurons in the LC. Because of low speed of neuronal impulses along unmyelinated axons, the activity of neurons in the LC can reach the cortex in 60–70 ms. Theoretically these responses can facilitate late stages[25] of information processing in sensory systems.

D. Norepinephrine as Modulator of Attention

Axons of neurons in the LC carry the only source of norepinephrine[26] (NE) to the cerebral cortex. The axons of NE neurons are unmyelinated and therefore slowly conducting. Moreover, NE may be released in extrasynaptic sites and, consequently, produces a non-local effect. These two features indicate that NE has a modulatory effect on target neurons. As we know, the modulatory synaptic effect of any modulator depends on the receptor. Both α_1 and α_2 adrenoreceptors are present in cortical areas. Their activation is associated with generating excitatory postsynaptic potentials in the target neurons and, consequently with decrease of thresholds of activation of those neurons[27]. Axons of the LC innervate the cortex non-homogenously. The mostly dense terminals are located in the parietal cortex and premotor/motor cortical areas (Fig. 11.7). Subcortical structures that are involved in attention (such as pulvinar and superior colliculus) also receive dense innervation from the LC. The role of NE in attention explains the interest of pharmaceutical approach in drugs that change the NE function. One of the recently developed drugs, Atomoxetine, is a NE reuptake blocker that lessens symptoms of attention deficit disorder[28].

VI. LATE POSITIVE COMPONENTS IN ERPS

From ERP studies we know that the time interval of 250–400 ms is associated with a family of late positive components usually united under the name "P300"

---

[25]Starting later than 200 ms.

[26]Norepinephrine has also another name – noradrenaline. The receptors of this modulator are often called adrenoreceptors.

[27]α_2 adrenoreceptors are dominant in LC itself and here serve a role of auto-receptors. Their activation is associated with inhibition – negative feedback in self-regulation of NA.

[28]Atomoxetine is classified as a norepinephrine reuptake inhibitor. It is manufactured and marketed in the form of the hydrochloride salt of atomoxetine under the brand name Strattera® by Eli Lilly Company. Strattera was originally intended to be a new antidepressant drug; however, in clinical trials, no such benefits could be proven. Since norepinephrine is believed to play a critical role in attention, Strattera was tested and subsequently approved as a treatment of attention deficit hyperactivity disorder (ADHD). It is the first non-stimulant drug approved for the treatment of ADHD. Its advantage over stimulants for the treatment of ADHD is that it has less abuse potential than stimulants and has proven in clinical trials to offer 24 h coverage of symptoms associated with ADHD in adults and children.

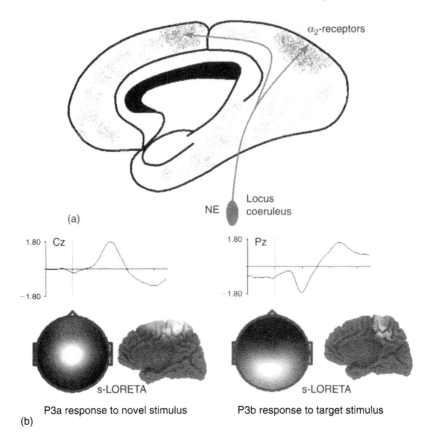

FIGURE 11.7 P3a and P3b components and their relationship to adrenergic innervation. (a) Cortical NE originates in the LC. Axons of LC neurons innervate the cortex widely (not shown) with the most dense projections to the parietal and motor/premotor areas (shown by gray scattered dots). (b) P3a and P3b components are elicited in a three stimulus oddball paradigm. In a typical experiment ERPs are recorded during an auditory oddball task in which infrequent (deviant) tones (targets) are interspersed among frequent (standard) tones and infrequent novel distracter sounds (such as a dog's bark) with the subjects task to respond to targets. In this task novel stimuli elicit P3a components while target stimuli generate P3b components. P3a and P3b have different topographies and different s-LORETA images.

or "P3" components. The P300 components are elicited by behaviorally meaningful stimuli. One of these components, P3b component is enhanced in response to targets, that is, to stimuli that are followed by motor or cognitive actions such as pressing a button or counting the number of targets[29]. An earlier component, P3a

---

[29]A typical experiment in which P3b is generated is an oddball task. For instance, in a auditory variant of the task two tones of different frequencies (say of 300 and 1000 Hz) are randomly presented to a subject with 500 ms intervals and with different probabilities (say and 90 per cent and 10 per cent). The subject is asked to press a button to rare tones.

component, is enhanced in response to a sudden and noticeable change in sensory stimulation and is associated with orienting to the stimulus change[30] (Fig. 11.7).

A. P3b Component

The first indications that P3b potentials might be associated with activity in the LC were found in monkey by Pineda et al. in 1989. In addition to it, the experimental evidence in humans indicate that both the LC phasic response and the P3 appear show similar features: (1) they both appear after target stimuli in odd-ball paradigms, and (2) both depend on the behavioral significance and attention paid to eliciting stimuli, (3) are greater for hits than for false alarms or misses in a signal–detection task. These considerations have led to a hypothesis that the P3b reflects the phasic enhancement of gain in the cerebral cortex induced by LC mediated release of NE (for a review see Aston-Jones and Cohen, 2005).

When in 1990s we studied ERPs in intracranial recordings in patients with implanted electrodes we were surprised by the observation that the P3b-like components could be found in many cortical and subcortical structures (Fig. 11.8)[31]. The pattern of response depended very much on the electrode location. Areas in the temporal cortex revealed MMN-like components that were of early (80–120 ms) peak latencies and did not depend on whether attention was paid to the stimuli or not[32]. In contrast, fronto-parietal cortical areas as well as the basal ganglia and thalamic nuclei evoked P3b-like components that were found only in the active condition when deviant stimuli required actions (pressing a button). These intracranial ERPs components were in the latency range of P3b scalp recorded component, but in contrast to the positive deflections in scalp were both of positive or negative polarities in intracranial recordings. The areas in which P3b-like activity was found were parietal and frontal (including lateral, medial parts, and anterior cingulate) cortical areas and the basal ganglia and the thalamic nuclei.

---

[30] A typical experiment in which P3a can be recorded is three stimulus task in which together with repeated standard tones and deviant tones (targets) novel stimuli (such as dog barking, of telephone ring) are rarely presented. The novel stimuli produces orienting response, shift of attention and generate P3a components.

[31] In these studies we used a three stimulus paradigm, in which standard (tones of 1000 Hz with probability of 80 per cent), deviants (tones of 1300 Hz with probability of 10 per cent) and novels (a random mixture of different tones) were interspersed with each other. In the passive variant of the task the patients read a book, while in the active variant of the task they had to press a button in response to deviants. When recorded from scalp electrodes, deviants elicited the mismatch-negativity (MMN) component with maximum amplitude in Fz in both passive and active task conditions, while in active condition in addition to the MMN component deviants elicited the parietally distributed P3b component. The P3b component was preceded by the N2 component.

[32] MMN was analyzed in detail in Part II Chapter 1 when we were talking about comparison operations in sensory systems.

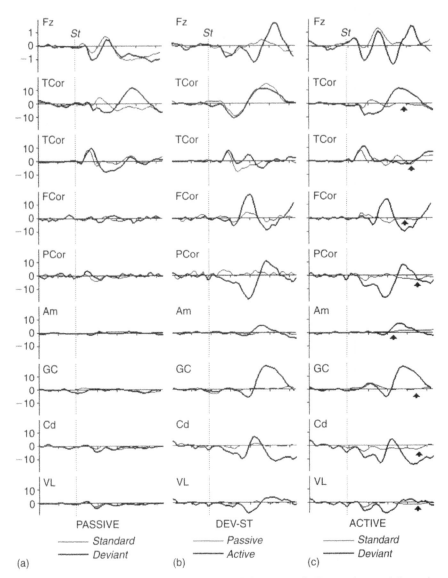

FIGURE 11.8 Variety of P3b-like activity recorded intracranially. Top- scalp recorded grand-average ERPs at Fz from a group of 20 patients with implanted electrodes. Amplitude scale 1 mcV Below the top graph – individual intracranial ERPs. Amplitude scale 10 mcV. ERPs were recorded in the acoustic oddball paradigm in which standard stimuli (tones of 100 ms and 1000 Hz) were randomly interspersed with rare deviant stimuli (tones of 100 ms and 1300 Hz). The patient's task was to press a button to deviants in Active condition (c) and to read a book and ignore auditory stimuli in passive condition (a). The difference wave between deviants and standards are presented in the middle (b).

More over, when recorded in one patient latencies and temporal dynamic of P3b-like components depended on the position of electrode indicating the existence not of one but several types of P3b activities generated in response to target stimuli within the latency of 200–400 ms after stimulus. We can conclude that the P3b component when recorded from scalp is distributed (according to s-LORETA) over parietal cortical areas, but when recorded intracranially it is found in a widely distributed brain system including parietal and frontal cortical areas working in concert with the basal ganglia and thalamus.

P3b component is the most studied in the scientific literature component both in theoretical and clinical fields. There were several reasons for that: First, the P3b is elicited in the odd ball task which is quite simple to perform for almost all categories of neurological or psychiatric patients. Second, the P3b is a relatively large component which is quite easy to discriminate as a difference wave between responses to target deviants and non-target standards. Third, the P3b seems to have a diagnostic power because the impairments of the P3b were found in several executive dysfunctions such as schizophrenia and attention deficit hyperactivity disorder (ADHD).

Several functional meanings of the P3b components were suggested. The most influential of them is a concept of working memory updating proposed by Donchin in 1981. The concept suggests that any target stimulus induces an action after which the brain updates the working memory – in his initial paper Donchin named this process "context updating"[33]. The concept was loosely defined at psychological level, was not associated with a neurophysiological circuit and cellular mechanisms and, consequently, was criticized[34].

B. P3a Component

Imagine you are driving a car and listening to a music enjoying the landscape around. But suddenly a slight change in the engine rhythmic noise attracts your attention. Something is wrong? You stop a car and take off the hood of the car to look and listen to the engine. This example shows that the brain constructs a model of sensory environment and maintains this model in the sensory system. When a sudden change occurs in the environment the system detects this new

[33]Unfortunately, this hypothesis was not supported by the following research. It was criticized in Verleger paper in 1988 (see also response to this critique by Donchin and Coles, 1988. Until now "context updating" hypotheses remains an attractive but unproven hypothesis.

[34]The experience obtained in our laboratory tells that that there are not one but several P3b-like components with different topographies and different temporal patterns. They are probably associated with different neuronal circuits having different functional meaning. We usually refer to the parietal P3b component as "engagement" component. The engagement component is considered as the result of activation of parietally and frontally distributed neurons needed for overt or covert execution of action. The activation of this parietal–temporal–frontal circuit seems to be a result of transformation of the sensory model of the brain into the action.

event and shifts attention toward the new object with a goal of exploring it more closely. This mechanism enables humans (and animals) to adapt in constantly changing situations by means of a so-called orienting response. Ivan Pavlov, to stress its involuntary nature, called it "orienting reflex."

Substantial insights into the nature of the orienting response have come from studies of scalp-recorded ERPs in humans. An ERP component associated with the orienting response – the P300a or P3a – was first described by Sutton and colleagues in 1965. Although the P3a has been studied most extensively in humans, "P3-like" potentials have been recorded from macaque and squirrel monkeys, cats, rabbits, rats, dogs, and dolphins, indicating that the P3a might represent processes that are conserved across mammalian species.

In a typical P3a experiment, a subject performs an auditory target detection task with simple pure tone stimuli, and occasionally hears a contextually novel sound (such as a dog bark) amidst these tones. Unlike the standard and target tones, these novel sounds elicit a scalp-recorded potential that peaks about 200–300 ms after the stimulus and that is largest over the central and frontal scalp electrodes[35] (Fig. 11.7).

It should be stressed here that neuronal circuits for generators of P3a are not limited by the premotor areas as indicated by s-LORETA images for P3a. As our own research and studies of Eric Halgren and his co-workers show, P3a-like activities can be found in a variety of cortical and subcortical structures, including prefrontal, parietal, lateral temporal, and medial temporal cortical areas as well as subcortical structures such as the basal ganglia and thalamus (Fig. 11.9). Obviously this heterogeneous network includes several systems with different functions. Some of these structures (temporal secondary and association auditory areas) are responsible for novelty detection by extracting features that are quite deviant from the background sensory stimulation. Some of these structures (such as hippocampal formation) are responsible for encoding contextually novel events and memorizing them. And finally, some of these structures (such as anterior cingulate and prefrontal cortex) are responsible for orienting attention in order to process the deviations from the background simulation in more detail.

In line with the heterogeneity of neuronal networks generated P3a, at least two different neuromodulators affect the P3a amplitude. They are noradrenaline (that is more densely distributed in the parietal and motor–premotor cortical areas) and acetylcholine that is the key mediator in memory-related hippocampal circuits.

---

[35]The functional characteristics of the novelty P3, and the cognitive processes it might index, have been a topic of active investigation. Results from these studies have shown four important features of P3a. First, P3a habituates across successive presentations of novel items, indicating that as these stimuli become more predictable, the magnitude of P3a decreases. Second, P3a is modality unspecific – similar P3a components have been observed for novel visual, auditory and somato-sensory events. Third, although P3a is typically elicited experimentally by complex sounds, similar potentials can be derived with simple stimuli, provided that they are contextually deviant. Fourth, P3a can be elicited in ignored channel provided that the novel stimuli deviate profoundly from the background stimulation.

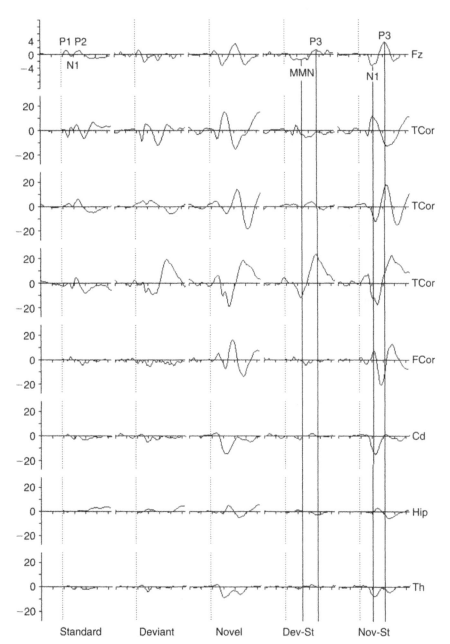

FIGURE 11.9   Variety of P3a-like activity recorded intracranially. Top – scalp recorded grand-average ERPs at Fz from a group of 20 patients with implanted electrodes. Amplitude scale 4 mcV. Below the top graph – individual intracranial ERPs. Amplitude scale 20 mcV. ERPs were recorded in the three stimulus paradigm in which standard stimuli (tones of 100 ms and 1000 Hz) were randomly interspersed with rare deviant stimuli and novel stimuli. The patients were reading a book. The difference waves between deviants and standards and novel and standards are presented in the right.

C. Diagnostic Values of P3a and P3b Components

P3a and P3b components are usually considered as indexes of attention and, for this reason, are widely used in diagnosing different brain disorders in which attentional systems are supposedly impaired. Most of the studies on ADHD report decrease of P3b component in ADHD population in comparison to norms.

In contrast to P3b applications, no consensus exists regarding usefulness of P3a component in diagnostic procedure. Some studies report no difference between ADHD and control groups (see, e.g., Jonkman et al., 2000), some studies report deviations from normality in P3a component indicating abnormal distractibility in ADHD children (see, e.g., Gumenyuk et al., 2004).

VII. SUMMARY

Attention from psychological point of view is associated with enhancement of relevant sensory information and suppression of irrelevant sensory information. Recordings of impulse activity of neurons in animal experiments showed that attention resolves the competition among multiple stimuli by counteracting the mutual inhibition between neuronal representations of simultaneously presented stimuli. In visual modality two types of attention – object-related and spatial – are implemented correspondingly in the ventral and dorsal visual streams. An impairment of spatial attention – called neglect – is associated with lesions in the right parietal cortex as a part of the dorsal stream. ERP studies in humans separate stages of information processing in the brain and show that early and late stages of the processing are modulated by attention in different ways. The early stages of information processing are associated with so-called selection negativities while the late stages are associated with so-called late positivities such as P3a and P3b components. The different modulatory effects of attention on different stages of information flow appear to be associated with tonic and phasic modes of firing of neurons in the LC. These neurons release a mediator called norepinephrine (NE). These noradrenalinergic neurons innervate the cortex widely thus modulating the early stages of sensory information flow by tonic activation of cortical neurons. This tonic modulation seems to be reflected in processing negativities of human ERPs. One of the recently developed drugs, Atomoxetine, is a NE reuptake blocker that lessens symptoms of inattention in ADHD. The NE neurons also develop strong connections with parietal and premotor areas of the cortex thus modulating the late stages of information flow by phasic activation of cortical neurons. This phasic modulation seems to be reflected in P3a and P3b components. The P3b and P3a components are widely used for discriminating the disordered brain from the healthy one.

CHAPTER 12

Executive System

*It ain't the roads we take; it's what's inside of us that makes us turn out
the way we do*

O'Henry – *The Roads We Take*

I. PSYCHOLOGY

A. Need for Executive Control

The term "executive functions" refers to the coordination and control of motor
and cognitive actions to attain specific goals. In neuropsychology, the term "executive functions" has long been used as a synonym for frontal lobe function. The
need for the executive control mechanism has been postulated for non-routine
situations requiring a supervisory system, for example, for situations for selecting
an appropriate action from variety of options, inhibition of inappropriate actions,
and keeping in working memory the plan of action as well as the results of actions.

The executive control is also needed for optimizing behavior. Deciding which
action to take is often biased by the anticipation of the action's outcome. The
mismatch between the anticipated and actual outcome is explored by the brain to
optimize and to correct behavior. For instance, if anticipated reward is not delivered the error is used for changing the previously learned behavioral pattern.

B. Types of Executive Operations

A modern view postulates several sub-components in the hypothetical executive mechanisms. In a frequently cited classification, Smith and Jonides (1999)

253

TABLE 12.1   Classification of Executive Operations

General operation	Executive function
Engagement operation	Activating neurons of the frontal–parietal cortex responsible for representation of a planned action with a goal to execute the action.
Disengagement operation	Suppressing neurons of the frontal cortex responsible for representation of a planned action with a goal to withhold from the action.
Working memory	Temporal storing the plans of actions for a few minutes to hours in order to actively use this information for engagement or disengagement operations.
Monitoring operations	Comparing the results of the executed action with a planned one with a goal to initiate a new action to eliminate the discrepancy.

distinguished between mechanisms relating to (a) attention and inhibition, (b) task management, (c) planning, (d) monitoring, and (e) coding. There is, however, no consensus regarding the number and the precise nature of the functional sub-components. Recent research has been concentrated on those sub-processes which are relatively well defined in both theoretical and empirical terms.

In this chapter we distinguish the following operations on actions: (1) selection operations such as engagement and disengagement procedures, (2) working memory, and (3) monitoring operations (see Table 12.1). These operations are well defined at psychological level. It is assumed that these different functions are subserved by different neuronal mechanisms and are reflected in different components of scalp-recorded potentials evoked by actions.

C. Association with Selection of Actions

Executive functions at neurophysiological level are defined as operations performed on representations of actions stored in the cortex. These representations are actually memories and plans of actions. The representations of actions are localized in neural networks of parietal–frontal cortical areas and, when activated, enable the access to the stored actions. Executive functions are viewed as computational procedures or algorithms of information processing that activate an appropriate action for the given time interval and for the given circumstance or suppress the representations of actions that are not needed in a given situation.

As any complex functions, the executive functions are implemented by a complex brain system that consists of several cortical and subcortical structures interconnected with each other. The cortical structures include the frontal and parietal areas. Neuronal activities in all these cortical structures are regulated by means of parallel circuits that map the corresponding cortical areas into a part of the basal ganglia, which in turn is projected to the corresponding thalamic nucleus that, in its turn, have reciprocal connections to the cortical areas.

II. BASAL GANGLIA AS DARK BASEMENTS OF THE BRAIN

A. Anatomy

The basal ganglia, as Kinnear-Wilson in the 1920s stated, have all the clarity of a dark basement. And so it has remained for the larger part of the century. Only recently mechanisms of the basal ganglia involvement in motor, cognitive, and affective actions clarified. According to the classic definition, the basal ganglia consist of five nuclei: the caudate nucleus, putamen, globus pallidus (external and internal parts), subthalamic nucleus, substantia nigra[1] (Fig. 12.1). The basal ganglia are the largest subcortical structures in the human forebrain. The input nuclei of the extended basal ganglia are the caudate nucleus and putamen (forming together the striatum) and the nucleus accumbens. These three nuclei receive inputs almost from the whole cortex except primary cortical areas. The output nucleus of the basal ganglia is the internal part of the pallidum. It sends the results of spatial remapping and temporal processing by the basal ganglia to the association thalamic nuclei. These thalamic nuclei in addition to the basal ganglia inputs receive inputs from the prefrontal cortex (PFC) and project back to the PFC. Briefly, the basal ganglia receive information from virtually all cortical areas, process it, and send the results of processing through the thalamus to the frontal cortex[2].

Each of the basal ganglia nuclei is profoundly important clinically. Degeneration of neurons in the striatum leads to Huntington's disease and related hyperkinetic disorders. Depletion of dopamine in the striatum (due to loss of dopaminergic cells in the substantia nigra) causes Parkinson's desease[3]. The excess of D2-receptors (receptors for dopamine in the striatum) is reported in schizophrenia. Attention deficit hyperactivity disorder (ADHD) is associated with excess of dopamine transporter (DAT) receptors – receptors responsible for reuptake of dopamine in the basal ganglia. The pallidum is the site of neurosurgical lesions (pallidotomy) and deep brain stimulation procedures used to relieve Parkinson's disease. The subthalamic nucleus

---

[1]The traditional boundaries of the basal ganglia had been extended in 1980 to include the nucleus accumbens (also called the ventral striatum) and the ventral pallidum.

[2]In addition to the feedback projection to the frontal cortex the basal ganglia send outputs to brainstem nuclei involved in motor control. For example, they project to the superior colliculus, which controls head and body axial orientation and saccadic eye movements.

[3]The substantia nigra, pars compacta contains dopaminergic neurons that regulate information flow through the striatum by setting neuronal thresholds.

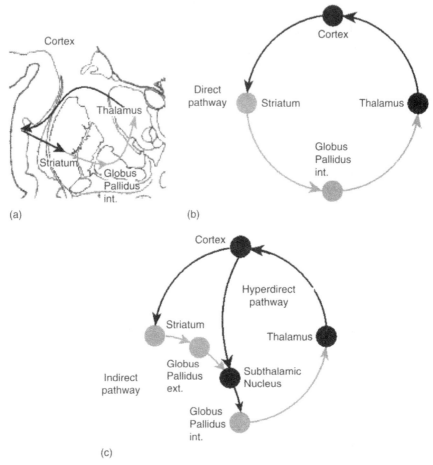

FIGURE 12.1   The basal ganglia circuits. (a) Anatomical localization of thalamus and basal ganglia at the coronal section. Basal ganglia consist of striatum and globus pallidus. Thalamus and basal ganglia are located close together. Connections between cortical areas, the basal ganglia, and thalamus are depicted by black arrows (for excitatory) and by gray arrows (for inhibitory connections). (b) A schematic representation of the direct pathway within the basal ganglia. (c) A schematic representation of indirect and hyperdirect pathways.

as a key structure controlling the function of the output nucleus of the basal ganglia (the internal part of the globus pallidus) is an increasingly favored site for deep brain stimulation in the treatment of Parkinson's disease.

B. Direct Pathway

Two pathways are separated within the basal ganglia: direct and indirect pathways. These two pathways perform different functions. The key function of the direct pathway (Fig. 12.1b) is to provide focused inhibition within output structures of the basal ganglia. The internal part of the globus pallidus as an output structure of the basal ganglia maintains inhibitory control over the thalamus (shown in Fig. 12.1a) and the brainstem motor nuclei and the superior colliculus (not shown in Fig. 12.1). In contrast to neurons in the striatum the background discharge rate of pallidal neurons is very high which provides strong inhibition to thalamic neurons[4]. The inhibition of this inhibitory effect (called disinhibition) gates thalamic neurons, that is, enables them to fire in response to external stimulation. Consequently, the direct pathway provides a positive feedback to the frontal cortex. Indeed, more activation at the frontal cortex creates more activation at the striatum and more inhibition of pallidal neurons which disinhibit thalamic neurons that in its turn creates more activation at the frontal cortex. At the thalamic level, the disinhibition operation can be compared with releasing "a brake" from the thalamic neurons. Thus the architecture of the direct pathway strongly suggests that its core function is to gate the thalamo-cortical pathway via the mechanism of disinhibition.

C. Intracranial Recordings in Patients

In our laboratory[5], we spent almost 20 years to study impulse activity of neurons and local field potentials in patients with Parkinson's disease, epilepsy, and obsessive-compulsive disorder. These investigations were performed for diagnostic and therapeutic purposes after stereotactic implantations of electrodes into target brain structures. Only those patients who did not respond to all conventional forms of treatment became subjects for stereotactic operations. Patients with implanted electrodes participated in different tasks designed to study executive functions.

When studying reactions of neurons in the basal ganglia, ventral thalamus, and the premotor cortex, we were stroked by abundance of preparatory components in those reactions, that is, components related to preparation to make a motor action or preparation to receive a stimulus. Those event-related neuronal responses were elicited only to stimuli that were of behavioral significance for subjects (Fig. 12.2).

---

[4]The spontaneous activity of neurons in the human globus pallidus is up to 200 spikes per second while the spontaneous discharges of neurons in the striatum are at very low rate – up to 20 spikes per second. This difference between the count rate of neurons is sometimes used for defining the area of the globus pallidus during stereotactic operations in order to make a lesion in the globus pallidus – the procedure similar (but more restricted) to pallidotomy.

[5]The laboratory in 1970–1990 belonged to the Institute for Experimental Medicine of the USSR Academy of Medical Sciences. Natalia Bechtereva, an outstanding Soviet and Russian neurophysiologist, initiated this field of research by combining several methods of brain research (such as recordings of impulse activity of neurons, local field potentials, and infraslow oscillations as well as observing the results of electrical stimulation on the human behavior) into a complex approach.

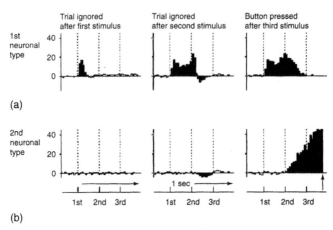

FIGURE 12.2   Two types of neuronal responses in basal ganglia–thalamocortical loop. (a) Example of neuron processing sensory information. (b) Example of neuron participating in motor preparation. Horizontal axis – time, vertical axis – frequency of neuronal discharge (relative values). In each trial of the behavioral task performed by the Parkinsonian patient with implanted electrodes, a set of three stimuli was presented (bottom): 1st – first stimulus defining whether the subject was to wait for the second stimulus or to ignore the whole trial; 2nd – second stimulus defining whether the subject should or should not press a button; 3rd – trigger stimulus serving as a signal for the subject to respond. Adapted from Kropotov et al. (1999).

The other striking feature of neuronal responses at the thalamic level was opposite responses observed in response to GO and NOGO cues. GO cues usually activated thalamic neurons with latencies longer than 200 ms, while NOGO cues inhibited the same neurons (Fig. 12.3). Those neuronal reactions were often accompanied by antagonistic fluctuations of local field potentials in response to GO and NOGO cues.

On the basis of the data obtained in our studies the theory of action programming was introduced (Kropotov, 1989)[6]. According to this theory the basal ganglia thalamo-cortical circuits play a critical role in action selection. Schematic representation of the theory is presented in Fig. 12.4.

D. The Model of Action Selection

Let us imagine a behavioral situation when it is necessary to select an action from the whole repertoire of possible actions – for example, to turn to the left or to

[6]An extensive review of the studies carried out in our laboratory is given in a paper published in 1999 (Kropotov and Etlinger, 1999). Dr. Susan Etlinger in those days was at the University of Vienna. She made her PhD studies concerning infraslow oscillations from implanted electrodes in neurological patients in our laboratory during 1984–1986.

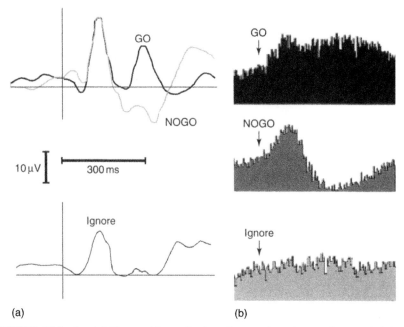

(a)   (b)

FIGURE 12.3   Local field potentials as reflection of neuronal reactions in the ventral thalamus. (a) Intracranial ERPs. (b) Responses of thalamic neurons to GO, NOGO, and Ignore stimuli in the three stimulus GO/NOGO paradigm (described in Fig. 12.2) At (a) Y-axis – averaged potentials recorded from an electrode implanted into the ventral part of the thalamus for GO (black line), NOGO (gray line), and Ignore (at the bottom) conditions. At (b) Y-axis – averaged impulse activity of neuron recorded from the same electrode. X-axis – time (unpublished data from the archive of the author's laboratory).

the right at a crossroad. The spatially distributed activities corresponding to cortical representations of the two actions (referred to as programs) are schematically shown in Fig. 12.4 (top, right). These activations are substantially overlapped in the premotor–motor cortical space (horizontal axis – spatial distance). As our data indicate, each distributed neuronal network corresponding to a distinct action is projected to a distinct area of the striatum[7]. In the figure, two programs overlapping at the cortical level are projected onto different zones of the striatum. Therefore, the striatum itself represents a map of actions.

Output neurons of the striatum are inhibitory. They are projected to the globus pallidus and at the same time send their collaterals to other striatal neurons thus performing lateral inhibition within the striatum[8]. The lateral inhibition allows

[7]This property is labeled as segregation of actions which means that representations of distinct actions are mapped into distinct parts of the striatum.

[8]From the theory of neuronal networks (see Methods of Part II) we know that the lateral inhibition, together with non-linear features of neurons, allows selecting a most activated input according to the principle "the winner takes all." As the data from our intracranial recordings show, striatal neurons

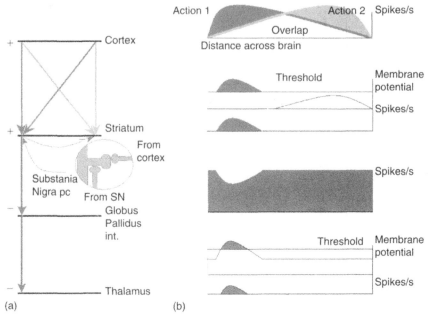

FIGURE 12.4   Action selection in the basal ganglia thalamo-cortical circuit. (a) Schematic representation of neurons in the cortex, striatum, globus pallidus, and thalamus with connections between them. +: excitatory connections, −: inhibitory connections. In insertion – dendrite of a striatal neuron with a distal synapse from a glutamatergic cortical neuron and proximal synapse from dopaminergic neuron of the substantia nigra. (b) Schematic representation of spatial activation patterns at different levels of the circuit. At the cortical level – overlapping representations of two actions are activated. At the striatal level – two overlapping programs are mapped into distinct parts of the striatum. Because of strong lateral inhibition in the striatum, only one of the programs is selected according to "winner takes all" principle. At the pallidal level – spontaneously active neurons corresponding to the selected program are inhibited. At the thalamic level the corresponding neurons are disinhibited and gate the thalamo-cortical pathway for intensifying the selected program of action. X-axis – space. Threshold – a threshold of firing neurons. Adapted from Kropotovand Etlinger (1999).

the striatum to perform a specific filtering according to the principle "winner takes all." The filtering selects only highly activated representations of potential actions and blocks less activated (i.e., less important for the current situation) ones.

E. Dopamine as Modulator in the Basal Ganglia

The threshold of spiking the output striatal neurons is defined by dopamine released in the striatum from neurons of the substantia nigra pas compacta. These

---

are almost "silent," exhibiting a low level activity, when a subject is awake. One of the reasons for such low spontaneous activity is strong feedforward and lateral inhibition generated by inhibitory striatal neurons. In Fig. 12.4 these inhibitory connections are shown by arrows within the striatum.

dopaminergic neurons in the substantia nigra project to the proximal parts of synaptic spines[9] and are in position to strongly modulate cortical inputs that are ended up at distal parts of the same spines (see insertion in Fig. 12.4). The dopamine receptors of the direct pathway are D2-receptors. They are excitatory receptors and slowly depolarize striatal neurons. The output neurons react only to the inputs that exceed the membrane threshold. The event of exceeding the threshold occur when the striatal neurons are selectively depolarized by inputs from the cortex (while the neighboring neurons are inhibited) and are globally depolarized by dopaminergic projections from substantia nigra[10]. Thus, by means of inhibitory lateral connections the striatum forms a basis for action selection. In its turn, the dopamine facilitates the selection operation by lowering the threshold of activation of striatal neurons. In particular, at Parkinson's disease this threshold is too high due to dopamine deficit so that initiation of action is quite difficult. On the contrary, at schizophrenia the threshold of the striatal neurons is abnormally low due to high concentration of dopamine receptors in the striatum, leading to simultaneous activation of several programs and to disintegration of consciousness[11].

F. Disinhibition of Thalamic Neurons

The striatal neurons belonging to the selected program project onto a corresponding area of the complex the globus pallidus/substantia nigra and inhibit its neurons. Neurons of the globus pallidus/substantia nigra in contrast to striatal ones, spontaneously discharge at a very high rate. Consequently, the selected action activates low rate striatal neurons and inhibits high rate neurons in the globus pallidus.

Neurons of the globus pallidus, in their turn, project on the thalamus. These projections are inhibitory. Since pallidal neurons are spontaneously active they have persistent inhibitory effect on thalamic neurons. When neurons of globus pallidus are inhibited, that is, their impulse activity reduced, thalamic neurons become disinhibited and thalamo-cortical path becomes opened. So, the thalamus functions as a gate to the cortex that is opened by the selected action. Using the searchlight metaphor of Francis Crick (Crick, 1984), we can say that the thalamus functions similarly to a searchlight that highlights, intensifies the selected program in the cortex.

---

[9]Spine is a little knob attached by smaller neck to the surface of dendrites.

[10]Recall that dopaminergic neurons in the substania nigra respond to behaviorally meaningful stimuli, in particular, to rewards, thus enabling only relevant programs to be selected. The phasic and tonic properties of dopaminergic transmission in the striatum are differently impaired in different brain diseases, such as Parkinson's disease, schizophrenia, and ADHD.

[11]The name schizophrenia comes from the Greek word schizophreneia, meaning "split mind." It is a psychiatric disorder that is characterized by impairments in the perception or expression of reality and by significant social or occupational dysfunction. A person experiencing schizophrenia is typically demonstrating disorganized thinking, delusions, or hallucinations.

Why the nature has created such a complicated mechanism for selecting actions? According to our theory (Kropotov, 1989) this mechanisms is a consequence of inability the brain to activate (highlight) one action and to inhibit another at the cortical level. The point is that all large scale intercortical connections are excitatory and cortical inhibition is performed only locally[12]. So, the brain uses an additional mechanism allowing it to perform selection at the subcortical level while the selected program is highlighted at the cortical level.

G. Indirect and Hyperdirect Pathways

The basal ganglia thalamo-cortical loops participate not only in initiating selected, relevant actions but also in inhibiting irrelevant actions. This operation is performed via the indirect pathway. These are pathways in the basal ganglia thalamo-cortical circuits that provide effects opposite to those of the direct pathway (Fig. 12.1). Their common function is to suppress irrelevant actions.

The key neuronal mechanism of the indirect pathway is to provide focused excitation within the output structures of the basal ganglia which maintain inhibitory control over executive subcortical and cortical structures. The excitation of the internal part of the globus pallidus can, for example, inhibit a prepared motor program directly by suppressing brainstem motor nuclei and superior colliculus and indirectly by inhibiting thalamic neurons that project to premotor cortical areas. The dopamine modulates the indirect pathway but in an opposite way in comparison to the direct pathway. In the striatum the starting point of the indirect pathway is controlled by D1 receptors (recall that the direct pathway involves D2 receptors). The D1 receptors work as inhibitory by hyperpolarizing the striatal neurons. Thus dopamine inhibits information flow in the indirect pathway (while facilitates information flow in the direct pathway).

The hyperdirect pathway conveys excitatory effects from the cortical areas to the globus pallidus, bypassing the striatum, with shorter conduction times in comparison to indirect pathway. Its function might be to suppress all irrelevant actions while selecting the relevant action via the direct pathway.

H. Output to the Brain Stem

Basal ganglia disorders are manifested not only by an inability to initiate and terminate voluntary movements, but also by an inability to suppress involuntary movements. In addition, the basal ganglia disorders are also characterized by an

---

[12]Recall that inhibitory neurons within the cortex have very short axons that can exert inhibition only locally.

abnormality in the velocity and the amount of movement, and an abnormal muscle tone. The basal ganglia seem to control the gate and muscle tone through the motor networks in the brainstem where fundamental neuronal networks for controlling postural muscle tone and locomotor movements are located.

I. Parallel Circuits

Almost any cortical area except primary sensory cortical areas projects to the striatum. The most dense projections are from the prefrontal areas. Roughly these cortical–striatal projections could be considered as topographic. However those projections are topographic only at first approximation. More detailed analysis shows that terminals of cortical axons directed from the cortex to the basal ganglia form local mosaic patterns in the striatum allowing any cortical neuron to project on spatially distinct areas of the striatum. At the same time, areas of the cortex that are connected functionally by means of intracortical connections project to the same zone of the striatum. In other words, the striatum represents a functional map of cortex rather than its topographic projection. In this functional map, neurons that are interconnected functionally are topographically projected on a certain area of the striatum[13].

Several functionally different parallel paths participating in cortical regulation in the basal ganglia thalamo-cortical circuits are selected. Each of these pathways is presented at the levels of the cortex, striatum, globus pallidus, and thalamus in specific and spatially distinct areas. Alexander and DeLong on the basis of their anatomical and physiological studies in 1980s separated the following parallel paths: motor, spatial, visual, and affective (Fig. 12.5). Each of these circuits occupies a specific portion in the striatum and receives multiple, partially overlapping inputs from several anatomically related cortical areas associated with the same function. According to their names the parallel pathways are involved in execution and planning of motor actions (motor), organization of spatial and object working memories (spatial, visual) and maintaining motivations and emotions (affective)[14].

The motor pathway regulates activity of motor, premotor, and supplementary motor cortical areas and surpasses through the putamen. It also receives inputs from the somato-sensory cortex. This circuit participates in initiation and suppression of

---

[13]The data obtained in my laboratory support this idea. Indeed, in our studies in patients with implanted electrodes we show that neurons responsible for sensory functions and those responsible for motor functions are spatially separated, or segregated, at the striatal level.

[14]As noted above, the processes maintained by the basal ganglia include planning of actions, initiation, and suppression of the corresponding actions, and storage of the results of actions in working memory. These operations altogether are unified by a single concept of executive functions and are implemented by the basal ganglia thalamo-cortical circuits parallel circuits.

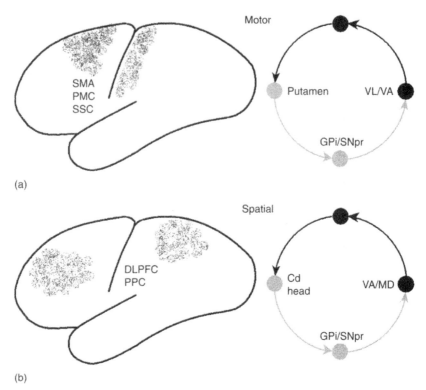

FIGURE 12.5   Parallel pathways in the basal ganglia thalamo-cortical circuits. From (a–c): motor, spatial, visual, and affective corticostriatal loops with the functions of execution and planning of motor actions (motor), organization of spatial and object working memories (spatial, visual) and maintaining motivations and emotions (affective). Abbreviations: SMA, supplementary motor area; PMC, premotor cortex; SSC, somato-sensory cortex; DLPFC, dorso-lateral prefrontal cortex; PPC, posterior parietal cortex; VLPFC, ventro-lateral prefrontal cortex; IT, inferior temporal cortex; ST, superior temporal gyrus; OFC, orbitofrontal cortex; CG, anterior cingulate; HC, hippocampus; Am, amygdala; VP, ventral pallidum; GPi, internal segment of the globus pallidus; SNpr, substantia nigra, pars reticulata; VP, ventral pallidum; VL, ventro-lateral thalamus; VA, ventral anterior thalamus; MD, mediodorsal thalamus; STN, subthalamic nucleus; GPe, external segment of globus pallidus. Note that distinct circuits involve different parts of the above mentioned nuclei. Adapted from Alexander et al. (1986).

motor actions, as well as in preparation of them. Sometimes the occulomotor circuit is separated from the motor cicuit. The occulomotor circuit regulates activity of the frontal cortex responsible for eye movements (frontal eye fields). It also receives inputs from the posterior parietal cortex (parietal eye fields). This path participates in enabling orientation of the eyes and body toward the selected source of sensory information.

The spatial pathway regulates activity of the dorso-lateral prefrontal cortex and posterior parietal cortex. This circuit seems to be responsible for maintaining working memory for spatial cues.

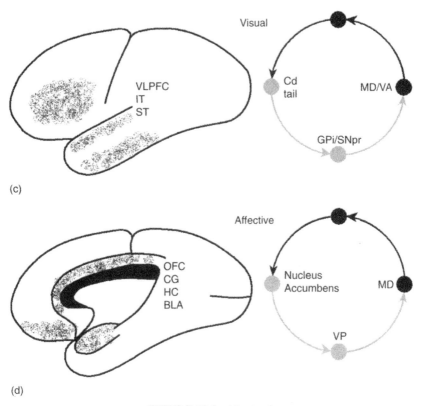

(c)

(d)

FIGURE 12.5   (*Continued*)

The visual pathway regulates activity in the ventro-lateral PFC and the lateral temporal cortex. This circuit seems to regulate working memory for objects, especially for visual objects.

Affective circuit regulates activity of the anterior cingulate cortex (ACC) and surpasses through the nucleus accumbens. It also receives inputs from the medial orbitofrontal cortex and the limbic allocortex (including hippocampus and entorhinal cortex). This circuit seems to be responsible for regulation of mood and emotional reactions.

Beside projecting to the ventral, dorso-medial, and anterior-ventral nuclei of the thalamus, the basal ganglia project also to the midline and intralaminar nuclei. In addition, these nuclei receive strong input from the cholinergic neurons of the brain stem reticular formation and project back to the basal ganglia as well as to widely distributed cortical areas. High frequency stimulation of the midline and intralaminar nuclei leads to desynchronization of the cortical electroencephalogram (EEG) accompanied by arousal. By contrast, low frequency stimulation of the same nuclei results in gradually developing slow waves and spindle bursts associated with inattention, drowsiness, and sleep.

J. EEG in Basal Ganglia Dysfunction

The basal ganglia circuits deal with actions. From theoretical point of view, activation of the corresponding parallel circuit in the basal ganglia thalamo-cortical pathway activates the corresponding frontal area and desynchronizes the cortical EEG. Vise versa, lesions in these circuits must lead to synchronization of slow oscillations in the cortical areas. These theoretical inferences are supported by experimental findings.

Indeed, lesions in the caudate nucleus and putamen of monkeys are shown to increase regular high amplitude waves with frequencies between 5 and 10 Hz. Similar findings are found in Parkinson's disease, irrespective of age or presence of dementia (Fig. 12.6). The degree of slowing of EEG is correlated with degree of motor disability in general and akinesia, in particular. Event-related desynchronization

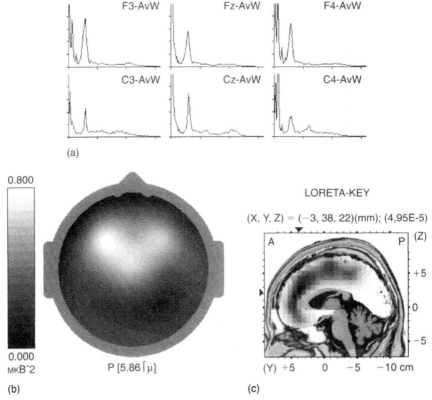

FIGURE 12.6   EEG spectra of a Parkinsonian patient. Power spectra (a) with peaks in the theta range, (b) a map, and (c) an LORETA image of theta rhythm (6 Hz) in a patient at early stage of Parkinson's disease.

(ERD) in response to voluntary movements in Parkinson's patients is also reduced. These changes are reversed by levodopa.

III. PREFRONTAL CORTEX AND EXECUTIVE CONTROL

A. Anatomy

The frontal lobes comprise about one third of the cerebral cortex in humans. The border with the parietal cortex is marked by the central sulcus, while the temporal lobe is separated by the Sylvian fissure. The frontal lobe is not a unitary structure. It consists of three broad subdivisions: the primary motor cortex (BA 4) – electrical stimulation of which produces muscular contractions and simple movements, the premotor and supplementary motor cortex (BA 6), anterior portion of the cingulate cortex and the remainder – the prefrontal cortex (PFC). The PFC is reciprocally connected with dorso-medial nucleus of the thalamus, the premotor cortex receives inputs and projects back to the lateral thalamic nuclei, the cingulate has reciprocal connections with the anterior nucleus of the thalamus.

Although it is clear that the PFC is important for higher cognitive skills, particularly in humans, it is still unclear how it achieves these functions. The neural architecture of human PFC is probably more sophisticated in comparison to other cortical areas to accommodate higher cognitive functions that are superior in humans than in other species[15].

The PFC receives multimodal sensory and limbic input from several pathways which project on discrete prefrontal subdivisions. Figure 12.7 schematically depicts information flow within the ventral visual pathway to the ventro-lateral PFC. In contrast to topographical projections between posterior cortical areas, projections to the prefrontal areas are not topographical in a strict sense. Instead, the same retinal location or eye movement direction is represented multiple times across the prefrontal cortical surface. Anatomical evidence suggests a highly regular pattern of axonal terminations from the posterior association cortices to the prefrontal areas, forming repeating, interdigitated stripes[16].

---

[15]The primate prefrontal cortex is defined as the cortex anterior to the arcuate sulcus. Roughly, it can be subdivided into three major divisions: lateral, medial, and orbital aspects. The lateral prefrontal cortex is further divided into: dorso-lateral PFC and ventro-lateral PFC. The medial prefrontal cortex is divided into anterior cingulate cortex and the medial frontal cortex. The orbitofrontal cortex is divided into medial, ventral, lateral, and frontopolar portions.

[16]Why would the representation of a stimulus or a motor target be replicated multiple times across the prefrontal cortex? Although no definitive answer is currently available, theoretical studies provide some possible explanations. The brain is able to flexibly generate variable responses to identical stimuli depending on the context in which they appear. The absence of a one-to-one correspondence between sensory stimuli and motor responses makes the replication of stimulus representations in the prefrontal cortex inevitable.

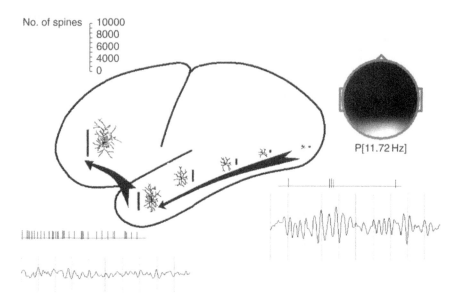

FIGURE 12.7   Increase of "complexity" from the visual to the prefrontal cortex. Neurons in monkey visual areas V1, V2, V4, temporal areas (TEO and TE) and PFC are illustrated to show differences in the size and branching patterns of their basal dendritic arbours. The number of individual dendritic spines of the "average" layer III pyramidal cell in each area is illustrated in solid vertical bars (with scale at the top). Adapted from Elston (2003). Neurons in occipital areas reveal activation in response to stimuli, while neurons in the prefrontal area show high frequency spontaneous activity. EEG of a human subject reveals alpha activity at occipital sites which is absent (or significantly reduced) at the prefrontal area.

B. Complexity of Wiring

Pioneers in comparative neuroscience were impressed by the similarity of the cerebral cortex in mammalian species. Unfortunately, "similar" was interpreted by many as the "same." As a result it became widely accepted during the latter part of the last century that the cerebral cortex is uniform in structure, the whole of cortex (with the exception of the primary visual areas) being composed of the same basic repeated units. In keeping with this dogma, regional differences in cortical function such as vision, somato-sensation, and hearing, were attributed solely to the source of their inputs and outputs.

The first evidence against equipotentiality came from studies in sensory systems. In 1980–1990 the research showed that monkeys have as many as 30 cortical visual areas. More recent research in the last 10 years showed that not only input/output connections characterize the specificity of information processing in these cortical visual areas. The information processing is also determined by the structure (such as spine density and branching patterns of dendrites and axons) of cells in these visual areas. Moreover, the intracortical structure was found to be different for different areas. For example, Layer III pyramidal cells in macaque area TE contain, on average, 11 times more spines in their basal dendritic arbors than those in macaque V1. The same is true for areas in the frontal lobe: pyramidal cells in PFC of man and macaques are, in general, more branched and more spinous than their counterparts in the occipital, parietal, and temporal lobes (Fig. 12.7).

C. Representation of Complex Actions

The PFC projects to motor areas and from this perspective might store complex representations of actions. The dorso-lateral PFC is thought to be evolved from motor regions. It seems reasonable, therefore, that the functions of the "newer" prefrontal regions would be related to those of the older motor areas. A recent discovery of mirror neurons, neurons that fire in response to both internally generated and observed actions preformed by other subjects, supports this view.

It should be stressed that the PFC is associated not with actions themselves but with executive functions, that is, functions that control execution of actions. The complexity of human behavior is associated with complexity of human actions. The extent to which subregions of the PFC are functionally differentiated, that is, the extent to which different cognitive functions can be mapped to discrete regions of PFC, remains controversial. On the one hand, situations that require cognitive control often elicit co-occurring activations in dorso-lateral PFC, ventro-lateral and medial PFC. On the other hand, at the risk of engaging in neophrenology, distinct subdivisions of PFC can be considered essential for implementing distinct cognitive control functions, which interact to facilitate task performance[17].

D. Hyperfrontality

Differences in neuronal structure specify properties of neuronal discharges. In monkey Joaquin Fuster (Fuster, 1990) revealed that the discharge properties of neurons in V1 differed from those in inferotemporal (IT) cortex, those in the former being characterized by phasic discharge properties whereas those in the latter are characterized by tonic activity[18] (Fig. 12.7). This persistent neural activity, associated with working memory, is manifested in a *hyperfrontality* – a feature that indicates more

---

[17]Yet, even when we acknowledge some degree of functional specialization within PFC, it cannot be a true statement claiming that any region within PFC maintains one function only. For instance, ventrolateral PFC has been argued to be involved in response inhibition, in task switching, procedural memory, and episodic memory retrieval.

[18]The first electrophysiological evidence of involving the prefrontal cortex in executive functions in the human was obtained by an English scientist Grey Walter in 1964 (see Walter, 1967). He discovered the contingent negative variation (CNV), a slow negative potential recorded from the anterior part of the head during preparation of subjects to receive a stimulus or to make a movement.

activation of the frontal lobe in comparison to the rest of the cortex. This feature was discovered by a Swedish scientist David Ingvar in 1970s (for review see Ingvar, 1985).

E. EEG Peculiarity

The differences between anterior and posterior regions are also observed in EEG (Fig. 12.7). Spectral characteristic of frontal and posterior EEG recordings are different. Idling alpha rhythms are observed only in central–posterior regions. In the normal brain alpha rhythms are absent in the frontal regions. Early (around up to 200 ms) ERP associated with visual information processing are found in occipital–temporal recordings, while late positive components associated with engagement operations and monitoring of actions are observed in frontal–parietal recordings.

IV. ENGAGEMENT/DISENGAGEMENT OPERATIONS

A. P3b Component as Index of Engagement Operation

P3b component or better to say P3b components[19] were analyzed in detail in Chapter 11 when we were talking about ERP components characterizing attentional networks. Although the highest density of generators of the conventional P3b component are located in the parietal cortex and strictly speaking in this respect the P3b component belongs to ERP indexes of attentional networks, a complex system including frontal/temporal/parietal areas together with the basal ganglia – thalamo-cortical circuits is involved in generation of the P3b component.

B. Sensory Comparison

In our daily life we always are looking forward[20] and are preparing to make further actions. However, the contextual content of the environment is rapidly changing, and in some cases the prepared action must be suppressed. The inhibition of prepared action is performed by a complex brain circuit with the lateral PFC as a part. As we learnt above, the PFC receives the sensory information from the sensory systems (visual, auditory, and somato-sensory) and is in position to make decision whether to GO or NOGO depending on the results. One can

---

[19]Note that P3b is actually a family of components that are elicited in response to targets. They have different distribution (from parietal to premotor and different dynamics).

[20]As a famous Russian poet Alexander Pushkin wrote "The heart lives in the future ..."

speculate that to inhibit a prepared action, the brain must first compare the current sensory situation with the sensory model and to detect the mismatch. From the above we learnt that the comparison operations of sensory signals take place in the posterior sensory systems. We can further speculate that the result of these comparison operations is transferred to the PFC to activate the circuits responsible for inhibition of the prepared action.

This speculation is supported by results of independent component analysis (ICA) performed on ERPs computed for GO and NOGO cues in the two stimulus GO/NOGO task (Fig. 12.8). As one can judge from Fig. 12.8 NOGO and GO cues evoke quite different components generated in the temporal and premotor areas. In the temporal cortex, NOGO cues evoke an additional component in comparison to GO cues while in the left premotor cortex NOGO and GO cues elicit opponent reactions. The difference in time dynamics of the two components for GO and NOGO cues shows that the components are functionally different. We can speculate that the first component characterized by positivity at the temporal area is associated with the sensory comparison operation – change detection (see also Fig. 10.16).

C. Motor Inhibition

We can also suggest that the second component generated in the left premotor cortex is associated with motor suppression. If one compares behavior of this component with time patterns of thalamic evoked potentials (see Fig. 12.3) one can notice striking similarity of this scalp recorded component with the local field potentials at the thalamic level. This resemblance, as well as location of the generators of this component, supports our suggestion[21]. Note that the motor inhibition component is negative in the frontal areas.

As we learned from the above, neuronal mechanisms of motor inhibition involve the basal ganglia circuits. The point is that within the cortex all long distance connections are excitatory while intracortical inhibition is of a local character and could not be responsible for suppression of action as a whole. The inhibition of the prepared action seems to be performed by means of the indirect pathway of the basal ganglia thalamo-cortical loop[22] with a cortical location in the premotor cortex.

---

[21]Note that the early part of the component (associated with the initial stage of motor suppression) increases in latency with aging.

[22]I recall a Parkinsonian patient in our clinic who was having difficulties in crossing the street at cross-roads with lights. He said "I know that I must stop at the red light" (so, the decision making was not impaired in him)"… but simply can not stop walking" (so, the suppression operation is impaired!!!) which is implemented partly through the basal ganglia-thalamo-cortical loop.

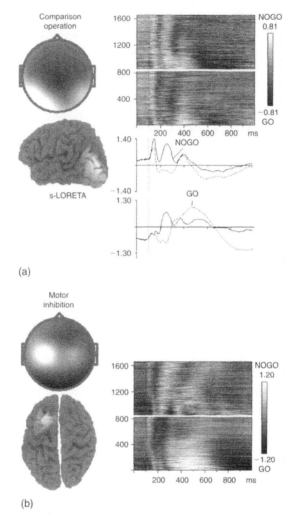

FIGURE 12.8   Reflection of sensory comparison and motor inhibition operations in ERPs independent components. ICA was performed on ERPs in GO and NOGO conditions in the visual two stimulus GO/NOGO task. ERPs of healthy subjects of age from 7 to 89 were taken from the Human Brain Institute Normative Database. (a) Comparison component. (b) Motor inhibition component. Vertically stacking thin color-coded horizontal bars, each representing the corresponding component for a single subject, are depicted for GO and NOGO conditions. Topographies, s-LORETA, images and time courses of components are depicted separately for each component and for GO and NOGO cues.

D. Action Suppression

The intriguing part of ICA of ERPs data in GO/NOGO task is the existence of the third component elicited by NOGO cues (Fig. 12.8). Spatial distribution, temporal pattern, and contrast to GO cues are different from the previous components. This component has only one prominent peak with latency of 340 ms. It is a symmetrical component with generators widely distributed over premotor and motor cortical areas. It is present only in NOGO condition. It is decreased in amplitude and increased in latency with aging. Note also that this component is negative in the frontal areas. We have named this component as the action suppression component to distinguish it from the asymmetrical motor inhibition component. We do not know why the brain generates this component after production of the specific motor suppression component. We also do not know whether it is generated by means of basal ganglia thalamo-cortical loops or generated purely within the cortex. But what we do know is that this component is almost 3 times larger than the motor inhibition component and, for this reason, seems to have a superior diagnostic power than the motor suppression component. There is also another explanation of this component: it might represent a P3a-like component which is elicited in unexpected condition.

E. Intracranial Recordings

In patients with implanted electrodes we were able to record intracranial ERPs in the two stimulus GO/NOGO task in auditory modality. Electrodes were implanted for diagnosis and therapy into different cortical and subcortical areas. In Parkinsonian patients electrodes were located in the basal/ganglia thalamus, in epileptic patients they were located in the medial (including hippocampus) and lateral temporal areas. In patients with obsessive-compulsive disorder electrodes were implanted into ACC and adjacent prefrontal areas. Figure 12.9 represents ERPs for two electrodes: one located in the temporal lobe and the other one located in the PFC. Patients performed an auditory version of the two stimulus GO/NOGO paradigm. As one can see the neuronal network in the temporal lobe responds to NOGO cues with a negative/positive component with corresponding latencies at 100 and 200 ms. The neuronal network in the frontal lobe also responds to NOGO cues with a similar pattern but with latencies 150 ms longer than in the temporal lobe. Note that ERPs in the temporal lobe reveal also components at latencies as early as 70 ms. However these early components did not differ between GO and NOGO cues and seems to be associated with sensory perception. In contrast, the frontal lobe exhibited only late components which were prominent only in response to NOGO cues[23]. Comparing intracranial data with scalp recorded ERPs we can conclude that in this particular case the local field potentials in the temporal lobe reflect comparison operation in the auditory modality while local field potentials in the prefrontal lobe reflect some late latency executive operation.

---

[23]Here we want to remind that intracranial ERPs (also called local field potentials) are quite local and may differ between each other at distances of few millimeters.

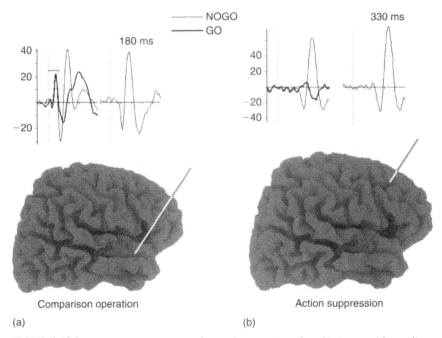

FIGURE 12.9   Comparison operation and executive operation reflected in intracranial recordings. Intracranial ERPs were recorded in patients to whom electrodes were implanted for diagnosis and therapy. Patients participated in the auditory two stimulus GO/NOGO task. Electrodes were located in the association auditory cortex (left) and in the dorso-lateral PFC (right). Intracranial ERPs for GO, NOGO and NOGO–GO conditions are depicted. Bottom – location of electrodes.

In humans, besides the GO/NOGO paradigm a stop-signal task (SST) is used to study action suppression. Similar to the GO/NOGO tasks the SSTs require suppression of ongoing actions only after presentation of the stop signal. Empirical imaging data obtained in the last years in these two paradigms indicate that the ventro-lateral PFC[24] plays a critical role in action inhibition. In ontogeny, it is the last brain area to develop, so that immature development of this part of the cortex might explain syndrome of impulsivity at least in some sub-groups of ADHD children. As studies by Adam Aron[25] from University of Cambridge, in UK show, extent of damage to the right ventro-lateral PFC, but not other regions, correlated with a response-inhibition measure (indexed by stop-signal reaction time): greater damage leads to slower inhibition.

[24]The ventro-lateral prefrontal cortex (sometimes named as inferior frontal cortex) in humans comprises Brodmann areas 44, 45, and 47/12.
[25]For review see Aron et al. (2004).

F. N200 Motor Inhibition Component

Research in neuronal mechanisms of motor inhibition started in 1970s. The most influential discoveries were made by Japanese scientists Gemba and Sasaki (Gemba and Sasaki, 1989, 1990). They found a specific premotor/motor cortical circuit involved in motor suppression. For example, they showed in monkeys that excitation of cells in the principle sulcus during regular responses yielded a decrease of activity in primary motor cortex and either a delay or the complete suppression of responses while direct electric stimulation of this area suppressed a prepared response to GO stimulus. In humans neural mechanisms underlying inhibitory processes were investigated by recording ERPs from the scalp. A frontally distributed negative ERP component, called N200 NOGO that peaks at about 200–260 ms poststimulus has been observed in numerous studies. This component had greater amplitude for NOGO in comparison to GO stimuli and was associated with response inhibition in GO–NOGO paradigms. A similar N2 component was also observed in response to stop signals. Note that in all classical studies the N2 component was separated simply as a difference between ERPs for GO and NOGO cues.

Below we are going to show that the classical N2 component is also found in our data. It is elicited after NOGO cues and expressed in frontally distributed negativity. Figure 12.10 represents ERPs recorded at Fz in the same group of healthy subjects as in Figs 12.8 and 12.11 in the two stimulus GO/NOGO paradigm. As one can see, NOGO cues elicit a strong negative wave with peak latency at 260 ms similar to one observed in the above mentioned classical studies. The minimum of the negative part of the difference wave is located near Fz. The negative fluctuation is followed by a positive component with the frontal distribution. If one compares the ERPs in this Fig. 12.10 with three independent components depicted in Figs 12.8 and 12.11 one can notice that the negative fluctuation in raw ERPs is actually a sum of negative fluctuations generated in three different components (Figs 12.8 and 12.11) revealed by ICA[26].

This association between raw ERPs and their independent components in this example allows us to make at least two conclusions. First, the power of ICA in discriminating separate psychological operations is superior to conventional methods of ERP analysis such as constructing ERP difference waves. The ICA provides decomposition of ERPs into several independent components each of them having specific temporal–spatial pattern and specific functional meaning. Second, independent components represent better endopenotypes than raw ERPs and might be used with a better success in diagnosis of different brain dysfunctions associated with impairments in specific operations such as comparison, motor inhibition, and action suppression operations.

---

[26]Note that only the motor inhibition and action suppression components are associated with negativity having minimum at Fz, while the comparison component is characterized by minimum of negativity at Cz.

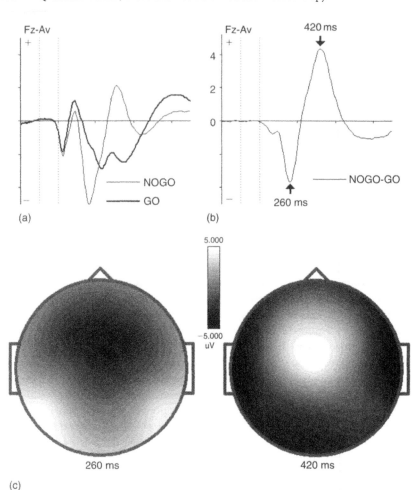

FIGURE 12.10   N200 motor inhibition wave. ERPs are averaged over the group of healthy subjects of age from 7 to 89 were taken from the Human Brain Institute Normative Database. (a) ERPs for GO and NOGO cues in the two stimulus GO/NOGO task for Fz location. (b) Difference wave (NOGO–GO). (c) Maps of ERPs difference waves computed for two different moments.

V. MONITORING OPERATION

A. P400 Monitoring Component in GO/NOGO Paradigm

NOGO-related independent components are not confined by the above mentioned components which are associated with activation of the temporal (for the

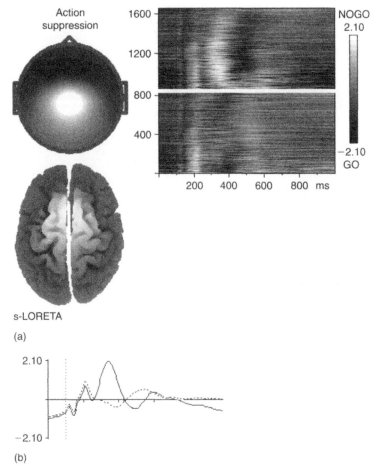

FIGURE 12.11   Reflection of action suppression in ERP independent components. ICA was performed on ERPs in GO and NOGO conditions. Healthy subjects of age from 7 to 89 were taken from the Human Brain Institute Normative Database. (a) Topography and s-LORETA image. Vertically stacking thin color-coded horizontal bars, each representing the corresponding component for a single subject, are depicted for GO, NOGO. The time courses of components are depicted at (b).

sensory comparison operation), premotor/motor (for the suppression operations) cortical areas. Actually, the largest in amplitude NOGO component is generated (according to s-LORETA) in medial prefrontal and anterior cingulate cortical areas (Fig. 12.12). It is a symmetrical positive component located centrally in the 2D space with maximum at Cz–Fz. The latency of the component changes with age significantly – from 370 ms at middle age to 420 ms at early age and 460 ms at older age.

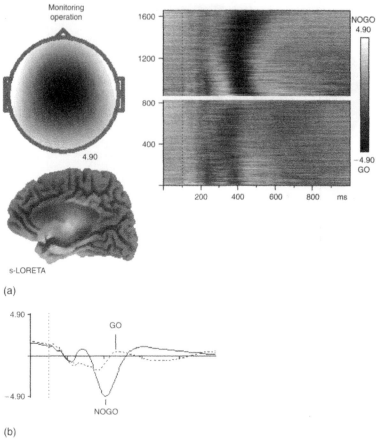

FIGURE 12.12   Monitoring operation reflected in ERPs independent component. ICA was performed on ERPs in GO and NOGO conditions. Healthy subjects of age from 7 to 89 were taken from the Human Brain Institute Normative Database. (a) Topography and s-LORETA image. Vertically stacking thin color-coded horizontal bars, each representing the corresponding component for a single subject, are depicted for GO, NOGO. The time courses of components are depicted at (b). Note that to get a scalp generated component we have to make a product of topography and time dynamics, which will result in positive component at Cz–Fz.

B. Function of ACC

The monitoring component is the one that is generated in the anterior cingulate cortex (ACC). So, it is the right place to discuss the anatomy and physiology of the ACC in detail. The ACC is not a homogenous structure. It consists of several fields with different internal morphology and different afferent (output) and efferent (input) connections. First of all, the ACC includes motor areas (see Fig. 12.13) that receive

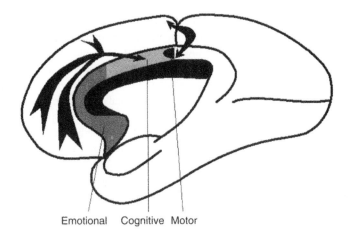

Emotional   Cognitive   Motor

FIGURE 12.13 Divisions and connections of ACC. The ACC receives reciprocal connection virtually from all areas of the PFC. The ACC is divided into three parts (marked by color) – emotional, cognitive, and motor parts.

inputs from the primary motor cortex, premotor, and supplementary motor areas. These motor areas thus store the precise image of a planned action. This part of the cingulate is also in position to initiate a new action. Second, the ventral part of the anterior cingulate receives inputs mostly from the affective (limbic) system directly (such as from the amygdala) or indirectly (via the anterior nucleus of the thalamus). For this reason the ventral portion of the ACC is called "limbic" part. Third, the dorsal part of the anterior cingulate has strong reciprocal connections with the lateral, anterior, and medial prefrontal cortical areas – areas presumably involved in cognitive functions. For this reason, the dorsal portion of the ACC is called "cognitive" part.

There is strong neuroimaging evidence supporting this anatomically based division of the ACC. Numerous positron emission tomography (PET) and functional magnetic resonance imaging (f MRI) studies show that the dorsal parts of the ACC are active in cognitive tasks while the ventral parts of the ACC are active during affective states defined by emotions and motivations. When, for example, a subject imagines angry or sad situation the ventral part of the ACC is activated[27]. On the other hand, when a subject makes an error or performing a Stroop task, the cognitive part of the ACC is activated.

C. Akinetic Mutism

In patients undergoing functional neurosurgery stimulation of the ventral part of the ACC could produce fear or pleasure depending on location, while the

[27]When, for example, phobic, OCD or posttraumatic stress syndrome patients are presented with stimuli that trigger their symptoms, these stimuli activate the ventral part of the anterior gyrus cingulate.

stimulation of the dorsal part produced a sense of anticipation of movement. Patients with medial frontal lobe lesions involving the cingulate cortex often show deficits in spontaneous initiation of movement and speech, and/or show an inability to suppress externally triggered motor subroutines[28]. Damasio and Van Hoesen have studied a series of stroke patients with large lesions of the ACC. Immediately following the stroke, such patients lie in their hospital beds saying or doing little. Antonio Damasio described one left anterior cingulate stroke patient 1 month after her stroke (Damasio, 1999): "The patient was remarkably recovered. She had considerable insight into the acute period of the illness and was able to give precious testimony as to her experiences then. Asked if she had ever experienced anguish for being apparently unable to communicate she answered negatively. She did not talk because she had nothing to say. Her mind was empty. She apparently was able to follow our conversations even during the early period of the illness, but felt no will to reply to our questions"[29]. Recently Cohen and his colleagues have studied a series of 18 patients who suffered from intractable pain and were treated with small bilateral lesions, 5 mm in diameter, in the anterior cingulated cortex. More than a year after the surgery they studied the behavior of these patients in comparison with a control group of chronic pain patients who had not received the cingulate lesions. They found that the cingulate-lesioned patients did gain relief from pain. They reported that the pain was still present but that it no longer bothered them as much[30].

D. Concept of Monitoring

What is the functional meaning of the cognitive part of the ACC? All available experimental findings indicate that the function of the dorsal part of the ACC is to monitor actions. The point is that flexible adjustments of human and animal behavior require the continuous assessment of ongoing actions and the outcomes of these actions. The ability to monitor and compare ongoing actions and performance outcomes with internal goals and standards is critical for optimizing decision making.

---

[28]Akinetic mutism, which is caused by bilateral lesions in the medial and anterior cingulate cortex, is an extreme example of this syndrome. Akinetic mutism is a medical condition of patients who tend neither to speak (mutism) nor move (akinesia). Unilateral lesions result in a milder version of mutism: spontaneous speech is scanty and, even on recovery, monotonous.

[29]I recall an attempt to record ERPs in a patient with bilateral lesions in the anterior cingulate cortex. The patient answered questions and appeared to be fully aware of her condition and hospital environment but could not perform any task. She just simply lost any interest in the task and fell asleep.

[30]The lesioned patients showed reduced levels of spontaneous behavior. They produced fewer verbal utterances during interviews than controls. In a written task, they also produced shorter statements. When asked to make objects from Tinker Toys, they produced fewer and simpler objects. Thus, the spontaneity of their behavior was reduced over the long term by these small lesions of the anterior cingulate.

This ability is called action monitoring. The ventral part of the ACC is suggested of being involved in this cognitive operation.

The concept of monitoring became highly influential in cognitive science during the last few years. The concept of monitoring must be distinguished from the concept of Attentional control. Attentional control refers to a top–down, limited-resource cognitive mechanism modulating *sensory* information processing, while the monitoring of actions refers to a cognitive mechanism that evaluates the quality of *executive* control and activates the executive system in the case of mismatch between expected and executed actions.

In order to associate a certain ERP component with the function of monitoring at least three requirements must be fulfilled. First, the component has to be of a long latency, i.e. appear after the neuronal signal for action initiation because the activation of the executed action has to be compared with the planned one. Second, the component has to be generated in an area that receives information from both the planned action and the executed one in order to compare these two signals. And, finally, the component has to occur in conflict situations when a prepared action has to be withheld because the current situation does not match the expected one or when an action has been executed but its outcome does not match the planned one. The late positive P400 component that occurs in NOGO trials, generated in the ACC fulfills these requirements and therefore can be considered as a "monitoring" component.

E. Error-Related Negativities

Monitoring operation is also studied in continuous performance tasks that are accompanied by errors in some trials[31]. Errors generate a component named error-related negativity (ERN) followed by a positive component. The negative wave is observed immediately following errors and has peak latency around 100 ms. It has a fronto–central distribution and dubbed as the error negativity (NE) or ERN. The ERN has repeatedly been modeled by a single dipole source, located in the vicinity of the ACC. In support of these dipole models, studies

---

[31]Actually, human research followed experiments in animals. In 1979 Niki and Watanabe recorded changes in the activity of single neurons of the anterior gyrus cingulate when a monkey made errors. Further studies in monkeys with recordings of single neuron activity showed that while some neurons in the anterior gyrus cingulus indeed respond when the monkey recognizes that it has made an error in the task performance some other neurons fire in response to decreasing reward in situations when the behavior must be switched to another behavioral pattern thus optimizing the receipt of reward. When neuronal activity in the ACC was temporally silenced by injection of GABA agonist (Shima and Tanji, 1998) monkeys failed to respond to decreasing in reward. These studies serve as an elegant prove of the involvement of the anterior cingulate cortex in monitoring performance and adjusting on the basis of the behavior to optimize payoff.

using fMRI have shown increased activation of the ventral part of the ACC during error trials relative to correct trials.

Error-related components in ERPs can be also observed in the mathematical paradigm. In this task subjects viewed brief presentations of a math operation on two numbers (such as 2 + 2) followed by a second number (say 4 or 5) with the subject's task to press a button if the second stimulus matches the result of mathematical operation (in this example, number 4) or to withhold from pressing in the

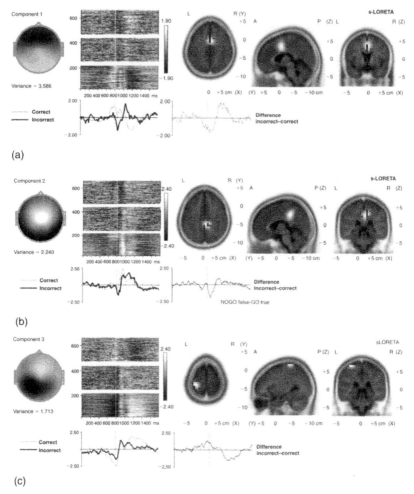

FIGURE 12.14   Error-related negativities. ICA was performed on a set of more than 200 individual ERPs taken from the Human Brain Institute Normative Database. ERP were triggered by correct and incorrect responses in the Mathematical task. The largest three independent components are presented from top to bottom. From left to right – topographies, individual color-coded vertically stalked components, and s-LORETA images. Below are components computed for superimposed correct trials (thin line), incorrect trials (think line) and separately for ERPs differences.

mismatch condition (in this example, number 5). To separate these components we need to compare two conditions: incorrect pressing to mismatch stimuli (commission errors) and correct pressing to match cues. Figure 12.14 represents the results of decomposing ERN into three independent components. The data are taken from the Human Brain Institute Normative Database. Subjects performed the mathematical task. The task is quite difficult to perform so that the subjects did a substantial number of errors. In each subject ERPs were computed for correct match trials[32] and incorrect mismatch trials[33]. Button pressing served as trigger events. The difference (incorrect–correct) waves were also computed. As one can see the ERN actually consists of two independent components, one is located in the dorsal anterior (cognitive) and the other one is located in the more posterior (motor) regions of the cingulate cortex. In addition to these two components elicited just after the incorrect motor response ERN also includes the component that starts before the motor response and is generated in the left sensory motor area of the cortex[34].

It should be noted here that the clinical use of ERN is limited for at least two reasons. First, the error is a very subjective event depending on a subject motivation, attention, and abilities of the sensory system. Because of that the number of errors in the same task but for different subjects differs substantially. Consequently, the number of "error" trials for averaging ERPs is not a constant value which has an effect on the individual parameter of ERN. Second, to get enough trials for a reliable ERN measurement the task must be quite difficult. But, some people (such as young children, Alzheimer patients) can not perform difficult tasks.

VI. WORKING MEMORY

A. Active Manipulation on Memory Trace

One of the most striking features of neurons in the PFC is their ability to fire over extended periods of time and across events, long after the event offset. This indicates that the PFC can maintain representations of stimuli and actions across time, enabling a subject to engage in behavior for achieving long-term goals. This function of the PFC is reflected in the concept of *Working Memory*. Working memory is a psychological process that enables the brain to maintain current plans of actions as well as the sensory information that is needed to execute these actions. The notion of working memory also implies an active manipulation with the temporary stored information which is the core of cognitive actions such as language, planning, decision making, etc.

---

[32]Recall that these are trials in which the second stimulus matched the sum of two numbers presented in the first stimulus and the subject correctly pressed a button.

[33]Recall that these are trials in which the second stimulus mismatched the sum of two numbers presented in the first stimulus while the subject incorrectly pressed a button.

[34]Recall that activation of the left sensory motor cortex corresponds to the fact that most of the subjected pressed the button by one of the right hand fingers.

B. Reciprocal Anatomical Pathways

From neurophysiological point of view, working memory is based on multiple reciprocal connections within the cortex. These reciprocal connections form a basis for reverberation of neuronal activity after the offset of a stimulus or an action. The connections include feedback and feedforward pathways within the cortex itself as well as feedback loops of the basal ganglia thalamo-cortical circuits. Although the ability to maintain information over extended periods of time is a general feature of the PFC, the information processors and, consequently neuronal networks, are divided into three modalities: visual-spatial, visual-shape, and color and verbal. The division of the working memory in three modalities is reflected in an influential model of the working memory proposed by Alan Baddeley in 1974 and revised in 2003[35].

C. Three Working Memory Systems

According to the model, the networks that maintain modality specific traces of the working memory consist of prefrontal regions and parietal–temporal association areas reciprocally connected with each other (see Fig. 12.15). These reciprocally connected networks maintain the plans of actions built up on the basis of synthesis of sensory information coming to the PFC by means of bottom–up pathways. These networks also intensify specific types of sensory information needed for selected action by means of top–down connections.

D. CNV as Correlate of Working Memory

Working memory is a slow process that last from several seconds to minutes. Consequently, it must be associated with slow components in ERPs. In two stimulus tasks, when the first stimulus in each trial serves as a warning stimulus and the second stimulus serves as imperative stimulus, a slow component evolving between the first and second stimulus presentations is found (see Fig. 12.16). In our joint studies with Risto Näätänen from University of Helsinki we recorded EEG (within the frequency range from DC to 70 Hz) in healthy subjects performing visual and auditory variants of the two stimulus GO/NOGO paradigm. In this paradigm subjects were instructed to press a button in response to the two designated stimuli and to withhold from pressing to other pairs.

---

[35]The concept of working memory was introduced by Baddeley and Hitch in 1974 in contrast to the concept of short-term memory first suggested by Hebb in 1949. The main difference is that working memory implies not only temporal storage but also an active manipulation of information during delay intervals. According to Baddeley (2003), the theoretical concept of working memory assumes that a limited capacity system, which temporarily maintains and stores information, supports human thought processes by providing an interface between perception, long-term memory, and action.

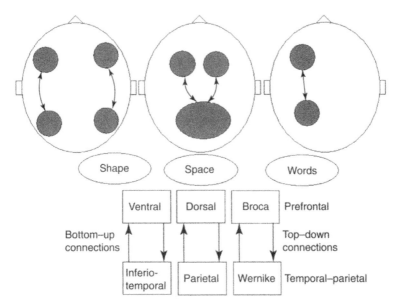

FIGURE 12.15   Three working memory systems. Right – verbal rehearsal system. It is the most efficient and predominant working memory in humans. It is implemented by predominantly left hemispheric network of premotor (Broca's) area and parietal (Wernike's) area. Middle – visual object working memory (e.g., working memory for shape, color ...). Left – visuospatial working memory system (e.g., working memory for spatial locations). Adapted from Baddeley (2003).

Figure 12.16 presents DC changes of cortical potential[36] during preparation to receive a stimulus in the trials when the first stimulus indicates that no motor response in these trials is required. The highest amplitudes of negative fluctuations are found in the left hemisphere at posterior temporal areas for visual modality and middle–posterior temporal areas for auditory modality. In contrast with those sensory-related contingent negative variations (CNVs), preparations to make a movement in both modalities are associated with negativities over the central areas. It could be speculated that the plan of the behavior in the given task is formed in the prefrontal areas. The higher level (prefrontal) areas through the frontal–temporal connections control the lower level (temporal) areas by depolarizing distal parts of apical dendrites of pyramidal neurons and thus preparing the pyramidal cells to respond fast to the prompting stimulus[37].

[36]These direct current (DC) changes were coined by Grey Walter as contingent negative variation – CNV.

[37]As we learnt from the previous, the pathways for these preparatory activities also include the basal ganglia thalamo-cortical circuits. To separate the effect of these subcortical circuits from the effect of the cortical (prefrontal–temporal, prefrontal–motor) appears to be impossible on the basis of ERPs analysis alone.

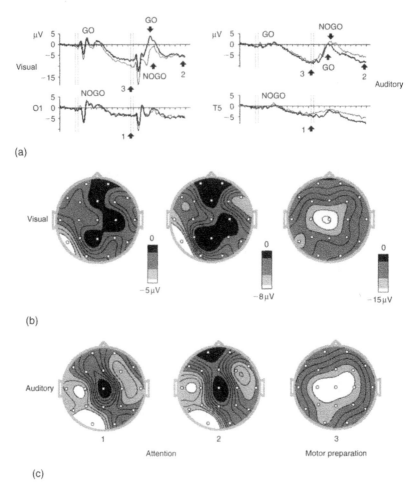

(a)

(b)

(c)

FIGURE 12.16   Slow shifts of potential (CNV) associated with preparation to receive a stimulus and preparations to make a movement. Potentials are averaged over a group of 10 healthy subjects performing the two stimulus GO/NOGO task in visual and auditory modality separately. Two categories of stimuli (defined conventionally as GO and NOGO) were presented in four different combinations of pairs with the subject's task to press a button to the pair of GO stimuli. In the visual modality digit 9 serve as GO stimulus, while digit 6 serves as NOGO stimulus. In the auditory modality, high tone (1300 Hz) serve as GO stimulus while low tone (1000 Hz) serve as NOGO stimulus. The subject task was to press a button in response to a pair of two GO stimuli. Moments 1 and 2 on the curve (marked by arrows) indicate the periods of preparation to receive a stimulus, while moment 3 indicates the periods of preparation to make a movement. Note that preparations to receive a stimulus are associated with negativities generated in the corresponding sensory modalities, while preparation to make a motor response are associated with negativities generated in the central regions of the cortex – around the somatosensory-motor strip.

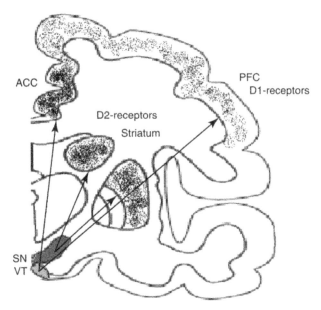

FIGURE 12.17   Distribution of dopamine receptors within the brain. The dopaminergic pathway from the substantia nigra (SN) innervates the striatum, while dopaminergic pathway from the ventral tegmental area (VT) innervates the PFC with highest density at the ACC.

VII. DOPAMINE AS A MEDIATOR OF THE EXECUTIVE SYSTEM

A. Cortical and Subcortical Distribution

The main mediator of the executive system is dopamine. It is found in the cortical areas of the prefrontal lobe as well as in subcortical structures of the executive system, such as the striatum. The distribution of dopamine receptors in the PFC and striatum is depicted in Fig. 12.17. The cingulate cortex (the core of the monitoring sub-system) receives the richest dopaminergic innervations of any cortical area.

B. Dopaminergic Systems

The complexity of dopaminergic system of the brain follows the heterogeneity of the executive system (Fig. 12.17). Most dopamine-containing cells develop from a single embryological cell group that originates at the mesencephalic–diencephalic junction. The cell group can be conventionally divided into two nuclei with different projections comprising different dopaminergic brain systems. The first one is called the nigrostriatal dopaminergic system. It originates in the zona compacta of the substantia nigra (SN) and is projected to the striatum. The other system is associated with the ventral tegmental area (VT) and is known as the mesocortical dopaminergic system. Cells in the medial ventral tegmental area project densely to the medial prefrontal and cingulate cortex[38]. Note that both tegmental and nigral cells receive feedback projections from the structures they innervate thus forming reverberation circuits in the corresponding (prefrontal and striatal) systems.

C. D1 and D2 Dopamine Receptors

The two dopaminergic systems are associated with different receptors for dopamine. The D1 family of dopamine receptors (D1 and D5) are an order of magnitude more abundant in the PFC than D2 family receptors (D2, D3, and D4), while D2 receptors are more prevalent in the striatum than in the cortex[39] (Fig. 12.18).

D. Functions of Dopaminergic Systems

Functions of the two dopaminergic systems (cortical and striatal) appear to be different. The nigrostriatal dopaminergic pathway sets the threshold of striatal neurons and, according to our theory, is involved in action selection and working memory. The mesocortical dopaminergic system modulates membrane potentials of neurons in prefrontal and ACC and is involved in maintaining functions of the corresponding cortical areas. As far as ACC concerns, one of its functions is associated with action monitoring. The other function is associated with a general quality of the prefrontal neurons – the ability to maintain a trace of action in the working memory[40]. Indeed, for more than 20 years dopamine is known as having a critical effect on working memory function of the prefrontal lobe. From studies

---

[38]The subset of neurons in the ventral tegmental area system projects to the nucleus accumbens, the septum, amygdala, hippocampus, and perirhinal cortex. This system is called the mesolimbic dopaminergic system and seems to be involved in memory consolidation.

[39]Receptor binding studies have shown that ligands specific to D1 family dopamine receptors bind with higher density in superficial layers (layers I–IIIa) and deep layers (layers V and VI) than in middle cortical layers (layers IIIb–IV). Experiments also suggest that D1 is more prevalent than D5 in the cortex of human and non-human primates.

[40]Here we need to mention that the other function of the anterior cingulate cortex is associated with emotions and motivations. In this context dopamine is associated with reward. In general terms, reward is a state of the brain in which a desired or expected action fits the real outcome of the current behavior. From animal experiments we know that rewarding stimuli such as food, water, lateral hypothalamic brain stimulation, and several drugs of abuse become ineffective as rewards if animals are given dopamine antagonists. We also know that midbrain dopamine neurons fire in response to rewards and to stimuli predicting rewards. The reward indicates the most efficient program of the current behavior. Thus, the release of dopamine in the striatum sets the lower threshold for the rewarded program.

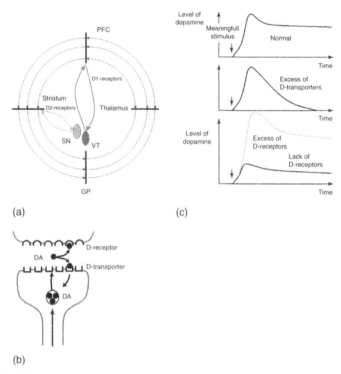

(a)   (c)

(b)

FIGURE 12.18   Dopaminergic pathways and dopamine circulation in neurons. (a) Schematic representation of dopamine pathways from the substantia nigra (SN) to the striatum with D2 receptors, from the ventral tegmental area (VT) to the PFC with D1 receptors. (b) Dynamics of dopamine (DA) in neuron – a meaningful stimulus releases a dopamine molecule from the vesicular, dopamine diffuses into the synaptic cleft and binds to the postsynaptic D-receptor. The dopamine in the synaptic cleft is "washed" out by re-uptake of the dopamine by presynaptic DAT-receptors. (c) In a normal brain any behaviorally meaningful stimulus evokes a trace that is partly defined by the time during which dopamine is kept in the synaptic cleft; with excess of D-transporters that re-uptake DA too fast, the trace of event is getting shorter; with a lack (excess) of D-receptors the amplitude of trace is reduced (enhanced).

in monkeys and rodents we know that too little or too much of dopamine receptor stimulation impairs performance in spatial memory tasks[41]. Optimal activation of D1-like receptors is necessary for persistent firing in neurons in the PFC, which is thought to be the cellular basis of information storage in working memory.

Recall, that contrary to glutamate (the main excitatory mediator of the brain) and GABA (the main inhibitory mediator) having quite fast effects lasting for

---

[41]Recall inverted U-shaped function that describes input–output relationship in neuronal systems (see Introduction). Working memory performance is influenced by dopamine activation of D1 family dopamine receptors in the prefrontal cortex: working memory performance is maximal at moderate stimulation of D1 family receptors and is reduced by either higher or lower levels of D1 stimulation.

several milliseconds, effect of dopamine in synaptic cleft can last for seconds or even tens of seconds. Duration of dopamine effect is defined by reuptake mechanism – receptors that reside on the presynaptic membrane and are known as dopamine transporters (DAT) (Fig. 12.18). The more receptors in the postsynaptic membrane of the dopaminergic neuron, the faster dopamine is consuming and, consequently, the shorter is the activation produced by a meaningful stimulus[42].

In contrast to DAT receptors defining dynamic properties of dopamine effect, D1, D2-receptor densities define the amplitude of dopamine effect. For example, decrease of dopamine receptors on the postsynaptic membrane is associated with low excitation of the striatal or cortical neurons (or with high threshold of activation of the corresponding neurons). Vice versa, excess of dopamine receptors on the postsynaptic membrane (such as in some forms of schizophrenia where increase of D2 receptors in the striatum is found) leads to lowering the threshold of activation of striatal neurons.

VIII. SUMMARY

The term "executive functions" refers to the coordination and control of motor and cognitive actions to attain specific goals. The need for an executive control mechanism has been postulated for non-routine situations requiring a supervisory system, for example, for situations for selecting an appropriate action from variety of options, inhibition of inappropriate actions, and keeping in working memory the plan of the action as well as the results of the action. The executive control is also needed for optimizing behavior. The executive functions are implemented by a complex brain system that consists of several cortical and subcortical structures interconnected with each other. The cortical structures include the prefrontal areas interconnected with the corresponding temporal–parietal areas. Neuronal activities in these cortical structures are regulated by means of parallel circuits that map the corresponding cortical areas into the basal ganglia. The basal ganglia are projected to the corresponding thalamic nuclei which, in their turn, have reciprocal connections to the cortical areas thus closing the circuit. The striatum as a key element in the subcortical circuits can be considered as a cognitive map of cortical representations of actions. The striatum performs selection of actions by means of long distance lateral inhibition. Frontal cortical areas reveal the highest level of complexity of neuronal wiring which is reflected in a so-called hyperfrontality – a

---

[42]In a subgroup of ADHD population an increase of DAT receptors in the striatum is found. This increase would eventually lead to shorten the "trace" induced by a meaningful stimulus (Fig. 12.18b,c). This in turn might lead to: (1) poor working memory, (2) inability to concentrate on the action for a long time (inattention), (3) a fast switch between different motor actions (hyperactivity), (4) a fast switching between visual objects and sounds (distractability), (5) a constant alteration in thoughts (impulsivity).

higher level of activation of the frontal areas in comparison to the posterior cortical regions. Together with the basal ganglia the prefrontal areas perform executive functions associated with engagement, disengagement, monitoring operations as well as with working memory. These operations are reflected in ERP components evoked in different paradigms such as oddball, GO/NOGO as well as in working memory tasks. Although the components associated with executive functions overlap in time and space, the recently developed ICA provides a powerful tool for separating them. Using the Human Brain Institute (HBI) normative database we were able to separate the following executive components in the two stimulus GO/NOGO task: the motor and action suppression components associated with frontal negativities at 200 ms (the conventional N2 inhibition component), the engagement component associated with parietal positivity at 300 ms (the conventional P3b component), the monitoring component associated with frontal–central positivity at 400 ms. According to s-LORETA the P3b engagement component is generated in the parietal cortical area, the N2 motor inhibition component is generated in the ipsi-lateral premotor, the P400 monitoring component is generated in the cingulate cortex. The ACC is also involved in generation of the ERN – a component that is elicited by erroneous compulsive actions in the mathematical task. Dopamine is the main mediator of the executive system. The dopamine is found in the cortical areas of the prefrontal lobe and exhibits its action by means of D1-family receptors. The dopamine is also found in the basal ganglia and exhibits its action by means of D2-family receptors. The drugs that effect different aspects of the dopaminergic modulation lessen executive dysfunctions in schizophrenia and ADHD.

CHAPTER 13

Affective System

*All happy families look similar to each other, every unhappy family is
unhappy in its own way*

Leo Tolstoy "Anna Karenina"

I. PSYCHOLOGY

A. Emotions Versus Reasoning

Emotions provide a dimension different from reasoning. Emotions play an important role in our life. The affective system of the brain is designed by nature for
surviving the organism in the world by using a dimension different from reasoning.
When reasoning is not enough for making decision, the brain relies on the affective
system. Just a simple example, we seldom rely on our reasoning when we choose
a wife or a husband, when we watch a football game played by a favorite teem,
or when we play with a family dog. Making some important steps in our lives
(like marriage, divorce, leaving a job…) we are usually driven by emotions. Another
example of the affective system functioning is releasing fundamental actions such as
seek for food, water, or a sexual partner.

The affective system produces certain habitual responses, called emotional
reactions, to certain events. These responses are produced when the brain detects
an emotionally competent stimulus[1]. The "habits of mind" – the routines of the

---

[1]This concept was introduced by Antonio Damasio. A popular version of his work is presented in
his recent book "The feeling of what happens," 1999.

affective system – enable us to associate those emotions (and feelings that follow them) with the corresponding experiences. The brain is prepared by evolution to respond to certain emotionally competent stimuli with specific repertoires of actions. However, while some of the emotionally competent stimuli are evolutionary determined, some can be learned through experience[2].

B. Punishers and Rewards

The emotional stimuli are usually divided into two basic classes – punishers and rewards. The two classes of the emotionally competent stimuli are associated with two different affective states: withdrawal and approach. The affective reactions associated with withdrawal and approach can be further divided into separate emotions such as fear, anxiety, happiness ... An attempt to classify emotionally competent stimuli and affective reactions is given in Table 13.1. Antonio Domasio, a world expert in the field of brain mechanisms of emotions, classifies emotions into three types: (1) background emotions, (2) primary emotions, and (3) social emotions.

1. Background Emotions

Background emotions are discouragement and enthusiasm. They are difficult to be discriminated from affective states. Primary (basic emotions) include fear, anger, disgust, sadness, surprise, and happiness. These emotions are easily identifiable in human being across several cultures and in non-human species. Most of what we know about neurobiology of emotions comes from studies of basic emotions. Fear leads the way. Social emotions include sympathy, embarrassment, shame, guilt, pride, jealousy, envy, gratitude, admiration, indignation, and contempt.

C. Drives and Motivations

When we talk about the affective system, we have to separate drives and motivations on the one hand and emotions and feelings on the other hand. The drives and motivations form the affective states which must be distinguished from emotional responses. Although some signs of affection can be perceived in birds, the limbic system (and emotions) only began to evolve in the mammals, being practically non-existent in reptiles, amphibians, and all other low species[3].

---

[2]So, an emotion is a complex collection of chemical and neuronal responses to certain external and internal events forming a distinctive pattern and reflecting in a certain behavior reaction (including facial expressions). The body responses (and particular facial expressions) can be perceived by other people and mimic, simulate a corresponding reactions in them by a specific brain system consisted of so-called mirror neurons. Emotions make us human. All arts (music, painting, literature ...) are about emotions.

[3]Paul MacLean used to say that "it is very difficult to imagine a lonelier and more emotionally empty being than a crocodile."

TABLE 13.1   Classification of Affective States and Emotions

Event (external and/or internal)	Affective state	Affective reaction (emotion)
Punishers	Withdrawal	Fear
		Anxiety
		Anger
		Disgust
		Sadness
		Contempt
		Embarrassment
		Guilt
		Shame
Rewards	Approaching	Happiness
		Joy
		Enthusiasm
		Pride
		Sexual love
		Maternal love

Major examples of drives and motivations are hunger, thirst, curiosity, attraction to an opposite sex. Motivations regulate our behavior by several mechanisms. A major role in motivational behavior is played by the hypothalamus. Neurons in the hypothalamus are very sensitive to different types of biochemical substances, while spike activity of these neurons reflects changes in concentration of some fundamental substances in blood and cerebrospinal fluid. The hypothalamic neurons in turn regulate release of various hormones in the pituitary gland (which is attached to the hypothalamus by a stalk) and acting on other parts of the affective system by releasing certain types of regulatory behaviors such as drinking, eating. Humans are driven not only by simple motivations to eat and to drink, but also by more complex and sometimes quite abstract drivers. Plans of those drivers seem to reside in the prefrontal areas.

II. ANATOMY

A. Limbic System

The affective system adds a new dimension (emotions/motivations), a new feature to our perceptions and actions. This new feature regulates the whole behavior by seeking for positive emotions and avoiding negative emotions. From information point of view, the affective system is designed to reinforce the trace of events that are crucial for human survival in association with emotional meaning of the events. As one can see the affective system[4] is defined from functional point of view.

[4]As well and all other systems in this book.

However, historically the first notion close to the affective system was the notion of the limbic system[5]. This concept was based on the anatomical, not functional, ground. According to the anatomic perspective, limbic system includes structures forming a border around the corpus collosum. In psychology and psychiatry the term "limbic system" became very popular and served as an explanatory concept to describe neuronal networks involved in generating emotions and affective states[6].

B. Papez Circuit

A scientific approach to the affective system of the brain started in 1937 when James Papez suggested that the limbic lobe works in cooperation with the hypothalamus which in those days was considered to have a critical role in expression of emotions. He made a special emphasis on the dorsal part of Broca's great limbic lobe called cingulum[7]. Indeed, the hypothalamus[8] sends signals to the cingulate cortex through the anterior thalamic nuclei by means of the fiber bundle called the mammilo-thalamic tract. In its turn, the hypothalamus receives input from the hippocampus via a bundle of axons called the fornix, while the hippocampus receives projections from the anterior cingulate cortex, thus closing the circle. According to Papez, the hypothalamus and the cingulate cortex form a reciprocal circuit that on the one hand allows emotions triggered by the hypothalamus to reach consciousness at the level of the cingulate cortex and on the other hand enable higher cognitive functions from the cingulate cortex to affect emotions. This hypothalamic–cingulum circuit was later coined as the Papez circuit (Fig. 13.1). Later on in a series of publications beginning in 1949, Paul MacLean extended the concept of the Papez circuit. He included into it some other anatomically related structures such as the amygdala, the septal area, nucleus accumbens, and the orbito-frontal cortex (OFC).

C. Cortical and Subcortical Elements

Modern anatomical and physiological research shows that from the functional point of view the limbic system can not be considered as a single entity, but rather

[5]Limbus in Latin means border. The term limbic lobe (le grand lobe limbique) was first introduced by Paul Broca in 1878 to define cortical gyri that form a ring around the corpus collosum. The limbic lobe according to his concept includes the cingulate gyrus and the hippocampus with adjacent cortical areas such as the parahippocampal gyrus and enthorinal cortex.

[6]In the same time, neuroscience focused on studying the variety of functions of anatomical structures in the border around the corpus collosum. For neuroscience emotion is one of many functions that are associated with limbic system. Executive and memory functions are other functions of the limbic system.

[7]This part of the cortex is called the cingulate cortex because it forms a cingulum or collar around the corpus callosum. It is in turn divided into anterior and posterior parts.

[8]Actually separate parts of the hypothalamus, called mamillary bodies.

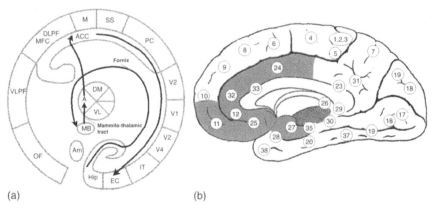

(a)　　　　　　　　　　　　　(b)

FIGURE 13.1　The Papez circuit. (a) Schematic connections between anatomical structures of the circuit. (b) Medial view of the human brain with the structures of the Papez circuit colored in gray. Abbreviations: VLPF, ventro-lateral prefrontal cortex; DLPF, dorso-lateral prefrontal cortex; M, motor areas of the cortex; SS, somato-sensory cortex; PC, parietal cortex; V1, V2, V4, cortical areas in the visual system; IT, inferior-temporal cortex; EC, enthorinal cortex; Hip, hippocampus; MB, mamillary bodies of hypothalamus; A, anterior nucleus of the thalamus; VL, ventro-lateral nucleus of the thalamus; DM, dorso-medial nucleus of the thalamus.

can be separated into different systems playing different functional roles associated not only with emotions/motivations, but with episodic memory and executive functions. First, in addition to previous concepts new evidence emphasizes that the hippocampus itself has reciprocal connections with the associated cortex of the sensory systems so that bilateral lesions to hippocampus produce both retrograde and anterograde amnesia. Second, the anterior gyrus cingulus was shown to be involved in attention and error correction – elements of executive functions[9].

In this book we consider the affective system as a complex of cortical and subcortical structures interconnected with each other to form a functional structure that enables a subject to generate and to feel emotional and motivational reactions to external and internal stimuli (Fig. 13.2)[10]. Cortical structures of the affective system are orbito-frontal cortex, anterior cingulate cortex, the insular cortex, and somato-sensory cortical areas. Subcortical structures include the amygdala, anterior hypothalamus, and ventral striatum (nucleus accumbens).

[9]The variety of functions that are attributed to the limbic system raises the question is it useful to use the term limbic, or to consider memory, executive, and affective systems as separate entities. In this book we follow functional organization of the brain and consider these systems separate. Here we have to remind the reader that any anatomical structure often has not one but many functions, while a certain brain function is maintained by a complex system of many brain structures.

[10]Note the affective system includes the Papez circuit as its major part.

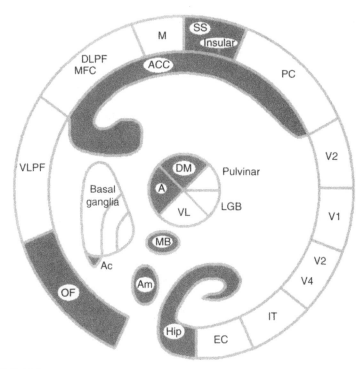

FIGURE 13.2   Anatomical structures of the affective system. Abbreviations are Am, amygdala; Ac, nucleus accumbens (ventral striatum). Cortical structures: OFC, orbito-frontal cortex; ACC, anterior cingulate cortex; SS/Ins, somato-sensory and insular cortical areas. Other abbreviations as in Fig. 13.1.

As one can see most of the anatomical structures of the affective system are located deep in the brain. The "internal" location of the affective system makes it difficult to record electroencephalogram (EEG) correlates of its functioning from the scalp.

III. PHYSIOLOGY

A. Orbito-frontal cortex as a Map of Rewards and Punishers

The orbito-frontal cortex (OFC) occupies the ventral part of the prefrontal cortex, including BA 11 and BA 47 (Fig. 13.1). Sometimes, BA 10 is refereed to the OFC, but it is more often considered as a single entity – anterior frontal cortex. One of distinct features of the OFC is its interindividual variability. The OFC receives polimodal inputs from all sensory systems. Visual, auditory, and somato-sensory systems convey information about external world, about status of our body, deep tissues, and viscera. Fundamental phylogenetically primitive modalities, such as the chemical senses bring signals to the OFC about smell and taste thus signaling pleasure or danger of food and drink. The amygdala sends the emotion-related information mostly associated with fear. The anterior cingulate cortex processes high level of cognitive and emotional information, especially when this information does not match the expected model. The OFC receives also pathways from other areas of the affective system, such as the hypothalamus. In addition, as any prefrontal cortical area, the OFC is self-regulated by means of the basal ganglia thalamo-cortical loop with the nucleus accumbens as the main part at the striatal level[11].

One of the most important symptoms of the OFC selective damage is a lack of effect[12]. In their textbook "An introduction to brain and behavior," Bryan Kolb and Ian Whishow described a patient who underwent a *frontal leucotomy*. As the authors report, the first thing that was noticed in this patient was a lack of emotion, and any sign of facial emotional expression. The patient was quite aware of her emotional deficit by saying that she no longer had any feelings about things or other people, she felt empty, much like a zombie. Patients with OFC damage are also impaired in identifying social signals such as emotional expressions of facial reactions and voice intonation (prosody). In addition, they exhibit profound personality changes, problems with self-conduct, social inappropriateness and irresponsibility, and difficulties making decisions in the context of their everyday life.

Meta-analysis of functional magnetic resonance imaging (fMRI) and positron emission tomography (PET) studies[13] showed that the OFC can be considered as a mapping instrument that represents rewards and punishers in a spatial (and, probably, temporal) pattern of activation of the cortex (see Fig. 13.3). The medial part of the OFC maps the reinforcers (rewards). Its close position and strong connection with the anterior cingulate cortex indicates that the medial part of the OFC plays a critical role in organizing behavior to approach rewards. The lateral part of the OFC maps the punishers. Its close position and strong connection with the lateral prefrontal cortex indicates that it might play an important role in suppressing behavior that is associated with punishers. According to this view, patients with damage in the OFC lost the ability to map effectively rewards (what is desirable) and punishers (what must be avoided) and consequently lost their ability to make appropriate decisions between selecting rewards and avoiding punishers.

---

[11]Recall that this basal-ganglia thalamic circuit is coined as the Limbic circuit with a function mediating regulation of emotions and motivations.

[12]A classic example of the OFC lesion (that also included damage in the anterior cingulate cortex is the case of Phineas Cage, whose frontal lobes were penetrated by a metal rode. After the accident Cage became a different person whose emotional processing and decision making had changed dramatically.

[13]Kringelbach and Rolls in their recent review of the functions of the human OFC performed a large meta-analysis of neuroimaging studies showing that different subregions of the OFC have different functions.

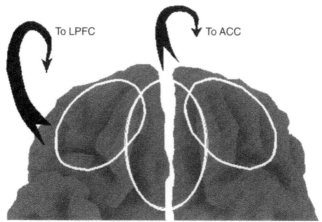

Punishers reinforcers Punishers

FIGURE 13.3   Maps of reinforcers and punishers in the OFC. Meta-analysis of the functions of the OFC (Kringelbach and Rolls, 2004) showed that the medial part of the cortex is related to processing reinforcers while the lateral part is related to processing punishers. The analysis also indicates that complex or abstract reinforcers (such as monetary gain and loss) are represented more anteriorly while less complex reinforcers such as taste are represented more posteriorly.

B. Positive Affect, Negative Affect, and Monitoring

It looks like that rewards and correspondingly positive emotional reactions to them constitute one dimension of the features of the affective system, while punishers and correspondingly negative emotional reactions to them constitute another dimension (Fig. 13.4). These two dimensions seem to form the neuronal basis of temperament[14]. However if we consider temperament in a more broader sense as reflecting not only emotional, motivational tendencies but also monitoring these affective states, we have to include another dimension (Fig. 13.4) – monitoring emotions, motivations, and drives[15]. The last dimension is actually an attribute of the executive system described in detail in the previous chapter. As was shown in previous chapter, the monitoring operation of the brain is maintained by a complex system with anterior cingulate cortex as a critical element. The dorsal part of the anterior cingulate cortex is involved in monitoring cognitive actions such as

[14]Do not mix temperament with personality. Temperament is mostly an attribute of the affective system, while personality is a broader term associated with combined attributes of all brain systems including affective, executive, attentional, sensory, and memory systems.

[15]These dimensions are very close to three fundamental dimensions of temperament – negative affectivity, positive affectivity, and constrain – introduced in a recent review of neurobiological basis of temperament by Sarah Whittle and her colleagues from University of Melbourne, Australia (Whittle et al., 2006).

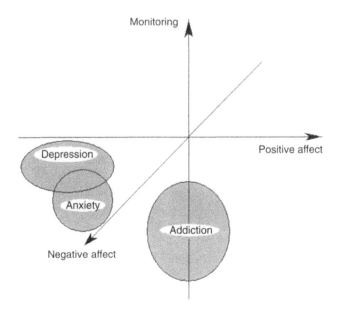

FIGURE 13.4   Three independent characteristics of affective system. Three characteristics (positive affect, negative affect, and monitoring) are schematically presented as a 3D space. A neutral emotional state corresponds to the origin of coordinates. Depression, anxiety, and addiction can be represented in this space (marked by gray color).

goal directed behavioral patterns and thoughts. In analogy with the monitoring concept of the dorsal anterior cingulate cortex we can suggest that the ventral part of this cortical area is associated with monitoring emotions.

Individuals high on positive affect are biased to experience a wide range of positive emotions such as joy, happiness, enthusiasm, and pride. Because of connection of the reinforcement-related activations of the OFC with the anterior cingulate cortex which monitors behavior the subjects high on positive affect are mostly engaged into active and positive social and family behavior. Some types of depression might be associated with low levels in this scale.

Individuals high on negative affect are biased to experience a wide range of negative moods such as fear, anxiety, sadness, and guilt. Because of the connection of the punishment-related activations to the lateral prefrontal cortex which inhibits behavioral patterns the individual high on negative affect are prone to avoid social communication and inhibit new and unknown endeavors. Anxiety, as a psychiatric disorder, might be associated with high values in this dimension.

Individuals high on monitoring dimension can effectively control their emotions and affective impulses, they have ability to wait (and sometimes for a long time) for gratification and reward. Individuals high on this dimension may be described as hard-working, persistent, reliable, and responsible. In contrast, individuals low on this index are impulsive and offensive, can not wait for reward and live in a moment. Addiction, as psychiatric disorder, seems to be associated with low level in this monitoring dimension. There is a general agreement that temperamental dimensions are genetically determined, are observed in infancy[16], and preserve across life span with moderate modulation by environmental factors.

The important functional feature of the orbital cortex is that as any frontal area it is self-regulated by means of the basal ganglia thalamo-cortical circuit. The cortical areas of the OFC are topographically mapped into distinct areas of the ventral striatum with a part called the nucleus accumbens. The neurons in the striatum are connected by strong lateral inhibitory connections that perform a "winner takes all" operation. Because of this lateral inhibition the activation of a certain representation (say the one of reinforcers) in the OFC would inhibit the representation of the opposite one (say the one of punishers). It indicates that any bias in emotional state (depression or mania) may be associated with a dysbalance of activation/inhibition at the cortical-basal ganglia network.

C. Asymmetry in Maps of Emotions?

The other important feature of the OFC concerns brain asymmetry of representations of emotions. In spite of extensive literature regarding MRI, fMRI, and PET indexes of brain asymmetry[17] we did not find any convincing evidence in favor of asymmetrical (left–right) distribution of the negative and positive emotions within the OFC, but there is an abundant evidence showing lateralization of negative and positive emotions in the lateral prefrontal cortex. The idea of lateralization of the affective system first came from clinical observation that lesions in the left prefrontal cortex are more often associated with induced depression in comparison to lesions in the right side[18]. The role of hemispheric laterality in emotion had become a source of debate for decades.

In 1993 Richard Davidson of the University of Wisconsin has proposed that the left frontal regions may be more active during the experience of approach-related (i.e., positive) emotions and the right frontal regions may be more active during the experience of withdrawal-related (i.e., negative) emotions, or,

---

[16]Except monitoring dimension, which evolves later in life due to delayed maturation of the executive system of the brain.

[17]Brain asymmetry has been observed in animals and humans in terms of structure, function, and behavior. This lateralization is thought to reflect evolutionary, hereditary, developmental, experiential, and pathological factors. We recommend a recent review of asymmetry studies by Arthur W. Toga and Paul M. Thompson (2003).

[18]In a study of Morris et al. (1996) patients with lesions involving left hemisphere prefrontal or basal ganglia structures had a higher frequency of depressive disorder (9/12; 75 per cent) than other left hemisphere lesions (1/12; 8 per cent) or those with right hemisphere lesions (5/17; 29 per cent), $p = 0.002$.

simplifying, the left hemisphere responds mostly to positive events, while the right hemisphere responds predominately to negative events.

Because the power of the EEG alpha band has been found to be inversely correlated to activation of the corresponding region of the brain, Davidson and his colleagues have contended that anterior alpha asymmetry measurements reflect relative differences in activity between the left and right hemispheres. Frontal alpha asymmetry has been found to be relatively stable over several week and months, enabling Davidson (Wheeler et al., 1993; Davidson, 1995) to suggest that this measurement reflects a trait-like tendency to respond differentially to positive (i.e., approach related) and negative (i.e., withdrawal-related) stimuli. Davidson and his collaborators have conducted several studies for providing support for this suggestion. They recorded baseline EEG from normal subjects, who then viewed film clips designed to elicit either amusement and happiness, or fear and disgust. They found that frontal EEG asymmetry was a stable characteristic of individuals and predicted positive affective responsivity, negative affective responsivity, and affective valence following presentation of the film clips. Asymmetry, however, was unrelated to baseline mood[19].

D. Amygdala

Amygdala is a relatively small nucleus that lies deep inside the anterio-inferior region of the medial temporal lobe[20]. Amygdala could be considered as an interface between sensory world[21] and emotions. Amygdala receives sensory information through the hippocampus from polimodal areas of the temporal and parietal cortex, extracts memories stored in the amygdala, and sends the results of the extraction to the prefrontal cortex through the dorso-medial nucleus of the thalamus.

Recordings in the human amygdala show that many neurons in it respond to unpleasant stimuli and few to pleasant stimuli. So the amygdala can be better described as a structure detecting threat or potential punishment and thus generating negative emotions such as fear and anxiety, in other words amygdala is

---

[19]Because alpha EEG power is inversely correlated with metabolic activation in the corresponding region of the brain, Davidson and his colleagues proposed the alpha asymmetry measurements as an index of relative differences in activity between the left and right hemispheres. This theory initiated a neurofeedback protocol for treatment depression called alpha asymmetry protocol (see Part III for more details).

[20]The concept of amygdala as a nucleus is a simplification. The structure and function of this part of affective system are better expressed in the notion of extended amygdala (Heimer and Van Hoesen, 2006). The extended amygdala consists of central and medial amygdaloid nuclei and their extensions to the subpalidal region and along the arc of the stria terminalis which link the centromedial amygdala to the bed nucleus of stria terminalis. The extended amygdala represents a strategic system that receives the polimodal input and coordinates activities in multiple regions of the limbic lobe.

[21]The main part of the sensory input to the amygdala comes from the visual and auditory systems.

supposedly to determine negative affective dimension. Patients with lesions in the amygdala do not feel fear and anger[22].

E. Medial and Anterior Nuclei of the Thalamus

Lesions or stimulations of the medial dorsal and anterior nuclei of the thalamus are associated with changes in emotional reactivity. However, these nuclei do not generate emotions by themselves but rather transfer emotion-related information to the prefrontal cortex. Indeed, the medial dorsal nucleus transfers the information from the amygdala to the OFC, while the anterior nuclei transfer the information from the mamillary bodies of the hypothalamus to the cingulate gyrus. It should be noted that the anterior thalamus lacks a sheet of neurons that surrounds the thalamus – the reticular nucleus. This anatomical feature seems to play an important role in the affective system. Indeed, the absence of the anterior part of the reticular nucleus is manifested in a lack of feedback inhibition that is provided by inhibitory neurons of the reticular nucleus. Thus a lack of inhibition leads in inability to block the flow of emotion-related information to the prefrontal cortex. Whatever happens in the outside world the emotional meaning will reach the cortex[23]!

F. Hypothalamus

Hypothalamus lies very deep in the brain, represents a small (less than 1 per cent of the human brain volume) nucleus without any selected direction of aligning neurons. Consequently the hypothalamus does not generate a collective local field potential that could be reliably recorded on the surface. This structure (at least some parts of it) regulates many fundamental programs such as keeping the body temperature, eating, drinking, and sexual behavior. Lesions of the hypothalamic nuclei interfere with several vegetative functions (such as thermal regulation, hunger and thirst) and some of the so-called motivational behaviors (such as sexuality, combativeness…).

The hypothalamus also plays an important role in emotion. Recall, that many of brain structures have not one but many functions. This is true for the hypothalamus. Indeed, lateral parts of the hypothalamus is involved in emotions such as pleasure and rage, while the median part is associated with aversion, displeasure, and

---

[22]Antonio Domasio in his book "The feeling of what happens" describes a patient who lost amygdala on both sides. Describing this patient he writes "… there was nothing wrong whatsoever with S's ability to learn new facts. … Her social history, on the other hand was exceptional. To put it in the simplest possible terms, I would say the S approached people and situations with a predominately positive attitude." In this patient, and in others with similar damages, the memories for fear and anger seem to be missing, at least for auditory and visual stimuli.

[23]Recall that a mother can be awaked from a deep sleep even by a brief cry of her child.

a tendency to uncontrollable and loud laughing. However, in general terms, the hypothalamus has more to do with the expression (symptomatic manifestations) of emotions than with the genesis of the affective states.

G. Ventral Part of the Anterior Cingulate Cortex

As was shown in the previous chapter the anterior cingulate cortex is divided into two parts affective (ventral) and executive (dorsal). For example, stimulation of the ventral part produced intense fear or pleasure, whereas electrical stimulation of the more dorsal part produced a sense of anticipation of movement. As far as emotions concern, the ventral part of the cingulate cortex participates in emotional reaction to pain, as well as in regulation of aggressive behavior[24]. The anterior cingulate cortex also receives a strong projection from the amygdala, which probably relays negative, fear-related, information.

H. Neuroimaging Patterns of Emotions

Antonio Domasio and his colleagues from University of Iowa College of Medicine in 2000 carried out a series of PET experiments aimed at investigating the neuro-biological basis of emotion and feeling (Damasio et al., 2000). Subjects recalled and re-experienced personal life episodes marked by sadness, happiness, anger, or fear while were placed in PET scans. The results show that all emotions engaged structures related to the affective system including the insular cortex, secondary somato-sensory cortex, cingulate cortex, and nuclei in brainstem tegmentum and hypothalamus[25]. These activation patterns provide distinctive "perceptual land-scapes" of the organism's internal state, while differences among those landscapes constitute the critical rationale why each emotion feels different.

Note that the low time resolution of PET does not allow analyzing temporal patterns of brain activation during separate stages associated with emotional reactions, feelings, and monitoring emotions. EEG and ERPs appear to present a tool that would enable us to study neuronal correlates of distinct stages of information flow in emotions. However, the anatomical evidence indicates that the most of the cortical structures of the affective system lie deep in the brain and, consequently,

---

[24]Wild animals, submitted to the ablation of the cingulate gyrus (cingulectomy), become totally tamed.

[25]For example, sadness induced bilateral, but asymmetric, activations of the insula cortex and the mixed activation–deactivation pattern in the cingulate cortex (activations anterior, deactivations posterior). Happiness induced activation of the right posterior cingulate cortex and suppression of the anterior third of the left cingulate, activation of the left insula cortex and the right secondary somato-sensory cortex.

can generate relatively week potentials at the scalp. In addition, nuclei of the affective system do not reveal a predominant orientation of neurons (such as pyramidal cells in the cortex) and provide small potentials outside the nuclei.

I. Frontal Midline Theta Rhythm and Emotions

However, in some subjects the activity from the cingulate cortex still can be reliably recorded from the surface of the head. A large body of EEG data shows that the anterior cingulate is the source of a so-called frontal midline theta rhythm[26]. This rhythm is manifested in short bursts of 5–8 Hz EEG signal recorded with maximal amplitude near Fz. This signal appears when the subject is performing a task requiring focused concentration and its amplitude increases with task load. When the subject is restless and anxious, the signal is reduced or eliminated; when the anxiety is relieved with drugs, the signal is restored. Sometimes, the frontal midline theta is associated with relief from anxiety. These data indicate that the anterior cingulate cortex is involved in regulating emotional state from restless anxiety to focused relaxation. This is also consistent with the common experience that focusing on a cognitive problem relieves anxiety[27].

IV. STAGES OF REACTIONS OF AFFECTIVE SYSTEM

The consecutive stages of processing emotionally significant stimulus are schematically represented in Fig. 13.5. The critical structures in this processing are: the areas in the temporal and parietal cortex that are responsible for recognition of face expressions and body movements, amygdala, ventral striatum (nucleus accumbens), and OFC that maps the stimulus into 2D space with one axis of negative affect (punishment) and the other axis of positive affect (reward); motor cortical areas that automatically react with emotional (body and face expression) response, somto-sensory and insular cortex that correspondingly map sensory-motor information of emotional reaction from face/body and visceral organs, and anterior cingulate cortex that by comparing the expected action and the real one generates a signal that through the motor part of the cingulate cortex modifies further behavior by escaping the punishment or approaching the reward.

---

[26]Recall that the incidence of frontal midline theta-emitting subjects reported by Japanese research groups is about 11–43 per cent depending on age.

[27]This fact can be explained by close location of the affective and executive parts of the anterior cingulate cortex. It appears that activation of the one part (say executive) of the anterior cingulate cortex due to the lateral inhibition at the level of the basal ganglia inhibits the other part (emotional) of the anterior cingulate cortex, and vice versa.

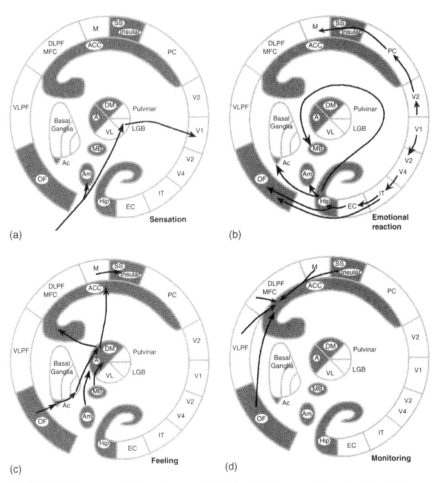

FIGURE 13.5   Stages of information processing in the affective system. See explanations in the text.

The stages can be classified into the representation (sensation) stage, the emotional reaction stage, the feeling stage and the monitoring (correcting) stage. In more detail the stages are as follows:

A. Sensation

Neuronal impulses generated by a stimulus almost simultaneously reach the amygdala[28] and the primary visual cortex. This is an early stage of a simple sensation of the stimulus.

[28]The short connections between ascending activation system and amygdala enable it to react in the punishers with short latencies which is important for survival in some dangerous situations.

B. Emotional Reaction

The visual information is processed in temporal[29] and parietal areas and reaches the motor cortex. It is also processed by hippocampus and from the hippocampus and the earlier stages of sensory processing reach the amygdala, OFC, and ventral striatum. This is a stage in which the stimulus is decomposed into spatial pattern in correspondence to the 2D affective space: positive affect and negative affect. This is also a stage in which motor system reacts (partly automatically) to the decomposed emotional stimulus.

C. Feeling Stage

During this stage information about emotional reaction reaches the somato-sensory cortex and insular. These cortical areas map the external (body/face) and internal (visceral) emotional reactions into distinct representations corresponding to distinct feelings such as feeling of happiness or feeling of joy[30].

D. Monitoring Stage

Finally, the expected emotion and the real emotional reaction are compared with each other in the anterior cingulate cortex. The results of this comparison operation via the motor part of the anterior cingulate cortex drive the body to avoid this discrepancy or to stay longer in the current state.

V. SEROTONIN AS MEDIATOR OF AFFECTIVE SYSTEM

In general, we know that brainstem nuclei modulate information processing in the brain systems. As far as the affective system concerns especially high concentrations of mediator – serotonin (5-hydroxytryptamine; 5-HT) are found in the anatomical structures of this system. In line with this evidence, central serotoninergic neurons and receptors are targets for a variety of therapeutic agents used in the treatment of disorders of the affective system.

---

[29]The fusiform gyrus of the temporal lobe, for example, plays a critical role in face discriminations and extracting emotional expressions from face images.

[30]So, by simply changing the expression of our face (say by smiling) we can perceive the emotion of happiness. I recall a story about a Tibetan monk who treated depressive states by forcing patients to smile. However, happiness is represented not only in face expression, but also in alterations of heart rate, speed of breathing, and other so-called visceral processes. These processes are mapped in a separate cortical areas including insular cortex.

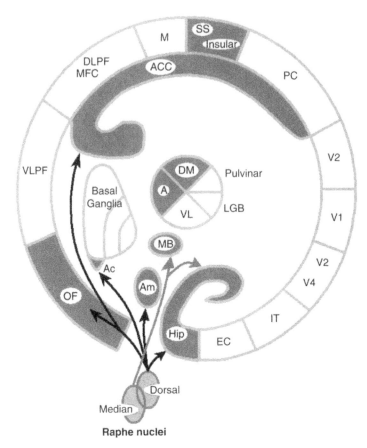

FIGURE 13.6   The dual serotoninergic system innervating the forebrain. Designed on the basis of data from Hensler (2006).

A. Functioning and Dysfunctioning of Serotoninergic System

The serotoninergic projections arise primarily from the dorsal and median raphe nuclei. They are composed of two distinct serotoninergic systems differing in their electrophysiological characteristics, topographic organization, morphology, as well as sensitivity to neurotoxins and perhaps psychoactive agents (Fig. 13.6). The thin varicose axon system arises from the serotoninergic cell bodies within the dorsal raphe nucleus with fibers that branch profusely in their target areas. They mostly innervate the prefrontal cortex, nucleus accumbens, amygdala, and ventral hippocampus. The thick, non-varicose axon system arises from the serotoninergic cell bodies within the median raphe nucleus with fibers that mostly innervate hypothalamus and dorsal hippocampus[31]. The serotoninergic modulation of the affective system suggests the monoamine hypothesis of depression. Indeed, several antidepressant drugs increased synaptic concentrations of serotonin, while reserpine, a catecholamine depleting drug, could cause depression-like symptoms.

VI. SUMMARY

From psychological point of view, the affective system adds a new dimension (emotions/motivations) to our perceptions and actions. This new feature regulates the whole behavior by seeking for positive emotions and avoiding negative emotions. From information point of view, the affective system is designed to reinforce the trace of events that are crucial for human survival in association with emotional meaning of the events. Anatomically, the affective system is a group of cortical and subcortical structures that are intimately interconnected with each other to provide a subject with ability to generate and to feel emotional reactions in response to sensory stimuli. Physiologically, some of these structures (such as the orbito-frontal cortex and amygdala) map external and internal sensory stimuli into categories of emotionally meaningful stimuli: rewards, punishments, motivations, and drivers, some of the structures express emotional reactions (such as face expressions) in response to the emotionally meaningful stimuli, and, finally, some of the structures (such as the insular cortex) are responsible for feelings of the emotional reactions and states. In 1993 Richard Davidson of the University of Wisconsin has proposed that the left frontal regions may be more active during the experience of approach-related (i.e., positive) emotions while the right frontal regions may be more active during the experience of withdrawal-related (i.e., negative) emotions, or, simplifying, the left hemisphere responds mostly to positive events, while the right hemisphere responds predominately to negative events. Because power in the EEG alpha band has been found to be inversely correlated to activation of the corresponding region of the brain, anterior alpha asymmetry measurements might serve as an index of depression and anxiety at least in some type of patients. The information flow in the affective system is modulated by serotoninergic enervation from the raphe nuclei of the brain stem. Some antidepressant drugs increase synaptic concentrations of serotonin in the brain.

---

[31]There are several types of serotonin receptors: 5-HT_{1A}, 5-HT_{2A}. While 5-HT_{1A} receptor is found only in the raphe nuclei where it serves as an autoreceptor regulating the firing of serotoninergic neurons by inhibiting them, 5-HT_{2A} receptors are found in high density in most of the structures of the affective system. The action of serotonin in the extracellular space is terminated by the serotonin transporter (SERT).

CHAPTER 14

Memory Systems

I. PSYCHOLOGY

A. Types of Memory

Few people know that the ancient Greeks, together with other arts, invented an art of memory, usually associated with "mnemotechnics." In the ages before invention of printing technique this art was vitally important. Although nowadays we rely on memories stored in books, computers, and Internet, the importance of our own memory is difficult to overestimate.

A major achievement of recent research on brain mechanisms of learning and memory is the recognition that there are several different types of memory involving different brain systems. One distinction can be made on the basis of temporal dynamics of the memory trace such as ultra-short (with duration of hundreds of milliseconds), short-term (with duration of several seconds), and long-term memories (up to periods comparable with life span). Long-term memories in turn can be divided into two broad categories depending on the type of stored information and neuronal mechanisms (see Table 14.1). They are explicit and implicit memories.

In general, explicit memory involves awareness of the memory whereas implicit memory does not necessarily involve being aware of the memory. Procedural memory as a type of implicit memory is based on learning and recalling motor

TABLE 14.1   Types of long-term memories

Category	Sub-category	What is the trace	Structures responsible for forming and storing
Declarative (Explicit)	Episodic	Personal events	Hippocampus – sensory multimodal – prefrontal
Declarative (Explicit)	Semantic	General facts without explicit reference to personal events	Hippocampus – sensory multimodal – prefrontal
Non-declarative (Implicit)	Procedural	Actions, such as speech production, or driving a car	Prefrontal cortex – basal ganglia–thalamic network
Non-declarative (Implicit)	Instrumental and conditioned reflexes	Association memory between conditional stimuli on the one hand and unconditioned responses (such as to rewards, punishers…) on the other hand	Sensory multimodal cortical, cerebellum, amygdala
Non-declarative (Implicit)	Priming*	Activating parts of particular representations in memory just before carrying out an action or task	Probably short-term modifications in synaptic connection of neurons of the neuronal representations of the stimulus
Non-declarative (Implicit)	Habituation	Non-associative memory trace resulted in decrease of response after repetitive presentation of a stimulus	Short-term depression in synapses

*Priming is an experimental technique by which a priming stimulus is used to sensitize the neuronal representation of the stimulus to a later presentation of the same or similar stimulus. For example, when a subject reads a list of words that includes the word "memory", and is later asked to name a word that starts with "mem", the list "primes" the subject to answer memory.

and cognitive skills. The distinction between implicit and explicit learning can be exemplified in language[1].

When an organism learns any information, a number of brain systems are engaged. However, in most cases there is one critical brain system, which when damaged causes permanent impairment in the particular form of learning and

[1]Memories for language can be divided into lexicon and grammar. The lexicon of the word-specific knowledge is stored in the temporal–parietal–occipital lobe junction and represents an example of declarative memory. This type of declarative memory underlies the storage and use of knowledge of facts and events expressed in words. The lexicon memory is compromised by lesions in the left temporal–parietal–occipital area and is known as Wernike aphasia. The grammar, which subserves the rule-governed combining lexical items into complex sentences, depends on a distinct neural system that includes frontal, basal-ganglia, parietal, and cerebellar structures. It represents an example of procedural memory. The grammar memory is compromised by lesions in the left frontal areas and subcortical structures. This type of aphasia is known as Broca's aphasia.

memory. Many readers will recall Lashley's (1950) pessimistic conclusion from his series of experiments and stated in his famous article, "In Search of the Engram." In all respect to Lashley's genius research, the existence of several different forms of memory with differing neuronal substrates was not recognized at his time nor were modern analytic techniques available then.

II. DECLARATIVE MEMORY

A. Anatomy

A classic case of severe amnesia in H.M. patient[2], indicates that the medial temporal areas play a critical role in consolidation of declarative memory. The medial temporal structures are hierarchically organized (Fig. 14.1): the hippocampal region is heavily connected with entorhinal cortex, which is strongly connected with both the perirhinal and parahippocampal cortices, which are in turn connected extensively with temporal and parietal neocortical regions. The hippocampus in its turn projects to the mammillary bodies of the hypothalamus and anterior nucleus of the thalamus. The last two structures are impaired in another amnestic syndrome named Korsakoff's syndrome[3]. High resolution functional brain imaging that was used to examine activity in these small, closely spaced structures located deep in the brain showed activation of the above mentioned structures in memory tasks. Animal studies have replicated and extended human findings, showing that the medial temporal lobe does not act as a single, homogenous structure in the formation of memories, but rather it functions through a complex interplay of many distinct subregions of the medial temporal cortex (see Fig. 14.1), with each subregion making a separate contribution to memory formation.

Modern view considers the medial–temporal complex as a complex system subserving several related memory functions, including the encoding, consolidation, and retrieval of new memories. It should be stressed that memories themselves are stored in temporal–parietal–frontal areas while the hippocampus serves as a reference to the memories. Memories eventually become largely independent of the medial temporal lobe structures, and dependent upon neocortical regions. For example, declarative memories of visual objects appear to be located in the "ventral" visual stream[4].

---

[2]The patient H.M. underwent a surgical operation as a treatment for medically refractory epilepsy that included removing left and right medial temporal areas (including hippocampus). From that day forth he was unable to form a new declarative memory for even the most salient of events.

[3]The Russian clinician Sergei Sergeievich Korsakov in 1887 was the first to describe amnesia (both retrograde and anterograde) that were associated with nutritional (thiamine) deficiency in alcoholics.

[4]This type of declarative memory is rooted in inferior and lateral temporal-lobe structures and underlies the formation of perceptual representations of objects. These representations are associated with recognition and identification of objects and the long-term storage of knowledge about objects. The ventral visual stream is thus a memory-based system, feeding representations into long-term (declarative) memory, and comparing those representations with new ones.

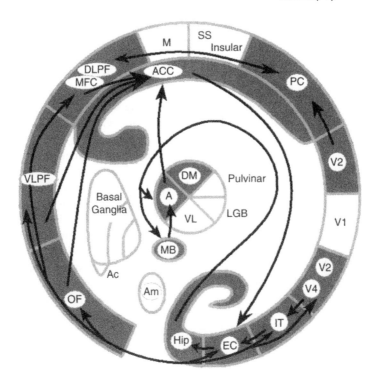

FIGURE 14.1   Components of the episodic memory system. Abbreviations as in Fig. 13.1 and 13.2.

A familiar object, face or scene might spontaneously trigger a memory trace, but most acts of remembering begin with a goal-directed active attempt to recall. The areas of the prefrontal cortex seem to be involved in this active recall operation. Indeed, on the one hand the prefrontal areas receive highly processed sensory information from the posterior cortical areas, store plans of actions, and perform executive functions such as working memory, action selection, action initiation, and action suppression. On the other hand, through the top–down connections the prefrontal cortex is in position to activate memories associated with a given action. Neuropsychological data support this theoretical inference: patients with frontal lesions are significantly impaired at free recall of memorized recent items[5].

---

[5]Moreover these patients are not using subjective organizational strategies, that is, healthy control subjects had a tendency to consistently group certain words together across retrieval trials (e.g., "spoon" and "plate"), frontal patients did so to a lesser degree, in essence recalling the words in a more random fashion. Having these difficulties with retrieval effort some of the frontal patients confabulate. This confabulation behavioral pattern is opposite to that typically observed in memory loss.

B. Encoding and Retrieval Operations

Memory as a single entity is manifested in three separate stages: encoding, storing, and retrieval. Storing can be divided into short-term and long-term memories. Mechanisms of long-term memory (permanent storing) are usually studied by cellular biology with emphasis on structural changes in neuronal synapses. The mechanisms of short-term (or working memory were reviewed in Chapter 12). In this chapter we focus on encoding and retrieval operations.

It is logical to suggest that to minimize efforts and resources memory is encoded and retrieved in the same areas that are responsible for presentation of sensory stimuli. Early evidence that sensory regions are associated with memory retrieval was obtained by Wilder Penfield from Neurological Institute of MacGill University in Montreal in 40–50s (see for example, Penfield and Perot, 1963). Penfield electrically stimulated regions of exposed cortex in awaked human patients undergoing surgery for epilepsy, and found that stimulation of regions of occipital and temporal cortex would sometimes elicit memories[6], and that the sensory modality of the elicited memories varied depending on the region of cortex stimulated.

The positron emission tomography (PET) and functional magnetic resonance imaging (fMRI) studies carried out in 1990s and later confirmed this inference. They provided direct evidence indicating that metabolic activations in encoding and retrieving stages of memory tasks significantly overlap with each other. For example, in a study by Wheeler et al. (2000) subjects memorized words paired with either sounds or pictures. At test, subjects were asked to recall whether the words had been previously associated with pictures or sounds, thus encouraging retrieval of vivid, modality-specific memories. Encoding resulted in increased activity in visual cortex (from calcarine to fusiform gyrus) for pictures, and in auditory cortex (from Heschl's gyrus to middle temporal gyrus) for sounds. Retrieval of pictures from memory was associated with reactivation of visual cortex near fusiform gyrus, whereas retrieval of sounds was associated with bilateral superior temporal gyrus near secondary auditory regions.

Retrieval operations were further decomposed into two sub-processes named as familiarity and recollection operations[7]. In a recent paper Michael Rugg and Andrew Yonelinas (2003) reviewed results from neuropsychological, event-related

---

[6]In these electrical stimulation studies, regions of superior and middle temporal lobes were associated with auditory memories ("I hear singing ... Yes, it is *White Christmas*") whereas regions of more posterior temporal and occipital lobes were associated with visual memories ("... I saw someone coming toward me as if he were going to hit me").

[7]To get the feeling of the difference between being familiar and being recollected, remember uncomfortable experience of recognizing a person as familiar, yet being unable to recollect any qualitative information about the person such as their name or where we met the person before. Such experiences suggest that recall from memory consists of two parts: (1) acontextual sense of familiarity, (2) recollection of detailed information about previous events.

potential (ERP), and functional neuroimaging studies to show that familiarity and recollection operations are supported by distinct neural mechanisms.

C. Neuronal Model

The most popular model of the hippocampus according to which the hippocampus encodes and temporally stores the compressed index of an episode (McNaughton, 1989) was presented in Chapter 4 of this book (see Fig. 4.5). Briefly, the sensory-related part of any episode is encoded in parietal–temporal lobes while the action-related part of the episode is encoded in the frontal lobe. Without the hippocampus, the trace of the episode in these areas can be kept only temporally in a form of reverberation of neuronal impulses in recurrent neuronal networks. Because of its electrical basis the temporal trace of the episode in the cortical neuronal networks is very sensitive to interference. The hippocampus is a place where the two spatially distributed representations of the episode (posterior and frontal) converge into a single activation pattern. The hippocampal trace is associated with long-term chemically based potentiation induced by a burst of the theta rhythm and, for this reason, lasts for longer time intervals. So, the hippocampus serves as a temporally storage mechanism for the episode. The hippocampal representation later becomes active either in explicit recall, or in implicit processes such as sleep. This gives rise to reinstatement of the corresponding neocortical memory, resulting in long-term adjustments of neocortical connections – long-term memory.

III. ACETYLCHOLINE AS MEDIATOR OF DECLARATIVE MEMORY

A. Septum as an Extension of Cholinergic Ascending System

The core element of the episodic memory system is the hippocampus. The hippocampus generates unique rhythms called the hippocampal theta rhythms. Generation of these rhythms is controlled by mediator acetylcholine (ACh). This mediator is produced in the septal nucleus and transported to the hippocampus via the septal–hippocampal pathway (Fig. 14.2). The intensity of cholinergic input to the hippocampus defines the amplitude of theta oscillations. It is important to stress here that the septum represents an extension of cholinergic ascending system located in the nuclei of the brain stem and receives a strong activation input from the brain stem.

The rest of the cortex excluding the hippocampus and including prefrontal, medial temporal, and insular cortical areas receives the cholinergic input from the nucleus basalis of Meynert. The basal nucleus in contrast to wide spread output

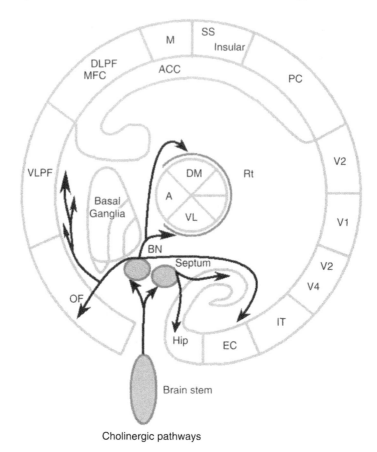

Cholinergic pathways

FIGURE 14.2   Cholinergic pathways of episodic memory. The basal nucleus of Meynert (BN) and the septal nucleus (septum) represent an extension of cholinergic neurons of the ascending reticular formation in the brain stem. Cholinergic neurons of the septal area project to the hippocampus and related cortical areas, while cholinergic pathways from the basal forebrain project more diffusely to the prefrontal areas and to the reticular nucleus (Rt) of the thalamus.

receives an input mostly from the limbic cortex and, consequently, can be considered as an interface between the limbic system and the entire cerebral cortex. The output of this nucleus is also directed to the reticular nucleus of the thalamus thus enabling the basal nucleus to modulate information flow through the thalamus to the cortex.

There are nicotinic and muscarinic receptors[8] for acetylcholine. The muscarinic receptors are diffusely distributed over the brain with M1 receptor being excitatory and M2 receptor being inhibitory. Nicotinic receptors are found more selectively in the brainstem.

[8]They are named so because of selectivity to the two alkaloids.

B. Hippocampal Theta Rhythm and Long-Term Potentiation

Theoretically, according to the scheme presented in Fig. 14.2 acetylcholine can modulate the episodic memory trace by two mechanisms: (1) by enhancing amplitude of theta rhythm in hippocampus and, consequently, by enhancing long-term potentiation in this region, and (2) by activating broad areas of the cortex in response to behaviorally meaningful stimuli through activation of the basal nucleus[9]. Numerous experimental studies support this theoretical inference. The studies show that any type of pharmacological manipulation within the cholinergic system in healthy adults affect declarative memory. For example, acetylcholine esterase inhibitors[10] improve declarative memory[11]. In line with this, administration of scopolamine, an anticholinergic agent, is associated with impaired learning of novel face–name associations and reduced the blood oxygen level dependent (BOLD) signal in ventro-lateral prefrontal, inferior temporal, and hippocampal regions. Finally, administration of scopolamine in humans also reduced the frontal P3a[12] component of ERP responses to infrequently occurring deviant stimuli. The association between the P3a and the level of acetylcholine in the brain shows that enhancement of neuronal responses to novel or contextually deviant stimuli is controlled by the cholinergic innervation.

IV. ERP INDEXES OF EPISODIC MEMORY

A. "Old–New" Effect in Recalling Stage

There are several paradigms to study neurobiological basis of episodic memory. In all of these paradigms stimuli are presented during the memorization stage and tested during the recalling stage. Different imaging parameters such as fMRI, PET,

---

[9]Recall that the basal nucleus receives most of its input from the limbic system thus forming an interface between the limbic system and the entire cortex.

[10]Note that acetylcholine esterase reuptakes the acetylcholine molecules from the synaptic cleft and consequently prolongs the excitatory effect of this modulator of the memory system.

[11]In contrast, systemic infusions of muscarinic cholinergic receptor antagonists produce an amnesic syndrome in humans, primates, and rodents. Disconnection of either the frontal or the temporal cortex from acetylcholine afferents leads to deficits in visual recognition memory and object–reward association learning. In addition, immunotoxic lesions of the basal nucleus lead to reductions in the level of acetylcholine in frontal and temporal cortices, the extent of which are correlated with concurrent behavioral impairments in a learning task.

[12]In Chapter 2 of the Part II devoted to the Attentional networks we mentioned the inherent structural heterogeneity of neuronal networks generated P3a. The attentional networks are interlinked with the memory systems. Attention enhances the response to the selected source of information and thus creates necessary condition for encoding and memorizing the trace of stimulus. So, the other mediator to elevate P3a component is noradrenaline – the mediator of attentional networks.

scalp electroencephalogram (EEG) have been used in healthy subjects. In few rare cases, intracranial local field potentials were recorded from electrodes inserted for diagnostic purposes into the brain of epileptic patients.

During the recalling stage of the old–new paradigm the imaging parameters are measured for two types of the presented items. The first type corresponds to the old items, that is, those items that were learned during the memorization stage. The second type of stimuli corresponds to the new items, that is, those items that are presented the first time to the subjects. The difference between ERPs to the old and new items is called "old–new" effect[13] and sometimes named Dm effect. The ERP difference wave is distributed over the left temporal–parietal area (Allan and Rugg, 1997) indicating involvement of the sensory systems in storing the episodic memories.

B. "Remembered–Forgotten" Effect in Encoding Stage

In the remembered–forgotten effect the imaging parameters are first measured during the encoding stage in which stimuli that will be memorized are presented. For example, EEG and ERP parameters are measured during the encoding (not recalling stage as in the old–new paradigm) for stimuli that are subsequently remembered or forgotten. The difference between the parameters is known as the "remembered–forgotten" effect. There are only few studies including intracranial recordings that dealt with this effect. The results of the studies are schematically presented in Fig. 14.3. As one can see, the remembered stimuli (1) elicit stronger responses in hippocampus, (2) higher coherences in gamma band between rhinal cortex (the polimodal entrance to the hippocampus) and the hippocampus, and (3) larger amplitude of scalp-recorded theta[14] oscillations.

V. PROCEDURAL MEMORY SYSTEM

A. Action-Related Memory Versus Sensory-Related Memory

The procedural memory system[15] is implicated in learning new composite actions. It is also involved in controlling the acquired sensory-motor and cognitive actions. Examples of sensory-motor actions are as follows: driving a car, playing tennis,

---

[13]The effect has never been described in ERPs elicited by old items incorrectly endorsed as new (misses), or by new items incorrectly judged old (false alarms). It therefore appears to be unrelated either to stimulus repetition per se, or merely to decision- or response-related factors.

[14]The functional role of hippocampal theta in memory formation see in Chapter 4.

[15]Note that we use the term "procedural memory" to refer only to one type of implicit, non-declarative, memory system (see Table 14.1).

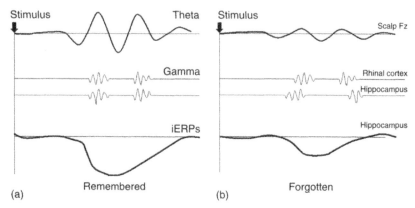

FIGURE 14.3   Remembered–forgotten effect. EEG responses to stimuli that will subsequently be remembered (a) or forgotten (b). Top – scalp-recorded EEG theta rhythms in healthy subjects. Middle – gamma coupling between rhinal cortex and hippocampus in epileptic patients with implanted electrodes. Bottom – intracranial ERPs from hippocampus in epileptic patients. Schematic representation of results from Klimesch (1999) (top), Fell et al. (2001) (middle), and Fernández et al. (1999) (bottom).

performing a piano, writing and typing, articulating words, singing…Such actions are also called skills, habits, routines[16]. The actions are mostly compound ones consisting of more simple actions that have been previously learned. One of the tasks of the procedural memory is to coordinate and to learn a complex sequence of simple actions. As we learned earlier, the brain could be roughly divided into two interconnected but separate parts: the sensory-related and action-related (executive) systems[17]. To simplify, we can say that the episodic memory is associated with the sensory-related system while the procedural memory is associated with the action-related system.

B. Anatomy of Procedural Memory

The action-related parts of brain deals primarily with actions. As is shown in Chapter 12 the striatum receives the input from anterior part of the cortex and

---

[16]I recall my good friend, a famous actor, used to say that all actors in their performance explore routines, templates and that a good actor differs from a bad one simply by the number of routines he or she learned in a class.

[17]Recall that the sensory-related part (sensory systems, attentional networks, and, partly, affective system) deals primarily with sensory information, stores this information in distinct element named chunks. The sensory-related memory system needs a special element – the hippocampus. Using the chunk metaphor we can say that the hippocampus creates the chunks associated with sensory episodes. The chunks are maintained in this system for a certain period of time before it is consolidated in the frontal–temporal–parietal areas of the cortex. Encoding the chunk into the hippocampal system needs a relatively short time that corresponds to a few oscillations of hippocampal theta rhythm.

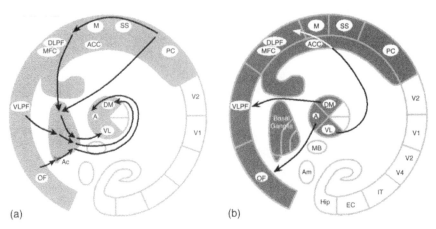

(a)   (b)

FIGURE 14.4   Pathways of procedural memory. The basal ganglia (1) map actions widely distributed in the frontal–parietal cortex, (2) project to the thalamus through direct and indirect pathways (a), (3) via the thalamus project back to the frontal lobe (b).

forms a map of actions. Acquiring a new action needs rearrangement of the map of actions. The mechanisms of these rearrangements represent the basis of procedural memory. So, procedural memory critically depends on the basal ganglia and related structures.

Procedural memory, unlike episodic memory, does not need a separate system for encoding and consolidating event. Memories reside in the executive system itself. An engram of procedural memory represents slowly changing synaptic connections in the executive system (Fig. 14.4). The system includes positive and negative loops in the frontal–basal ganglia–thalamo-cortical circuits. So, besides the executive functions the basal ganglia are involved in learning sensory-motor contingencies, organization of sequential movements, reinforcement-based learning (including emotionally competent award-based learning), motor planning particularly if it involves precise timing, and multiple motor programs[18]. In addition to the executive system of the cerebrum the procedural memory appears to include the cerebellum (not shown in our scheme in Fig. 14.4)[19].

---

[18]I recall a Parkinsonian patient in a clinic of the Institute of the Human Brain with severe impairments in learning a simple GO/NOGO task. It was impossible for him to learn a simple contingency: to press a button to GO cues and to withheld from pressing to NOGO cues.

[19]The cerebellum has additionally been implicated in coordination of complex implicit and imaginative hand movements and in mental rotation. The cerebellum has important timing functions, and seems to be involved in coordination sequences of actions. Similar to the basal ganglia, the cerebellum projects via the thalamus to frontal cortex, with each cerebellar region projecting to particular frontal regions.

C. Basal Ganglia and Language

As we know from Chapter 12 the basal ganglia receive mapping projections from frontal–parietal–temporal areas which are parallely processed in segregated circuits. These parallel circuits have the same network structure and perform the same general functions such as action selection, action initiation, and action suppression. For example, Broca's area is projecting to the striatum in the similar way as other cortical areas. This indicates that the basal ganglia participate in all functions ascribed to Broca's area including procedural learning of grammatical rules[20]. It seems logical that damage to Broca's area produces a common difficulty known as agrammatism. For those patients speech is difficult to initiate, it is non-fluent, labored, and halting while language is reduced to disjointed words with great difficulty to construct an appropriate sentence[21]. Similar speech disturbances are observed in damage or electrical stimulation of all parts of the basal ganglia thalamic circuits. For example, George Ojemann, a scientist from University of Washington, reported that electrical stimulation of the dominant ventro-lateral thalamus can produce deficits in language processing that are not seen after similar stimulation of the non-dominant ventro-lateral thalamus. The nature of the language deficit varies, depending upon the location of the stimulation site (Johnson and Ojemann, 2000)[22].

D. Gradual Memorization

Unlike fast encoding subserved by the declarative memory system, learning in the procedural memory system is gradual and needs many associations of the contextual information with the acquiring action. Recall of how long it took you to learn to play tennis or drive a car and compare it with a few seconds event, such as a car accident, that was imprinted in your episodic memory for ever. In the same way recalling from the episodic memory is associated with conscious recollection and takes at least few hundred milliseconds depending on the type of sensory information. Recalling from a procedural memory is faster and could be done without any conscious recollection, automatically.

---

[20]A child learns the grammar of his mother language from the environment gradually and without efforts. However, when we learn a new language it takes us tremendous efforts to acquire a new vocabulary, but the most difficult is to use grammatical rules in fluent speech.

[21]For example, this is how a Broca's aphasic patient is trying to explain how he came to the hospital: Yes...ah...Monday...er...Dad and Peter H...(his own name), and Dad....er...hospital...and ah... Wednesday...Wednesday, nine o'clock...and oh...Thursday...ten o'clock, ah doctors...two...an' doctors...and er...teeth...yah. (Goodlas and Geschwind, 1976).

[22]A Russian Professor Vladimir Smirnov (with whom the author worked for 15 years) wrote a book "Stereotactic neurology" (Smirnov, 1976) where he summarized his observations during electrical stimulation of subcortical sites in patients with electrodes implanted for diagnosis and therapy.

E. ERP Correlates of Recalling from Procedural Memory

ERP correlates of recalling from procedural memory in comparison to conscious recollecting are presented in Fig. 14.5. Recalling from procedural memory is presented by the frontal lateralized P2 component elicited by GO cues in the two stimulus visual GO/NOGO task. An example of conscious recollection is presented by P3b component which we associate with engagement operation (see Chapter 12). As one can see recalling from episodic memory is at least 100 ms faster than conscious recollection of the event.

VI. MEDIATORS OF PROCEDURAL MEMORY

Theoretically we can separate two main mediators of the procedural memory system – (1) dopamine that is transported to the striatum from the substantia nigra and (2) acetylcholine that is produced by specific cholinergic cells within the striatum itself (Fig. 14.6). These two mediators modulate information flow in the basal ganglia. The dopamine from the substantia nigra changes the threshold of excitation of the striatal neurons while the acetylcholine produced by a certain type of neurons within the striatum itself activates or deactivates the neighboring output neurons of the striatum[23].

The following studies support this theoretical inference. Parkinsonian patients with depletion of dopamine in the striatum display a lower performance on procedural learning tasks supporting the involvement of dopamine in the procedural memory. In a recent study Yasuji Kitabatake from Kyoto University Faculty of Medicine and his colleagues (Kitabatake et al., 2003) showed that selective ablation of cholinergic neurons in the striatum impairs procedural learning in the tone-cued T-maze memory task thus supporting the involvement of acetylcholine in episodic memory.

VII. SUMMARY

There are several different types of memory which involve different brain systems. One distinction can be made on the basis of temporal dynamics such as ultra-short (hundreds of milliseconds), short-term (several seconds), and long-term memories (up to periods comparable with life span). Long-term memory in turn can be divided into two broad categories depending on the type of stored information and neuronal mechanisms. They are explicit or declarative memory (which in turn is divided into episodic and semantic subtypes) and implicit or procedural memories (which is divided into procedural memory, instrumental, and conditioned reflexes).

---

[23]Recall that dopamine has been viewed in this book as the main mediator of the executive system while acetylcholine has been viewed as the main mediator of the episodic memory system.

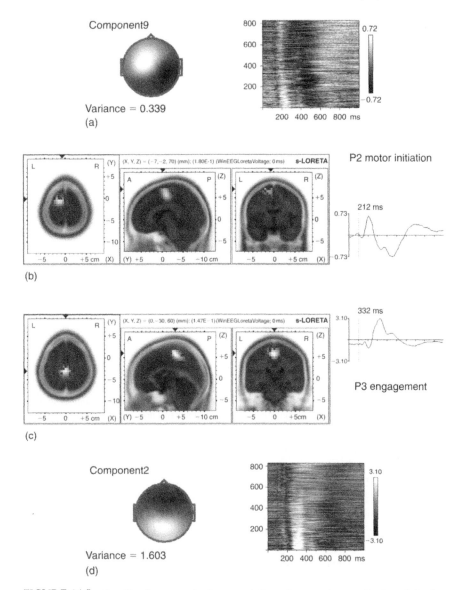

FIGURE 14.5   Recalling from procedural memory is faster than conscious recollection of stimulus. Two independent components in response to GO stimuli in the two stimulus GO/NOGO task are contrasted – (a, b) the component representing recall from the episodic memory and (c, d) the component associated with conscious recollection of the GO event. The subjects trained 20 trials before the testing and performed the task with few errors. The first component is generated in the premotor cortex of the frontal lobe, while the second component (P3b) is generated in the parietal cortex. For each component, topography, s-LORETA image, time dynamics and age dependence in a sample of over 800 healthy subjects of age 7 to 89 are depicted in the same way as in Fig. 10.7. ERPs are taken from the HBI normative database.

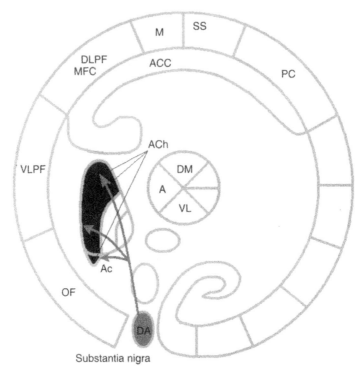

FIGURE 14.6   Mediator pathways of procedural memory. The main (projection) neurons of striatum (the core element of the procedural memory shown in black color) receive dopaminergic input
from the substantia nigra and cholinergic input from local cholinergic neurons of the striatum itself.

The declarative memory system includes hippocampus and related structures such as
the mammillary bodies of the hypothalamus and the anterior nucleus of the thalamus.
PET and fMRI studies show co-activation of these areas in encoding and retrieving
stages of episodic memory. Hippocampal theta rhythm samples the encoding information into chunks that are memorized due to long-term potentiation of hippocampal neurons. "Old–new effect" of the recalling stage and "remembered–forgotten"
effect of the encoding stage constitute ERP correlates of the episodic memory.
The power of the theta rhythm is modulated by mediator acetylcholine. This mediator is produced in the septal nucleus and transported to the hippocampus via septal–hippocampal pathway. The procedural memory system is associated with learning
new motor and cognitive actions and critically depends on the basal ganglia and
related structures. Recalling from the procedural memory is faster than recalling
from the episodic memory. The recalling from procedural and episodic memories
are reflected in different ERP components elicited in response to GO cues of the
GO/NOGO task. There are two main mediators of the procedural memory system:
dopamine that is transported to the striatum from the substantia nigra and acetylcholine that is produced by specific cholinergic cells within the striatum itself.

CHAPTER 15

Methods: Neuronal Networks and Event-Related Potentials

I. INFORMATION PROCESSING IN NEURONAL NETWORKS

A. Analytic Approach

One way of studying information flow in the brain is an analytic approach. The main idea of the approach is to decompose a complex system to elemental parts and to analyze those parts separately[1]. The analytic approach has been used with a good success in studies of the sensory systems. This approach considers perception as a brain operation that can be separated from movement. Moreover, perception is viewed as a sequence of *computational operations* performed by neurons located at different hierarchical levels of sensory information processing.

The basics of this analytic approach in studies of information processing in the brain were laid down in the late 1950s when several laboratories employed the method of recording impulse activity of single neurons and explored how those neurons

---

[1]The analytic approach is opposed to the synthetic approach which studies how new properties of complex systems emerge as the result of collective behavior of the elements of the systems.

respond to stimuli in different modalities. Hubel and Wiesel[2] became famous for their pioneering research in visual modality, Vernon Mountcastle – for his research in somato-sensory modality. Their approach extended the concept of receptive field introduced by Steve Kuffler in 1950s. Kuffler described the organization of receptive field of ganglion cells in retina in a form of ON center OFF periphery circles and introduced the concept of lateral inhibition. Hubel and Wiesel showed that receptive fields in the primary visual cortex (area V1) were more complex having elongated ON and OFF regions and enabling neurons to respond selectively to orientation of visual lines and to spatial frequencies of 2D gratings.

When the properties of single neurons were roughly described researchers were inspired by the idea to study how interaction of single neurons in the brain would allow the emergence of new properties such as memory, gestalt recognition, and even consciousness. Mathematical and computational models of neuronal structural and functional organization appeared as a theoretical, synthetic approach in neuroscience. This approach was laid down by MacCalloch and Pits in 1943 and was coined "neuronal networks"[3].

B. Networks with Lateral Inhibition

Lateral inhibition is a structure of a network in which neurons inhibit their neighbors (see Fig. 15.1a). This type of neural nets was first discovered by Keffe Hartline and his colleagues at Rockefeller University in their studies of the compound eye of the horseshoe crab, *Limulus*.

Neurons in the network receive input $F_i(x)$, where x is a coordinate of a particular neuron. They send inhibitory connections to neighboring neurons with weight distributed according to a function $W(y - x)$. W is called a connectivity function and shows how the strength of connections between neurons changes at

---

[2]Torsten Nils Wiesel and David H. Hubel received in 1981 the Nobel Prize in Physiology and Medicine, for their discoveries in information processing in the visual system. In one experiment they recorded impulse activity of neurons in the primary visual cortex of an anesthetized cat while projected different patterns of light and dark on a screen in front of the cat. They discovered that some neurons fired rapidly when presented with lines of a certain angel. These responses were quite different from responses of neurons in the retina and the geniculate body of the thalamus. Hubel and Wiesel called the cortical neurons that reacted to lines as "simple cells." Other neurons, which they termed "complex cells," responded best to lines or gratings positioned at a certain angle and moving in a certain direction. Further, Hubel and Wiesel showed that different types of neurons in the visual cortex are not randomly scattered over the cortex but instead form organized columns, slabs (e.g., occular dominance or orientation columns).

[3]Simulation of neuronal networks is a dynamically evolving approach in neuroscience. This approach has two goals: (1) to build up a general theory of information processing in the brain and (2) to apply theoretical findings to practical applications in computer science (approach called neuro-computing) as well as in technical vision, robotic sensing, etc.

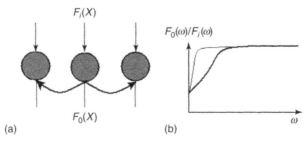

$F_i(X)$

$F_0(\omega)/F_i(\omega)$

$F_0(X)$

(a)

(b)

ω

FIGURE 15.1   Spatial filtration in the neural net with lateral inhibition. (a) Structure of a neural net with lateral inhibition. Circles schematically depict neurons. Each neuron in location x receives the input $I(x)$ and sends inhibition to neighboring neurons. (b) Amplitude–frequency characteristic of the response of the network to sinusoidal ($\sin \omega x$) inputs. Vertical axis – $F_0(\omega)/F_i(\omega)A$ – output/input ratio, Horizontal axis – ω – spatial frequency of the input. The broader is the lateral inhibition (thin line) the sharper is the amplitude–frequency characteristics.

a distance between them. Usually this distribution is modeled by a Gaussian (normal) distribution (see formula below), which has two parameters: amplitude A and radius of action σ, where large A means a higher peak, large σ means a broader spread of the Gaussian curve.

$$W(y - x) = A \exp(-(y - x)^2/2\sigma)$$

C. Spatial Filtration in Neuronal Networks

If a cell linearly transfers the input to the output (it is a good approximation when potentials of membrane of neurons are kept near the threshold), then for the output function $f_0(x)$ of a neuron at a location x we can write the following equation:

$$f_0(x) = k[f_i(x) - \int w(x - y)f_0(y)dy]$$

sign $(-)$ before the integral means that the cells receives inhibitory connections from neighboring neurons, f_0 is the output signal, k is the coefficient of transformation of the input signal to the output signal.

In a spatial frequency domain (using the so-called convolution theorem) this equation looks like:

$$F_0(\omega) = k[F_i(\omega) - W(\omega)F_0(\omega)]$$

Where $F(w)$ is a Fourier transform of a function $f(x)$.

Solving this equation, we get:

$$F_0(\omega) = kF_i(\omega)/(1 + kW(\omega))$$

In other words, this type of network with lateral inhibition works like a high frequency filter – it suppresses the low frequencies and leaves the higher frequencies. The Fourier transform for the Gaussian function is:

$$W(\omega) = \sqrt{2\pi}\sigma \, \exp(-4\pi^2\omega^2/\sigma^2)$$

So, if the lateral inhibition is local, then σ is small and filtration is quite ineffective because besides low frequencies it suppresses the higher frequencies. If the lateral inhibition is global it effectively suppresses only low frequencies (Fig. 15.1b).

This type of network seems to be implemented in the striatum with its long-distance inhibitory interconnections. Thus, we can suggest that the striatum (the input structure of the basal ganglia)[4] can be considered as a filter. This filter is modified during procedural learning and thus can be tuned for mapping newly learned actions.

D. Enhancing Higher Spatial Frequencies in Visual System

One of the functions of the neural net with lateral inhibition is to enhance (to get it more prominent) the most remarkable information. In the frequency domain the enhancement of the important information looks like suppression of low frequencies of the spatial signal. The low frequencies are of less importance because in the visual modality they are associated with information about general luminosity of the visual scene. The high frequencies of the spatial signal are associated with small details of the image which are crucial for recognition of complex objects. The functioning of the network with lateral inhibition can explain some visual illusions (see, e.g., Fig. 15.2).

A more realistic, two layer network is presented in Fig. 15.3. In this network together with lateral inhibition there is also a lateral excitation. If the radius of inhibition is wider, then we get enhancement of the specific frequencies defined by the following equations:

The output function $f_o(x)$ of a neuron at a location x in the case of the network presented in Fig. 15.3 is defined by the following equation:

$$f_o(x) = k\left[f_i(x) + \int w_{ex}(x - y)f_i(y)dy - \int w_{in}(x - y)f_o(y)dy \right]$$

In the frequency domain this equation can presented as follows:

$$F_o(\omega) = kF_i(\omega) + kW_{ex}(\omega)F_o(\omega) - kW_{in}(\omega)F_o(\omega)$$

---

[4]Recall that the striatum receives inputs from the cortex. At the cortical level representations of distinct actions are overlapped with each other but on the striatal level they become segregated (for the experimental evidence see Chapter 12).

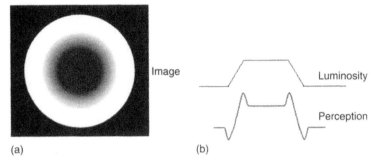

(a)   (b)

FIGURE 15.2   Example of lateral inhibition (Mach band) in the visual system. (a) The Mach image – the luminosity changes as follows: the outside annular area is white, the inner circle is black, and between them brightness changes linearly. We perceive, however, a brighter narrow ring at the outside border and a darker narrow ring at the inside border. (b) The perception curve that is obtained if we apply the spatial filter of the lateral inhibition to the image.

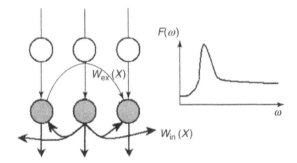

FIGURE 15.3   A neural net with lateral inhibition and lateral excitation. The interplay between excitation and inhibition produces an amplitude–frequency characteristic depicted at the right.

That gives the following relation between the input and output:

$$F_o(\omega) = kF_i(\omega)/[1 + k(W_{in}(\omega) - W_{ex}(\omega)]$$

The dependence of the output/input function on the frequency of the input signal is presented in Fig. 15.3 at right. One can see that the network with combination of lateral inhibition and lateral excitation with a smaller radius of connectivity performs as a band filter that enhances the signal only in a relatively narrow band of frequencies. All through the visual pathway, but especially at the retina and lateral geniculate body – the early stages of visual information processing – lateral inhibition mechanisms enable us to enhance the most remarkable information about sensory images.

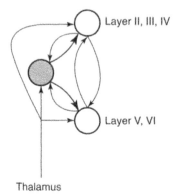

Thalamus

FIGURE 15.4   Canonical cortical circuit. Block diagram of a circuit that successfully models the intracellular responses of cortical neurons to stimulation of thalamic afferents. Three populations of neurons interact with each another: one population is inhibitory neurons (gray circles), and two are excitatory neurons (white circles), representing superficial (layers II and III) and deep (layers V and VI) pyramidal neurons. The layer IV spiny-stellate cells (layer IV) are incorporated with the superficial group of pyramidal cells. Neurons within each population receive excitatory inputs from the thalamus. Self-regulating feedback connections are not shown. Adapted from Douglas and Martin (1991).

E. Canonical Cortical Circuit

There exists a widely accepted general model of the neuron such as Hodgkin-Huxley[5] model but so far there is no model of the cortex that would be admitted by most of neuroscientists. However, many of them do except the basic idea that cortical circuits are organized in recurrent excitatory and inhibitory pathways and that that this organization leads to a number of important emergent properties. This general model was first proposed by Rodney Douglas and Kevan Martin in 1989 (Douglas et al., 1989; Douglas and Martin, 1991) and is known as a canonical cortical circuit (Fig. 15.4).

According to this model, four populations of cortical neurons interact with each other. One population is inhibitory, GABAergic neurons, and three other are excitatory representing stellate cells of layer IV, pyramidal neurons in superficial (layer II, III) and deep (layer V and VI) pyramidal cells. According to the model, inhibition and excitation are not separable events. Only interplay between inhibition and excitation provides the cortex with its unique characteristics. Synchronous electrical activation of neurons in the cortex inevitably set in motion a sequence of excitation and inhibition events. The temporal form of this response depends on the cortical

[5]The Hodgkin-Huxley model of neuron is a set of non-linear differential equations that describe how action potentials in neurons are initiated and propagated. Alan Lloyd Hodgkin and Andrew Huxley won in 1963 the Nobel Prize in Physiology or Medicine for this work they had done in 1952.

layer in which the neuron is located. The temporal dynamics of excitation/inhibition seems to be reflected in positive/negative components of event-related potentials (ERPs).

F. Inhibition as Cause of High Frequency Oscillations

As one can judge from Fig. 15.4 excitatory connections dominate in the cortical canonical circuits. These excitatory connections are reciprocal ones forming positive feedback loops which serve as a basis for reverberation of activity within local neuronal circuits. Indeed, the more the excitatory neurons fire, the more they send postsynaptic potentials to the neighbor neurons, that is, the more neurons are depolarized, and consequently the more they discharge. These excitatory interconnections induce a kind of avalanche behavior – exponentially increasing activity of neurons.

This avalanche is stopped by inhibitory connections. Inhibitory neurons hyperpolarize neighbor neurons and prevent them from firing. So, neurons stop firing for a period of inhibitory postsynaptic potentials, start firing again when the inhibition decays, and so on. This temporal sequence of excitation followed by inhibition produces oscillations with a frequency defined by the duration of inhibitory postsynaptic potentials[6]. Intracellular recording of Douglas and Martin combined with ionophoresis of GABA agonists and antagonists showed that intracortical inhibition is mediated by $GABA_A$ and $GABA_B$ receptors. The $GABA_A$ component occurs in the early phase of the impulse response. It is reflected in the strong hyperpolarization that follows the excitatory response and lasts about 50 ms. This type of hyperpolarization probably is reflected in oscillations of about 20 Hz which is in the beta frequency range. The $GABA_B$ component occurs in the late phase of the response, and is reflected in a sustained hyperpolarization that lasts some 200–300 ms.

G. Synaptic Depression as Source of Low Frequency Oscillations

The other source of preventing avalanche behavior lies in synaptic depression. The synaptic depression is a more slow process in comparison to the duration of inhibitory postsynaptic potentials. It lasts a few hundreds of milliseconds (400–500 ms). Consequently, the synaptic depression, in theory, can produce oscillations in delta frequency band. In our laboratory in 1990s we modeled behavior of the realistic neuronal network with interconnections imitating synaptic depression. In computer simulations it was shown that under certain conditions the network starts producing oscillations with a frequency defined by the time constant of synaptic

---

[6]As was shown in Part I, Chapter 3, the interplay between excitatory and inhibitory processes within the canonical cortical circuit forms a basis for beta oscillations.

depression[7]. A result of these studies is presented in Fig. 15.5. One can see that the network of cells interconnected by synapses exhibiting depression in course of continuous stimulation can produce oscillations. The frequency of the oscillations is determined by the time constant of the synaptic depression.

H. Canonical Cortical Module

In 1980s in our laboratory we developed a mathematical model of a so-called canonical cortical module (Kropotov and Kremen, 1999). The basic idea was a suggestion that the cortex is organized in small modules[8]. Each module corresponds to approximately a 500 × 500 square microns cortical area. The module is supposed to exhibit the full array of operators that are implemented in the primary visual cortex. These operators include encoding all orientations and all possible spatial frequencies which are extracted in the cortical area at a given eccentricity. The model relies on the following basic principles of cortical organization:

1. *Opponent Cell Principle*: According to this principle neuronal circuits include opponent cells selectively encoding complementary (opponent) features of the input. An example of opponent neurons is given by a pair of ON and OFF segregated channels in the retino-geniculo-striate system. The ON and OFF channels include neurons that are selectively excited in response to the two opponent features of the visual image: lightness for ON cells[9]) and darkness for OFF cells.

2. *Assembly Principle*: According to this principle, cells with similar features are gathered into assemblies. Examples of such assemblies are found in somato-sensory, auditory, and visual cortical areas. In the striate cortex eye dominance slabs have a form of parallel bands, while spatial frequency slabs are organized in the pinwheel patterns.

3. *Canonical Cortical Circuit Principle*: The principle states that different parts of the same cortical area (such as the primary visual cortex) have the same basic microcircuitry. Several components and connections dominate in

---

[7]It is not clear, however, if such conditions can be met in real cortical networks. We can only speculate that in the case of a disconnection of the cortical area from the thalamus (induced, e.g., by tumor) these conditions are met and the corresponding cortical area starts generating rhythmic activity in a low (delta) frequency band.

[8]The organization of modules may depend on the location of the cortical area and may be different for the primary visual area and the inferior temporal cortex. Our goal was to simulate information processing in the primary visual cortex. I was inspired by the work that in those days was performed in the laboratory of Vadim Gleser at the Pavlovian Institute of Physiology in St. Petersburg. In his studies he showed the existence of opponent sub-fields in receptive fields of simple and complex cells in the visual cortex of cats. He also suggested that these cells perform local Gabor transformations of the retinal image.

[9]Lightness (darkness), by definition, is a local incremental (decremental) deviation in luminosity from the averaged global luminosity.

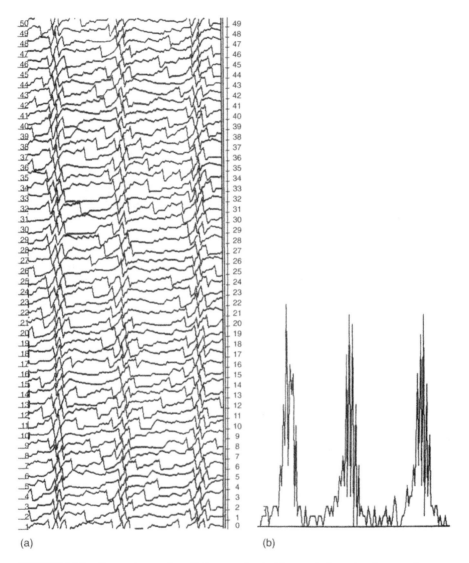

(a)   (b)

FIGURE 15.5   Neuronal network oscillations associated with synaptic depression. A neuronal network with synaptic depression is simulated on the computer. Fifty neurons with strong lateral connections compose the network. (a) Changes of membrane potentials of all 50 neurons. Note that they almost synchronously exceed the threshold of their membranes. (b) Averaged discharge rate of neurons. Note periodic bursts of spikes (Kropotov and Ponomarev, unpublished data).

most cortical areas. They are summarized in a so-called canonical cortical circuit (see Fig. 15.4 above).

4. *Modular Principle*: According to this principle the cortical areas are divided into modules with the same internal structure. In 1974, Hubel and Wiesel

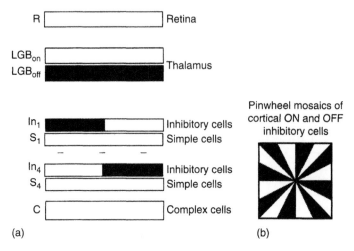

(a)   (b)

FIGURE 15.6   The canonical cortical module. (a) Layers of the canonical cortical module. R – retina, LGB – the lateral geniculate body of the thalamus, $In_1 \dots In_4$ – the layers of inhibitory neurons within the cortex, $S1 \dots S4$ – the layers of cortical simple cells, C – the layer of complex cells. (b) – the distribution of ON and OFF cells in an inhibitory layer of the canonical cortical module – a pinwheel mosaic. White color defines locations of neurons that receive inputs from the ON channel, black color defines locations of neurons that receive inputs from the OFF channel. ON neurons respond with activation to a light spot in the image, while OFF neurons respond to a dark spot of the image. Adapted from Kropotov and Kremen (1999).

were the first to introduce the concept of the hypercolumn as the elementary functional unit of the visual cortex[10].

Taking into account these principles, we can construct a basic architecture of the canonical cortical module in the primary visual cortex. As one can judge, the principles do not provide a unique solution of the cortical organization. It is quite possible that different visual areas (such as areas 17, 18, 19) are organized in a different manner for a better performing of their specific functions. One of the solutions is presented in Fig. 15.6.

Let us describe the basic operations performed by the canonical cortical module in Fig. 15.6. An input signal at the retina is described as a function $s(x,y)$. According to the *opponent cells principle* at the level of the thalamus, the input activity is encoded by activation of two channels of opponent cells. For simplification of further calculations, let us define a new variable: $S(x,y) = s(x,y) - s_{average}$ (where $s_{average}$ is a luminosity averaged over the whole retina and $S(x,y)$

[10]The hypercolumn represents all set of possible orientations in the corresponding local visual field. The hypercolumns are organized in the repetitive fashion within the visual cortex.

determines the fluctuation of a local input activity s from an average background activity $s_{average}$. Then, the ON channel encodes $S(x,y)$, if $S(x,y) \geq 0$. The OFF channel provides excitatory signal for a local decrease in $S(x,y)$, that is, it encodes $|S(x, y)| = -S(x, y)$, if $S(x, y) < 0$ [11].

We further suggest that at the thalamic level ON and OFF cells have uniform distribution located in two different layers. When the outputs of the ON and OFF cells converge in the cortex in the inhibitory layer, according to the *assembly principle*, they form a specific mosaic. Theoretically, many different ON/OFF mosaics might be suggested. Among all possible spatial patterns here we describe the pinwheel pattern (Fig. 15.6b) [12].

According to the *canonical cortical circuit* principle the excitatory cells in the cortical layer of simple cells receive positive inputs directly from the thalamic neurons and inhibitory inputs from the cortical inhibitory cells. We simulated a model with four pinwheel layers of inhibitory neurons, shifted in relation to each other by $\pi/2$. The densities of inhibitory neurons distributed in four different layers In_i $(i = 1...4)$ are represented as follows:

$$n_{In(i)on} = 1 - \sin(\omega\psi + \pi i/2)$$
$$n_{In(i)off} = 1 + \sin(\omega\psi + \pi i/2) \tag{15.1}$$

where ω – circular frequency determining the number of "pins" in the mosaic; ψ – polar angle of inhibitory neuron in the plane In_i.

Each module has also four layers of simple cortical neurons (S_i, $i = 1...4$) and one layer of complex cortical neurons (C). The cells in the complex layer integrate inputs from the corresponding cells in the four simple cells layers. The complex cells layer is considered as the output layer of the canonical cortical module.

I. Gabor Filtration in the Canonical Cortical Model

We do not want to present here all mathematical transformations that we made, but the mathematically advanced readers can produce a final formula by themselves. This formula represents the output of the complex cell layer in dependence on the retinal input. Using this formula, we obtained spatial frequency and orientational characteristics for complex neurons located in different parts of the module.

---

[11]Note that brain uses both ON and OFF channels instead of one because information is conveyed within the nervous activity by discharge rate of neurons which is of a positive value.

[12]Several years later after our publication of the pinwheel modular organization of the cortex, the iso-orientation domains were explored in primary visual cortex of monkey by newly developed optical imaging. High-resolution maps revealed that the most prominent organizational feature of orientation preference was a radial arrangement, forming a pinwheel-like structure surrounding a singularity point (Bartfeld and Grinvald, 1992). Thus these experimental finding confirmed our theoretical solution.

These characteristics are presented in Fig. 15.7. One can see that the canonical cortical module performs a spatial frequency decomposition of the input by mapping different frequencies and orientations into spatially separated different output areas of the module.

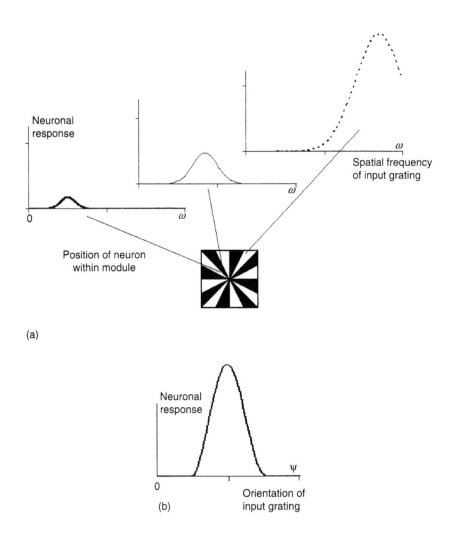

FIGURE 15.7 Spatial frequency and orientational selectivity of complex cells in the canonical cortical module. (a) Spatial frequency characteristics of a complex neuron – response of the neurons with different polar radii to sine-wave gratings of different spatial frequencies ω. (b) Orientational characteristics of a complex neuron – response of the neuron to different orientations (ψ) of the input grating. Adapted from Kropotov and Kremen (1999).

J. Texture Encoding by the Canonical Cortical Module

The model of the canonical cortical module can be used in different practical applications in computer vision. One of the apparent properties of the model is that it performs a piecewise Gabor decomposition of input textures[13]. In our computer simulations we tested the model by using different textures as inputs and observed the output as activity of the complex cells (Fig. 15.8). As illustrated in Fig. 15.8, different textures (that remarkably overlap at the input level) are mapped into distinct (non-overlapping) parts of the canonical cortical module.

From the above, we can generalize that neural nets with complex spatial patterns of excitation and inhibition can perform complex spatial filtrations of the input signal and can map overlapping inputs to non-overlapping outputs. In the visual cortex, small (500 × 500 squared microns) modules perform local Gabor decomposition of visual images. This inference of the model is supported by numerous experimental studies of receptive fields of neurons in the primary visual cortex.

K. Hierarchical Organization

Information flow within the cortex is hierarchically organized. For example, during viewing a behaviorally meaningless visual object, the sensory information propagates through the hierarchically organized cortical system from the primary sensory areas to the higher cortical regions. The latencies of neuronal responses in different areas of the visual hierarchy have been experimentally measured in monkeys. In a study by Mathew Schmolesky and his colleagues from Utah University (Schmolesky et al., 1998), onset latencies from many primate visual areas using the same experimental and analytical techniques were obtained. The results demonstrated that the two major functional streams in the primate visual system respond with quite different latencies. Neurons in the dorsal stream that arises from the

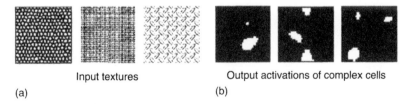

Input textures   Output activations of complex cells
(a)   (b)

FIGURE 15.8   Texture discrimination by the canonical cortical module. (a) Input textures. (b) The complex layer outputs of the canonical cortical module for the corresponding textures. Adapted from Kropotov and Kremen (1999).

[13]A texture is considered as a set of elements filling a surface in a more or less periodic manner. Thus the texture itself can be interpreted as a superposition of small elements with different spatial frequencies and orientations.

magnocellular neurons in distinct layers of the lateral geniculate body of the thalamus deal mostly with perception of spatial relationships and motion[14] and respond with shorter latencies than neurons in the ventral stream. Neurons in the ventral stream arise from the parvocellular neurons in the layers of the lateral geniculate body distinct from the magnocellular layers. The neurons in the ventral visual stream deal mostly with object recognition and color coding and respond with longer latencies.

L. Feedforward and Feedback Connections

The hierarchically organized dorsal and ventral streams in addition to feedforward synaptic connections conveying information from "the bottom to the top" have strong feedback connections returning information from "the top to the bottom." The feedforward and feedback connections can be distinguished by the cortical layers from which they originate and in which they terminate, as illustrated in Fig. 15.9.

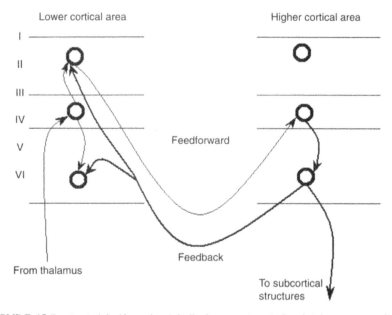

FIGURE 15.9   Cortical feedforward and feedback connections. Left and right – correspondingly lower and higher level cortical areas with numbers depicting layers of the cortex. Feedforward connections are depicted in thin lines. Feedback connections are depicted in thick lines. See explanations in the text.

[14]This pathway is also feeding information to the frontal and parietal lobe visual areas (including eye fields) for navigation and manipulation with visual objects.

The feedforward connections between two cortical areas (the low level and the high level) are formed by the axon projections of pyramidal cells from the lower cortical area to the higher cortical area. These projections terminate predominantly in layer IV of the higher region (as do inputs from the thalamus). The main targets for these feedforward projections are spiny-stellate cells which, in turn, target the basal dendrites of pyramidal cells in layers II and III.

The feedback connections between the two cortical areas are formed by the axon projections from pyramidal cells in the layers V and VI of the higher cortical area. These projections terminate mainly in layers I and VI of the lower cortical area and also terminate at the subcortical structures, such as basal ganglia. The main targets of the feedback projections terminating in layer I are the apical dendrites of pyramidal cells with somata in layers II, III, and V[15].

As one can see, cortical regions tend to be reciprocally connected by feedforward and feedback connections. This type of connectivity is called recurrent or re-entrant (according to Edelman, 1987[16]) pattern. Despite of the fact that these connections are known since early years of neuroscience, the functional meaning of the feedback connections is not clear. There are many speculations regarding their role. One of those speculations suggests that that the top–bottom connections are critical for attention and working memory. The other speculation about the role of feedback connections in the visual pathway concerns the enhancement of contrast in figure background separation.

M. Reflection of Recurrent Connections in ERPs

In monkey, average latencies of neuronal responses of the visual system vary from 76 to 110 ms depending on cortical location. These latencies are smaller than the peak latencies of components in ERPs recorded from the human brain. In Fig. 15.10 we present independent components (and their s-LORETA images) extracted from a set of ERPs computed for healthy adult subjects (selected from the Human Brain Institute Database) in response to presentation of irrelevant visual stimuli. The peak latencies of average neuronal responses to visual stimuli in monkey are presented in ovals. Although the comparing results were obtained in different groups (monkeys and humans) and different techniques (measuring

---

[15]Recall, that negative slow cortical potentials recorded from the scalp during anticipation of the sensory stimulus or the prepared action considered in Chapter 1, Part I as the results of such feedback connections. Through these connections neurons at the higher cortical areas depolarize the apical dendrites and form the sink (negativity) for electrical current in the superficial layers of the cortex.

[16]Gerald Maurice Edelman (the Nobel Prize in Physiology or Medicine in 1972 for his work on the immune system) proposed a theory of consciousness which he named Neural Darwinism or The Theory of Neuronal Group Selection (Edelman, 1987, 1993). The basic concept of his theory is "re-entrant signaling." According to his view the re-entrant signaling is more than a feedback process that corrects errors, it is also a mechanism capable of constructing new groups of neurons responsible for actions.

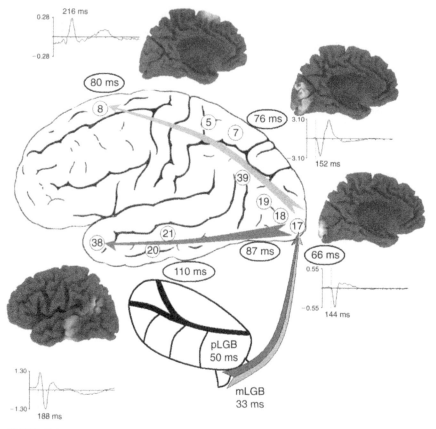

FIGURE 15.10   Latencies of hierarchical information processing in the visual system. Middle – schematic representation of the dorsal and ventral streams in the visual system with the average latencies of neuronal responses in milliseconds to visual stimuli. Average latencies are obtained from monkey experiments of Schmolesky et al. (1998). Latencies are schematically depicted near the corresponding thalamic or cortical area in thick ovals. For comparison 3D s-LORETA images and time dynamic of independent components are depicted. The independent components are extracted from array of 576 ERPs computed for healthy subjects in response to the second stimulus in PP-pair in the two stimulus visual GO/NOGO task. Peak latencies of main fluctuation in ERPs are depicted near the corresponding components.

impulse activity of single neurons on monkey and using independent component analysis[17] in human) the comparison is very useful from didactic point of view. First, we see that a ERP independent component is a sum of positive and negative fluctuations reflecting sequential involvement of excitatory and inhibitory

---

[17]For details see section in Methods, Part II below.

postsynaptic potentials in the cortical areas. It should be noted that the polarity of components depends on three factors: (1) on type of postsynaptic potentials (excitatory or inhibitory) that are dominant in the given time interval, (2) on location, and (3) orientation of the cortical surface that produces the corresponding component a well as (4) on the cortical layer in which postsynaptic potentials are generated. Although these factors are difficult to estimate, it is a temptation to associate positive parts of the visual-related components with excitatory postsynaptic potentials while negative parts of the components with inhibitory postsynaptic potentials. Second, it is difficult to estimate onset latencies from ERPs because we can reliably measure only peak latencies of the ERP components which might be longer than average latencies of responses of impulse activity of neurons. Third, and the most important, negative fluctuations in ERP components do reflect differences in the speed of information flow in the ventral and dorsal streams – the dorsal stream responds faster than the ventral stream.

II. NEUROTRANSMITTERS AND NEUROMODULATORS

A. Fast Transmitters

As we learned in this part of the book, information processing in the brain is performed by means of transformation of spike activity of the presynaptic neurons to slower fluctuations of membrane potentials[18] of the postsynaptic neurons. In its turn information processing can be divided into two different classes of neural net operations: information flow and information modulation[19]. These two operations are maintained by two different classes of neuromediators. They are fast acting and slow acting mediators. These two classes of mediators play different functional roles in information processing.

Neuromediators that are responsible for information flow are fast in their action (Fig. 15.11). They are named neurotransmitters, because it takes them a few milliseconds to bind to receptors of the postsynaptic membrane and to transmit the information. These receptors are usually ligand-gated channels. They open very fast in response to a presynaptic signal. So, in a few millisecond time window after arriving of a spike to the terminal of the presynaptic neuron the flux of ions of the postsynaptic neuron is gated (opened or closed) by the neurotransmitter binding

---

[18]Such as postsynaptic excitatory and inhibitory postsynaptic potentials.

[19]Information flow is the fast process of transformation of activity of presynaptic neurons to activity of postsynaptic neurons. This process is modulated by slower processes in membrane potentials which are united in this book under a common name of modulatory processes, or simply, information modulation.

to the postsynaptic membrane. Two examples of such "fast acting" are given by mediators glutamate and gamma-aminobutyric acid (GABA)[20].

B. Slow Modulators

Neuromediators that are responsible for information modulation are slower in action (Fig. 15.11). It takes them hundreds of milliseconds or even several seconds to change the membrane potential of the postsynaptic neuron. They are usually called neuromodulators to emphasize the fact that the function of these mediators

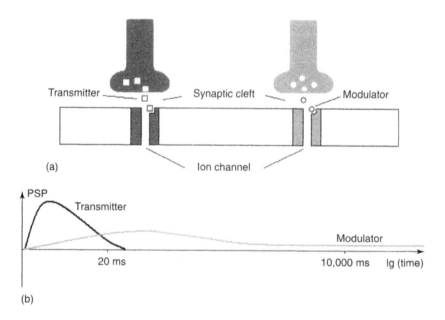

FIGURE 15.11   Neurotransmitters and neuromodulators. (a) Schematic presentation of action of the two types of neuromediators. In both cases the neurotransmitter is released in the synaptic cleft by arriving of spike to the presynaptic terminal. Both neurotransmitter and neuromodulator open the corresponding ion channel. However, action of the neuromodulator is much longer that the action of the neurotransmitter. (b) Time dynamics of postsynaptic potentials induced by correspondingly the neurotransmitter and the neuromodulator.

[20]Glutamate is a common excitatory neurotransmitter in the brain. It activates Na^+ channels on the postsynaptic membrane and depolarizes it. GABA is a common inhibitory neurotransmitter. It activates Cl^- channels and hypopolarizes the membrane. These two neurotransmitters relay sensory information about the external and internal milieu to hierarchically organized sensory cortical areas and are also responsible for execution of actions in response to the constantly changing internal and external conditions.

is to modulate (to change slowly) the action of fast acting transmitters. The action of neuromodulators can be longer (but weaker) than action of the fast acting neurotransmitters because the cascades that they trigger can last for days. Examples of neuromodulators are monoamines (such as norepinephrine, dopamine, and serotonin), acetylcholine, and neuropeptides[21].

C. Modulator Systems

There are four modulator systems in the brain: the cholinergic, noradrenergic, serotoninergic, and dopaminergic systems. All of them are characterized by the following common features: (1) they originate in relatively small parts of the brain stem and the basal forebrain, (2) they project to reticular nucleus of the thalamus, (3) they widely innervate cortical areas, the basal ganglia, as well as the cerebellum[22] and the brain stem centers[23].

The cholinergic and monoaminergic neurons of the brain form a global network. Although the cholinergic and monoaminergic neurons originate in local regions of the brain, occupying regions in the spinal cord, brain stem, and basal telencephalon (Fig. 15.12), they innervate large subcortical and cortical areas and modulate information flow in these regions. These neurons operate as a unified network generating widespread patterns of activity in concert with the states of the brain such as sleep and wakefulness, as well as in concert with different moods such as happiness and sadness, and in association with cognitive gestalts such as focused attention and meditation.

Cholinergic neurons are clustered in the midbrain nuclei, in the basal forebrain nuclei as well as in the basal ganglia. From the septal area, cholinergic neurons project to the hippocampus. From the basal forebrain, cholinergic neurons project to the reticular nucleus of the thalamus, to the orbitofrontal cortex as well to other cortical areas. The cholinergic system is thought to control a general arousal and play an important role in memory formation by activating hippocampal system. The power of hippocampal theta rhythm is determined by the acetylcholine, while death of the acetylcholine neurons is thought to be related to Alzheimer's disease. Drugs that increase the level of acetylcholine in the brain (such as inhibitors of acetylcholine esterase) are now used in elderly patients with failing memory (e.g., Alzheimer's patients).

Most of the noradrenergic[24] neurons of the brain are located in the brainstem in an area called the locus coeruleus. The neurons in this nucleus project to the

---

[21]In analogy with computers we can simplify that transmitters perform in the processor for computing the information while modulators provide a power supply to the main processor.

[22]This innervation is not uniform and equally spread, however. Each mediator has some areas in the brain that are more densely innervated than the others.

[23]These brain centers are responsible for fundamental functions such as respiration, heart beating, etc.

[24]Another name of noradrenaline is norepinephrine.

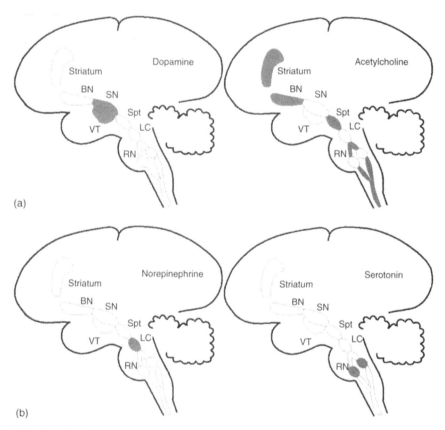

FIGURE 15.12   Cholinergic and monoaminergic neurons in the brain. Note that these clusters of neurons are organized in a continuum that extends from the spinal cord to the basal telencephalon. Projections from these relatively small number of neurons innervate the entire brain and all peripheral muscles, organs, and glands. See text for further details.

frontal cortex thus modulating the mood through beta 1 receptors. Those projections, mediated by alpha 2 receptors are associated with attention and working memory. Noradrenergic neurons project also to the limbic cortex thus modulating emotions, to the cerebellum modulating motor actions, and to the cardiovascular centers of the brain stem modulating blood pressure. Decreases in norepinephrine activity are thought to be related to depression, whereas increases are thought to be related to mania.

Most of the serotoninergic neurons of the brain are located in the brainstem in an area called the raphe nuclei. The neurons from this nucleus innervate the frontal cortex and the limbic system thus modulating mood and emotions (particularly involving in anxiety and pain). The neurons of raphe nuclei also innervate the basal ganglia thus modulating movements, as well as obsessions and compulsions. Serotoninergic projections to the hypothalamus modulate appetite and eating behavior, while serotoninergic projections to the sleep centers in the brainstem are responsible for modulating states of sleep and wakefulness.

There are three different dopamine pathways in the brain that include the mesolimbic dopamine pathway, the mesocortical dopamine pathway, and the nigrostriatal dopamine pathway[25]. The nigrostriatal dopamine pathway projects form the substantia nigra to the basal ganglia, the key element of the system responsible for action selection. The mesolimbic dopamine pathway projects from the ventral tegmental area of the brainstem to the nucleus accumbens, a part of the basal ganglia participating in the limbic circuit and playing an important role in emotional behaviors, such as pleasurable sensations, the powerful euphorea of drugs of abuse. The mesocortical dopamine pathway projects from the ventral tegmental area of the brainstem to the dorso-lateral prefrontal cortex and cingulate (limbic) cortex. During 30 years of pharmacological research the drugs that change concentration of dopamine of the brain were found. It was also shown that drugs increasing the concentration of dopamine produce positive psychotic symptoms, while drugs that decrease the level of dopamine reduce these symptoms. For example, stimulants such as amphetamine and cocaine, that increase the level of dopamine, can cause a paranoid psychosis similar to schizophrenia. On the other hand, all known antipsychotic (reducing psychotic symptoms) drugs block dopamine receptors, particularly D2 receptors. These facts enabled some scientists to suggest a theory of psychosis referred to as the dopamine theory of schizophrenia.

III. METHODS OF ANALYZING ERPS

A. Averaging Technique

In the vast majority of behavioral paradigms invented to study responses of the brain to stimuli and actions, the waveforms of so-called ERPs are isolated from the background electroencephalogram (EEG) by means of averaging procedures. It is tempting to think of the averaging procedure as an operation that extracts a constant signal

---

[25]There is also the tuberoinfundibular dopamine pathway that originates in the hypothalamus and projects to the anterior pituitary gland thus controlling prolactin secretion.

[26]However, theoretically, if the signal changes during the task (e.g., during habituation or learning) the averaged ERP may provide a distorted view of the single-trial waveforms. This is a reason why usually researchers, before recording EEG, ask a subject to perform a short testing task to make sure that the subject understands the task correctly, can do it as fast as needed, and that the orienting response has been extinguished.

associated with information flow in the cortical networks[26] from a background EEG. It is also tempting to view the background EEG as a physiological parameter reflecting modulation processes. Figure 15.13 shows EEG recorded during different sequential trials of the two stimulus GO/NOGO task. The subject was selected

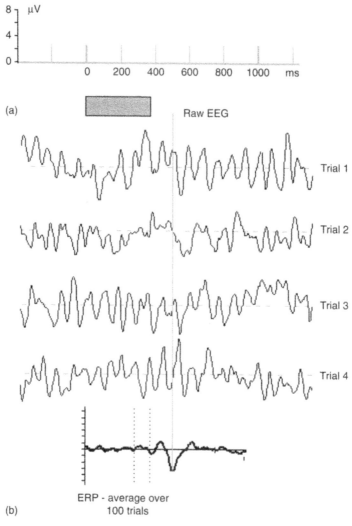

FIGURE 15.13 Averaging technique of ERP computation. (a) EEG recorded from Fz during four so-called ignore trials (presentations of plant–plant pairs which the subject had to ignore) of the two stimulus visual GO/NOGO task. The time course of the trial is schematically presented on the top as a gray box. (b) ERP computed by averaging 100 trials. The ERP reflects, with high temporal resolution, the pattern of neuronal activity evoked by a visual stimulus at Fz electrode position. The EEG was taken from the Human Brain Institute Normative Database – a healthy subject of age 32 was selected.

randomly from the normative database while electrode position was deliberately selected at Fz – an area where no prominent high amplitude alpha oscillations are observed. One can hardly see any changes of EEG pattern in response to stimulus. To observe this small change many trials must be averaged[27]. The averaging technique sums up EEG patterns time-locked to the stimulus presentation. Because trials are not time-locked to EEG oscillations and are presented randomly irrespective of the phase of the current EEG, negative and positive fluctuations preceding the stimulus cancel each other so that the prestimulus interval can be approximated by a straight line with an averaged zero potential.

B. Number of Trials

After averaging EEG fragments over trails of the same category, an ERP for a given electrode represents a waveform of several peaks and troughs (see Fig. 15.13). The amplitude of the peaks and troughs in ERPs varies from $1\mu V$ up to $15-20\mu V$ depending on the task, subject, subject's age, and montage. Recall that amplitude of children EEG recorded in reference to linked earlobes at posterior site may be around $70\mu V$, while amplitude of adult EEG may be around $50\mu V$. Figure 15.13 represents background EEG and ERPs in a healthy women of 32 years old. Note that in this case the amplitude of the spontaneous background oscillations in Fz areas is higher than the average amplitude of the ERP components.

The fluctuations of averaged EEG prior to stimulus represent a noise[28] while averaged ERPs after the stimulus onset represent a signal. Intuitively we feel that the signal to noise ratio depends on the number of trials: the more the trials, the higher is the ratio. The number of trials needed to obtain an optimal signal-to-noise ratio depends on the amplitude of ERP components (the signal) and the background oscillations of the EEG[29]. Moreover, because the signal (s) is assumed to be unaffected by the averaging process, the signal-to-noise (s/n) ratio increases with increasing the number of trials N (see Fig. 15.14). It can be theoretically shown that the ratio depends on N as $\sqrt{N}$. For example, imagine an experiment in which you are measuring the amplitude of the P3 wave, and the actual amplitude of the P3 wave is $20\mu V$. If the EEG noise is $50\mu V$ on a single trial, then the s/n ratio on a single trial will be $20/50$, or 0.4, which means that the noise exceeds the signal. If you average five trials together, then the s/n ratio will be increased by only a factor of 2.2 (which is again not satisfactory). But when you average 100

[27]This is a situation where simple visual inspection can't help. One needs a special computational procedure (averaging) to extract a signal from the background spontaneous EEG activity.

[28]Ideally the prestimulus fluctuations in ERPs must be zero which can be obtained by averaging over a very large number of trials. Practically the prestimulus ERPs differ from zero. The power of these deviations measures the noise.

[29]Experience is the best guide in selecting the number of trials. In the HBI database the rule of thumb is that we need 100 trials per category of stimulus in the task.

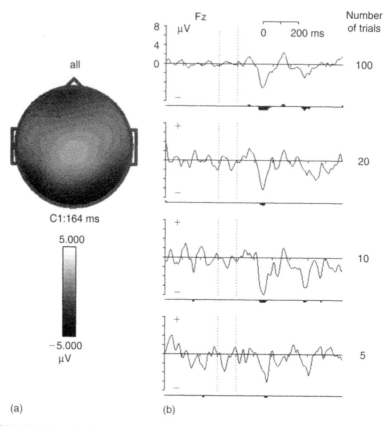

(a)   (b)

FIGURE 15.14   Signal-to-noise ratio of ERP depends on the number of trials as the square root of the number. (a) Topography of the component measured at 160 ms. (b) ERPs averaged over 5, 10, 20, and 100 trials. EEG was recorded from Fz in the healthy subject from Fig. 15.13.

trials the s/n will be increased by a factor 10. This relationship between the number of trials and the s/n ratio is rather disappointing, because it means that achieving a substantial increase in s/n ratio requires a very large increase in the number of trials. For example, to get a reasonable s/n for mismatch negativity – a component that is just 1–4 μV in amplitude – we need to present at least 2000 standard auditory stimuli and 200 deviants.

There are at least three two factors that determine the signal to noise ratio: (1) variations in the background spontaneous EEG activity (such as alpha, theta, and beta oscillations), (2) changes in signal itself, such as due to habituation, fluctuations in arousal level, etc., and (3) non-EEG artifacts (such as eye movements, muscle activity...). An appropriate design of task is needed to minimize the first two factors. To minimize the third factor, several methods of artifact correction have been suggested (see Chapter 8).

C. Single Trial Representations of Independent Components

There is a general agreement that the averaged ERP in cognitive tasks can be represented as a sum of separate components generated by distinct sources in the cortex. If a signal-to-noise ratio is high enough, there is a theoretical possibility to decompose single trial EEG epochs into separate components. In the Human Brain Institute Normative Database, this possibility is provided by a specific computational procedure that employs the algorithm of ICA (see Chapter 8). Figure 15.15 depicts the results of application of the ICA algorithm to a set epochs of EEG recorded during sequential single trials in GO/NOGO task. The task was performed by the same normal subject as in Fig. 15.13.

As one can see the individual P1/N2 component observed in the averaged ERP of this subject is actually decomposed into two separate components: the one that is generated by the left inferior temporal lobe and the one that is generated by the right inferior temporal lobe (see s-LORETA images of the components at the right). Note that the P1/N2 component at the averaged ERP is very small (just only 2.3 μV at negative peak at Fz). However, application of the ICA method have been able to decompose it into two separate components. Moreover these two components can be seen in single trials as is depicted in the middle of Fig. 15.15[30].

In the above mentioned approach the sequence of procedures is as follows. First, we perform the ICA procedure on stimulus-locked single trial EEG fragments recorded from 19 electrodes from a single individual. Second, using topography of the extracted components we calculate generators of the components using s-LORETA. Another approach is also possible. This approach is as follows. First, we perform the ICA on the 19-channel EEG recorded during the whole task (not time-locked to the stimulus) and extract components associated with separate EEG oscillations (such as frontal midline theta, occipital and parietal alpha rhythms, mu-rhythms). Second, using spatial filters built up on the basis of the corresponding topographies we extract the EEG component. And finally, for the extracted EEG rhythm we compute ERPs[31].

---

[30]A similar approach had been recently reported from the Scott Makage group in University of California, San Diego (Tsai et al., 2006). In this study they proposed a statistical framework for estimating the time course of spatiotemporally independent EEG components simultaneously with their cortical distributions. Within this framework, they implemented Bayesian spatiotemporal analysis for imaging the sources of EEG features on the cortical surface. The framework allows researchers to include prior knowledge regarding spatial locations as well as spatiotemporal independence of different EEG sources. The method was named the electromagnetic spatiotemporal ICA (EMSICA) method.

[31]This approach was implemented by the same group of scientists from University of California, San Diego.

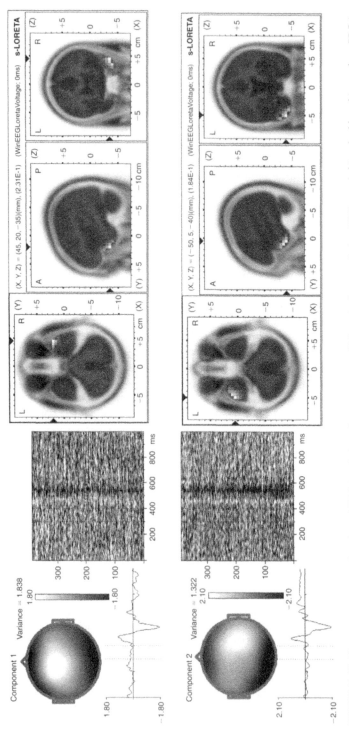

FIGURE 15.15 Decomposition of single trial EEG into independent components. ICA method was applied to EEG recorded in a healthy subjects whose ERP in the two stimulus GO/NOGO task is presented in Fig. 15.13. Two independent components corresponding to the P1/N2 component of the averaged ERP are presented at the top and bottom of the figure. Left – topographies and time courses of the components. Middle – vertically stacking thin color-coded horizontal bars, each representing a single trial. 400 trials are presented. Right – s-LORETA images of the two components.

D. Alpha Ringing

An example of the second methodological approach is presented in Fig. 15.16. EEG data were recorded from a subject performing a two stimulus GO/NOGO task. By means of the ICA method an independent component in raw EEG has been selected. Note that this component is different from the components extracted from time-locked EEG fragments corresponding to separate trials. The topography and s-LORETA image of the extracted component of the background EEG suggests its source in the parietal lobe. Further on, we computed ERPs on the EEG filtered by the extracted component. An example of the ERPs recorded at Pz is presented in Fig. 15.16. The ERP shows that in the prestimulus time interval the averaged fluctuations in EEG are quite small, while presentation of the visual stimulus reset the phase of the fluctuations which results in increase of ERP amplitude after the stimulus presentation – the effect called alpha ringing. A similar approach was implemented by the Scott Makage group from University of California in San Diego (see Jung et al., 2001).

E. ICA Decomposition of Grand Average ERPs

An ERP waveform for a single subject consists of a series of peaks and troughs. These averaged voltage deflections reflect the sum of several components. The components are supposed to be generated by the distributed generators and are associated with certain psychological operations (factors). It should be pointed out that these components are not necessarily to be associated with peaks (positive deflections), and troughs (negative deflections)[32] on ERPs waveforms.

The idea of decomposing ERPs into separate component is equivalent to the idea of reducing multi-dimensional ERPs into a smaller number of waveforms. It is presumed that the decomposed waveforms represent distinct psychological operations performed in specific cortical locations with specific time dynamics. The idea is similar to the one of decomposing a raw EEG signal into distinct oscillations with different cortical locations and frequencies (see paragraph on Blind source separation and ICA in Chapter 8). Methods for implementing these ideas are also similar.

A first attempt of decomposing ERPs into separate components was made as early as in 1970s[33]. A principle component analysis (PCA) was applied. As we

---

[32]Recall that in this book positive fluctuations in EEG are depicted upward while negative fluctuation of potential are depicted downward.

[33]I recall that in our laboratory we were using PCI in order to extract physiological meaningful factors from responses in the discharge rate in impulse activity of neurons. It took me the whole night of computations at the French computer IN-110. In those days it was a usual thing to use the computer time for computations during nights.

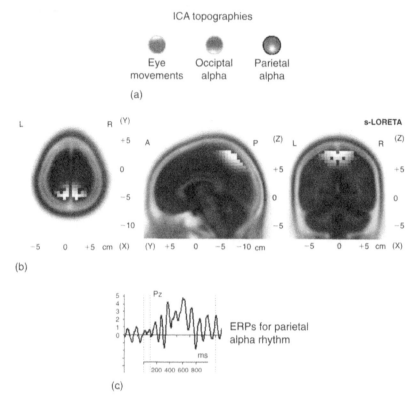

FIGURE 15.16   Alpha ringing in ERP. EEG was recorded from a healthy subject that had a high amplitude parietal alpha rhythm. The subject performed the two stimulus task visual GO/NOGO task. Only ignored (PP) trials were analyzed. Responses to the first stimulus are presented. This rhythm was extracted by the ICA from the raw EEG. (a) Topographies of the three most powerful components. (b) s-LORETA image of the component corresponding the third component – the parietal alpha component. On the basis of the topography of this component a spatial filter was obtained and applied to the raw EEG. ERPs were computed by using the conventional averaging technique (c). Note that rhythmicity is hardly evident in the prestimulus interval, while the rhythmicity changes its phase which is expressed in a substantial increase of ERP in amplitude after the stimulus presentation.

know from Chapter 8, the method of PCA provided only orthogonal components[34]. However, physiologically meaningful components are not necessarily orthogonal. In our laboratory we tried to use the PCA for neurophysiological data in 1980s without any success. The main difficulty was physiological interpretation of the components.

---

[34]In the 2D or 3D space orthogonal vectors are the vectors that are perpendicular (forming an angle of 90°) to each other.

Only recently, a good solution for component dissociation was introduced. This solution is given by the ICA[35]. A brief description of the ICA method is given in Chapter 8. Assumptions that underline the application of ICA for analysis of averaged individual ERPs are as follows: (1) summation of the cortical electric currents induced by separate psychological operations is linear at the scalp electrodes; (2) spatial distribution of components' generators remains fixed across time; (3) different operations and consequently their scalp-recorded generators are temporally independent from each other; (4) distribution of potentials is not Gaussian. These assumptions are difficult to test experimentally and the only prove for correctness of the whole method seems to be a practice. So far, application of ICA method for ERP analysis not only has been in agreement with the whole bulk of previous experimental finding but also has given new insights in understanding the principles of information processing in laboratory settings and has provided new tools for diagnostic purposes in the clinical environment.

An example of application of ICA for the array of ERPs obtained in more than 800 healthy people is presented in Fig. 15.17. The independent components are depicted from the top to the bottom depending on the latency of the largest peak in the component's temporal pattern. As you can see only few components could be approximated by a single dipole[36] (the parameter RRE is below 0.1). The other components are most likely generated by distributed neuronal circuits and could not be described by single dipoles. Low Resolution Electromagnetic Tomography (LORETA) appears to be a more adequate method for assessing spatial distributions of current density of elemental dipoles generating the component.

In Fig. 15.18 s-LORETA images of the components are presented instead of dipole approximations. Peak latencies of the components are marked by vertical lines with numbers corresponding to the latencies of the corresponding components. One can clearly track the information flow in the cortex in the NOGO condition. The flow evolved in several stages. First: the occipital areas around primary visual cortical area are activated at peak latency of 116 ms. This component represents the sequence of recurrent excitations in the occipital area. Second, the temporal–occipital area in the ventral visual stream is activated with latency of 144 ms. The corresponding component reflects change detection: physical at the

---

[35]Both PCA and ICA methods use the correlational structure of an ERP data set (so-called covariation matrixes). Therefore the methods are supposed to extract components that are based on functional relationships between them. We have to stress here that any correlation-based method has limitations. One limitation is that when two separate cognitive processes covary, they may be captured as part of a single component even if they occur in different brain areas and represent different operations. For example, if change detections in physical and semantic modality correlate with each other the ICA decomposition would give a superposition of two component rather than two separate components with different time courses and topographies. The other limitation of the method is that when the same component varies in latency across conditions the ICA will treat this single component as multiple components.

[36]The residual relative energy (RRE) in such cases must be less than 10 per cent (RRE $<$ 0.1).

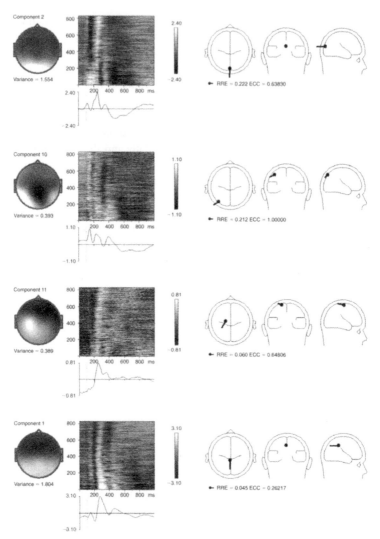

FIGURE 15.17   ICA for grand average ERPs. Independent components were extracted from an array of more than 800 individual ERPs in NOGO condition (AP pair, second stimulus presentation) in the two stimulus GO/NOGO task. Components are presented in order that corresponds to the latency of the component that was computed for the largest peak in the component. Left – topographies of the components with numbers below corresponding to the variance of the component. Middle – vertically stacking thin color-coded horizontal bars, each representing the corresponding component for a single subject with time courses of the components below. Right – dipole approximations of the components. The quality of approximation is given by relative residual energy (RRE). Scales are presented near corresponding pictures.

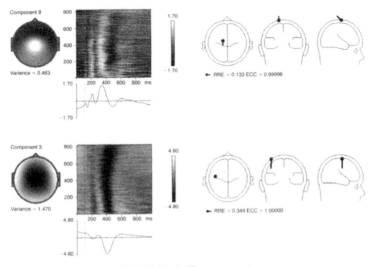

FIGURE 15.17   (*Continued*).

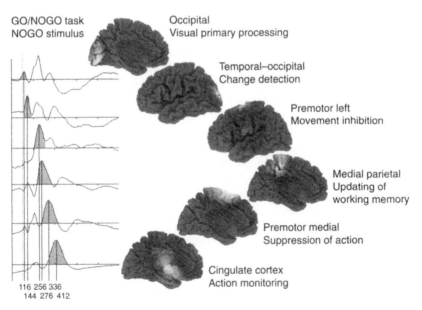

FIGURE 15.18   s-LORETA images of independent components. The same components as in Fig. 15.17 are presented together with their s-LORETA images. The names of cortical areas corresponding to the highest density of ERPs component are presented near s-LORETA images. Note stages of the flow of information from the occipital cortex to the cingulate cortex.

first peak and semantic at the second peak. The third component takes place right after semantic change detection and is associated with activation of the left premotor area. This component reflects activation of neurons responsible for inhibition of the prepared movement. Fourth, the medial parietal area becomes active with latency of 276 ms that corresponds to conventional P3b component and is associated (according to Donchin) with operation of updating the working memory. The fifth component is generated in the medial premotor cortex with latency of 336 ms and is associated with suppression of action as a whole. This component is clearly different from the third component associated with motor inhibition. And finally, all information about the current behavior converges in the cingulate cortex and the mismatch between the expected action (press a button) and the real one (withhold from pressing) activates neurons in the cingulate cortex.

IV. PHARMACO-ERP

In Introduction of this book we briefly described a so-called pharmaco-EEG approach. The main idea of this approach is to apply quantitative parameters of EEG to measure brain responses to pharmaceutical substances. Numerous studies during the last 50 years showed that different classes of pharmaceutical agents differently effect spatial–temporal parameters of background EEG. However individual QEEG profiles of responses for distinct classes of drugs overlap with each other so that the size effects are too small to be used in the clinical practice for diagnostic and treatment purposes. This is one of many hurdles that limit the clinical application of pharmaco-EEG. However, there is a hope that independent components of ERPs might be better endophenotypes for assessment functioning of brain systems and, consequently, might have a bigger size effect. This new line of pharmaco-EEG research emerged only recently and needs further investigations. Here we present a methodology that can be used in this so-called pharmaco-ERP research.

This approach consists of the following stages. First, ERPs for a certain task are recorded in a representative group of healthy subjects (norms). Second, the grand average ERPs in this control group are decomposed into separate components that are generated in different locations of the cortex, exhibit different time dynamics, and are independent of each other. This decomposition may be performed by a recently developed ICA method. Third, the patient is asked to perform the same task before taking a drug and some time after the pharmacological intervention. Fourth, the individual ERPs are decomposed into the components by means of spatial filtration built up on the basis of topograms of the components obtained for the control group. Fifth, the deviations from normality before taking the drug are determined and the most abnormal component is separated. Sixth, the response of this component to the drug is observed.

An example of application of this approach is shown in Fig. 15.19. A subject was an attention deficit hyperactivity disorder (ADHD) boy who initially had a strong deviation from normality selectively in N1/P2 auditory-related component.

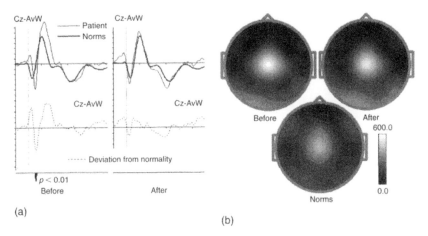

FIGURE 15.19 Pharmaco-ERPs. (a, top) N1/P2 novelty ERP component (thin line) recorded in an ADHD boy before and 1 h after taking Ritalin in comparison to the independent component extracted from a group of healthy subjects (thick line). (a, bottom) – difference wave (dotted line) between the patient's novelty component and the component obtained in the normal group. (b) Maps of theta/beta ratio computed for the control group and for the patient before and after taking Ritalin.

This component is found in response to the second stimulus in pairs (plant, human + novel) and is suggested to reflect a novelty effect – the response of the brain to an unexpected novel stimulus. As one can see, 1 h later after taking Ritalin the ERP component of this patient became almost normal. Note also that no statistically significant deviations from normality, or any significant changes in response to taking Ritalin are found in the inattention index (theta/beta ratio) computed from EEG spectra in this patient.

V. BEHAVIORAL PARADIGMS

A. Classification of Paradigms

Below we are going to present short descriptions of some tasks that are used in ERP studies. The tasks are divided into categories. The list (see Table 15.1) of the tasks is not complete but it gives an overall view of attempts that were made in order to analyze stages of information processing in different brain systems.

In more detail the paradigms are as follows.

B. Sensory and Attention Systems

1. Odd Ball Paradigm

In the odd ball paradigm two types of stimuli are sequentially and randomly presented to the subject. They are standard stimuli (St) and deviant stimuli (Dev)

TABLE 15.1 Tasks for Studying Information Processing in the Brain

System	Behavioral paradigm (scheme)	Description	Name	Components in ERPs
Sensory and attention systems	St St Dev St St Dev	Standard (St) and deviant (Dev) stimuli are presented sequentially, in a random order and with different probabilities (i.e., 90 per cent for standards and 10 per cent for deviants). In the active mode subjects are required to respond with an action such as pressing a button to deviants or counting the number of deviants. In the passive mode (mostly in auditory modality) subjects are asked to perform another task while ignoring the stimuli.	Oddball	MMN in the passive mode. P3b in the active mode.
	St St Dev St St Nov	Standard (St), deviant (Dev), and novel stimuli (Nov) are presented sequentially, in random order and with different probabilities (i.e., 80 per cent for standards, 10 per cent for deviants, and 10 per cent for novels). In the active mode subjects are required to respond to deviants.	Oddball with novels	MMN, P3b, and P3a.
	St St Dev St St St Dev / St St Dev St St St Attended location / Unattended location	Two streams of stimuli are presented in two different spatial locations with the subjects' task to attend to one location and to press a button to deviant stimuli coming from this source of sensory information.	Dichotic listening paradigm and its visual analogs.	Processing negativity (PN).
	Color 1 Color 2	In the visual modality the attended stimuli are of one color, while the stimuli of a different color are to be ignored. ERPs are recorded to attended (relevant) stimuli as well as to unattended (ignored) stimuli.	Selective attention (non-spatial) tasks.	Selection negativity (SN).
	Valid Invalid — Cue Target Cue Target	In each trial the target (in this example, +) can appear either in the left or right part of the visual field. It is cued by a warning stimulus (in this example by an arrow). The targets in different trials can be either validly or invalidly cued.	Spatial-cueing paradigm (Posner's task).	Validity effect – difference between validly and invalidly cued targets.

Executive system	Presentation of a stimulus (test stimulus) is followed by a delay, after which a probe stimulus is offered and the subject has to decide (and to respond correspondingly) whether the probe stimulus matches the test stimulus or not.	Delayed matching-to-sample paradigm.	CNV is recorded during delay period.
	In this task the subject is presented with a series of stimuli and is required to respond when the stimulus on the current trial matches the one that was presented N trials ago.	N-back task.	Correlates of working memory.
	Subjects had to react as quickly and as accurately as possible to the central letter of the five letter string with the index finger of the left (H) or right (S) hand.	Conflict paradigm (Eriksen flanker task, Stroop task – not shown).	ERN is elicited in erroneous trials.
	Two types of stimuli (GO and NOGO) are presented in a random order and with equal probabilities. Interstimulus interval is long enough for a subject to prepare a response.	GO/NOGO paradigm (the two stimulus GO/NOGO task is a variant of this paradigm).	N2 NOGO is elicited in response to NOGO stimuli. P400 monitoring is also elicited for NOGO stimuli.
Affective system	Memory prompts, derived from a person's experience are played through head-phones to a subject. Facial expressions (happy, sad, or neutral) are presented afterwards.	Mood provocation paradigm.	Happy–sad difference.
Episodic memory	In this paradigm a day before testing subjects are given a list of words to memorize. During testing on the next day subjects are presented "old" (memorized) and new items.	Old/new paradigm.	Old–new effect.

appearing in random order and with quite different probabilities: standard stimuli are presented more often than deviant stimuli. Usually the probabilities are 90 per cent for standards and 10 per cent for deviants. Deviants are "odd balls," consequently the paradigm is named the "oddball" paradigm. In this paradigm stimuli are presented with relatively small interstimulus intervals so that they can be perceived as a monotonous stimulation. Occasionally, a standard stimulus is substituted by a deviant one, and monotonous stimulation is interrupted. Usually, the deviant stimulus differs from the standard in one dimension and the deviation is relatively small.

For example, the auditory modality standards could be tones of 1000 Hz of frequency and 100 ms of durations. Deviants could be tones of 1,100 Hz with the same duration as for standards. In the visual modality, a standard stimulus could be the digit 6 while a deviant stimulus could be the digit 9. The interstimuli intervals are usually around 1 s either regular in some experiments or irregular in others.

The oddball paradigm is usually an "active paradigm," that is, the behavioral task requires an action from the subject, such as pressing the button in response to deviants or counting silently the number of deviants. But in auditory modality the oddball paradigm is often used in the passive mode, that is, in the situation when subjects are instructed to do another task, such as viewing a movie or reading a book. This mode is perfectly suited for eliciting mismatch negativity – a small component that is present in ERPs to deviant stimuli as a negative additional (in relation to the ERPs of standard stimuli) component recorded at Fz.

2. Oddball with Novels

This task is a useful extension of the oddball paradigm. In this task, together with frequent standards and rare deviants, quite different stimuli (called novels – Nov) are occasionally presented. Novels are usually unique stimuli, such as a key ring, dog barking …and are intended to shift attention of the subject. Similar to the oddball paradigm this paradigm can be performed in two modes: active and passive. In the passive one, subjects are required to perform another task, while in the active paradigm they respond to deviant stimuli with action. The active paradigm is often used to record the two P3 components: P3a that appears in response to novels and P3b that appears in response to targets, that is, deviant stimuli followed by actions.

3. Spatial Selective Attention Paradigm

The common methodology of the selective attention paradigm is to present two distinct streams that are coming from two distinct sources and differ between each other in some basic parameters of the stimuli[37]. Attention of the subjects is selectively

---

[37]These streams could be from two distinctive spatial locations or could differ in some non-spatial simple feature such as color.

directed only to stimuli from one source of stimuli. In the auditory modality a simple variant of this paradigm is a dichotic listening task. The dichotic listening task was designed in 1950s to study a so-called "cocktail partly" phenomenon. In one variant of the task, competing speeches are delivered to the two ears through headphones while subjects are asked to attend either to the left or the right ear. In ERP studies, two different sequences each consisting of a mixture of standard and deviant sounds[38] are presented independently to two ears.

The dichotic listening task is an active paradigm, in which subjects are instructed to press a button or to perform some other action in response to deviants presented only to one ear. The attended ear is announced to be left in one session of the experiment and right in another session. For each ear, ERPs to standards in the unattended ear are subtracted from ERPs to standards in the attended ear. The difference wave is associated with selected attention to the corresponding location[39]. In the auditory modality this difference is of negative value in frontal leads and therefore is named processing negativity (PN).

It is easy to implement a visual analog of the dichotic listening task. One just needs to present visual stimuli in two distinct spatial locations, such as left or right part of the visual field and ask subjects to attend to each of these locations in different sessions.

4. Spatial-Cuing Paradigm

Spatial-cuing paradigm is designed to assess selective attention in spatial domain. A general idea is that target stimuli are preceded by cue stimuli. The cue stimuli are of two types: those that validly indicate the location of the following target (valid cues) and those that invalidly indicate the location of the subsequent target (invalid cues). The difference in speed and accuracy of responding to targets between invalid and valid trials (so-called validity effect), is assumed to reflect the spatial attention on the cued location. An example of spatial cuing paradigm is a Posner's task. In this task a subject fixates on the central point and has to detect briefly presented targets appearing in the periphery. These targets appear a few hundred milliseconds after presentation of a directional (peripheral or central) cue. The reaction time (RT) to validly cued targets is shorter than the one to invalidly cued targets, while the difference between reaction times are associated with spatial attention to a cued location[40].

---

[38]The parameters of sounds (such as loudness, duration or frequency of acoustic stimuli) differ between ears making discrimination of two currents easier.

[39]Note that spatial attention is one of many types of selective attention.

[40]The spatial cuing paradigm enables the researchers to measure attention effect as a difference between reaction times, but reveals difficulties in analyzing ERPs. Indeed the ERPs to valid and invalid cues include the motor-related component which are different to validly and invalidly cued targets and which mask the effects of attention per se.

5. Non-spatial Selective Attention Tasks

Non-spatial selective attention can be studied by presenting a sequence of stimuli different from each other in one visual parameter (such as color, direction of motion …). For example, in visual modality the attended stimuli could be of blue color, while all yellow ones are to be ignored. ERPs are recorded to attended (relevant) stimuli as well as to unattended (ignored) stimuli. The difference wave between these ERPs measures the effect of the selective attention to a particular color. Such difference waves are usually called "selection" components.

C. Executive Functions

1. Delayed Matching-To-Sample Paradigm

To study the working memory, namely operations of encoding, retention, and recalling, a so-called matching-to-sample paradigm is often used. In this paradigm presentation of a stimulus (test stimulus) is followed by a delay, after which a probe stimulus is offered and the subject has to decide (and to respond correspondingly) whether the probe stimulus matches the test stimulus or not.

2. N-Back Task

In this task the subject is presented with a series of stimuli and is required to respond when the stimulus on the current trial matches that presented on N trials ago. The memory load can be increased by increasing N. The subject has a dual task: to encode the current stimulus and to compare it with that presented on the N-to-last trial.

3. Conflict Paradigm

Tasks of the conflict paradigm are designed to study monitoring operation of the executive system. This operation seems to be performed by a complex network with the anterior cingulate cortex as a critical part. Most of the conflict tasks activate this part of the cortex. One of the conflict paradigm tests is the Stroop task. This task was designed by a doctoral student J.R. Stroop in 1935 and became one of the most popular tasks in cognitive psychology. In this task, a list of words is presented and the subjects are instructed to name the color of each stimulus as fast as possible. It is easy to do this task when the words match the ink colors. If the word (say word GREEN) does not match the ink in which it is written (say ink RED) two representations – one, the word, and the other, the color, compete with each other and responses are delayed as well as the number of errors increases.

Another test of the conflict paradigm is an Eriksen flanker task. This task has been applied in many studies of error-related negativity in ERPs. It was published in 1979 (Eriksen and Eriksen, 1979). In this task, after a warning cue one of four string letter combinations (HHHHH, HHSHH, SSHSS, or SSSSS) is presented. Subjects had to react as quickly and as accurately as possible to the central letter of the five letter string with the index finger of the left (H) or right (S) hand.

4. GO/NOGO Paradigm

A general idea of GO/NOGO paradigm is to create conditions that would enable researchers to study one of the executive operations – action suppression. So, in this paradigm, the subjects are supposed to prepare to make an action (GO) for each trial, but have to suppress the prepared action in some (NOGO) trials. Note that in the oddball paradigm subjects also have to make actions to some stimuli and withhold from actions to other stimuli, but the low probability of deviant stimuli and small interstimulus intervals does not allow the subjects to prepare the action for each stimulus. Rather standard stimuli in the oddball paradigm create a background on which deviant (GO) stimuli rarely appear. In contrast to the odd-ball conditions, the GO/NOGO conditions require longer interstimulus intervals and higher probability of GO stimuli.

A simple GO/NOGO task consists of sequential and random presentation of two stimuli (e.g., of red and green colors) that follow with interstimulus intervals of about 2 s and appear at equal probabilities. The subject's task is to press a button in response to one stimulus named GO stimulus (e.g., stimulus of green color) and to withhold from pressing to another (e.g., red) stimulus named NOGO stimulus.

In the C-X version of the GO/NOGO paradigm, subjects are presented with rapid sequences of letters. 20 per cent of the stimuli are the letter C, which is fol-lowed 50 per cent of the time by an X, and 50 per cent of the time by another let-ter (e.g., R,V,T, etc.). Subjects are instructed to withhold their response when they see an X following a C (NOGO stimulus) but to respond when any other letter follows the letter C (e.g., C-R, C-V, etc., GO stimuli).

In another version of GO/NOGO paradigm (named the stop-signal task) sub-jects are presented with a series of trials that begin with either the letter A or the letter B. On each of these, subjects perform a two-choice RT task, responding to the A with one button and the B with a second button. On 25 per cent of the trials a stop signal (the letter S) follows the A or B by a variable time interval (e.g., 200–600 ms, stop-signal interval), and the subject must withhold his/her response on that trial. For healthy subjects, for the shorter stop-signal intervals (e.g., 200–400 ms) it is easier to inhibit responding, while at the longer stop-signal intervals (400–600 ms) it is substantially more difficult to do so and the probability of inhibition is much lower. Probability of inhibition (Y-axis) is plotted against stop-signal time interval to give a measure of inhibition control (for more details Pliszka et al., 2000).

Two stimulus GO/NOGO tasks represent a subtype of the general GO/NOGO paradigm. An idea is to present stimuli in pairs so that the subject would implicitly be able to prepare to make a response after the first stimulus in the pair and to respond as fast as possible after the second stimulus presentation. There are two variants of the tasks. In the first variant, the first stimulus in the trials serves as simple warning stimulus. In the second variant, the first stimulus in turn can be either the "continue" or "discontinue" trial. The second variant of GO/NOGO paradigm was designed for our studies. It was also implemented in the Human Brain Institute Normative Database (for more details see Chapter 12).

D. Affective System

The tasks to study the affective system usually deal with two basic emotions: happiness and sadness. To induce these emotions two categories of emotionally competent stimuli are usually presented: so-called sad and happy pictures. They may be happy or sad expressions of human face, happy or sad scenes from the human life. It must be taken into consideration that expressing and feeling emotion needs time. Consequently interstimulus intervals are supposed to be quite long. More over, emotions are very subjective, and the same picture sometimes can produce a positive emotion in one subject and negative emotion in another subject. So, the pictures must be individually tailored for a subject. The paradigm that fits these requirements is the mood provocation paradigm.

1. Mood Provocation Paradigm

The task relies on two presumptions[41]: (1) People are different and episodes elicited positive emotions in some people can be neutral or even negative for others. Consequently, individually tailored pictures must be selected for presentation in the tasks. (2) Perception of emotional expressions of other people as well as perception of different life scenes strongly depend on the background emotional state of perceiving subject: We know from our experience that when we are in a bad mood everything appears in gray colors, but when we are in a high mood all "the troubles seem so far away." Moreover, one needs time to switch from one mood to another mood. In the task, all individuals completed a life events questionnaire asking them to describe five positive, five negative, and five neutral previous life experiences that had made them feel particularly happy, sad, or emotionally indifferent, respectively. Memory prompts of up to 8 s duration, derived from the above procedure, were prerecorded. They were designed to be played prior to the presentation of mood congruent facial expressions. Prompts took the form "Use the following sad faces to remember how you felt at your father's funeral when your mother cried." Facial expressions (100 per cent happy, 100 per cent sad or neutral) were selected from a standardized series (Ekman and Friesen, 1976). All subjects

---

[41]It was implemented by a group of researchers from University of Pittsburgh Medical School and Institute of Psychiatry in London (Keedwell et al., 2005).

participated in two 6 min experiments in which they were exposed to ten 36 s alternating blocks of emotional (sad or happy) or neutral stimuli. The order in which the two experiments were conducted was fully counterbalanced, as was the order of the emotional and neutral conditions within each experiment.

E. Episodic Memory

1. Old–New Paradigm

In this paradigm a day before testing subjects are given a list of words or other items to memorize. During night those items are supposed to consolidate into episodic memory. During testing on the next day subjects are presented with "old" (memorized) and new (different from memorized) items. ERPs recorded for new and old items are subtracted from each other to reveal an "old–new" effect.

CHAPTER 16

Practice: ERP analysis

I. INTRODUCTION

The book is equipped with the educational software. Some methods for spectral analysis of spontaneous electroencephalogram (EEG) has been presented in the previous part of the book. The basic idea of spectral analysis is decomposing EEG pattern into simple components – sinusoidal waves. As was shown in Part I, EEG oscillations in different frequency bands reflect different modes of cortical self-regulation. The decomposition of the background EEG into simple components is performed by means of Fourier analysis, wavelet transformations, and independent component analysis (ICA). Here we present basic methods of analysis of event-related potentials (ERPs). The ERPs represent a different window of looking at the brain. ERPs reflect stages of information flow within the neuronal networks while the background EEG reflects modulation of this information flow. In spite of this qualitative difference the basic idea of ERP analysis is similar to the basic idea of the background EEG analysis. The basic idea of ERP analysis is decomposition of ERPs into simple elements – independent components each reflecting a specific operation in the information flow in the brain.

Methods of ERPs computing and processing can be divided into the following categories: (1) constructing psychological tasks, (2) preprocessing EEG, such as setting a montage, correcting, and eliminating artifacts, (3) applying ICA for a set of EEG fragments in single trials of a given individual subject[1], (4) averaging EEG fragments over trials of a given category for an individual[2], (5) arranging the obtained ERPs for a given group of subjects or patients into the built-in database so that single ERPs can be viewed, and the whole set of ERPs can be processed by averaging technique or ICA[3], (6) obtaining grand average ERPs by averaging single subject ERPs from the database, (7) extracting independent components that are common for the whole set of subjects and for given task conditions by means of ICA, and constructing spatial filters for each component on the basis of topographies of the components, (8) comparing individual ERPs or ERP components with the normative data computed for a representative group of healthy subjects of the same age and gender, (9) compiling reports, that is, presenting the results of processing in a short and meaningful form with conclusions and recommendations for therapy.

These categories of ERP processing are schematically presented in Fig. 16.1. They are all implemented in the Human Brain Institute Normative Database. Many commercially available EEG systems (such as Neuroscan, Nicolet ...) have some of these categories, the other categories of ERPs processing can be obtained in Matlab (EEG-lab) software package. It should be stressed that in this book we are not going to present a complete system. Rather the goal of the educational software is to enable the user to learn basic methods of ERP processing.

II. DESIGNING TASK

The educational software includes *Psytask* program[4]. *Psytask* is a program that enables the researcher to design a psychological task and run it simultaneously with EEG recording. So *Psytask* works together with an EEG acquisition software and provides a synchronous time mark to the recorded EEG. Two computers are connected via *COM* ports. The one that records EEG is named *Main computer*, and the one that presents stimuli to the subject on the computer screen is named *Slave computer*. *Psytask* can be also used as stand-by software for measuring reaction time, omission, and commission errors in psychological tasks.

---

[1]Although this method has been realized in our basic software, its practical application is not clear yet. We are going to skip this method of analysis in the following description and in the educational software.

[2]For example, obtaining ERPs for a single subject for all electrodes separately in GO/NOGO task for GO trials.

[3]For example, arranging ERPs in GO/NOGO task for a group of ADHD patients of inattentive subtype into a distinct database.

[4]This program was written by Valery Ponomarev – a senior research fellow from the author's laboratory at the Institute of the Human Brain of Russian Academy of Sciences in St. Petersburg. It is free software.

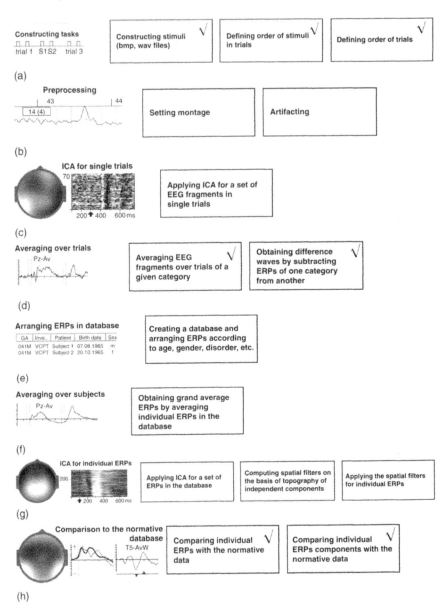

FIGURE 16.1   Steps of ERPs analysis. Rows from top to bottom – (1) constructing psychological tasks, (2) preprocessing EEG, (3) ICA on EEG in single trials for a given subject, (4) averaging EEG fragments over trials, (5) arranging files of computed ERPs in the individual database, (6) averaging ERPs over subjects (grand average), (7) ICA on ERPs computed for a group of subjects, (8) comparing individual ERPs or ERP components with the normative data. Items that are present in EdEEG software are marked.

After installation of *Psytask*[5] the following window will appear (Fig. 16.2). The button *Start New Task* is used to start a new psychological task by selecting it from the list tasks. The button *Display Database* is used to open the built-in database to display results of testing. The button *Display List of Tasks* is used to run the built-in editor of task protocols. This is the button you have to press in order to create your own task. The button *Switch to Slave Mode* is used to start the waiting mode of the slave computer in which *Psytask* is waiting for control and synchronization commands from the EEG acquisition software that is working on another computer connected to the slave computer via COM port. The button *Setup Database* is used to modify the database pathname to open another existing database or create new one. The button *Modify Synchronization Parameters* is used to change parameters of COM port that is used for synchronization. The button *Quit* is used to close *Psytask* program.

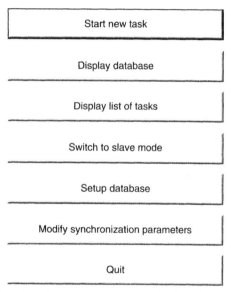

Start new task

Display database

Display list of tasks

Switch to slave mode

Setup database

Modify synchronization parameters

Quit

FIGURE 16.2   Psytask window. From top to bottom: (1) Start New Task from the list of standard tasks, (2) Display the Database which stores results of psychological testing, (3) Display List of Tasks which include standard tasks supplied with the program, (4) Switch to Slave Mode – used to start the waiting mode of the slave computer, (5) Setup Database of behavioral parameters (number of errors, reaction time), (6) Modify Synchronization Parameters that are used for synchronization of the slave computer with the main computer, (7) Quit PSYTASK program.

---

[5]The software is stored in a zipped form and are provided via a web site created and hosted by Elsevier, and accessed through this one common URL: www.elsevierdirect.com/companions/9780123745125. There are two different pieces of software – EdEEG and Psytask. They are available separately in compressed zip files. After downloading, the user will need to extract the zip file and run "Setup.exe" to install the software. We presume that EdEEG program has been already installed by the reader as described in Chapter 9 of Part 1.

The central concept of Psytask is *Presentation protocol* of the task. The protocol defines stimuli that are going to be used in the task. The protocol also defines timing of stimuli in trials, sequence of trials, and the way of the subject's responding to the stimuli in the trials. All this information excluding stimuli is stored in files (so-called stimulus presentation protocols) with extension .*PRO*[6]. The protocols together with the files corresponding to the stimuli are stored in separate folders. Visual stimuli are pixel images stored as ★.BMP or ★.JPEG files. Sounds are acoustic traces stored in standard ★.WAV files. The task is defined by *Name* (e.g., GONOGO), *Name of folder* (e.g., GONOGO). The folder corresponding to a task is created in the root folder of *Psytask* program (Fig. 16.3). The root

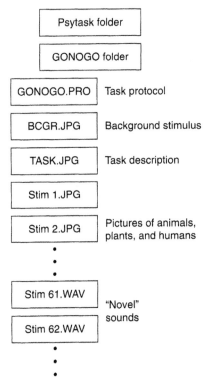

FIGURE 16.3   Arranging files for the protocol of the two-stimulus GO/NOGO task. The Psytask folder includes descriptions of all tasks in the corresponding subfolders. The subfolder of GONOGO task is presented as an example. The parameters of the task such as the stimuli list, timing of stimuli in trails and sequence of trials are presented in the file GONOGO.PRO Stimuli – images and sounds – are presented in separate files.

[6]Note that files with extension. *PRO* are simple text files (ASCII) that could read and edited by any text editor.

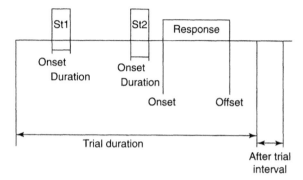

FIGURE 16.4   Parameters of a trail. Parameters of a two stimulus task are presented as an example. These parameters are determined by the user of the Psytask program.

folder also includes the descriptions of all tasks written in the file *PSYTASK. CFG*. The protocol of the task is automatically created in Psytask from *Display List of Task → New* window. It includes the following prompts: *Task property* (Task name, subfolder name, Protocol name, Screen Resolution), *Stimuli List, Trials List, Presentation Order, Response Processing*[7].

To create a Stimuli List one must first prepare images and sounds of stimuli that are going to be used in the task. Second, these stimuli must be inserted in the Task folder by command *Add* in the *Trials List* prompt. The parameters of trials in the two stimulus GO/NOGO task are schematically presented in Fig. 16.4.

In the *Presentation Order* prompt one must define (1) the order in which trials will be presented in the task, delays (after trial intervals) and (2) the number of category of trials (e.g., number 1 for trials of GO category, number 2 for trials of NOGO category). In the *Response Processing* prompt the following parameters have to be defined: (1) the source of the subject response – it could be a microswitch (mouse) with left and right buttons, it could be some keys on the keyboard of the slave computer, (2) the time interval of the correct response (e.g., 200, 1000 ms so that only responses within this interval will be considered as correct), and (3) the way of responding (e.g., *Press Left Button, Don't press Left Button*).

For example, a protocol for the two stimulus GO/NOGO task from the Human Brain Institute Normative Database is presented in Fig. 16.5. For more details see the Psytask Manual that can be found in Psytask sub-folder *DOC*.

During learning the methods for ERPs analysis pursue the following steps. To practice open file S3_VCPT (or S4_VCPT) from the folder EdEEG/DATA and perform the following steps of the EdEEG software.

---

[7]In some cases there is a need to transfer the task created on another computer to your own *Slave* computer. In order to do this procedure in *Display List of Tasks* window press *Add from* button and find the protocol you want to add.

```
TaskName "VCPT"
StimuliList
  Image S1 STIM1.JPG
  Image S2 STIM2.JPG
  Image S3 STIM3.JPG        List of all stimuli:
                            Images, Sounds,
  Image BkGr BkGr..JPG      Background and
  Image Task Task..JPG      Task desription
                            in a picture

  Sound S62 STIM3.WAV
  Sound S63 STIM4.WAV
EndStimuli
                            List of all trials:
  Trial T1 3000             Name, Duration
    S1 300 100              First stimulus in
    S1 1400 100             a trial, onset from
  EndTrial                  the beginning of trial,
                            duration
  Trial T2 3000             Second stimulus in
    S2 300 100              a trial, onset from
    S2 1400 100             the beginning of trial,
  EndTrial                  duration


PsyTest 640x480xTrueColor
  LeftTop                   Presentation order
    ShowPicture Task        of Task description,
    SetBackground BkGr      setting background,
    Wait 3000               trial sequence
    T62 200 4               with after trial
    T2 200 1                interval and the number
    T23 200 3               of trail category
  EndTest


ResponseProcessing
  "Go" 2 100 1000 VK_RIGHT Press None None 1
  "Nogo" 2 100 1000 VK_RIGHT Skip None None 2
  "Ignore1" 2 100 1000 VK_RIGHT Skip None None 3
  "Ignore2" 2 100 1000 VK_RIGHT Skip None None 4
EndProcessing    Reaction to trals that are considered as correct:
                 Name of trial category, Time window for respose,
                 Action for 3 buttons, Number of trial category
```

FIGURE 16.5   An example of a protocol of the two stimulus GO/NOGO task. This is the GONOGO.PRO file from Fig. 16.3. The file includes description of stimuli, description of trails, and description of the sequence of trails in the task.

III. EdEEG SOFTWARE

Step 1. Opening EEG file: Install the EdEEG software according to conventional procedure described in Practice of Part I. Start EdEEG.exe program. In the main window you can see *Menus: File, View, Analysis, Setup.* Each menu has its own

Commands. In addition to the main Window two smaller windows are depicted – *Map Window* and *Dipole Window.* From the *File* menu select the button *Open file* in order to view 19-channel raw EEG recorded during the two stimulus GO/ NOGO task.

Step 2. Viewing EEG record: The EEG window is used for viewing the recorded EEG. It has three bars: the *Channel Names bar* placed on the left side, the *Status bar* placed in the bottom, and the *Filters Bar* placed on the top. Above traces of EEG there are marks of trials depicted as boxes with the number of trial and the stimulus category (in Fig. 16.6, e.g., 23[1] within the top-left box mean that this mark corresponds to trial number 23 of category number 1-GO trials). The left side of the box corresponds to the beginning of the trial. On the bottom of the window, a mark of the *Button* pressing is presented. The left side of the button pressing mark corresponds to beginning of subject's response.

Step 3. Preprocessing EEG record – setting montage: The recorded EEG is stored on the disk in the linked ears montage within the full bandwidth of EEG amplifies. For viewing and analyzing the data other montages can be selected. This can be done by pressing *Select Montage* in View menu. The *Montage Parameters window* will pop up. In the Human Brain Institute database we use three different montages: linked ears montage, common average montage, and local average montage according to Lemos. For the particular example depicted in Fig. 16.6 we select the local average montage.

Step 4. Preprocessing EEG record – eye movement correction: In Part I we have presented three methods of artifacting: (1) manual delete (*Clear*), (2) Automated *Marking artifacts*, and (3) automated *Artifact correction* by means of spatial filtration. For more information the reader is referred to Chapter 9 of the book.

Step 5. Computing ERPs by averaging EEG fragments: Individual ERPs are computed by averaging EEG fragments time locked to the beginning of trials. Figure 16.7 represents ERPs averaged over around 90 trials for a healthy subject (recall that trials with artifacts and incorrect responses - which are different for different categories of trials – are discarded). ERPs are computed for Cz electrode for two conditions (GO and NOGO) in the two stimulus GO/NOGO task. Note that before the second stimulus ERPs are almost identical because the first stimulus in GO and NOGO trials is the same – a picture of animal. The similarity between two ERPs for GO and NOGO conditions within the time window from the first to the second stimuli represent a so-called test/retest index. This index can be used as a measure of defining reliability of ERPs obtained in a particular subject.

To implement averaging, go to *Analysis menu* and click *Compute ERP.* The following window will appear (Fig. 16.8). In the top a sub-window *Groups of trials* is located. For two stimulus GO/NOGO task (shown as an example in Fig. 16.8) the following categories (or groups) of trials are to be computed: GO trials (AA) labeled by number 1, NOGO trials (AP) labeled by number 2, Discontinue visual trials (PP) labeled by number 3, and Discontinue auditory trails (PH) labeled by number 4. We also combined groups 1 and 2 to get a so-called Continue (with name "+" and number 5) group. We combined groups 3 and 4 to get a

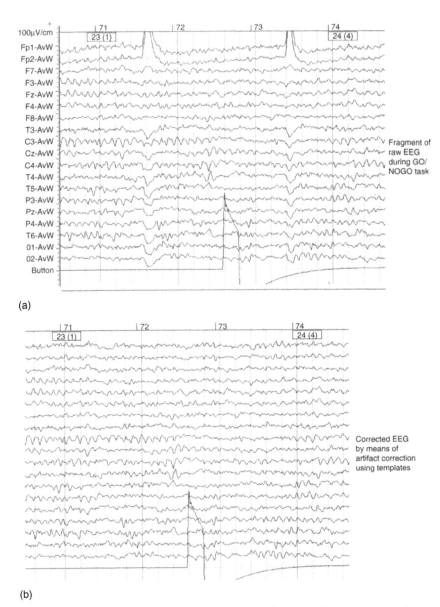

(a)

(b)

FIGURE 16.6 Eye movement correction. An Example of 19-channel EEG recorded in the two stimulus GO/NOGO task before (a) and after (b) correcting eye blinks.

Discontinue group (with name "−" and number 6). During averaging the program will compute the number of correct responses, the number of incorrect responses (omission and commission errors), and the number of trails with artifacts (see Artifacting section). We are also going to compute ERP differences that are useful

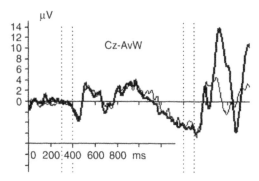

FIGURE 16.7   ERPs in GO and NOGO trials for a healthy subject. An example of ERPs averaged over GO (thin line) and NOGO (thick line) trials in the two stimulus GO/NOGO task. ERPs are computed for Cz. Note that ERP patterns before the second stimulus look similar for GO and NOGO trials because the first stimulus in these trails is the same – an image of animal.

Groups of trials

No	Name	Labels	Correct		Incorrect		Artifact
1.	a-a GO	1	0	.	0	.	0
2.	a-p NoGO	2	0	.	0	.	0
3.	p-p	3	0	.	0	.	0
4.	p-h	4	0	.	0	.	0
5.	+	1, 2	0	.	0	.	0
6.	-	3, 4	0	.	0	.	0
7.			0	.	0	.	0
8.			0	.	0	.	0

Group differences

2-1, 4-3, 6-5   Choose

Artifact processing
Level: 100   uV
Channels: Only EEG ▾
Thresholds for channels

Synchronization
Type: Stimulus ▾
Stimulus: #1 ▾
Button channel: Not selected ▾

Subject responce processing
Defined
Define
Compression: Off ▾

Time interval before (ms): 0   Time interval after (ms): 0

☑ Calculate statistical significance   ☑ Use as default
     0%   100%

Load   Save   Load from database   OK   Cancel

FIGURE 16.8   Window for computing ERPs. The user defines the names of categories of trials such as GO for category (label) "1", the differences between categories such as "2-1" for the difference between ERPs for GO and NOGO trails. Note that the labels are defined in the Psytask protocol. In addition the user sets the timing of correct responses and synchronization type, that is, the way of ERP averaging starts – by stimulus or by subject's response. Note that for computing ERP in a task of the HBI reference database one simply needs to load the parameters from the database.

in extracting components associated with distinct psychological operations[8]. These differences are listed in a sub-window *Group differences*. You can choose any combination of difference waves from the full list by clicking the button *Choose*.

The other three sub-windows are *Artifact processing*, *Synchronization*, and *Subject's response processing*. The artifact elimination procedure is based on comparison of the current amplitude of EEG signal with a preset threshold. The recommended value of the threshold is 100 μV. Note, that *Only EEG channels* must be selected for artifact elimination, otherwise all trials with subject's response will be thrown away.

Usually *Synchronization* by first stimulus of the trial is recommended. Another setting of synchronization parameters can be used if two or more stimuli in the trials are presented with different intrastimuli intervals and there is a need to synchronize ERPs by the second or third stimuli. ERPs can be also synchronized by button pressing, that is, by initiation of the subject response to the stimuli.

The parameters of *Subject's response processing* are defined in a separate subwindow. The parameters include: (1) *Time interval* within which the response of the subject is considered as a correct one, (2) *Groups of trials* after which the response is expected, (3) *Stimulus* after which the response is required, (4) Category of *Left or Right button* responses (*Press button, Don't press button*, and *No* – not applied). Note that in our version of the hardware there are many devices that could be used to computing reaction times, so the one that has been actually used must be defined in *Left (Right) Button Channel*.

Once you have defined all parameters of ERP computations you can save these parameters in a separate file (with ★.par extension) and can download them again when needed. The parameters for computing ERPs in all tasks of the Human Brain Institute Normative Database are saved in a separate folder (*Parameters*).

When using the Human Brain Institute Normative Database, the user does not need to worry about parameters of processing: they have to be downloaded from the database by simply clicking the button *Load from database*.

Step 6. Comparison with the normative database: Now when we have computed ERPs in the task for the individual patient, we want to know how his/her ERPs differ from the normative data obtained from a group of healthy subjects of the same age. There are two ways of making the comparison: (1) to compare the

---

[8]Some 5–10 years ago computing difference waves was the only method for extracting ERP components. It was assumed that because of specific design of the task a certain psychological operation was present in one group of trials and absent in the other group of trials, so that subtracting ERPs would give an electrophysiological correlate of this psychological operation. For example, it can be speculated that in the two stimulus GO/NOGO task described in the book hypothetical operation of motor inhibition is present only in NOGO trials so that subtracting ERPs to GO trials from ERPs to NOGO trials gives an index of motor inhibition. However, GO trials in turn elicit operations (such as motor execution and engagement operations) that might be absent (like motor execution) or developed differently (such as engagement operation) in NOGO trials. These operations overlap in time and space with the operation of motor inhibition. Consequently, ERPs differences between GO and NOGO trials represent not one but several overlapping psychological operations.

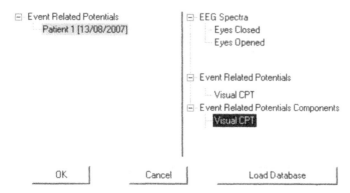

FIGURE 16.9   Window for comparing individual ERPs with the normative database. This window is opened after pressing the command "Comparison of Results" from Analysis menu and after Loading the database.

individual ERPs with the grand average ERPs of the normal group, (2) to compare the individual ERP components with the grand average ERP components extracted from the normative database by means of ICA. In both cases you go to *Analysis* menu and select *Comparison of results* option. In this option select the *Load Database* key. The following window will appear (Fig. 16.9).

As one can see there are two options for the comparison of ERPs in GO/NOGO task. You can select either *Event Related Potentials / Visual CPT* option for comparison of ERPs, or you can select *Event Related Potentials Components/Visual CPT* option for comparison of ERPs components extracted from the ERPs of the patient by applying spatial filtration[9].

Let us start with simple comparison of raw ERPs. Figure 16.10 represents a part of the window that is opened up after pressing OK in the *Comparison* window. The names of categories of ERPs are presented on the top of Fig. 16.10. By clicking at ▼ you can select different categories of stimuli (*Active Groups*) for which ERPs have been computed such as "a-a GO," "a-p NOGO" … A symbol in squared parentheses at the right of the name of the category means the following: "[1]" – an individual for whom ERPs were recorded, "[2]" – the normative database, "[D]" – difference between the individual ERPs and the normative database.

[9]Note that the spatial filters are based on the topographies of components derived from the independent component analysis of the large number of individual ERPs of the healthy control subjects. It should be also noted that a priori the topographies may be different for different age groups. However, comparison of the topographies computed for the children and adults collected in the Human Brain Institute Database showed that these two distinct groups revealed independent components with similar topographies while dynamics of components changed dramatically with age for some components and did not show age dependency for other components. Thus it looks like that the spatial distribution of a specific psychological operation associated with a specific component is a quite stable characteristic while timing of the operation may depend of age.

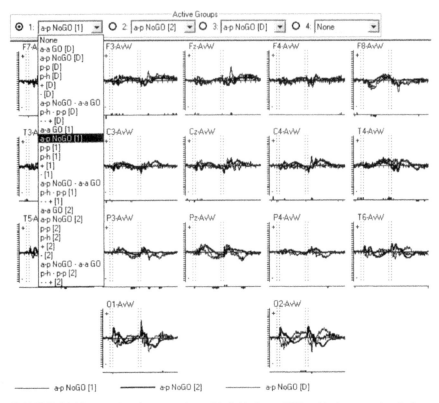

FIGURE 16.10   Window for comparison of individual raw ERPs with the normative database. The window is opened up after pressing OK in the *Comparison ERPs* window. The comparison can be made by depicting ERPs for a separate category of trail (GO, NOGO, ...) for a subject, for the database and ERPs differences. "[1]" – a subject, "[2]" – the normative database, "[D]" – difference between the individual ERPs and the normative database.

Besides comparing raw ERPs the EdEEG provides the reader with an option of comparing independent components extracted from individual ERPs with the independent components for people from the normative data with the same age. Figure 16.11 represents a part of the window that is opened up after selecting *Event Related Potentials Components/Visual CPT* option in the *Comparison* window. The names of categories of ERP components are presented on the top of Fig. 16.11. By clicking at ▼ you can select different categories of independent components that were extracted for the two stimulus GO/NOGO task such as P3GO, P3NOGO, P2NOGO ... A symbol in squared parentheses at the right of the name of category means the following: "[1]" – an individual for whom ERPs independent components were computed, "[2]" – the normative data, "[D]" – difference between the individual ERPs independent components and the normative data.

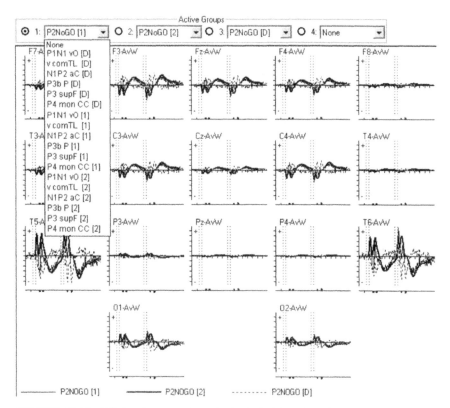

FIGURE 16.11   Window for comparison of individual ERPs independent components with the normative database. The window is opened up after pressing OK in the *Comparison ERP components* window. The comparison can be made by depicting ERPs components (P3b GO, P3NOGO ...) for a subject, for the database as well as ERPs differences. "[1]" – a subject, "[2]" – the normative database, "[D]" – difference between the individual ERPs components and the normative database.

An example of comparing two individual ERP components (comparison and monitoring) with the normative data is presented in Fig. 16.12.

Fig. 16.12 depicts two independent components computed for a patient. They are the comparison component, presented in the top row, and the monitoring component, presented at the bottom row. Thin lines correspond to ERP components for the patient, thick lines correspond to ERP components for the group of healthy subjects, while dotted lines correspond to deviations of the patient's components from the "normal" ERP components. Topographies of the two components are presented at the right. Note dramatic deviations from normality in the comparison component and no significant difference in the monitoring component. Vertical bars below the difference waves correspond to the significant level of deviation from the normative data.

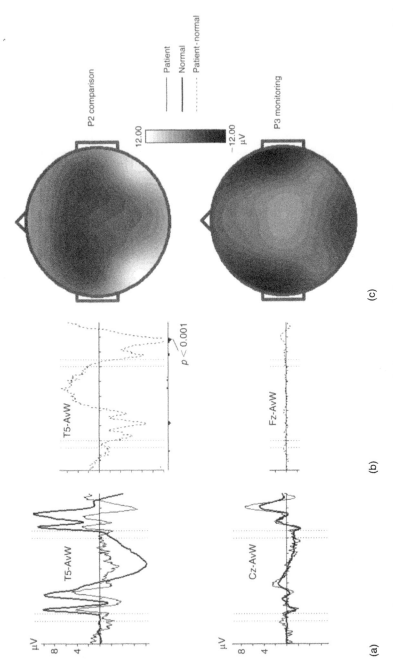

FIGURE 16.12   Comparing two individual ERPs components with the normative database. Top row – comparison component. Bottom row – monitoring component. (a) ERPs components for the patient (thin line) and for the group of healthy subjects of the same age (thick line). (c) Topographies of the comparison and monitoring. (b) Deviation from normality. Vertical bars below the difference wave – time intervals in which the deviation is significant at $p < 0.001$.

IV. EXERCISES

The EdEEG software is provided with two EEG files recorded in a healthy subject and in a patient during the two-stimulus GO/NOGO task. Both subjects
belong to the same age group of 13–14 years old.

We suggest the reader to exercise with the two files and to answer the following questions:

1. Which file corresponds to a healthy subject and which one corresponds to
   a patient?
2. Which independent components are within the normative range and
   which are abnormal?
3. What type of brain dysfunction is found in the ERPs of the patient?
4. What brain disorder (ADHD, OCD, or dyslexia) can be associated with the
   observed brain dysfunction?

To answer these questions perform the steps of ERPs computation and analysis
described above. Briefly the actions are as follow:

1. Start *EdEEG.exe* program.
2. From *File menu* click *Open File* command.
3. Open file from *EdEEG* folder *Data* subfolder (which if installed Typical is
   located on Disk C). There are two files S3_VCPT and S4_VCPT. Analyze
   each of the files separately.
4. Use buttons from the Input Control toolbar (■ ◀◀ ◀ ▶ ▶▶) to
   view the record. These buttons correspond to Stop, Fast rewind back, Slow
   rewind back, Slow play back, Fast play back. You can also view the EEG
   at different time intervals by moving the scroll bar located below the EEG
   record.
5. From *View menu* click *Select Montage* and in the window *Montage Name*
   select *DataBase Version 1 montage*. This montage name is the last in the list
   of montages. By clicking *References* dialog box in the *Montage parameters*
   window make sure that it is the *Weighted average by Lemos* montage. Then
   press *OK*. The EEG record will appear in the selected montage.
6. By visual inspection find artifacts of vertical and horizontal eye movements.
7. Select the whole record. This is done by clicking *the left button* of the mouse
   at the beginning of the record and *the right button* – at the end of the record.
   Clicking must be done within the *time bar* located above the record. After
   clicking the right button the time bar will become yellow.
8. From *Analysis menu* click *Artifact correction* command. The program will
   automatically decompose the EEG fragment into 19 components by
   means of the Principle Component Analysis (PCA). From *Method* menu
   (presented at the bottom) select ICA (Independent Component Analysis)
   and click OK. The program will start iteration procedure of extracting

independent components from the EEG fragment. The procedure usually takes more than 20 seconds and consists of 100 iterations or more. In topographies presented on the right of the appeared window the first (from the top) topography is highlighted by a red circle. This component is the most strong and corresponds usually to eye blinks. Make sure that this is the case and click *OK*. The software will filter out this type of artifacts from the whole EEG record. By visual inspection of the record make sure that the corresponding artifact is corrected.

9. From *Analysis menu* click *Mark Artifacts* command. Load the parameters of artifact rejection from the database by clicking command *Load from database*. After pressing *OK* the software will mark the artifacts that fit the criteria.

10. From *Analysis menu* click *Compute ERP* command. Load the parameters of ERP computation from the database by clicking command *Load from database*. The software will compute ERPs for *VCPT*[10] *(visual continuous performance task)* for all categories of trials and for each electrode separately and present them in a form of 19 graphs located in a way similar to which the electrodes are located on the scalp.

11. From *Analysis menu* click *Comparison of results* command. The window named *Processing Results comparison* will appear. To load ERPs from the normative database click *Load Database* bar. At the left of the window the name of subject's ERP is present while at the right one can see two options: *Event Related Potentials* and *Event related Components computed* for VCPT condition.

12. First compare raw ERPs with the normative data. To do it, click the subject's file from *Event Related Potentials* from the left and then click *Event Related Potentials/visual VCPT* from the right. Press *OK*.

13. The ERPs for GO trails for the subject [1}, the database [2], and the difference ERPs [3] for (subject-database) will appear in *Comparison Window* (an example is presented in Fig. 16.10). Note that the confidence level of deviation from normality is presented in a form of small vertical bars below the ERPs. To view ERPs and ERP differences in the same graphs for a different task condition (e.g., NOGO) do as follows: (a) press ▼ for the first *Active Group* and select condition *a-p NOGO[1]* – ERPs for NOGO condition of the patient, (b) press ▼ for the second *Active Group* and select condition *a-p NOGO[2]* – averaged ERPs for NOGO condition of healthy subjects of the same age, (c) press ▼ for the third *Active Group* and select ERPs difference-condition *a-p NOGO[D]*. Note that the scale, time interval, and base line correction for ERP analysis can be selected from the right window. For example, to view the responses to

the second stimulus type "1400" for Time interval/From (ms), and type "700" for duration (ms).

14. Second, compare ERPs independent components with the normative data. To do it, from *Analysis menu* click *Comparison of results* command. The window named *Processing Results comparison* will appear again. To load ERPs from the normative database click *Load Database* bar. At the left of the window the name of subject's ERP is present while at the right one can see two options: *Event Related Potentials* and *Event related Components* computed for VCPT condition.

15. Select the second option. Click the patient's file from *Event Related Potentials* from the left and then click *Event Related Potentials Components/ visual VCPT* from the right. Press *OK*.

16. The ERPs for the first independent component P1N1 for the subject [1}, the database-P1N1 [2] and the difference ERPs-P1N1 [D] for (subject-database) will appear in *Comparison Window* (an example is presented in Fig. 16.11). Note that the confidence level of deviation from normality is presented in a form of small vertical bars below the ERPs. To view ERPs and ERP differences in the same graphs for a given independent component (e.g., P3b) do as follows: (a) press ▼ for the first *Active Group* and select condition *P3b P[1]* – ERPs for the P3b component of the patient, (b) press ▼ for the second *Active Group* and select condition *P3b P[2]* – averaged ERPs for the P3b independent component of healthy subjects of the same age, (c) press ▼ for the third *Active Group* and select ERPs difference-condition *P3b P[D]*. The names of the components correspond to the psychological operations described in the book as follows: P1 N1 – for the visual processing in the occipital lobe, N1P2 aC – for the auditory processing, v com TL – for the comparing operation in the left ventral stream, S3 sup – for operation of action suppression, P4 mon – for monitoring operation. Note that the scale, time interval, and base line correction for ERP analysis can be selected from the right window. For example, to view the responses to the second stimulus type "1400" for Time interval/From (ms), and type "700" for duration (ms).

Do the same analysis with the second file and try to answer the questions presented above.

PART III

Disorders of the Brain Systems

I. INTRODUCTION

As was shown in Part II, the brain can be divided into systems. These brain systems consist of separate cortical and subcortical anatomical structures and play different functions in processing sensory information and organizing actions. The systems we have analyzed in the previous part are: sensory systems, attentional networks, executive system, affective system, and memory systems. We presume that dysfunctioning of a separate brain system is associated with a separate class of brain disorders.

However brain disorders are classified not on the basis of neurophysiological data but on the basis of behavior. There are two main classification manuals: DSM-IV and

ICD-10[1]. The two manuals rely only on behavioral symptoms. Although research is advancing and several objective diagnostic parameters[2] have been suggested for specific disorders, no reliable biological markers or endophenotypes of distinct disorders are accepted so far. This part of the book holds the following closely related goals: (1) analyzing dysfunctions of the above mentioned systems in connection with known psychiatric and neurological disorders, (2) associating the dysfunctions of the brain systems with QEEG/ERP markers described in Parts I and II of this book, (3) suggesting an appropriate neurotherapy for correcting dysfunctions of the brain systems.

From Part II we have learnt that distinct brain systems are controlled by separate neuromodulators in the brainstem. Consequently, the brain systems can be corrected by pharmacological[3] interventions on these mediators. The interventions include increasing or decreasing the action of neuromodulators (1) by feeding the brain with biochemical precursors of mediators (such as with L-dopa – a precursor of dopamine), (2) by blocking the postsynaptic receptors (such as with antipsychotic drugs that have affinity to dopamine receptors), (3) by blocking the reuptake mechanisms (such as with Ritalin that suppresses the dopamine reuptake mechanisms), or changing the cellular mechanisms of neurotransmission in other ways[4].

It should be noted here that before 1950s, scientists tried several nonpharmacological interventions such as electrical invasive and non-invasive

[1]The Diagnostic and Statistical Manual of Mental Disorders (DSM) is a handbook that lists different categories of mental disorder and the criteria for diagnosing them, according to the American Psychiatric Association. It is used worldwide by clinicians and researchers. The DSM has gone through several revisions since 1952. The last major revision was the DSM-IV published in 1994. The DSM-V is currently in preparation, due for publication in approximately 2011. The mental disorders section of the International Statistical Classification of Diseases and Related Health Problems (ICD) is another commonly used guide, and the two classifications use similar diagnostic codes.

[2]Such as the inattention index (theta beta ratio) in EEG spectra for diagnosis of attentional dysfunctions.

[3]Pharmacology (from Greek *pharmakon* - drug and *lego* – to tell about) studies effects of different biochemical substances on function in the leaving organs. If substances have medical properties, they are called pharmaceuticals. The field includes compositing drugs, studying their properties, and observing their medical applications. Neuro- and *psychopharmacology* (effects of medication on behavior and nervous system functioning) are considered as sub-fields of pharmacology.

[4]Although different plants were the source of medication for centuries, modern western medicine utilizes purified bioactive compounds, rather than an entire sample of plant matter. The real breakthrough period in psychopharmacology started in 1950s by introduction of the first set of psychotropics and new methodological approaches in pharmacology. Treatment of heterogeneous disorders such as mania, schizophrenia, depression, bipolar disorder, became available.

intrusions, as well as anatomical destructions including neurosurgical and stereotactic operations. Most of the attempts were abandoned after the revolutionary events in psycho-pharmacology. However, 50 years of using psycho-pharmacology brought some dissatisfaction and controversy. One part of this controversy is associated with a failure to find a certain geno-type as a pathological mechanism for a certain disease[5]. Recent attempts of medical genetics have indicated that most of psychiatric disorders do not follow a simple Mendelian rule and that no single gene could be attrib-uted to a single disorder. This led some scientists to introduce the concept of endophenotypes as biological markers of disease that are non-molecular but closer to the genotype than behaviorally defined classification of dis-eases. Some QEEG parameters and ERP components have been suggested as candidates for endophenotypes of at least some of brain diseases.

Renaissance of non-pharmacological methods of treatment started recently as a rebound effect of exponentially increasing use of pharmaco-logical substances to treat various brain diseases. The non-pharmacological methods include neurofeedback and electromagnetic stimulation methods such as transcranial direct current stimulation (tDCS), transmagnetic stim-ulation (TMS), deep brain stimulation (DBS), and electroconvulsive ther-apy (ECT). They are united under a common name "neurotherapy."

So, in this part of the book we are going to present the most common brain diseases in association with QEEG and ERP indexes of the brain systems that are supposed to be involved in pathogenesis of the diseases. The diseases we are going to discuss in this pat of the book are listed in Table PIII.1. The brain systems that are associated with these dysfunctions are marked. The table simplifies the reality. It does not show complex inter-actions between systems[6] and heterogeneity of distinct diseases. Still, the concept depicted in the table may serve as a starting point for presenting

---

[5]The other part of controversy is associated with more practical issues. First of all, pharmacother-apy does not help everyone: some patients remain unresponsive to the pharmacological interventions. Moreover, selection of the appropriate medication (especially in depression) is a matter of trial and error. Because the effect of some substances needs few weeks to be exhibited and there are many potential drugs that might treat the disease, the trial and error procedure could last for many months and is very expensive both in monetary expression and in human resources. On the top of that most of the drugs have undesirable side effects.

[6]In the dysfunctional brain different systems interact with each other so that dysfunction, for example, of executive system might cause the dysfunction of the affective system and vice versa. This interaction complicates the behavioral pattern of disease in a particular patient.

TABLE PIII.1   Association Between Psychiatric/Neurological Diseases and Impairments of Brain systems

Disease/System	Sensory	Affective	Memory	Executive
Dyslexia	————			
Neglect	————			
Depression		————		
Anxiety		————		
Alzheimer's			————	
Parkinson's				————
Schizophrenia				————
OCD				————
ADHD				————
Addiction		————	————	————

data and ideas regarding QEEG/ERP markers of brain disorders and neurotherapeutical approaches for correcting these disorders.

We have learnt in this book that operations of the brain systems are maintained by complex neuronal networks that include subcortical and cortical anatomical structures. Let us consider some generally defined neuronal network[7]. The network is characterized by two parameters: (1) by activation level of the network and (2) by response of the system to an elemental increase of the input to the system. As we have shown in Introduction to the book the relationship between the response of the network and its activation level is described by the inverted U-curve (Fig. PIII.1).

We presume that the response of the neuronal network is approximated by the corresponding ERP independent component generated in by the network in an adequate psychological condition[8]. One can see that the maximum of ERPs amplitude corresponds to the optimal level of activation of the neuronal network. From Part I we know that the increase of the optimal level of activation of the cortex is associated with the excess of beta activity in the background EEG generated by the corresponding part of the

---

[7]For example, the network subserving monitoring operation includes several cortical areas of the frontal cortex with the anterior cingulate cortex as a key element.

[8]For example, the response of the monitoring network is measured by the amplitude of P400 monitoring component in two stimulus GO/NOGO task.

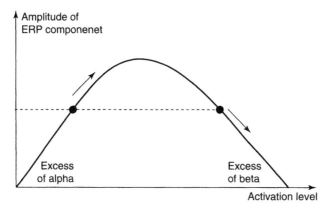

FIGURE PIII.1   Response (amplitude of ERP component) versus activation level of a hypothetical neuronal network. Horizontal axis – overall activation of neuronal network. Vertical axis – response of the system to a relevant stimulus measured in amplitude of evoked potential. Lower level of activation is characterized by excess of alpha activity while higher level of activation is characterized by excess of beta activity in the EEG.

cortex, while decrease in the level of activation is associated with the excess of alpha activity[9]. Note that both extremes are associated with decrease of amplitude of ERP components. The decrease of ERPs amplitude is associated with decrease of reactivity of the system when the system moves away from its optimal performance point[10]. Consequently, the excess of beta activity as well as excess of alpha activity is accompanied by low amplitude of ERP components that are associated with poor performance of the system. These theoretical considerations show necessity of simultaneous measurement of ERP components and background EEG characteristics.

II. GLOSSARY

Addiction is a compulsive, out-of-control drug use despite serious negative consequences.

---

[9]Recall the relationship between metabolic activity of the cortex and alpha and beta activity generated in the corresponding local cortical area (see Fig. PIII.1). According to this relationship, excessive (in comparison to norms) beta in EEG corresponds to increase of metabolic activity, while excessive alpha corresponds to decrease of metabolic activity in the local cortical area.

[10]For example, decrease in the monitoring component may be associated with excessive activation of the monitoring network as well as with decrease of its activation.

ADHD is the most common developmental disorder that affects 3–8 per cent of children worldwide according to conservative estimation and includes children displaying developmentally inappropriate levels of inattention, hyperactivity, and impulsivity that begin in childhood and cause impairment to school performance, intellectual functioning, social skills, driving, and occupational functioning.

Alzheimer's disease is a degenerative brain disorder that at the first stage starts with progressive memory loss and at later stages develops into a generalized dementia. The loss of cholinergic cells in the basal forebrain appears to be responsible for the first stage.

Antipsychotic drugs are pharmacological agents that are used to treat psychosis.

Anhedonia is loss of interest or pleasure in almost all activities.

Cognitive-behavioral psychotherapy is a form of psychotherapy that aims to strengthen self-esteem and provide the patient with support and understanding. Cognitive-behavioral psychotherapy emphasizes the analysis of the problems at hand, and the definition of concrete goals and solutions so that the patient can recognize progress.

Compulsions are actions repeated over and over in ritualistic, stereotyped succession.

DC (direct current) is a flow of electric charge that does not change direction and value. Applying to a cortical tissue, DC polarizes neurons, that is, changes membrane potentials of cells.

Depression (or major depression) is a disorder of the affective system characterized by low or depressed mood, anhedonia, and low energy or fatigue.

Diagnostic and Statistical Manual of Mental Disorders (DSM) is a handbook that lists different categories of mental disorder and the criteria for diagnosing them, according to the American Psychiatric Association. It is used worldwide by clinicians and researchers. The DSM has gone through several revisions since 1952. The last major revision was the DSM-IV published in 1994. In Europe, the mental disorders section of *the International Statistical Classification of Diseases and Related Health Problems (ICD)* is more often used.

Electroconvulsive therapy (ECT), also known as electroshock, is a psychiatric treatment in which seizures are induced by means of strong electrical current.

Effect size is a measure of a certain effect that is defined as the difference between the means of a measured parameter for the experimental and control groups, divided by the standard deviation of the control group or the average standard deviation of both groups. The effect size is a standardized measure and allows comparing the effects found in different studies with different parameters.

Endophenotype is a biological marker of a disease.

Monoamine oxidase is an enzyme located on the outer mitochondrial membrane, which catalyses the hydrolysis of biogenic amines such as catecholamines and serotonin.

Morbidity is the incidence or prevalence of a disease in a population.

Neurofeedback is a technique of self-regulation by means of EEG-based biofeedback. In this technique, neurofeedback parameters of EEG currently recorded from a subject's scalp (such as an EEG power in a given frequency band) are presented to the subject through visual, auditory, or tactile modality with the task to voluntarily alter these parameters in a desired (leading to a more efficient mode of brain functioning) direction.

Obsessions are thoughts that repeat over and over again, unwanted but insistent.

OCD is a disorder characterized by recurrent obsessions and compulsions causing marked distress or significant impairment.

Oppositional defiant disorder (ODD) is associated with taking unsafe risks, breaking laws, refusing to follow instructions or directions.

Psychosis includes distortions in thinking, such as delusions (false beliefs that are firmly held in the face of contradictory evidence), and perceptual disturbances, such as hallucinations. Auditory hallucinations, usually experienced as voices distinct from one's own thoughts, are most common in schizophrenia.

Psychopharmacology is a subfield of pharmacology that in particular studies effects of different biochemical substances on behavior and nervous system functioning.

Psychosurgery is a type of surgical ablation or disconnection of brain tissue with the intent to alter affective or cognitive states caused by mental illness.

Schizophrenia is a psychiatric disorder characterized by (1) impairments in the executive system such as disordered thoughts, disorganized speech, inability to plan, initiate, and regulate goal directed behavior, as well as by (2) impairments in the sensory systems such as hallucinations, and by (3) associated symptoms of the affective system, such as blunted emotions.

Learning disability (LD) is a difficulty in mastering language, reading, or math.

tDCS – transcranial direct current stimulation – a neurotherapeutic technique of application of direct current to the brain by means of electrodes placed on the head. Because of polarizing effect on neuronal cells, tDCS in 1960–1970s was called polarization technique.

Tourette's syndrome is associated with having tics – uncontrolled movements like eye blinks, or facial twitches, or vocal sounds.

Tricyclic drugs are molecules that inhibit biogenic amine reuptake, therefore prolonging the period during which these neurotransmitters are active at the synaptic cleft.

CHAPTER 17

Attention Deficit
Hyperactivity Disorder

I. DESCRIPTION OF BEHAVIOR

A. Executive Operations and ERP Components

We start with disorders of the executive system. The basic operations of the executive system are the maintenance of working memory and attention, the engagement operation, the inhibition of actions, and the monitoring operation. The event-related potential (ERP) components reflecting these operations and tasks in which the components are generated, are listed in Table 17.1. Recall that an ERP component reflects the response of a certain brain sub-system (such as monitoring neuronal network) to an adequate stimulus in an appropriate behavioral paradigm. As one can see no single task could be chosen as a gold standard for assessment of the executive system. However some variants of the two stimulus GO/NOGO tasks might be considered as a good approximation of the gold standard.

B. Symptoms of ADHD in DSM-IV and ICD-10

Imagine yourself living in fast-moving kaleidoscope, where objects around you are constantly shifting and your mind drives from one image, sound, thought to the next. Imagine also yourself easily distracted by unimportant sights and sounds,

TABLE 17.1   ERP Components as Indexes of Operations in the Executive System

Executive operation	Engagement	Working memory/ attention	Response inhibition	Monitoring
ERP component and psychological task	P3b to targets in the oddball and GO/NOGO tasks	P2 comparison component in the GO/NOGO task. CNV in the delayed response tasks	N2 for Stop stimulus in the Stop-signal tasks or the motor inhibition component for NOGO stimuli in the GO/NOGO tasks	P4NOGO monitoring component in the GO/NOGO tasks, ERN in the CPT tasks

feeling bored, yet helpless to complete the tasks you need to accomplish. This is how ADHD children feel[1].

ADHD is one of the most prevalent conditions in child psychiatry[2]. The other labels of the disorder introduced in the past are attention deficit disorder (ADD), hyperactivity, hyperkinesis, hyperkinetic syndrome, minimal brain dysfunction, and minimal brain damage[3]. DSM-IV distinguishes three subtypes of ADHD: predominately inattentive type, predominately hyperactive-impulsive type, and combined type. This classification is based on three groups of symptoms: inattention, hyperactivity, and impulsivity[4]. Evidence for the validity and clinical use of these subtypes is mixed and controversial. Current work has not yet resolved the controversy about whether a purely inattentive subtype must be considered separately from ADHD or not.

Along with being the most common disorder ADHD is, undoubtedly, the most controversial. The controversy can be seen, for example, in the differences between US diagnostic criteria for the disorder, as defined by the DSM-IV and the European diagnostic criteria for hyperkinetic disorder (HKD), as defined by the ICD-10.

---

[1]Literature is full of descriptions of such characters. As long ago as in 1845, Dr. Heinrich Hoffman, a German physician, wrote "The Story of Fidgety Philip" as a portrait of an ADHD boy. Another good example of an ADHD child was described by a famous Russian writer Nikolai Nosov in his beautiful book "Adventures of Dunno and his Friends." Dunno was contrasted to Doono which we would call a normal healthy boy. The most amazing thing to mention is that every child in Russia liked Dunno not Doono.

[2]At conservative estimation it affects 3–7.5 per cent of children worldwide.

[3]DSM-IV description of ADHD is given, for example, in http://en.wikipedia.org/wiki/DSM-IV_Codes.

[4]Inattentive children have a hard time keeping their mind on any one thing, may get bored with a task after only a few minutes, have difficulty in voluntary focusing, in organizing and completing a task. Hyperactive children always seem to be in motion, can't sit still, may touch everything or talk incessantly, may feel intensely restless, may try to do several things at once bouncing from one activity to another. People who are impulsive are unable to curb their immediate reactions, can't think before they act, have hard time in waiting for things they want or in taking their turn in games.

Both classifications include children displaying developmentally inappropriate levels of inattention, hyperactivity, and impulsivity that begin in childhood and cause impairment to school performance, intellectual functioning, social skills, driving, and occupational functioning. But ICD-10 criteria are more restrictive than the DSM-IV diagnosis of ADHD because they need a greater degree of symptom expression[5]. The male-to-female sex ratio for the disorder is greater in clinical studies than in community studies. This difference is probably because of ADHD being less disruptive in women than in men as well as because of increased exposure of mails to environmental sources of cause, such as head injury.

Although both DSM-IV and ICD-10 provide well structured, criterion-based diagnoses for ADHD and HKD, they have several weaknesses. The diagnostic criteria do not provide developmentally sensitive definitions for helping doctors to differentiate ADHD symptoms from developmentally healthy levels of inattention, hyperactivity, and impulsivity. Clinicians often receive diagnostic data from multiple informants (e.g., from parents and teachers) but both diagnostic manuals provide no guidelines of how to integrate this information. The weaknesses of the diagnostic system have led to critics of ADHD diagnosis as subjective and have initiated a search of objective markers or endophenotypes of this disease[6].

II. GENETIC AND ENVIRONMENTAL FACTORS

A. Complex Genetic Disorder

Research shows that ADHD runs in families and approximately one-half of parents who have had ADHD have a child with this disorder. According to twin and adoption studies, genes have a substantial role in the familial transmission of ADHD. These data estimate the heritability of ADHD to be 0·76. In the same time, genetic studies show that ADHD, similar to the most of psychiatric disorders, fails to follow Mendelian patterns of inheritance and must be classified as a complex genetic disorder[7].

---

[5]In this way DSM-IV ADHD is more prevalent than ICD HKD, because it includes inattentive subtype. This diagnostic difference has sometimes been misinterpreted to mean that ADHD is more common in the United States than in countries using ICD criteria. However, when the same diagnostic criteria are used the prevalence of ADHD is similar worldwide.

[6]The first attempt to introduce endophenotypes as neuroscience based markers of ADHD was done Xavier Castellanos and Rosemary Tannock in 2002. They proposed three endophenotypes that would correspond to the causes of ADHD: (1) a specific abnormality in reward-related circuitry that leads to shortened delay gradients, (2) deficits in temporal processing that result in intra-subject internal variability, and (3) deficits in working memory (Castellanos and Tannock, 2002).

[7]The abnormalities in the dopamine-transporter gene on chromosome 5 were found in children with severe forms of ADHD. We know that stimulant drugs which are effective in ADHD block the dopamine transporter. This fact led to suggestion that the dopamine D4 and D5 receptors and the genes related to their expression might be associated with ADHD.

B. Environmental Risk Factors

Although the idea that particular foods or food additives might cause ADHD received much attention in the media, systematic studies have shown that this theory in general is not correct. However, by contrast with the mostly negative studies of dietary factors, lead exposure has been implicated in the pathophysiology of the disorder.

Several studies indicate that pregnancy and delivery complications raise the risk for ADHD. The basal ganglia, which are commonly implicated in ADHD, are one of the most metabolically active structures in the brain, and are particularly sensitive to hypoxic insults. Many studies confirm that prematurity, as indexed by low birth-weight, is a risk factor for ADHD. Prospective studies of infants show that fetal exposure to maternal alcohol use leads to behavioral, cognitive, and learning problems that could be represented as ADHD. In a similar way, exposure of the fetus to nicotine (e.g., due to maternal smoking) can damage the brain at critical points in the developmental process. The other environmental factors include severe early deprivation, family psychosocial adversity, traumatic brain injury, and stroke, particularly when the basal ganglia are affected.

C. Co-morbidity

Much work from both clinical and epidemiological studies shows that the disease puts children at risk for co-morbidity with other psychiatric and substance use disorders. For example, some studies suggest that ADHD can put adults at risk for personality disorders. At all ages, ADHD is associated with functional impairments such as school dysfunction, peer problems, family conflict, poor occupational performance, injuries, antisocial behavior, traffic violations, and traffic accidents. Follow-up studies have shown that ADHD persists into adulthood. There is clearly an age-dependent decline in symptoms, but even when symptoms are not prominent enough to prompt a diagnosis, they are frequently associated with clinically significant impairments.

ADHD is often accompanied by other disorders such as specific learning disability (LD), oppositional defiant disorder (ODD), Tourette's syndrome, anxiety and depression (Fig. 17.1). Only ODD and Tourette's syndrome are considered as disorders of the executive system. Anxiety and depression are associated with the affective system, while learning disabilities (such as dyslexia) are associated with sensory systems.

III. IMAGING CORRELATES

A. PET and MRI

Is ADHD merely the extreme of a healthy variation worsen by adverse environmental factors or is it a brain disorder with impairment in certain brain systems?

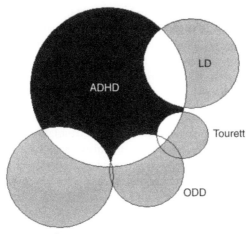

FIGURE 17.1   Co-morbidity of ADHD. See text.

Neuroscience-based methods help us to answer this question. However, as with any other brain disease, the initial phase of research of neurobiology of ADHD has been purely descriptive by design. In this design neuroanatomical and neurophysiological parameters of the ADHD brain were statistically compared with a control group of healthy subjects. Most of attention of the researchers was attracted to the basal ganglia and prefrontal cortical areas. This research has revealed the following facts:

1. Magnetic resonance imaging (MRI) studies observed smaller sizes of the caudate nucleus, globus pallidus and pre-frontal cortical areas. For example, in a study by a group of researchers from the National Institutes of Health (NIH) in Bethesda, USA (Castellanos et al., 2003) the authors obtained MRI scans of monozygotic twins discordant for ADHD. The affected twins were observed to have significantly smaller caudate volumes[8]. These results provide support for involving the striatum as a part of the basal ganglia in ADHD pathophysiology. It is also noteworthy to mention another MRI study of a joint group of scientists from the NHI and John Hopkins Medical Institutions in Baltimore (Herskovits et al., 1999). The study was made on children without prior history of ADHD. Their MRI images were obtained 3 months after closed-head injury. Children who developed

[8]For example, one of affected twins was found to have an unsuspected focal abnormality in the left caudate, left putamen, and adjacent white matter.

secondary (closed-head injury-induced) ADHD revealed more lesions in the right putamen than children who did not develop secondary ADHD[9].

2. In line with functional magnetic resonace imaging (fMRI) studies of positron emission tomography (PET) research found lower glucose consumption in the ADHD group in comparison to norms in the frontal lobe and basal ganglia, especially during demanding tasks.

Although the effect sizes of MRI and PET comparison studies were qualitatively (statistically) significant they were quite small quantitatively. Indeed, the group difference between ADHD and normal populations in MRI studies was about 6 per cent which is comparable with the standard deviation in the normal group. At the same time, nearly two decades of studies in psychiatric genetics were also quite unsuccessful. These unsatisfactory results initiated interest in studies of EEG and ERPs quantitative indices of the disease liability, termed endophenotypes. The endophenotypes are supposed to predict the risk of ADHD in the same way as appearance of spikes in raw EEG predicts the risk of epilepsy. Such endophenotypes should be continuously quantifiable and should predict disorder probabilistically.

B. QEEG

Below, we are going to review the literature and our own studies within the framework of theoretical constructs presented in Part II of the book. We presume that the main brain system impaired in ADHD is the executive system. The executive system is characterized by two parameters: the level of overall activation of the system and the amplitude of response associated with four different operations in the system: working memory, action selection, action inhibition, and action monitoring. Let us start with description of spontaneous electrical activity in EEG which can be considered as an index of the overall activity of the executive system and, consequently, as a background for executive operations.

As we learnt from Part I of this book, EEG recorded in eyes open and eyes closed resting state conditions is a good indicator of metabolic activity in the cortex. Increase of slow activities and decrease of beta activities in local EEG indicate low metabolic activity in the area that generates the corresponding EEG. These types of abnormalities are the most common to be observed in ADHD population.

---

[9]The basal ganglia appear to be not the only structures involved in pathogenesis of ADHD. For example, in a recent study from Stanford University School of Medicine (Tamm et al., 2004) a group of ADHD adolescent boys participating in GO/NOGO task was compared with healthy controls using event related fMRI. Individuals with ADHD showed marked abnormalities in brain activation during NOGO trials including hypoactivation of the anterior/mid-cingulate cortex extending to the supplementary motor area.

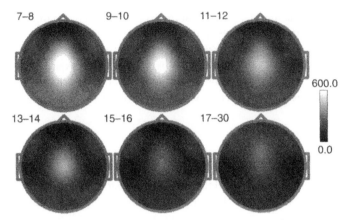

FIGURE 17.2 Mapping inattention index. The data are taken from the Human Brain Institute Normative Database. Local average montage (Lemos) is sued. The index is defined as theta/beta power ratio, where theta: 4–8 Hz, beta: 13–21 Hz.

C. Theta Beta Ratio as Inattention Index

Most of the quantitative electroencephalogram (QEEG) studies have reported that ADHD population as a whole shows elevated levels of slow wave power in comparison to normal children[10]. Taking into account that absolute values of spectra exhibit a big variation depending on several brain unrelated features (such as thickness of the skull) a relative parameter defined as the theta beta ratio has been used instead of absolute values. The theta beta ratio was labeled as inattention index by a group of participants in multi-center studies in the USA (Monastra et al., 1999)[11]. Our experience of assessing QEEG in more than 1000 ADHD children shows that computing the inattention index gives a good measure of the background EEG at least for a part of ADHD population. However, mapping this index in normal population tells us that the location of the maximum of this index changes significantly with age: from central–parietal location at 7–8 years old children to frontal–central location in adults (Fig. 17.2). This observation shows that for better

[10]One of the earliest studies to identify EEG abnormalities in children with minimal brain dysfunction (a synonym of ADHD in 1930–1950s) was as early as in 1938 (Jasper et al., 1938). Similar studies were made later in 1950s and 1960s all using visual evaluation of paper recordings of the EEG.. The most common qualitative finding was an increase in EEG activity in the delta and theta bands. This finding was confirmed by quantitative EEG analysis in 1970s and later years.

[11]A so-called inattention index is defined as a ratio of theta EEG power (measured within the 4–8 Hz frequency band) and beta EEG power (measured within the 13–21 Hz frequency band). The EEG is recorded at a single place Cz in reference to linked ears. At the age of 6–11 years this ratio was found to be 3 times higher in ADHD inattentive and combined types in comparison to norms. Sensitivity of this index (the percentage of ADHD children testing positive regarding QEEG index) was found to be 86 per cent, and specificity of this index (the percentage of non-ADHD testing negative regarding this index) was found to be 98 per cent (Monastra et al., 1999).

results in discriminating ADHD population from healthy subjects this index has to be measured in different electrode positions depending on age.

As far as coherence measure concerns, Robert Barry and his colleagues from University of Wollongong, Australia on the basis of their own experience and literature search concluded that there are insufficient studies to evaluate the reliability of coherence measurements in discriminating ADHD children (Barry et al., 2003)[12].

IV. ERP CORRELATES

There is a vast amount of empirical knowledge regarding ERPs in ADHD. As the studies of QEEG indexes of ADHD, the ERP studies until recently were mostly descriptive. The basic idea was (1) to select a behavioral paradigm that is supposedly associated with processes thought to be impaired in ADHD, (2) to choose an ERPs component that is computed as a subtraction wave between two task conditions[13], (3) to measure this component in the two groups (ADHD versus controls) or in the subtypes of ADHD such as the inattentive type and the combined type versus controls, (4) to assess the size effect, that is, relative differences between mean values computed for the selected groups.

ERP studies in ADHD started in 1970s with the work of Satterfield and his group (Satterfield et al., 1972). Enormous number of ERP papers in ADHD gave a variety of results, sometimes inconsistent. A full review on this subject was recently published in *Clinical Neurophysiology Journal* (Barry et al., 2003). In this book we present only typical studies with consistent results. These studies are grouped according to psychological operations that are supposedly impaired in ADHD.

A. Selective Attention

Spatial-cuing paradigms are the ones to assess selective attention. Recall, in this paradigm target stimuli are preceded by cue stimuli which either validly or invalidly indicate the location of the subsequent target. The validity effect measured as the difference in speed and accuracy of responding to targets between invalid and valid trials is assumed to reflect the process of focusing attention on the cued location. However, behavioral results of studies that used this paradigm with ADHD children

---

[12]Note that from statistical point of view there is a systematic error in assessing the coherence values. This error depends on the number of epochs that are used for calculating the parameter. So, strictly speaking, to make statistically reliable assessments of coherence measures and to be able to compare these measures with the database one needs an equal number of EEG epochs both in the normative database and in the subject whose EEG is comparing with the database.

[13]For example, the difference waves can be obtained as deviant-standard difference ERPs in the oddball paradigm, attended-ignored difference in the selective attention paradigm, or NOGO–GO difference in GO/NOGO paradigm.

are not consistent. Recently Huang-Pollock and Nigg (2003) conducted a meta-analysis of experimental findings and concluded that there was no indication of a reliable deficit of visual–spatial orienting in ADHD in general or in one of ADHD subtypes in particular.

Another paradigm to study selective attention is the dichotic listening task or its visual analogs. Recently, high resolution spatio-temporal mapping of ERPs in the visual selective attention paradigm revealed abnormalities in ADHD population (Jonkman et al., 2004)[14]. ADHD children lack the so-called frontal selection negativity – the ERP component reflecting sensory-related selection operation. However, in an earlier study that used the processing negativity as an index of selective attention no difference between ADHD sub-groups and healthy subjects were observed (Rothenberger et al., 2000). The inconsistency in studies of selective attention mechanisms in ADHD might be explained by heterogeneity of ADHD population. We can only speculate that there might be a relatively small ADHD subgroup that is associated with impairment in selective attention mechanisms.

B. Working Memory

As we learnt from Part II of the book the working memory is executive operation maintained by a complex system with the basal ganglia as an element of the system. In a very rough simplification (that we make here only for didactic purposes), working memory can be considered as an active trace which is characterized by the amplitude and the rate of decay (Fig. 17.3). The larger is the amplitude of the trace and the longer it lasts, the better is the working memory. We suggest that in ADHD population the initial trace in the working is the same as in healthy controls but the decay is much faster than those for the norms (Fig. 17.3)[15].

There are several ERP indexes of working memory. They are: (1) contingent negative variation (CNV) in the two stimulus tasks as a measure of preparatory activity in the brain[16], (2) mismatch negativity (MMN) in oddball tasks as a probe of

---

[14]In this study, participants viewed random sequences of red and yellow rectangles. They were instructed to monitor rectangles of only one color for occasionally deviating orientations, and to ignore rectangles of the other color. Shortly after 100 ms, control children exhibit attentional modulation of stimulus-related activity, which persists over some hundreds of milliseconds – the phenomenon called frontal selection negativity.

[15]There are few facts supporting this suggestion. One of them is an increase of DAT receptors in the striatum found in a sub-population of ADHD children. The increased density of DAT receptors leads to the fast washout of the dopamine from synaptic cleft. The fast decay of the striatal dopamine could lead to the fast decay of the working memory subserved by the basal ganglia thalamo-cortical feedback circuits.

[16]Recall that CNV can be decomposed into two components: the one associated with preparation to receive a stimulus and the one that is associated with preparation to make a movement. These two components are not discriminated in ADHD studies, the fact that can create inconsistency in these studies.

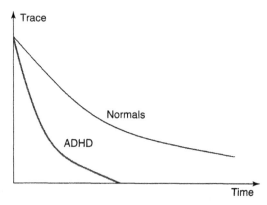

FIGURE 17.3   Hypothetical trace decays in the working memory of normal and ADHD population.

attention memory trace of the repetitive sound in the auditory cortex, (3) P2 comparison component in GO/NOGO tasks as an index of change detection of the current stimulus in comparison to the memory trace stored in working memory.

Few studies have directly examined CNV amplitude in children with ADHD, and their results are conflicting, some studies showing reduction of CNV amplitude in ADHD subjects compared to controls, while other studies failed to find differences. The studies of MMN in ADHD that are available in the current literature are also inconsistent. Although some studies reported a reduction of MMN in ADHD group in comparison to healthy controls, other studies failed to observe the differences. Note however that the MMN can be considered only as indirect measures of working memory, or, better to say, of its automatic part[17].

Another indirect index of working memory is given by the comparison component elicited in the two stimulus GO/NOGO task. This component is observed in response to the second stimulus in NOGO trials when the presented stimulus does not match the expectation. The component is associated with change detection in sensory physical and semantic modalities. In our study we analyzed 150 children who were diagnosed as ADHD. Spatial filters for P2 comparison component were derived from the set of 500 ERPs (GO and NOGO) computed for a group of healthy children. Further, the spatial filtration was applied to each ADHD children and the resulting P2 component for each patient was compared with the normative data separately for different age groups. The results of such comparison for one patient are shown in Fig. 17.4. Four independent components are presented, P2 comparison, N1/P2 auditory to novel stimuli, P3b and P4 monitoring. Note that for this patient only one component (P2 comparison) is selectively

---

[17]The MMN is associated with comparison of the incoming auditory stimulus with a memory trace. The trace is attention independent and is supposedly formed automatically.

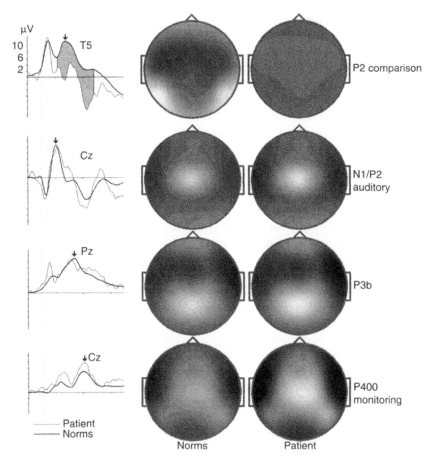

FIGURE 17.4   Selective impairment of P2 comparison component in an ADHD child. Left –
superposition of ERP waveforms for four independent components, from top to bottom, P2 comparison, N1/P1 auditory, P3b and P4 monitoring. In the superposition, thin line – individual components
for the ADHD child, thick line – grand average component for a group of healthy subjects of the corresponding age. Right – maps of the components for the patient and for the group of normal subjects.

decreased. This selective decrease of the comparison component might serve as
an index of reduction of the stimulus trace in the working memory. Indeed, the
reduction of the memory trace would presumably lead to decrease of the change
detection and, consequently, to decrease of the P2 comparison component[18].

---

[18]From the whole group of 150 patients 36 (25 per cent revealed selective decrease in the P2 comparison component. We still do not know how this sub-group of ADHD children differs behaviorally
from the norms.

C. Engagement Operation

The engagement operation from neurophysiological point of view is associated with activation of cortical and subcortical structures that are involved in execution of the selected action. From psychological, functional point of view the engagement operation is associated with combining all brain resources for the action to be accomplished. This operation is manifested in the P3b component. The oddball paradigm is the simplest and the most used behavioral task for eliciting the P3b component. In this task, the P3b is defined as the difference wave between ERPs to target stimuli (i.e., stimuli that are followed by actions) and standard stimuli (i.e., stimuli that are simply perceived by the subject without any subsequent response). It would not be an overstatement to say that most of the clinically oriented ERP studies in ADHD are associated with the oddball paradigm[19].

Most of the studies reported decrease of P3b component in ADHD population in comparison to healthy controls (see, e.g., one of our early studies Kropotov et al., 1999). From the deductive point of view, it is worth to mention a study that contrasted the P3b component with the P3a component while assessing differences between ADHD population and healthy controls (Jonkman et al., 2000). In this study a three stimulus visual odd ball task (presentation of standards, deviants, and novels) served as the background of the two visual tasks that varied in task difficulty. P3b and P3a components have been computed as difference waves. P3b component was shown to increase in the hard task in controls but not in ADHD and was smaller in the ADHD group. In contrast, P3a component decreased in hard task in both groups and did not differ between groups. Methylphenidate increased the P3b component, but did not affect the P3a component. It was concluded that ADHD children do not suffer from a shortage in attentional capacity which seems to be associated with the P3a component[20].

D. Response Inhibition

The response inhibition from neurophysiological point of view involves a separate circuit in the right ventral prefrontal cortical–basal ganglia–thalamic loop. The

---

[19]It should be noted here that the auditory oddball paradigm has been more often used. The only advantage of using the oddball paradigm in the auditory modality is fewer number of eye movements during the task. However, application of the spatial filtration methods to artifact correcting enable us not to worry about eye movement artifacts in EEG. Moreover, ERP components in the visual modality (including the P3b component) are larger than corresponding components in the auditory modality, probably because larger cortical areas are involved in visual processing than in auditory processing. Consequently the visual oddball tasks must be considered as favorable for studying the P3b component.

[20]In the terms of our theory the results show that the shift operation, that is ability to shift attention to a new stimulus, is not impaired in the ADHD population while the engagement operation, that is, ability to combine brain resources to execute an action, is indeed impaired.

ventral prefrontal cortex receives the information from sensory-related systems that detect mismatch between expected and real sensory stimulus. For example, it receives input from visual areas of the ventral stream. The ventral prefrontal cortex also receives inputs for the anterior cingulate cortex, the area where the executed action is compared with a prepared one. In both cases, the ventral prefrontal cortex is active when there is a need to stop or inhibit the ongoing behavioral pattern. The inhibition operation also involves the corresponding basal ganglia thalamo-cortical circuit. Since 1970s when Japanese scientists Gemba and Sasaki discovered electrophysiological correlates of inhibition operation in monkey and in humans, the frontal N2 component elicited in GO/NOGO task was thought to reflect this operation[21].

Impairment in response inhibition has been conceptualized as a core of ADHD by many authors including Russel Barkly, the leading figure in the field of ADHD. However attempts to test this hypothesis experimentally have been controversial. An international team from University of Goettingen in Germany and University of Zurich (Banaschewski et al., 2004) recently reported a failure to find any deviations from normality in an ADHD group in N2 component of ERPs in a variant of GO/NOGO paradigm – CPT-A-X task (see task descriptions in Methods of Part II). In contrast, in a study at University of Texas ERPs in another variant of GO/NOGO paradigm – stop signal task – showed a remarkable decrease of N2 component in ADHD group in comparison to healthy subjects. In response to all stop signals, control participants produced a large negative wave at 200 ms (N200) over right inferior frontal cortex, which was markedly reduced in ADHD children. The N200 amplitude was significantly correlated across subjects with response – inhibition performance. According to this study, ADHD children appear to have an abnormality in an early-latency, right inferior frontal processing component critical to the initiation of normal response inhibition operations.

The controversy between the above mentioned studies again shows importance of selecting an adequate paradigm to observe reliable size effects. In general, it is a common case in ERP studies that some tasks (either too easy to perform or generating too small component associated with a given psychological operation) are not able to reveal differences between a patient group (such as ADHD) and healthy controls, while other tasks (either difficult enough or generating larger and more reliable components) do reveal statistically significant deviations from normality[22].

---

[21]It should be stressed that independent component analysis of ERPs data from the Human Brain Institute Normative Database revealed not one but several components supposedly associated with inhibition of prepared action (for details see Chapter 12).

[22]Recall, that some defects in the car functioning can be observed only if the car is driven at a highest speed. This metaphor shows the importance of selecting the appropriate task for observing a reliable size effect when comparing a patient group with the healthy control subjects. In general the task must be difficult enough, while trials must elicit quite large components that must reveal a good test–retest reliability.

E. Monitoring Operation

Monitoring operation is an executive operation that is needed, for example, for correcting errors. The monitoring operation from neurophysiological point of view seems to be based on a common neuronal mechanism of comparing the expected event with the real one. The only difference is that in case of monitoring operation the expected action but not a sensory trace (as in the case of P2 change detection component) is compared with the actual behavioral response. If the executed or inhibited action does not fit the expectation, the result of comparison initiates a change in behavioral pattern in order to correct this discrepancy. This operation can be directly measured by error-related negativity (ERN) and following positivity (Pe) – ERP components that are elicited by the brain right after an error[23].

Another index of monitoring operation is given by the late P400 component elicited in response to NOGO trials and generated in the anterior cingulate cortex. In our study we analyzed 150 children who were diagnosed as ADHD. Spatial filters for P4 monitoring component were derived from a set of 500 ERPs (GO and NOGO) computed for a group of healthy children. Further, spatial filtration was applied to each ADHD children and the resulting P400 component for each patient was compared with the normative data separately for different age groups. The results of such comparison for an ADHD patient are shown in Fig. 17.5. Four independent components are presented, P2 comparison, N1/P2 auditory, P3b and P4 monitoring. Note that for this patient only one component (P4 monitoring) is selectively decreased. Note that the monitoring component has similar topographic distribution as the ERN and, according to LORETA, is generated in the anterior cingulate cortex.

V. DOPAMINE HYPOTHESIS OF ADHD

One of the basic mediators of the executive system is dopamine. As we showed in Chapter 12 the dopamine sets up the threshold of striatal neurons and consequently plays a critical role in action selection. The dopamine hypothesis of ADHD is a very popular one and receives an increasing scientific support. The hypothesis is based on solid experimental evidence such as the fact that symptoms

---

[23]Recently scientists from Ghent University in Belgium (Wiersema et al., 2005) used a GO/NOGO task with 25 per cent of NOGO trails to study ERPs differences between ADHD and normal groups. The authors showed that ADHD children made twice as many errors as healthy control subjects and fail to adjust their speed of responding after making an error. Exploring the error-related potentials revealed that the error-related negativity (ERN) was the same for the two groups, but that children with ADHD showed diminished error positivity (Pe). Based on these findings, the authors concluded that children with ADHD are normal in early error monitoring processes related to error detection, but show abnormal response strategy adjustments and were deviant in later error monitoring processes associated with the subjective emotional and conscious evaluation of the error.

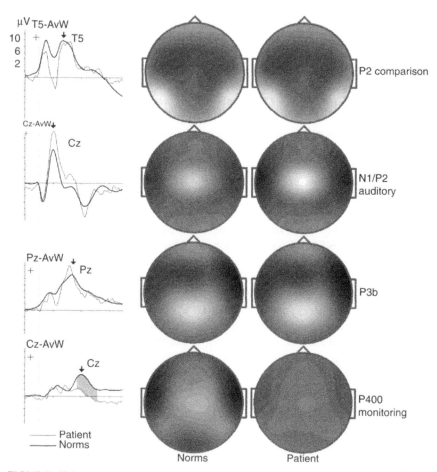

FIGURE 17.5   Selective impairment of P400 monitoring component in an ADHD child. Left – superposition of ERP waveforms for four independent components, from top to bottom, P2 comparison, N1/P2 auditory, P3b and P4 monitoring. In the superposition, thin line – individual components for the ADHD child, thick line – grand average component for a group of healthy subjects of the corresponding age. Right – maps of the components for the patient and for the group of normal subjects.

of ADHD respond well to treatment with stimulants by blocking the dopamine reuptake mechanism, and the fact that children with severe cases of ADHD have abnormalities in the genes that are responsible for dopamine regulation.

A. Increased Level of DAT

To test the dopamine hypothesis of ADHD directly, several single photon emission tomography (SPECT) and positron emission tomography (PET) studies have been performed in children, adolescents, and adults. Using SPECT and different radio-ligands, three independent groups have reported increased dopamine transporter (DAT) density in the putamen and the caudate nucleus in adults and children, however, these findings have not been replicated by another two independent groups reporting unaltered DAT binding. This inconsistency of results might indicate heterogeneity of the ADHD population where some subtype of ADHD might be associated by increased level of dopamine reuptake receptors while the other subtypes do not depend on dopamine regulation[24].

B. Noradrenalin Transporter

Here is the right place to mention that while the executive system of the brain is modulated by dopamine, attentional networks per se are modulated by mediator noradrenalin (NE), different from dopamine by its distribution and functional action. In the same way as the level of dopamine in the synaptic cleft is controlled by the DAT, the level of noradrenalin is controlled by the noradrenalin transporter (NET). The premotor cortex and the parietal areas of the brain have the highest density of the NET in the cortex[25]. During the last three decades some scientists suggested that dysregulation of noradrenalinergic systems might be critical to the pathophysiology of ADHD. The discovery of the drug atomoxetine that is now used for treatment of ADHD seems to support this suggestion. Indeed atomoxetine has an approximately 300-fold selectivity for the NET over the DAT and mostly affect the noradrenalinergic system of the brain.

VI. TREATMENT

A. Psychostimulants

Most of the pharmacological agents that lessen behavior symptoms of ADHD affect the dopaminergic or noradrenalinergic systems. Psychostimulant medication[26] has been used safely in clinical practice for the short treatment of ADHD symptoms for more than 60 years. The psychostimulants efficacy was confirmed in many randomized, double-blind, placebo-controlled clinical trails. Methylphenidate is the most commonly used psychostimulant. It blocks the reuptake of the dopamine

---

[24]For those who are interested in this research we recommend a paper by Klaus-Henning Krause and his colleagues from Ludwig-Maximilians-University (Krause et al., 2000).

[25]Recall also that the cortical level of noradrenalin is much higher than its density in the striatum.

[26]Psychostimulants are a class of drugs that enhance locomotor behavior. Examples of psychostimulants include amphetamine, methamphetamine, cocaine, and methylphenidate. Psychostimulants often affect the regulation of the modulator dopamine in the brain.

(and partly noradrenalin) by their transporters DAT and NET. Amphetamines also stabilize dopamine and noradrenalin transporters. The decrease of symptoms starts about 30 min after oral consumption. Intravenous injections of methylphenidate, in contrast to oral ingestions, induce euphoric sensations indistinguishable from those induced by cocaine.

Although stimulants have been shown to be quite effective in the treatment of ADHD, estimates indicate that as many as 30 per cent of children with ADHD either do not respond to stimulant treatment or cannot tolerate the treatment secondary to side effects. In addition, ADHD is frequently co-morbid with other psychiatric disorders. For these complicated cases, stimulant medications may actually worsen the symptoms of the co-morbid condition, particularly in children with mood disorders. In spite of their long-term use, stimulants do have side effects. Most common side effects include headaches, abdominal pain, appetite suppression, irritability, insomnia, and hypertension[27].

B. Neurofeedback

The fact that 30 per cent of ADHD population cannot be treated by psychostimulants motivated researchers to search for alternative forms of treatment. The rationale for EEG biofeedback is derived from substantial neurophysiological research and QEEG assessment in ADHD population. One of the leading scientists in this field, Barry Sterman in his review (Sterman, 1996), indicated that "variations in alertness and behavioral control appear directly related to specific thalamo-cortical generator mechanisms and that such variations are evident in distinctive EEG frequency rhythms that emerge over specific topographic regions of the brain." He hypothesized that neuropathology (such as ADHD) could alter these rhythms and that EEG feedback training directed at normalizing these rhythms may yield sustaining clinical benefits.

The QEEG abnormalities of ADHD population are presented above in this chapter. Roughly, there are four different subtypes of QEEG deviations from the normative multi-spectra[28]: (1) abnormal increase of slow activity (in delta–theta frequency range) centrally or centrally–frontally, (2) abnormal increase of frontal midline theta rhythm generated with maximum at Fz within the frequency range of 5.5–8 Hz in long (more than 1 s) bursts and increased with task load; (3) abnormal increase of beta activity within 13–30 Hz frontally; (4) excess of alpha activities at posterior, central, or frontal (quite rare) leads such as abnormal mu-rhythms at C3, C4 – "monkey face" pattern of the spectra as it was labeled

---

[27]Controversy remains over the possible association of stimulants with suppression of growth.

[28]The inferences are made on the basis of our experience of using the Human Brain Institute (HBI) Normative Database for assessing electrophysiological correlates of ADHD.

by Barry Sterman[29]. Note, that the first two groups mentioned above reveal an elevated level of the theta beta ratio, but not the third group. As one can see, each of these ADHD subgroups reveals a specific way of cortical dysregulation and, consequently, needs a specific protocol of neurofeedback. The need of QEEG-based tailoring protocols was recognized quite early in the field but only recently it became a gold standard.

Retrospectively, based on extensive research during the last decade we now recognize the existence of QEEG subtypes in ADHD and understand the need of different neurofeedback protocols to correct QEEG abnormalities in ADHD subtypes, but historically some of the protocols at the first years of neurofeedback era were obtained more empirically than on the basis of subtyping ADHD. Usually, selected patients participated in one type of training procedures in which they were reinforced (via tone or visual display) for producing a specific change in cortical activity (e.g., reducing the amplitude of activity at slower EEG frequencies; increasing activity in faster frequencies). The patients had to maintain this desired change for a period of 0.5 s in order to be "rewarded."

As we mentioned before, the main hypothesis behind neurofeedback approach was that if patients could "normalize" the QEEG pattern in regions responsible for attention and behavioral control, they would begin to demonstrate developmentally appropriate abilities to attend and maintain behavioral control. The initial demonstration that biofeedback could yield changes in cortical activity and that such modifications resulted in observable improvements in behavior/functioning was provided by Sterman and his colleagues[30].

Most of the neurofeedback protocols we are now using for ADHD were invented and tested in laboratories of the USA. Those protocols use the conventional EEG in the frequency range higher than 0.1 Hz. EEG at lower frequencies (called slow cortical potentials – SCP) was used in studies of a German group of scientists in the University of Tuebingen. Training (shifting DC potentials in negative or positive direction) was used for optimizing the frontal lobe functioning in ADHD children[31].

---

[29]On the basis of literature analysis as well on his own experience Barry Sterman (Sterman, 1996) separated the following abnormalities in QEEG of ADHD children: (1) A localized excess of 4–8 Hz theta activity in prefrontal, frontal, and sensory-motor cortex; (2. A generalized excess of theta or slowed alpha activity in all cortical areas, often exaggerated during task engagement; (3) A significant excess of normal alpha rhythm activity mostly in anterior cortical areas; (4) A significant reduction of normal 12–20 Hz rhythmic activity in the sensory-motor area; (5) EEG hypercoherence between left and right frontal recordings and between frontal/temporal regions within each hemisphere as well as interhemispheric power asymmetry in left and right posterior temporal and parietal regions.

[30]Barry Sterman summarized his experience of assessing QEEG abnormalities in ADHD children and of constructing neurofeedback protocols, as well as of making recommendations for pharmacotherapy in his review paper (Sterman, 1989, 1996).

[31]As well as for decreasing the frequency of seizures in epileptic patients.

C. Beta Enhancement/Theta Suppression Protocol

This protocol is associated with the name of Barry Sterman. In his experiments with cats in 1960s he identified the "sensory-motor rhythm" (or SMR), which is generated over the Rolandic cortex. The "peak activity" of the SMR in cats was found at 12–14 Hz[32]. Barry Sterman and his co-workers found that cats could be trained to produce this rhythm voluntarily. Further on they applied this type of operant conditioning for the treatment of individuals with a specific type of epilepsy. As reviewed by Sterman (1989, 1996), this application of EEG biofeedback was particularly helpful in the treatment of seizure disorders in patients who have not responded to pharmacological treatments. The initial application of SMR training for treatment of patients with ADHD was made in Joel Lubar laboratory in 1970s. His demonstration of clinical response in hyperactive children stimulated considerable interest in SMR training as a potential treatment for ADHD.

Subsequently in 1980s, in response to experimental evidence of excessive cortical slowing over central, midline, and frontal regions in ADHD patients, Lubar and his colleagues expanded their EEG biofeedback protocols to include rewarding of EEG activity in a faster frequency range (beta: 16–20 Hz), while suppressing activity at lower frequencies (theta: 4–8 Hz)[33]. This protocol was later on applied in several controlled group studies of EEG biofeedback in the treatment of ADHD[34]. Recordings were obtained at Cz with linked ear reference (for review see Monastra et al., 2005)[35].

D. Relative Beta Training Protocol

As one can see, a common procedure for above mentioned protocols is enhancing activity in a higher frequency band and inhibiting activity in a lower frequency band. Figure 17.6 top schematically represents comparison between power spectra of ADHD children and normal controls. EEG recording is made over Fz–Cz area. The spectrum of EEG recorded in a patient from the most common (theta

---

[32]Note that in humans alpha-like activity reflecting the idling state of the sensory-motor cortex is within 9–13 Hz in children and adults (observations from the HBI Normative Database).

[33]Typically, recordings are obtained from one active site, referenced to linked earlobes, with a sampling rate of at least 128 Hz. Auditory (tones) and visual feedback (counter display; movement of puzzle pieces, graphic designs, or animated figures) is provided based on patient success in controlling the power or amplitude of the corresponding rhythm or controlling the percentage of time that these rhythms are below (or above) pretreatment "thresholds."

[34]Although recent QEEG findings of a beta excessive subtype of ADHD patients, characterized by excessive "beta" activity over frontal regions, have prompted interest in the developing protocols to suppress excessive beta in this type of patients, no controlled group studies examining this type of EEG biofeedback have been reported.

[35]In some variants of the protocol bipolar montages are used such as FCz-PCz or Cz-Pz.

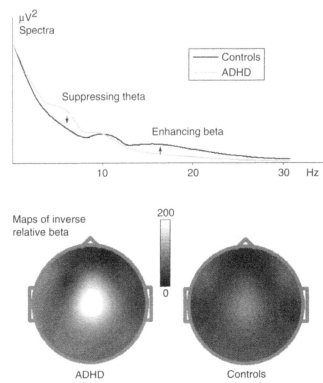

FIGURE 17.6   Rational for the relative beta protocol. EEG spectra for controls (black line) and ADHD population together with the corresponding theta/beta ratio maps are schematically presented.

excess) subtype of ADHD is schematically depicted. As you can see, the ADHD subtype is characterized by access of EEG power in the lower (theta) band and a lack (in comparison to norms) of EEG power in the beta frequency band. This pattern of deviation from normality results in decrease of the relative beta activity. This illustrated at the bottom of Fig. 17.6 where the maps of the inverse relative beta for the ADHD and control groups are presented.

E. Normalization of Executive ERP Components

In our recent study (Kropotov et al., 2005) we used the relative beta[36] as a neuro-feedback parameter. The EEG was recorded bipolar from C3 and Fz electrodes in

---

[36]In more detail, the neurofeedback parameter was a ratio of EEG power in beta frequency band (15–18 Hz) and EEG power in the rest of the EEG band, that is,. in 4–14 Hz frequency band, and 19–30 Hz frequency band.

the standard 10–20 system. A typical training session included 20 min of relative beta training. The biofeedback procedure consisted of the following computations: power spectrum was calculated for a 1 s epoch every 250 ms using fast Fourier transformation. Visual feedback was provided by a bar against a background on a computer screen. The height of the bar followed the dynamics of the biofeedback parameter. Patient's task was to keep the bar above a threshold determined at the pre-training 2 min interval.

In addition to the simple visual feedback, a so-called video mode was used. In this mode, the biofeedback parameter controlled the level of a noise generated by a separate electronic unit called Jammer (the unit was designed specifically for this purpose in our laboratory). The amplitude of the noise was maximal if the biofeedback parameter was minimal, and decreased gradually up to zero while the parameter approached a threshold. The noise was mixed with the video-signal of a video-player and was fed to a TV-set. Thus the patient actually controlled the quality of the picture on the screen by his/her brainwaves: when the biofeedback parameter was higher than the threshold, the picture on the screen was clear, otherwise the TV picture was blurred by the noise.

Usually during the first 5–8 sessions, patients performed training in the simple visual mode with the bar to be able to get a feeling of the procedure. Then training in the video mode started[37]. The threshold for the biofeedback parameter was defined by the pre-feedback baseline mean measure taken during 2 min of feedback-free period with eyes open at the beginning of each session. The threshold was typically set in the range of about 0.03–0.05 and 0.05–0.1 for junior and senior age groups, respectively. The dynamics of the biofeedback parameter (training curve) was obtained for each patient and for each session. Figure 17.7a shows a typical training curve for a single patient taken at the 15th session. One can see that the patient was able to elevate the parameter during periods of training while the parameter dropped at the pre-training level during rest periods.

Figure 17.7b shows comparison of mean values of relative beta power (averaged across 22 patients) at 19 electrodes between rest and training periods. The recordings were made during one session at the end of treatment. A registration of EEG from 19 electrodes during a biofeedback training session is a time-consuming

---

[37]The patient was instructed about the rationale of the procedure, as well as about the dependence of the biofeedback signal on the brain activity and attention. Before the procedure, the patient tried to relax, decrease muscular tension, and maintain regular diaphragmatic breath. Patient was asked to assess his or her own internal state and feelings when the biofeedback parameter surpassed the threshold and to reproduce this state. Different patients used different strategies with a common numerator of concentrating on a particular external object. The number of training sessions for each patient depended on several factors such as age, type of ADHD, learning curves, parent reports, and varied from 15 to 22 (mean 17). The termination criteria was: (1) stabilization of training performance during the last 3–5 sessions, and (2) stabilization of patient's behavior according to parents reports. Sessions were administered 2–5 times per week for 5–8 weeks.

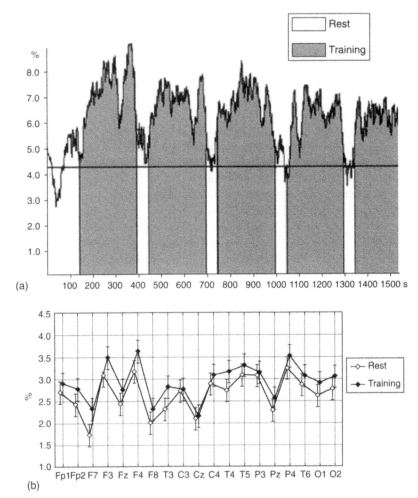

FIGURE 17.7   Relative beta training. (a) Training curve for a single session in ADHD children (vertical axis – neurofeedback parameter, horizontal axis – time of training in seconds). (b) Mean values of relative beta power at rest and training periods computed in 19 electrodes for a single session and averaged over 22 patients. Adapted from Kropotov et al. (2005).

procedure; therefore, we randomly selected only 22 patients for this investigation. One can see a statistically significant difference of EEG power in beta range between rest and training periods. Although widely distributed, the increase was the largest at the frontal areas.

It should be noted that not all patients were able to reliably elevate the relative beta activity even after 10–20 sessions. The quality of patient's performance, that is, the ability of a patient to increase the neurofeedback parameter during training periods, was assessed. We considered the training session to be successful if a patient was able to increase the biofeedback parameter during training periods at more than 25 per cent in comparison to resting periods. Patients were referred to as good performers if they were successful in more than 60 per cent of sessions. Seventy-one patients (82.5 per cent) were assigned to the good performance group. Those patients who had less than 60 per cent successful training sessions were referred to as bad performers. Fifteen patients (17.5 per cent) were assigned to the bad performance group. This group was considered as a control group in the following data analysis.

To test the functioning of the executive system, ERPs in the auditory two stimulus GO/NOGO task were recorded before and after all sessions of neurofeedback. ERPs to NOGO cures superimposed on each other in "before" and "after" recordings are presented in Fig. 17.8. One can see enhancement of the positive component at the frontal leads after 20 sessions of the relative beta training.

The grand average ERP differences and their maps computed by subtraction of the ERPs made before any interventions from those made after 20 sessions of the relative beta neurofeedback are presented in Fig. 17.9. For a comparison, the data for the groups of good and bad performers are presented. Note a statistically significant increase of ERPs in response to NOGO cues in the group of good performers, while no reliable changes in the group of bad performers are observed. In our study, we used the auditory two stimulus GO/ NOGO task for objective assessment of parameters of attention. It should be noted that the relative beta training does not change early (with latencies of 80–180 ms) components of ERPs but leads to significant enhancement of later positive components. Thus, our data indicate that relative beta training does not affect auditory information processing in the human brain, while significantly changes the functioning of the executive system reflected in the late ERP components.

Theoretically, our protocol differs from conventional protocols, because elevation of the biofeedback parameter in our study could be achieved by increasing beta power, and/or by decreasing theta as well as alpha power. However, as the results of our study indicate, the application of the relative beta protocol turns out to be as effective as conventional protocols. Indeed, 80 per cent of our patients were able to significantly increase their neurofeedback parameters in more than 60 per cent of sessions. Moreover, according to parents' assessment by SNAP-IV, neurofeedback significantly improved behavior as reflected in the corresponding changes of indexes of inattention and impulsivity.

F. Transcranial Direct Current Stimulation

In our laboratory in addition to the neurofeedback training we are using transcranial direct current stimulation (tDCS) for correcting symptoms of ADHD. The history of development of this method goes back to 1960s when cathodic micropolarization was first applied to switch off the pathological rhythmic firing of neurons

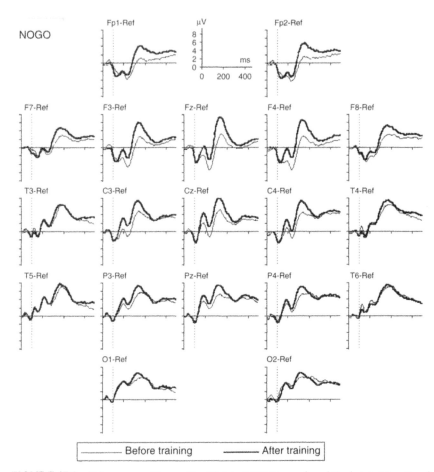

FIGURE 17.8   Enhancement of late positive ERPs to NOGO cues after relative beta training. Grand average ERPs in response to NOGO stimuli in the two stimulus auditory GO/NOGO test for the group of good performers before and after 20 sessions of the relative beta training. Thin line: ERPs taken before training; thick line: ERPs taken after 20 sessions of training. Adapted from Kropotov et al. (2005).

in subcortical structures of patients with Parkinson's disease[38]. Several years of experiments on dogs and cats in 1970s confirmed that application of negative DC potentials to the electrodes implanted in the deep structures induced suppression of impulse activity of neurons located near the electrodes, while application

---

[38]I recall that in those days we injected electric current through implanted electrodes in patients with Parkinson's disorder to whom those electrodes were implanted for diagnostic and therapeutic reasons. Recording impulse activity of neurons from the same electrodes showed the decrease of spiking rate of multi-units when electrode served as cathode and increase of spiking when electrode served as anode. Professor Bechtereva suggested to use this method for diagnostic purposes.

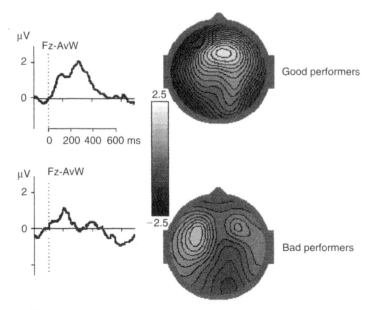

FIGURE 17.9   Enhancement of late positive ERPs associated with neurofeedback training is found only in the group of good performers. Top – ERPs differences (left) and their map (right) induced by 20 sessions of neurofeedback in the group of good performers. Bottom – ERPs differences (left) and their map (right) induced by 20 sessions of neurofeedback in the group of bad performers. Adapted from Kropotov et al. (2005).

of anodic currents produced an opposite effect[39]. After experiments on dogs and cats the method was introduced into the clinical practice for treatment of different neurological dysfunctions in adults. Recently, we started using a low anodic current stimulation for ADHD in children.

In the studies of one my colleagues, Sergei Saraev[40], in 1990 the anode electrode was placed over the F8 site while the cathode was placed near the Fp2 location. The direct current was between 700–1000 μA tailored individually so that the patients could not feel the current. Sessions of tDCS lasted for 20 min and repeated every 2–3 days with the total number of 7 sessions. An EEG coherence between different electrodes in the alpha frequency band was used as a parameter for assessing the brain function. The average coherence was computed for each electrode as a mean value of coherence of a given electrode with all others electrodes. Figure 17.10 represents the results of the study. One can see that 7 sessions of tDCS normalized the

[39]I want to mention names of Ivan Danilov, Georgy Galdinov, and Genrich Vartanian who made a major contribution to our understanding of neurophysiological mechanisms of micro-polarization technique.

[40]Unfortunately Sergei died in a car accident and was not able to publish his studies. Here I present the results of our unpublished paper that we prepared with him just before his death.

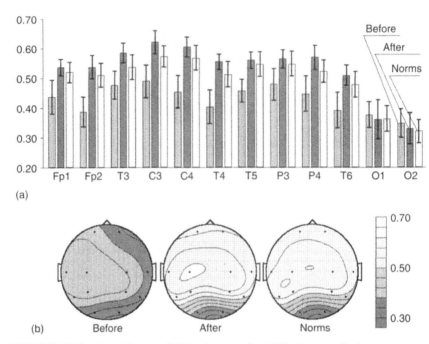

(a)

(b)   Before   After   Norms

FIGURE 17.10   Normalization of EEG coherence after tDCS. (a) Averaged coherence measures for a group ($N = 12$) of ADHD children of 7–12 years old. The coherence between EEG for a given electrode and the rest of electrodes was averaged for each patient and then again averaged over all 12 patients. (b) Maps of averaged coherence before and after 7 sessions of tDCS in comparison to the control group (unpublished data from Kropotov et al., 2002).

coherence values. In addition, psychological assessment of attention (by SNAP-IV questionnaire and the letter cancellation task) showed improvement of indexes of attention in the ADHD group. We continue using the tDCS in our laboratory not only for ADHD children but also for children with delays in speech and cognitive development. This work is done by a neurologist Leonid Chutko who modified the method suggested by Sergei Saraev. The electrodes positions are F7 – left mastoid and F8 – right mastoid.

VII. SUMMARY

ADHD is one of the most prevalent conditions in child psychiatry. DSM-IV distinguishes three subtypes of ADHD: predominately inattentive type, predominately hyperactive-impulsive type, and combined type. This classification is based on three groups of symptoms: inattention, hyperactivity, and impulsivity. Genetic studies show that ADHD fails to follow Mendelian patterns of inheritance and is classified as a complex genetic disorder. Environmental factors such as pregnancy and delivery complications raise the risk for ADHD. ADHD is often accompanied by other disorders such as specific LD, ODD, Tourette's syndrome, anxiety and depression. MRI studies in ADHD found smaller sizes of the caudate nucleus, globus pallidus, and pre-frontal cortical areas while PET and fMRI studies showed lower metabolic activities in these structures. Most of QEEG studies have reported elevated levels of slow wave power in ADHD population in comparison to normal children. As a consequence, the theta beta ratio (labeled as inattention index) is increased in ADHD. Few studies have directly examined CNV amplitude in children with ADHD, and their results are conflicting. The studies of MMN in ADHD are also inconsistent. The P2 component elicited in the two stimulus GO/NOGO task and associated with change detection was shown to be selectively suppressed in a group of ADHD children. The P3b component as an index of engagement operation has repeatedly been shown to be reduced in ADHD. Methylphenidate increases the P3b component, but does not affect the P3a component. Some studies found reduction of the N2 component of ERPs in GO/NOGO task which can be interpreted as a dysfunction of motor inhibition in ADHD population. Suppression of the P400 monitoring component was found in a subtype of ADHD children. The dopamine hypothesis of ADHD is based on the fact that symptoms of ADHD respond well to stimulant treatment by blocking dopamine reuptake receptors. Most of the pharmacological agents that lessen behavior symptoms of ADHD affect the dopaminergic or noradrenalinergic systems. Psychostimulant medication has been used in clinical medicine for the short treatment of ADHD symptoms for more than 60 years. However, the fact that 30 per cent of ADHD population cannot be treated by psychostimulants motivated researchers to search for alternative forms of treatment. They are neurofeedback and tDCS. The rationale for EEG biofeedback is derived from substantial neurophysiological research and QEEG assessment in ADHD population. Several protocols of neurofeedback have been suggested such as beta enhancement/theta suppression protocol and relative beta protocol. They were shown to lessen symptoms of ADHD as well as to normalize spectral characteristics of EEG and executive components of ERPs.

CHAPTER 18

Schizophrenia

I. DESCRIPTION OF BEHAVIOR

A. Involvement of Three Brain Systems

Schizophrenia[1] is a psychiatric disorder that describes a mental illness characterized by impairments in three brain systems: (1) impairments in the executive system, such as paranoid or bizarre delusions[2] or disorganized speech and thinking, (2) impairments in the sensory systems, such as auditory hallucinations, and (3) impairments in affective system such as blunted emotions. Due to involvement of different brain systems in pathogenesis of the disorder there is debate regarding whether the diagnosis represents a single disorder or a number of discrete syndromes. For this reason, Eugen Bleuler[3] termed the disease *the schizophrenias* (plural) when he

---

[1]The name "schizophrenia" comes from the Greek word meaning "split mind."

[2]Delusion is a false belief .... In psychiatry delusions typically occur in mental illness. Although they have been found in many pathological states, delusions are of particular diagnostic importance in schizophrenia.

[3]Paul Eugen Bleuler is a Swiss psychiatrist who coined the term "schizophrenia" in 1908. He is also known for treating famous Russian ballet dancer Vaslav Nijinsky.

coined the name. Schizophrenia is a devastating illness that affects approximately 0.4–0.6 per cent of the world's population. Affected individuals frequently come to clinical attention during late adolescence or early adulthood. About 10 per cent of those diagnosed with schizophrenia eventually commit suicide and most experience a lifetime disability such as long-term unemployment, poverty, and homelessness. As a result, schizophrenia is associated with a substantial burden for the families of those affected.

B. Dysfunction of Executive System

Although psychosis presents the most striking clinical aspect of schizophrenia, it is not diagnostic of the disorder per se. Of the many clinical features of schizophrenia, disturbances in the executive system such as impairments in attention, the ability to plan, initiate, and regulate goal directed behavior, apparently represent the core of the illness. Cognitive abnormalities have been found throughout the life span of individuals with schizophrenia, including childhood and adolescence. The unaffected relatives of patients with schizophrenia show similar, although milder, cognitive deficits which clearly indicates involvement of genetic factors in schizophrenia. At present, no findings from laboratory procedures, neuroimaging methods, or psychological tests are diagnostic of schizophrenia. Schizophrenia, as any other psychiatric disorder, is diagnosed purely on the basis of the clinical syndrome[4]. For the purpose of diagnostic reliability, these features have been formulated into specific criteria[5].

II. GENETICS AND ENVIRONMENTAL FACTORS

A. Multiple Genes are Involved

Genetic factors play an important role in developing schizophrenia[6]. Several susceptibility genes for schizophrenia have been identified with a small value of the

[4]In psychiatry the term syndrome refers to the association of several clinically recognizable features, signs (discovered by a physician), and symptoms (reported by the patient) that often occur together.

[5]The first diagnostic criterion requires the presence of two or more of the following clinical features: delusions, hallucinations, disorganized thinking and speech, grossly disorganized or catatonic behavior, and negative symptoms such as flat affect, poverty of speech, and inability to initiate and persist in goal-directed behavior. The second diagnostic criterion requires evidence of social or occupational dysfunction, such as deterioration in interpersonal relationships, work habits, or personal hygiene. Third, the signs of the disturbance must be continuously present for at least 6 months. Fourth, it must be clear that the clinical features are not attributable to another disorder such as substance abuse.

[6]Estimates of the heritability of schizophrenia vary owing to the difficulty of separating the effects of genetics and the environment. However, twin studies have suggested a heritability as large as 80 per cent.

risk factor for each gene[7]. Moreover, for most genes the biological basis of the increased risk for illness is unclear. All these facts indicate that genetic liability alone is not sufficient to cause the clinical features of the illness. It is likely that schizophrenia is a condition of complex inheritance, with several genes possibly interacting to generate risk for schizophrenia. Recent work has suggested that genes of the risk for schizophrenia are non-specific, and may also raise the risk of developing other psychotic disorders such as bipolar disorder.

B. Environmental Risk Factors

Living in an urban environment is one of the strongest environmental risk factors for schizophrenia. Social adversity, racial discrimination, family dysfunction, unemployment, and poor housing conditions have been proposed as contributing factors. For this reason, being a first or second generation immigrant is a strong risk factor for schizophrenia. Childhood experiences of abuse or trauma have also been implicated as risk factors for schizophrenia. There is also evidence that prenatal exposure to infections increases the risk for developing schizophrenia later in life[8].

III. IMAGING CORRELATES

A. Magnetic Resonance Imaging

As we previously noted, the main deficit in schizophrenia concerns the executive system. For example, schizophrenic patients have problems with directing attention. The three stimulus oddball paradigm that includes presentation of standard, deviant, and novel stimuli is traditionally used to study functioning and dysfunctioning of the executive system. Recently a group of scientists from University of Pennsylvania School of Medicine in Philadelphia studied blood oxygen level dependent (BOLD) changes in magnetic resonance imaging (MRI) signals in the three stimulus oddball paradigm in schizophrenia patients (Gur et al., 2007). In particular, they found that for targets, the schizophrenic patients in comparison to healthy subjects had diminished activation in superior temporal and frontal gyri, cingulate, thalamus, and basal ganglia. This data demonstrate a hypoactivation of the executive system in schizophrenia.

---

[7]A risk factor is a variable associated with an increased risk of disease. Risk factors are correlational and not necessarily causal, because correlation does not imply causation.

[8]Amphetamines that promote the release of dopamine in the brain worsen schizophrenia symptoms. Schizophrenia can be also triggered by heavy use of other stimulants as well as by hallucinogenic drugs.

B. Quantitative Electroencephalogram

Research of quantitative electroencephalogram (QEEG) in schizophrenia has been quite inconsistent. While some studies have reported increase of beta and reduction of alpha EEG power, other research has shown no differences and even opposite results. This inconsistency is due to several interacting factors: (1) heterogeneity of population of patients with schizophrenia; (2) small number of patients, (3) low size effect. In some studies patients were under medication that changed the QEEG pattern.

Although no reliable index of background EEG for schizophrenia was found, EEG correlates of psychosis as a certain state in schizophrenia have been observed. For example, hallucinations were associated with increase of beta power in EEG over the left temporal areas (Lee et al., 2006).

C. Mismatch Negativity

Mismatch negativity (MMN) is thought to be an automatic response of the temporal cortex to a rare change in a repetitive sound. The MMN is associated with a cortical operation of comparing the sensory input with the memory trace. The most consistence observation in event-related potential (ERP) research on schizophrenic population was a reduction of amplitude of the MMN in schizophrenics in comparison to healthy control subjects. Some studies report the reduction of about 50 per cent from the normal mean value (McCarley et al., 1997). Noteworthy, the size effect in MMN reduction in schizophrenic patients versus healthy controls depends on parameters of the oddball paradigm (in particular on interstimulus interval with the size effect larger at longer intervals)[9]. It is important to note here that differences in MMN depend not only on parameters of behavioral task but also on a selected group of schizophrenic patients. For example, first-episode patients do not show reduction of MMN (Umbricht et al., 2006) in contrast to recent-onset and chronic schizophrenics.

D. Contingent Negative Variation

As we learnt in Part II, the working memory depends on the dorso-lateral prefrontal cortex and associated basal ganglia thalamo-cortical circuits. Individuals with schizophrenia tend to perform poorly on working memory tasks and show reduced activation of the dorso-lateral prefrontal cortex (as reflected in PET and

---

[9]A complete review of clinical applications of MMN in schizophrenia and other psychiatric and neurological disorders can be found in an article by Risto Näätänen (Näätänen, 2003).

fMRI studies) when attempting to carry out such tasks. Moreover, the amount of deficit in activation of the dorso-lateral prefrontal cortex, but not of other cortical regions, during working memory tasks predicts the severity of cognitive symptoms in schizophrenia. This hypoactivation of the dorso-lateral prefrontal cortex seems to be specific for schizophrenia because other psychotic disorders or major depression show normal activation of the dorso-lateral prefrontal cortex during working memory tasks. Therefore, working memory deficits might be a central feature of schizophrenia, and identifying the pathological dysfunction of the dorso-lateral prefrontal cortex is essential for understanding pathophysiological mechanisms of schizophrenia.

Working memory as a preparatory activity is reflected in contingent negative variation (CNV) – a slow component of ERPs elicited in two-stimulus tasks. As was shown by a German group from University of Konstanz (Klein et al., 1996) schizophrenic patients revealed reduction in the CNV amplitude and enhancement of so-called postimperative negative variation – another slow wave that followed the imperative stimulus.

E. Engagement Operation

Engagement operation of the executive system is reflected in P3b component of ERPs generated in many paradigms requiring active engagement and action performance of subjects in the tasks[10]. In schizophrenia the P3b amplitude reduction has been replicated many times since the pioneering work of Roth and Cannon in 1972 that was done few years after discovery of this component. The decrease of the P3b component of ERPs has been classified as a vulnerability marker of the disease. The reduced P3b seem to reflect decrease in amount of resources needed for action execution in schizophrenic patients[11].

The meta-analysis of papers published between January 1994 and August 2003 was recently performed by a group of scientists from Institute of Psychiatry from London (Bramon et al., 2004). The standardized effect size for the P3b amplitude defined as the difference between the mean values in two groups (patients with schizophrenia versus healthy controls) divided by their pooled standard deviations was assessed to be 0.85[12].

In a recent study by a group of researchers from Albert-Ludwigs-University from Freiburg, Germany (Olbrich et al., 2005) ERPs in GO/NOGO task for schizophrenics patients and healthy controls were subjective to independent component

---

[10]To study the P3b component tasks of the oddball paradigm are the most frequently used, however both types of stimuli in GO/NOGO paradigm produce similar P3b components.

[11]For review of P3b research see paper by Judith Ford in 1999 (Ford, 1999).

[12]For latency of P3b component the pooled standardized effect size was smaller estimated as −0.57.

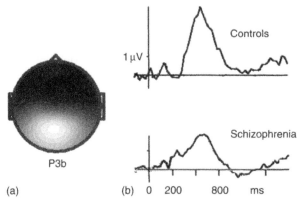

FIGURE 18.1   Reduction of P3b component in schizophrenic patients. (a) Topographical map of P3b component extracted by means of ICA for ERPs to GO stimuli in the GO/NOGO task for healthy controls (data from the Human Brain Institute database). (b) Activation time curves separately displayed for GO responses for a group with schizophrenia and for a control group. Adapted from Olbrich et al. (2005).

analysis (ICA). The P3b was one of the components extracted in this analysis. It had a parietal distribution with slightly longer duration for GO cues in comparison to NOGO cues[13]. The study showed that P3b component was significantly reduced in the schizophrenic patients in comparison to healthy controls (Fig. 18.1).

F. Monitoring Operation

Monitoring operation in the executive system is reflected in the P400 NOGO component of ERPs elicited by NOGO stimuli in the two stimulus visual GO/NOGO paradigm. As we showed in Part II this component is separated by the ICA. S-LORETA imaging shows that the component is generated in widely distributed areas of cingulate cortex including anterior and sub-colossal parts. The ICA methods enabled the above mentioned group of German scientists (Olbrich et al., 2005) to separate a P3 component that had the larger amplitude in response to NOGO trials and named as P3ng. This component had a central–frontal distribution and was similar in both spatial and temporal parameters to the P400 monitoring component separated in our own studies with Human Brain Institute Normative Database. The studies of the German group showed that the P3ng component was reduced in schizophrenic patients.

In a recent study by a group of researchers from Stanford University, California headed by Judith Ford fMRI and ERPs were recorded in a simple GO/NOGO task. P3 component to NOGO cues was found to be smaller in schizophrenic

---

[13]The P3b component extracted in this study was virtually the same as observed in our ICA made on GO and NOGO. ERPs obtained in the Human Brain Institute Normative DataBase.

patients. The corresponding metabolic activation as measured by functional magnetic resonance imaging (fMRI) was restricted only to anterior cingulate cortex in schizophrenic patients, while in normal subjects the activation occupied larger areas including the dorsal lateral prefrontal cortex, and right inferior parietal lobule and caudate nucleus.

IV. DOPAMINE HYPOTHESIS OF SCHIZOPHRENIA

A. Excess of Striatal Dopamine Receptors

Relative hyperfunction of the subcortical dopamine systems has been suggested to be one of the key pathophysiologic mechanisms in schizophrenic psychosis. In spite of the fact that research in this field was rather contradictive, dopamine hypothesis of schizophrenia still remains the most popular one. It continues to receive a strong empirical support.

The empirical evidence obtained so far can be summarized as follows. First, recent studies on a variety of animal models of psychosis such as sensitization of animal behavior by amphetamine show that those animals were associated with a marked behavioral supersensitivity to dopamine and a marked rise in the number of dopamine D2 receptors in the brain. Second, in humans psychostimulants such as amphetamine and cocaine increase levels of dopamine in the brain and, after prolonged use, cause psychosis (named as amphetamine or cocaine psychosis) that is virtually indistinguishable from the positive symptoms associated with schizophrenia. Third, antipsychotic drugs block D2 dopamine receptors and reduce positive psychotic symptoms.

A recent positron emission tomography (PET) study of a Finnish group from University of Turku gives an additional evidence to the dopamine hypothesis of schizophrenia (Hirvonen et al., 2005). Using the carbon 11 labeled racropride (a substance with affinity to D2 receptors) they studied mono and heterozygotic twins with and without history of schizophrenia. They found that unaffected monozygotic co-twins had increased caudate D2 density compared with unaffected dizygotic co-twins and healthy control twins. Higher D2 receptor binding in the caudate nucleus was associated with a poor performance on cognitive tasks related to schizophrenia vulnerability in the whole sample. The authors concluded that the caudate dopamine D2 receptor upregulation is related to genetic risk for schizophrenia.

B. Neural Net Model

According to our theory of action selection within the basal ganglia thalamocortical circuits (see Chapter 18) the striatum serves as a map of actions in which

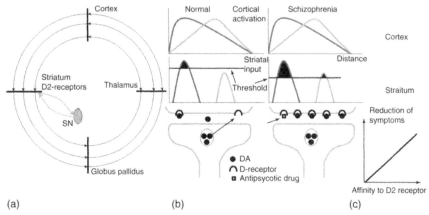

FIGURE 18.2   Impaired action selection in the striatum of schizophrenic patients. (a) Parallel basal ganglia thalamo-cortical loops with the dopaminergic modulatory input from the substantia nigra to the striatum. (b) Two overlapped representations of potential actions overlapped in the cortex, but segregated at the striatal level. Excess of modulatory dopaminergic activation from the substantia nigra due to the excess of density of postsynaptic dopamine receptors in schizophrenia leads to a condition in which the irrelevant action (depicted as a lower amplitude bell shape) is selected together with the relevant action (giving the largest input to the striatum) – the state called as "split of consciousness." DA – dopamine, D-receptors – postsynaptic striatal receptors to DA, antipsychotic drug – a schematic representation of a molecular of an antipsychotic drug that blocks the D-receptors and lessen symptoms of schizophrenia. (c) The schematic relationship between the affinity to D2 receptors of antipsychotic drug (the ability to block D2 receptors) versus reduction of psychotic symptoms.

representations of different actions are mapped into separate locations. The selection of the relevant representation of action is performed within the striatum by means of long distance lateral inhibition according to "winner takes all" principle. In line with the model, the representation of an action is selected if its activation exceeds some threshold (Fig. 18.2). The threshold of activation of striatal neurons[14] is set by the mediator dopamine. The effect of dopamine is defined by density of dopamine receptors at the postsynaptic membrane of striatal neurons.

In healthy subjects the threshold is high enough so that only currently important actions are selected while others are suppressed. The selected action is performed and comes into consciousness. In schizophrenic patients the density of D-receptors is high and consequently the threshold is low. The low threshold enables selection of several actions simultaneously. The selected actions compete

---

[14]The threshold defined in this context is the minimal amount of excitatory postsynaptic potentials coming from the activated cortical representation to trigger firing of striatal neurons. It differs from the classically defined threshold of a neuron (which is constant) because in this context the input to the neuron is divided into two parts: fast acting activation from the cortical neurons and long lasting modulatory activation from dopaminergic neurons in the substania nigra. Consequently, increase of the modulatory input would decrease the amount of the cortical input needed to activate the striatal neuron.

with each other and create "the split of consciousness"[15]. Blocking D2-receptors by antipsychotic drugs increases the threshold for action selection and restrains psychosis. Note that the ability of a drug to lessen symptoms of psychosis strongly correlates with the affinity of the drug molecules to the D-receptors, that is, with the ability of the drug to block the D-receptors (Fig. 18.2c). The amount of cortical resources allocated by the brain to execution of the selected action is reflected in the P3b component of ERPs. If the resources are split among competing actions the P3b component decreases. This explains why schizophrenic patients exhibit lower amplitudes of P3b component in comparison to healthy controls.

V. TREATMENT

A. Antipsychotic Agents

All pharmacological treatments currently used for schizophrenia primarily suppress the psychotic symptoms but not cognitive deficits. Drugs that are used to treat psychosis are called antipsychotic agents. They are in use for more than 50 yeas. The discovery of one of the antipsychotic drugs, chlorpromazine, was made by chance in 1950s. This discovery dramatically reduced the number of patients held in mental institutions. Antipsychotic medication remains the mainstream for treatment of schizophrenia. This treatment provides symptomatic relief from the positive symptoms of psychosis. Most medications take around 7–14 days to have an antipsychotic effect. The two classes of antipsychotics are generally thought equally effective for the treatment of the positive symptoms but atypical antipsychotics have fewer extrapyramidal side effects. Typical antipsychotics have the affinity the D2 dopamine receptors and block them. The affinity of different antipsychotic agents strongly correlates with the reduction of psychotic symptoms produced by these drugs. This correlation was first reported by Philip Seeman and his colleagues in 1975 (Seeman et al., 1975, 1976). It should be stressed here that despite the clinical importance of cognitive abnormalities, there are still no approved treatments for these deficits.

B. Electroconvulsive Therapy

Electroconvulsive therapy (ECT), also known as electroshock, is a controversial psychiatric treatment in which seizures are induced by means of strong electrical

---

[15]In some situations (such as scientific research) it is good to allow non-trivial (and consequently, less activated) actions to be selected. I recall my classmate from the St. Petersburg Lyceum for Physics and Mathematics (famous school 239) who was one of the best in math in our school. He later graduated from Department of Mathematics of St. Petersburg State University and became a famous mathematician. Half of his time he spends in a psychiatric clinic for treatment of schizophrenia, the other half he writes papers for prestigious mathematical journals.

current. ECT was invented in Italy in 1937 and became widespread in the 1940s and 1950s. It is widely accepted that ECT carried out in a modern way does not cause brain damage. Now, ECT is most often used as a treatment for severe major depression unresponsible to other forms of therapy, but it is also occasionally used in the treatment of schizophrenia. As noted in (Fink and Sackeim, 1996), ECT is effective early in the course of treatment of acutely psychotic patients, especially in first-break psychotic patients.

C. Psychosurgery

Psychosurgery is a type of surgical ablation or disconnection of brain tissue with the intent to alter affective or cognitive states caused by mental illness. Psychosurgery was first introduced as a treatment for severe mental illness by Egas Moniz in 1936. At that time, no satisfactory pharmacological treatment options existed. At the height of enthusiasm, psychiatric neurosurgery was recommended for curing schizophrenia, depression, criminal behavior, and some other mental disorders. It is estimated that over 50,000 procedures were performed in the United States alone between 1936 and the mid-1950s. These operations were associated with many complications including intellectual impairment, personality change, seizures, paralysis, and death. Despite these complications, the operations were helpful in the majority of patients and Moniz was awarded the Nobel Prize in Medicine in 1949 "for his discovery of the therapeutic value of prefrontal leucotomy in certain psychoses." With the introduction of antipsychotic drugs in 1954 the role of surgery declined. Nevertheless, some patients failed to respond to appropriate pharmacological therapy and referrals to specialized centers for neurosurgical intervention continued.

Nowadays psychosurgery is used for treatment of Parkinson's disease, epilepsy, and obsessive-compulsive disorder (OCD) – brain disorders with known (to some extent) pathophysiology[16]. However the biological basis of most psychiatric disorders remains poorly understood and biological markers of mental or psychic symptoms are still a matter of research. These circumstances limit application of psychosurgery for treatment of schizophrenia. Meanwhile, introduction of PET, fMRI, and QEEG/ERPs as biological markers of psychiatric disorders as well as

---

[16]Those are types of patients who might be accepted as candidates for stereotactic neurosurgery in our Institute of the Human Brain in St. Petersburg. My subjective experience of working with these patients tells that the operation was the only chance for them to be treated because they did not respond to other conventional forms of treatment. After mild stereotactic interventions quite many of them showed remarkable reduction of symptoms and felt that the operation was successful. For more details see (Anichkov et al., 2005).

the tendency of the modern neurosurgery to use less invasive techniques[17] open new horizons in the treatment of schizophrenic patients who are unresponsible to all pharmacological forms of therapy.

D. Neurofeedback

There were few attempts to treat schizophrenia by means of neurofeedback. Besides severity of the disorder, the fact that no statistically significant and clinically discriminative deviations form normality in EEG spectra have been found does not provide any scientifically based rationale for treatment. However, regulation of slow cortical potentials appeared to be dysregulated in schizophrenia. Indeed, schizophrenic patients revealed reduction in CNV amplitude and enhancement of so-called postimperative negative variation – another slow wave that followed the imperative stimulus[18].

On the basis of these observations it was concluded that schizophrenic patients might have a failure in regulating cortical excitability (reflected in slow cortical processes) rather than reduction of excitability per se (any signs of which must be present in EEG spectra). In a study of a group of scientists from University of Tuebingen, Germany (Schneider et al., 1992) medicated schizophrenic patients were compared with healthy subjects. Although the patients were able to learn the self-regulation technique of slow potentials (however it needed more sessions for them to learn than for healthy controls) they had difficulties in transferring this ability for situations in the absence of feedback.

Later another group of researchers from Imperial College School of Medicine at Charing Cross Hospital in London (Gruzelier et al., 1999) used a similar technique to train schizophrenic patients to shift negativity from one hemisphere to another. It was hypothesized that left–right asymmetry was associated with mental overactivity and affective delusions, while the right > left asymmetry characterized a withdrawal syndrome in schizophrenia. These studies showed that despite executive dysfunctions schizophrenic patients could learn self-regulating neurofeedback techniques. However, no indication that these methods could lessen symptoms of schizophrenia has been obtained so far.

---

[17]One of such techniques is stereotactic neurosurgery. With a special technology (named stereotactic apparatus) it can be used to reach the most inaccessible areas of the brain, without extensive opening of the skull and unnecessary destruction of normal brain areas lying above the target. The stereotactic apparatus allows the precise positioning of the patient's head inside a geometrical coordinates system, so that each structure inside the brain can be reached from the outside. The neurosurgeon needs only to make a small opening in the patient's skull, under local anesthesia and to insert a thin probe into the target area of the brain.

[18]Recall, that CNV paradigm consists of presentation of trials of two stimuli: a warning stimulus that is to prepare the subject for further actions and an imperative stimulus that trigger the prepared action.

VI. SUMMARY

Schizophrenia is a psychiatric disorder that is characterized by impairments in the executive system, such as paranoid or disorganized speech and thinking, impairments in the sensory systems, such as auditory hallucinations, and impairments in affective system such as blunted emotions. Due to involvement of different brain systems there is debate regarding whether the diagnosis represents a single disorder or a number of discrete syndromes. Although genetic factors play a substantial part, the etiology of schizophrenia apparently requires an interaction between genetic susceptibility and environmental risk factors. This interaction is thought to alter neurodevelopmental processes that occur before the onset of symptoms. All pharmacological treatments currently used for schizophrenia primarily suppress the psychotic symptoms but not the cognitive abnormalities. BOLD fMRI studies demonstrate hypoactivation of the executive system in schizophrenia. Investigations of QEEG abnormalities in schizophrenia are inconsistent: some studies have reported increase of beta and reduction of alpha EEG power in schizophrenia, other research has shown no differences and even opposite results. The most consistence observations in ERP research on schizophrenic population are: reduction of amplitude of the MMN, reduction of the CNV, and reduction of the engagement of P3b component. Some studies reported reduction of the late positive monitoring component elicited to NOGO cues in the GO/NOGO paradigm and generated in the anterior cingulate cortex. Relative hyperfunction of the subcortical dopamine systems has been suggested to be one of the key pathophysiologic mechanisms in schizophrenic psychosis and is reflected in the dopamine hypothesis of schizophrenia. PET studies as well as the ability of antipsychotic drugs to block dopamine receptors seem to support this hypothesis. According to our model schizophrenia might be associated with impairment of selection of actions in the striatum of schizophrenic patients. The discovery of antipsychotic drugs in 1950s significantly reduced the number of electroconvulsive therapeutic interventions and completely abolished the use of psychosurgery for treatment schizophrenia. There were few attempts to treat schizophrenia by means of neurofeedback.

CHAPTER 19

Addiction

I. DESCRIPTION OF BEHAVIOR

A. Symptoms

Addiction is an extreme state of drug abuse[1]. Addiction is defined as a compulsive, out-of-control drug use despite serious negative consequences. The behavioral pattern of an addicted person becomes progressively focused on obtaining, using, and recovering from the effects of drugs. It continues despite illness, disrupted relationships and failures in life. Compulsive actions could be misinterpreted by frustrated family members as deliberate self-destruction.

Important character of addiction is the high risk of relapse to drug use. The potential for relapse maintains even in abstinent addicts long after they stop taking drugs. The relapse is caused by two factors: cues and stress. Drug-conditioned cues can be environmental or interoceptive. For example, the risk of relapse is elevated when addicts encounter people or places associated with earlier drug use. Stress

---

[1]In its turn, *substance abuse* is a behavioral pattern in which people rely on drug excessively, so that the drugs eventually occupy a central part in their life.

also plays a significant role in relapses in addicts[2]. Current treatments for addiction are helpful to some patients, but far from satisfactory.

From the theory presented in Part II, addiction can be conceptualized as impairment in monitoring operation that is resolved in uncontrolled, compulsive patterns of drug use. In this definition addiction appears to be similar to obsessive-compulsive disorder (OCD) (see Chapter 20). Indeed, clinical descriptions of both OCD and addiction are associated with inability to inhibit intrusive repetitive thoughts (obsessions or cravings, respectively) and ritualistic behaviors (compulsions or active drug-seeking/taking, respectively).

B. Substances of Abuse

There are many types of substances of abuse. They are listed in Table 19.1.

C. Tolerance, Dependence, and Withdrawal

In addition to addiction the drugs of abuse can produce tolerance, dependence, and withdrawal symptoms[3]. It should be stressed, that tolerance, dependence, and withdrawal can be observed in response to other, non-addictive drugs (e.g., drugs for treatment of asthma and hypertension). Not all drugs of abuse produce physical

TABLE 19.1   Substances of Abuse and their Action

Substance of abuse	The main action on cellular level
Opioids (morphine, heroin)	Perform as agonists to opiate receptors
Psycho-stimulants (cocaine, amphetamines)	Inhibit dopamine transporters
Barbiturates and benzodiazepines	Enhance conductance of Cl⁻ channels in neuronal membrane, perform as GABA receptor agonists
Nicotine	Agonist of acetylcholine receptors
Alcohol	Facilitates GABA receptors

[2]A debate continues as to whether cues initiate relapses through sub-conscious classical conditioned reflexes or by the mediation of intense consciously experienced urges. However, cue-initiated relapses occur even in individuals who have strongly resolved never to use drugs again, sometimes without any insight into what is happening to them.

[3]*Tolerance* is a decrease in the effect of a drug despite a constant dose, or a need for increased dosage to maintain a stable effect. Some drugs can also produce *sensitization* (enhancement) of drug responses. *Dependence*, narrowly defined, refers to an adapted state of the brain that occurs in response to excessive drug stimulation. After drug cessation, this adapted state can result in the production of cognitive, emotional, or "physical" *withdrawal* symptoms.

dependence: cocaine and amphetamine are examples of such drugs. For psycho-stimulants physical withdrawal symptoms are absent, while emotional withdrawal symptoms are variable and can be mild. Physical dependence and withdrawal are clinically significant, but do not constitute the mechanisms for "psychological" dependence (addiction) as a compulsive drug use with late relapses.

II. IMAGING CORRELATES

A. PET and MRI

Several studies of responses to drug-conditioned cues using positron emission tomography (PET) and functional magnetic resonance imaging (fMRI) consistently showed activation of several brain areas such as prefrontal cortical regions, the nucleus accumbens in the striatum, and the amygdala in the limbic system[4]. For example, a group of researchers from School of Medicine at Emory University, used PET to localize alterations in synaptic activity related to cue-induced drug craving (Kilts et al., 2001). In their approach, script-guided imagery of autobiographical memories were used as individualized cues to internally generate a cocaine craving state and two control (anger and neutral episodic memory recall) states. Compared with the neutral imagery control condition, imagery-induced drug craving was associated with bilateral activation of the amygdala, the left insula and anterior cingulate gyrus, and the right subcallosal gyrus and nucleus accumbens area.

B. Increased Level of Dopamine in Nucleus Accumbens

Recent research shows that addictive drugs directly (such as cocaine) or indirectly (such as opiates) increase the levels of synaptic dopamine in the nucleus accumbens, for example, by blocking dopamine receptors (Fig. 19.1b). Moreover, the increase of dopamine in the striatum positively correlates with the "high" induced by methylphenidate (or cocaine)[5] (Fig. 19.1c). Recall that dopamine is generally required for reward and reinforcement. So, dopamine appears to be critical for acute reward and initiation of addiction.

The current literature also suggests that in addition to the brain's reward system, two frontal cortical regions (anterior cingulate and orbito-frontal cortices), critical for the control over reward-related behavior, are dysfunctional in addicted individuals. These are the same regions that have been implicated in compulsive conditions characterized by deficits in inhibitory control over maladaptive behaviors,

---

[4]Note that activation areas are detected as the difference between response to drug-related cues in comparison to neutral cues.

[5]See a recent review by Peter Kalivas and Nora Volkow (2005).

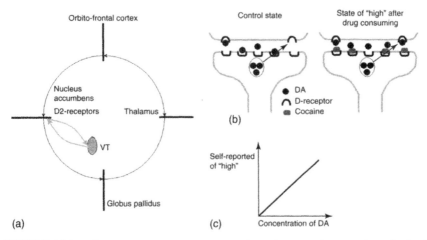

FIGURE 19.1   Effect of cocaine on the dopamine in the nucleus accumbens. (a) The limbic basal ganglia thalamo-cortical circuit with the dopaminergic modulatory input from the substantia nigra to the nucleus accumbens. (b) Cocaine blocks dopamine transporters (DAT) which increases the concentration of dopamine in the nucleus accumbens. (c) The level of dopamine concentration strongly correlates with self-reported of "high" of cocaine addicts. DA – dopamine, D-receptors – postsynaptic striatal receptors to DA.

such as OCD (see Chapter 20). In a study by Steven Forman (Forman et al., 2004) from University of Pittsburg, event-related fMRI was used to study individuals with opiate dependence and healthy control individuals performing a Go/NOGO task. Compared with controls, opiate addicts exhibited an attenuated anterior cingulate cortex error signal and significantly poorer task performance.

III. STAGES OF ADDICTION

A vast amount of empirical and theoretical knowledge in the neurophysiology of addiction enables us to suggest that addiction is a complex psychological process that evolves during several stages each having its own neuronal mechanism.

A. Expectation Stage

At the first stage – an expectation, a *motivation* for initial drug use often comes from normal desires to elevate mood or to experience new feelings. Indeed, in majority of cases initial drug use produces a desirable affect – a positive subjective experience – a pleasure, a high. Neuronal mechanisms of this stage are conventional mechanisms of motivational behavior.

B. Consolidation Stage

At the second stage – memorization of drug consuming, the subjective experience associated with drug consumption is consolidated as an emotionally significant event – reward. As any learning procedure, this stage links the reward with mental representation of objects and actions related to consuming the drug. During this association learning any object or action linked to drug consuming in future becomes a cue eliciting a pleasure. Neuronal mechanisms involved in this stage are common mechanisms of learning – a complex process that probably involves both procedural and episodic memories. What differs learning in addiction from normal learning is the extraordinary *emotional context* (an elevated level of pleasure, a "high") that constitutes initial drug consuming. But the most important factor seems to be the direct effect of the drug on synaptic transmission associated with enhancing release of dopamine into synaptic clefts. As we know from neuroscience (see Chapter 13) the orbito-frontal cortex receives strong connections from multi-modal areas of the cortex and from the limbic system. It is a cortical site where representations of rewards as emotionally meaningful events are stored. From neuroscience we also know that dopamine is a modulator that enhances the memory trace formed in the corresponding cortical area. So, at the second (consolidation) stage the drug consumption produces an extremely intensive memory of a new drug-associated reward in the orbito-frontal cortex[6].

C. Habituation/Sensitization Stage

At the third stage (habituation/sensitization), the effects of drug itself (pleasure or release of dysphoric moods) start to habituate. For drugs such as alcohol, nicotine, and heroine, pleasure can be markedly reduced over time by medical complications. Heroin addicts often report that they feel miserable, that they do understand that drugs ruin their lives, but they still want them. Drug addicts sometimes describe their continuing drug use as an attempt to re-experience remembered "highs," often without success. A question arises, why drug addicts continue to take drugs even if the drug itself does not produce pleasure anymore? To answer this question Robinson and Berridge in 1993 proposed incentive-sensitization (or simply, wanting–liking) theory. According to this theory, a drug at the second (consolidation) stage produces a certain amount of "wanting" and "liking" – activities in different brain systems. After several drug takings the tolerance to drug increases and liking decreases, habituates. In the same time, "wanting," that is now associated not with drug itself but with pleasure giving by cues related to the drug-induced positive sensations increases.

---

[6]The circuit that is responsible for the second stage of addiction includes: the limbic system with amygdala as a nucleus responsible for emotional component, the ventral striatum with nucleus accumbens as an element responsible for memorizing the behavioral pattern, and the orbito-frontal cortex as a cortical place of representation of the whole event as a significantly emotional reward.

D. Neural Net Model

According to the theory of brain functioning introduced in this book (Part II), neuronal mechanisms of different stages of addiction could viewed as follows (Fig. 19.2).

During the expectation stage most of the prefrontal cortical areas activate the motor cortex to initiate a new and possibly pleasurable action.

During the consolidation stage the orbito-frontal and anterior cingulate cortical areas receive strong and emotionally meaningful inputs from the limbic system. The representation of the reward in the orbito-frontal cortex is strongly consolidated due to normal mechanisms, such as enhancement of synapses in the circuit orbito-frontal cortex → nucleus accumbens → globus pallidus → anterior nucleus of the thalamus. Under normal circumstances, this dopaminergic circuit is a crucial substrate for rewarding and reinforcing effects of positive natural stimuli associated with survival, such as food and reproductive opportunities. During drug consumption, the release of dopamine is dramatically enhanced due to the direct or indirect drug effect. High concentrations of dopamine at the dendrites of cells in the nucleus accumbens enhance activity of striatal neurons and "imprint" the representation of the reward and the behavioral pattern associated with it. Thus addicted drugs stimulate brain reward circuitry with a strength, time course, and reliability that exceeds almost any natural stimulus, powerfully consolidating responses to drug-associated stimuli. After the memory of the reward has been stored in the limbic circuit, any cue (either internal, just a subjective recall from memory, or external, associated with the drug) activates this critical circuit[7].

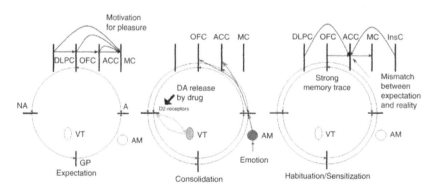

FIGURE 19.2   Neuronal networks and stages of drug addiction. See explanation in text.

[7]The critical circuit for the consolidation stage includes the limbic system (with the amygdala as a critical element for generating emotions), the nucleus accumbens as a critical element for learning behavioral patterns associated with drugs, and the orbito-frontal cortex as a cortical map for representation and storing rewards. Whether related to drug taking or survival, actions that increase synaptic dopamine in this brain "reward" circuitry tend to be repeated.

At the habituation/sensitization stage the activity from the orbital–frontal cortex recalled from the memory about the reward (e.g., how wonderful it was during the first drug consumption...) is compared with the representation of the real situation (e.g., life is boring and grey) in the anterior cingulate cortex. The result of the comparison reflecting this inconsistency activates the basal ganglia thalamo-cortical loop associated with the anterior cingulate cortex. In its turn, the activation of the anterior cingulate cortex starts drug-seeking behavior by activation of premotor and motor areas of the cortex.

IV. TREATMENT

A. Stereotactic Anterior Cingulotomy in Heroin Addicts

The prediction of the model described above is that addiction at its final stage is associated with high level of activation of neurons in the anterior cingulate cortex. This hyperactivation is due to constant mismatch between the reality[8] and the strong memory trace of the drug consuming behavior. This constant hyperactivation of the anterior cingulate cortex constantly drives the drug addict's behavior to search for a drug. The hyperactive state of the anterior cingulus is similar to the corresponding state in the OCD.

In the Institute of the Human Brain in St. Petersburg a stereotactic operation for restraining compulsive behavior in heroin drug addicts has been suggested. More than 300 drug addicts have been operated with a good success. Figure 19.3 represents the results of study in our laboratory with a group of drug addicts. Scalp-recorded event-related potentials (ERPs) in the visual two stimulus GO/NOGO task were taken before (thin line) and after (thick line) stereotactic operation of anterio-cingulotomy in 13 patients with heroin drug addiction[9]. The P400 monitoring component was found to be selectively suppressed after the operation[10]. This data indicate that this component is a good indicator of functioning of the anterior cingulate cortex and could be used for examining the results of stereotactic operation. The outcome of operations also shows that compulsive component is very strong in addiction and that destruction of this "compulsive" circuit is a very powerful tool in the treatment of addiction.

---

[8]The information about reality is coming to the anterior cingulate cortex from several sources including the insular and sensory motor cortical areas, while information about the highly activated program for drug consumption is probably coming from the orbito-frontal cortex.

[9]The study was approved by the ethical committee of the Institute of the Human Brain. Patients gave a written consent for undergoing a stereotactic operation as well as for participating in the study.

[10]Recall that this component is generated in the anterior cingulate cortex.

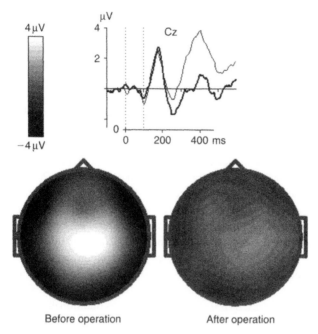

FIGURE 19.3   ERPs in addiction. Grand average ERPs in the two stimulus GO/NOGO task for a group of heroin drug addicts before (thick line) and after (thin line) a stereotactic destruction of a part of the anterior cingulate cortex. Note, that operation selectively diminishes the P4 monitoring NOGO component.

B. Neurofeedback

The most known neurofeedback protocol for addiction uses alpha–theta biofeedback. This technique involves the simultaneous measurement of occipital alpha (8–13 Hz) and theta (4–8 Hz) and the feedback[11] for each band for the spectral power that exceeds the preset thresholds[12]. The subject is encouraged to relax and increase the amount of time for each signal.

Alpha–theta feedback training was first used and described by Green et al. in 1975 at the Menninger clinic. This method was based on Green's observations of single-lead electroencephalogram (EEG) during meditative states in practiced meditators. When the separate and independent auditory feedback of alpha and theta signal was given to subjects in eyes closed or self-induced relaxed conditions, states of profound relaxation and trance were reported to occur. As meditational states progressed, an increased theta amplitude was observed following an initial increase

[11]The feedback is presented by separate auditory tones separately for each band.

[12]Note that EEG activity in the alpha band is highest in posterior regions of the cortex during eyes closed condition, while EEG in the theta band increases in deeply relaxed states. The alpha–theta protocol is accomplished in eyes closed condition with the auditory feedback.

of alpha amplitude, at the next stage the drop of the alpha amplitude (theta–alpha crossover) was usually observed. Whereas the EEG changes are similar to stage 1 sleep, the subjects are maintained in a relaxed yet focused condition, subjectively similar to a hypnotic trance with a sense of timelessness. Those effects may be non-specific to the alpha–theta brain wave biofeedback method and may be achievable with other biofeedback techniques or with meditational techniques alone.

Note that alpha–theta neurofeedback in addiction is not used alone. Green and colleagues applied this technique for augmenting effects of psychotherapy. The first studies of alpha–theta biofeedback for addictions focused on augmenting therapy experience in alcoholics engaged in psychotherapy and 12-step model programs in a Veterans Administration hospital setting. Daily 20 min alpha–theta EEG biofeedback sessions (integrated with EMG biofeedback and temperature control biofeedback) were done over 6 weeks and resulted in free, loose associations, heightened sensitivity, and increased suggestibility. Patients discussed their insights and experiences associated with biofeedback in therapy groups several times a week, which augmented expressive psychotherapy.

Peniston and Kulkosky reported a randomized and controlled study of adult chronic treatment resistant alcoholics treated with alpha–theta EEG biofeedback (Peniston and Kulkosky, 1989). Compared with a traditionally treated alcoholic control group and non-alcoholic controls, alcoholics who received brain wave and temperature biofeedback did show significant increases in percentages of EEG record in alpha and theta rhythms. In addition, the experimentally treated subjects showed reductions in Beck Depression Inventory scores compared with the control groups. 13-month follow-up data indicated sustained prevention of relapse in alcoholics that completed alpha–theta brainwave training. The alpha–theta protocol has become known as the "Peniston-Kulkosky Protocol."

V. SUMMARY

Addiction is defined as a compulsive, out-of-control drug use despite serious negative consequences. The behavioral pattern of an addicted person becomes progressively focused on obtaining, using, and recovering from the effects of drugs. Addiction is a complex psychological process that evolves during several stages such as expectation, consolidation, and habituation/sensitization stages each having its own neuronal mechanism. Recent research shows that addictive drugs directly (such as cocaine) or indirectly (such as opiates) increase the levels of synaptic dopamine in the nucleus accumbens. The level of the dopamine concentration strongly correlates with self-reported of "high" of cocaine addicts. So, dopamine appears to be critical for acute reward and initiation of addiction. In later stages the anterior cingulate cortex interconnected with the nucleus accumbens becomes overactive. The anterior cingulate cortex plays a critical role in monitoring behavior, so that its hyperactivation is resolved in uncontrolled, compulsive patterns of drug seeking. According to our theory addiction at least in some patients can be conceptualized as impairment in monitoring operation. This inference was supported by our recordings of ERP components in the GO/NOGO paradigm in heroin drug addicts before and after stereotactic cingulotomy performed in these patients to relieve their obsessive thoughts and compulsive actions. The P400 monitoring component was selectively suppressed by lesions in the anterior cingulate cortex in these patients. Theoretically, any relaxation protocol of neurofeedback might be helpful in drug addiction. The most known of them is alpha–theta or Peniston-Kulkosky protocol. This technique involves the simultaneous measurement of occipital alpha and theta activity while the subject is encouraged to relax and increase the amount of time of each signal.

CHAPTER 20

Obsessive-Compulsive Disorder

I. DESCRIPTION OF BEHAVIOR

A. Symptoms

The name, obsessive-compulsive disorder (OCD), comes from symptoms of the disease, which affect both cognition (flow of thoughts) and motor behavior (action). *Obsessions* are thoughts that repeat over and over again, unwanted but insistent. *Compulsions* are actions repeated over and over in ritualistic, stereotyped succession. Usually, particular compulsive acts are carried out in response to a particular obsession to neutralize the anxiety associated with that obsession. However, there are some patients who suffer mainly obsessions, and, there are patients who suffer mainly compulsions.

People with OCD are usually aware that the obsessions and compulsions are senseless, but, despite great effort, they cannot control them. A common type of obsessions and compulsions is checking, that is, going back over and over in response to obsessive self-doubts whether it was done, and done just right. Other types of OCD are washing, ordering.... The obsessions and compulsions can go on for hours. For example, a "checker" checks again and again, and the question "what if?" dominates, and there is no behavioral closure. These recurrent obsessions or compulsions "are severe enough to be time consuming or cause marked distress or significant impairment" (Diagnostic and Statistical Manual of Mental Disorders, Fourth edition)[1]. The repeated doubt and subsequent checking that surround actions is particularly the salient features of OCD. Within the framework of the brain model described in the book, these intrusive obsessions and subsequent compulsions can be viewed in terms of dysfunctional response monitoring. However, because these obsessions/compulsions are also associated with anxiety, OCD may also be associated with affective system.

OCD is estimated to affect 1–3 per cent of the population. Prevalence is similar throughout countries and cultures. Symptoms generally begin in childhood or adolescence and are associated with dramatic impairment in social and occupational functioning. In a 1998 World Health Organization study, OCD was among the top 10 leading medical or psychiatric causes of disability in developed countries. Even when the most aggressive medical and behavioral therapies are applied, an estimated 10 per cent of the OCD population remains severely affected.

II. GENETICS AND CO-MORBIDITY

A. Poor Heritability

Twin studies strongly suggest that vulnerability to the OCD can be inherited, but a positive family history is absent in many patients. Only 10 per cent of the parents of children with OCD have the disorder themselves.

B. Co-morbid Disorders

Patients with the OCD often suffer from other (co-morbid) disorders, including depression, anxiety and Tourette syndrome. Major depression has a lifetime prevalence of 60–70 per cent in OCD patients while 90 per cent of patients with Tourette syndrome have OCD.

III. IMAGING CORRELATES

A. PET, MRI

Theoretically, the OCD might be associated with impairments in different operations in the executive system, such as (1) impairment in inhibition operation, that

---

[1]We all have habits, mannerisms, and sometimes expose superstitious behavioral patterns. But in many cases these are not disturbing behaviors. They give us certain personality features forming a background for our cognitive and motor activities. In people who suffer from OCD such habitual patterns are out of control.

is, inability to suppress unwanted action or (2) impairment in selection operation, that is, inability to switch to another action, or (3) impairment in monitoring operation, that is inability to compare the executed action with a desired one
and to complete the action. All these operations are associated with the frontal
cortex–basal ganglia–thalamo-cortical circuits (Fig. 20.1).

In line with these theoretical considerations, the majority of brain imaging (positron emission tomography – PET, functional magnetic resonance imaging – fMRI)
studies in subjects with the OCD has shown an abnormal activation of the fronto-
striatal system including the following anatomical structures: (1) at the cortical level:
the orbito-frontal (OFC), dorso-lateral prefrontal (DLPFC), and anterior cingulate
cortex (ACC); (2) at the striatal level: the ventro-medial striatum (including nucleus
accumbens), the globus pallidus/substantia nigra pars reticulata complex, (3) at the
thalamic level: anterior and medio-dorsal thalamic nuclei. For example, increased
activity was shown consistently in the OFC and the caudate nucleus, under resting
conditions as well as under symptom provocation. This hyperactivity was correlated
with the symptomatology and normalized after therapy.

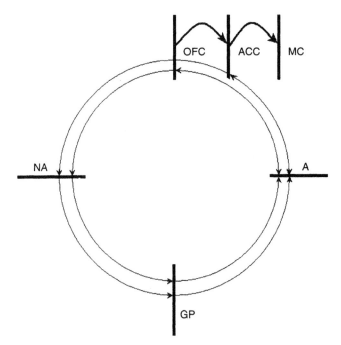

FIGURE 20.1   A neuronal network of OCD. Inputs from the prefrontal cortical areas (including the
orbito-prefrontal cortex) strongly activate the ACC. The ACC in turn drives the motor cortex either
directly through cortico-cortical pathways or indirectly through the ACC → NA → GP → A circuit,
where ACC stands for anterior cingulate cortex, NA – for nucleus accumbens, GP – for the corresponding part of the globus pallidus, A – for the anterior nucleus of the thalamus. These pathways from
the prefrontal cortex drive the motor areas to perform compulsive actions.

B. QEEG

In a recent study researchers from University of Naples in Italy (Bucci et al., 2004) used quantitative electroencephalogram (QEEG) to show the signs of hyperactivation of the frontal cortex in the OCD. They found a decrease of the slow alpha band power mainly in the frontal areas in OCD patients as compared to healthy subjects. In addition, significant negative correlation between the slow alpha band power and the time to complete a neuropsychological test exploring executive functions was found: the more reduced the slow alpha band power, the slower the performance on this test. This relationship was accompanied by positive correlation between the beta band power and the characteristic of OCD. However, as this hyperactivity was found not only in patients with OCD, but also in specific phobias and post-traumatic stress disorder under symptom provocation, it has been argued that hyperactivity might reflect anxiety component of the OCD more than its specific neuronal correlates. Leslie Sherlin and Marco Congedo from Novatech using low resolution electromagnetic tomography (LORETA) imaging found an excess of current source density of beta activity in the cingulate cortex in OCD patients as compared with healthy subjects (Sherlin and Congedo, 2005).

C. Monitoring Component of ERPs

As we know, the ACC is involved in monitoring operations manifested in P400 monitoring component elicited in response to NOGO cues in the two stimulus GO/NOGO task. We also learnt that the hyperactivation of the system may result in reduction of the event-related potentials (ERPs) component similar to reduction caused by the hypoactivation of the system[2]. The results of a group from University of Wurzburg, Germany (Herrmann et al., 2003) are in line with this theoretical consideration. In this study patients with OCD and healthy controls performed a cued GO/NOGO task, while ERPs were registered with multiple electrodes. The authors showed a reduction of P3 NOGO component in OCD patients in comparison to healthy controls. The reduction of P3 NOGO component was manifested in a so-called anteriorization parameter computed as the difference between the location of the positive centroid in the GO and NOGO conditions. This parameter was negatively correlated with the symptomatology as measured by the Yale-Brown Obsessive-Compulsive Scale. In summary, hyperactivation of the ACC could be considered as a core of the disease. Because this cortical area is involved in both the executive and affective system, both basic mediators seem to be effective in treatment of OCD.

---

[2] Recall inverted U-relationship between activation of the system and its functional ability.

IV. MEDIATORS

There is strong evidence that the serotoninergic system modulates symptoms of the OCD. Potent inhibitors of serotonin transporter function (serotonin reuptake inhibitors) are unique among antidepressants in producing at least some clinical benefit in most patients with the OCD. Interestingly, both the serotonin transporter and some serotonin receptor subtypes implicated in the OCD are highly expressed in the ventral striatum where they could influence the functioning of the basal ganglia–thalamo-cortical circuits. In theory, other neurotransmitter systems within these circuits may play a role in susceptibility, course, or response to OCD treatment. For example, dopaminergic mechanisms have been implicated by controlled studies demonstrating that neuroleptics, ineffective as monotherapy in OCD, are beneficial when added to ongoing serotonin reuptake inhibitor treatment.

V. TREATMENT

A. Stereotactic Anterior Cingulotomy

Fulton (1951) was the first to suggest that the anterior cingulum would be an appropriate target for psychosurgical intervention. Ballantine et al (1987) subsequently demonstrated the safety and effectiveness of cingulotomy in a large number of patients[3]. Cingulotomy has been a surgical procedure of choice in the North America over the last 30 years and currently is used for treatment of the OCD[4].

B. QEEG/ERPs Assessment in an OCD Patient

Cingulotomy is used for the treatment of OCD in the Neurosurgery clinic of the Institute of the Human Brain in St. Petersburg. Recently, we started using QEEG and ERP for localizing the source of cortical hyperactivation in OCD patients who were unresponsive to all conventional forms of treatment and therefore recommended for stereotactic operation. The results of assessment of one of such

---

[3]Although the patient may experience an immediate reduction in anxiety just after the operation, there is generally a delay to the onset of beneficial effect on OCD. This latency may be as long as 6–12 weeks. The results of bilateral cingulotomy in 198 patients suffering from a variety of psychiatric disorders were reported retrospectively by Ballantine et al in 1987. In patients with OCD approximately 56 per cent were found to have undergone clinically significant improvement. A recent retrospective study evaluating cingulotomy in 33 patients with refractory OCD demonstrated that using very strict criteria for successful outcome, at least 25–30 per cent of patients benefited substantially from the procedure. (Jenike et al., 1991). An independent analysis of patients who underwent cingulotomy demonstrated no significant intellectual deficits as a result of the cingulate lesions themselves.

[4]As well as for refractory major affective disorder and chronic anxiety states.

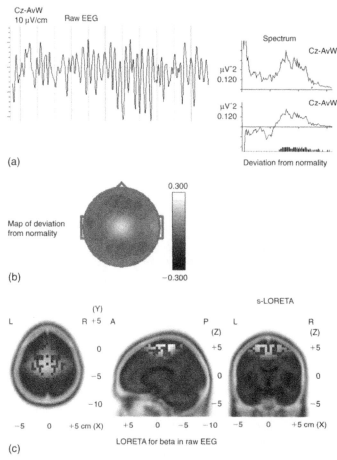

(a)

(b)

(c)   LORETA for beta in raw EEG

FIGURE 20.2   QEEG/ERP assessment of an OCD patient. A young OCD patient was scheduled for stereotactic anterior cingulotomy at the Neurosurgical clinic of the Institute of the Human Brain of Russian Academy of Sciences. (a) A fragment of raw EEG and corresponding spectrum in eyes open condition recorded at Cz. (b) The results of comparison of the spectrum at Cz with the normative data: the map of deviation and the difference spectrum. (c) s-LORETA image of raw signal in beta frequency range. (d) Superposition of ERP components of the patient (thin line) with the normative data (thick line), P400 monitoring component at the left and P2 comparison component at the right. (e) s-LORETA image of the P400 monitoring component.

OCD patients are presented in Fig. 20.2. As one can see, this patient is characterized by strong ($p < 0.0001$) access of beta activity in central medial regions with maximum at Cz that according to s-LORETA is generated in the areas of the middle prefrontal cortex and ACC. In addition, independent analysis of ERP components shows a selective statistically significant ($p < 0.02$) deviation from normality in the P4 monitoring component while no significant deviations in other

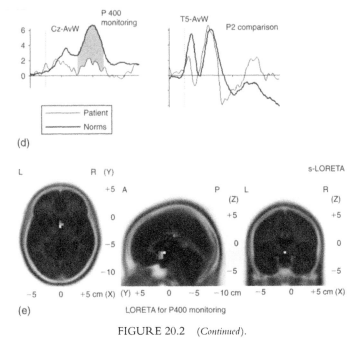

FIGURE 20.2   (*Continued*).

independent components are found. All these findings consistently show hyperactivation of the cortical area that is located around ACC. Note also that the effected area overlaps with the prefrontal area that is involved in inhibition of actions.

C. Neurofeedback

A review of the literature on the neurofeedback treatment of anxiety disorders was made by Moore in 2000 (Moore, 2000). He was able to identify two published studies of application of neurofeedback in the OCD. Both studies used alpha enhancement training, without positive results. Viewed from a modern perspective, these studies, which were published in the mid-1970s, used a simplistic treatment approach of only doing alpha enhancement training. Literature since that time has shown that there are at least two subtypes of EEG patterns found in OCD. Recent reports are available on the successful treatment, with lengthy follow-ups, of three consecutive cases of OCD. In each of these cases, neurofeedback protocols were individualized to the unique neurophysiologic characteristics of each patient through a QEEG assessment.

VI. SUMMARY

The name, obsessive-compulsive disorder (OCD), comes from symptoms of the disease, which affect both cognition (flow of thoughts) and motor behavior (actions). Obsessions are thoughts that repeat over and over again, unwanted but insistent while compulsions are actions repeated over and over in ritualistic, stereotyped succession. People with the OCD are usually aware that the obsessions and compulsions are senseless, but, despite great effort, they cannot control them. The majority of brain imaging (PET, fMRI) studies in subjects with OCD showed an abnormal activation of the fronto-striatal system including the OFC, DLPFC, and ACC, nucleus accumbens, and anterior thalamic nuclei. QEEG studies found overactivation pattern in the frontal cortex, while ERP studies revealed reduction of NOGO monitoring component in OCD patients in comparison to healthy controls. Cingulotomy has been a surgical procedure of choice and currently is used for the treatment of OCD. Alpha neurofeedback protocols performed in the mid-1970 did not show positive results. Recent protocols of the successful neurofeedback treatment were individualized to the unique neurophysiologic characteristics of each patient through a QEEG assessment.

CHAPTER 21

Depression

I. DESCRIPTION OF BEHAVIOR

A. History

The word "melancholia" (derived from Greek melaina chole – black bile) is known as the first description of depression by Hippocrates 24 centuries ago. In the end of the 19th century Emil Kraepelin created a new nosological system to classify psychiatric disorders in which the term "involutional melancholia" was introduced. From a historical perspective, there have been large swings in the classification systems, ranging from descriptive strategies, such as those of Kraepelin, to interpretative-based approaches, such as Freud's ideas who viewed depression as the manifestation of internalized anger or loss. In most of the western countries the Kraepelinian, descriptive approaches have always prevailed.

B. Symptoms

Major depression is a disorder of the affective system[1]. Major depression is characterized by a triad of symptoms: (1) low or depressed mood, (2) anhedonia

---

[1]Other disorders of the affective system include dysthymia (chronic intermittent minor depression), bipolar disorder (manic–depressive illness), and cyclothymia (a mild form of bipolar disorder).

(loss of interest or pleasure in almost all activities), and (3) low energy or fatigue. Other symptoms, such as sleep and psychomotor disturbances, pessimism, guilty feelings, low self-esteem, suicidal tendencies, and food-intake and body-weight dysregulation, are also often present. The prevalence of depression is consistently high worldwide and affects about 7–18 per cent of the population on at least one occasion in their lives, before the age of 40. The disease is more prevalent in women – the female/male ratio can be as high as 5:2. Typically, the course of depression is recurrent; patients go through periods with symptomatic episodes and periods of recovery[2]. Depression is one of the top 10 causes of mortality. Suicide, which is usually a consequence of depression, is one of the leading causes of death all over the world[3].

C. Subtyping Depression

It is a common understanding that there is no one structure that is responsible for the symptoms of depression and that there are several subtypes of depression depending on the brain structures involved. Positron emission tomography (PET) and functional magnetic resonance imaging (fMRI) studies indicate the heterogeneity of brain structures that are dysfunctional in the illness[4]. This heterogeneity is expressed in diversity of symptoms, variability of the course, and highly individual responses to available treatments. The heterogeneity of major depression enables most experts to view depression as a syndrome, not a disease, assuming that different neuronal circuits in the brain might be responsible for symptoms of depression.

D. Heritability

Depression is highly heritable with roughly 40–50 per cent of the risk for this illness being genetic. However, specific genes that underlie the risk have not been identified. The remaining 60–50 per cent of the risk are also poorly defined. Early childhood trauma, emotional stress, physical illness, and even viral infections have been suggested as non-genetic risk factors.

---

[2]However, about 20 per cent of patients have a chronic course without remissions.

[3]The rate of suicide depends on age: in the United States, suicide is the fourth leading cause of death in the 25–44 age group and the third leading cause of death in the 15–24 age group. The incidence of major depression is increasing and nowadays the onset occurs at a younger age in comparison to previous generations.

[4]Numerous neuroimaging studies indicate the impairment of hippocampus and prefrontal cortical areas (involving probably in producing cognitive symptoms), amygdala (in producing emotional symptoms), and the hypothalamus (in producing symptoms related to appetite, sleep, and circadian rhythms abnormalities).

E. Need for Objective Diagnostic System

A key problem in diagnosis is that existing classification systems are solely based on the subjective descriptions of symptoms. Such detailed phenomenology includes the description of multiple clinical subtypes; however, there is no biological feature that separates one subtype from another. The distinction between depression and everyday sadness is based on the inexorable nature of depression and the accompanying disability. Because each of symptoms of major depression is not qualitatively different from experience that all of us have at some points in our lives, depression is frequently not detected or misdiagnosed, and, at the same time, overdiagnosed. An objective method for depression is needed.

II. IMAGING CORRELATES

A. PET, MRI

Early influential studies that examined resting cerebral glucose metabolism and blood flow with PET in patients with depression found decreased prefrontal activity. This decreased activity was correlated with severity of depression and was reversed upon recovery from depression. These initial imaging findings were confirmed later by fMRI studies as well by EEG studies that demonstrated increased alpha power (alpha power is thought to be inversely related to neural activity) in left frontal regions of the brains of depressed patients.

From clinical experience we know that depressed patients preferentially focus on sad events (low mood) and fail to respond with pleasure to happy events (anhedonia). One of the echologically valid approaches for studying the affective system is to observe metabolic or EEG responses of the brain to emotionally meaningful (happy and sad) events. A study of researchers from University of Pittsburgh Medical School and Institute of Psychiatry in London (Keedwell et al., 2005) employed this paradigm (see Methods of Part III) to compare the responses of the brain to positively and negatively valenced stimuli[5]. The main finding was a double dissociation of response of the ventro-medial prefrontal cortex to different stimuli in a group of depressed patients in comparison to a group of healthy subjects: relative increase of response of this cortical area to happy stimuli compared to sad stimuli in depressed patients, but an inverse pattern − relative decrease of response of happy stimuli compared with sad stimuli in healthy individuals[6].

---

[5]They used blood oxygenation level dependent (BOLD) functional magnetic resonance imaging (fMRI) as an index of metabolic activity.

[6]Simultaneously with decrease of metabolic activity mostly in the ventral parts of the prefrontal cortex hyperactivation (excess of metabolic activity) was found in dorsal parts of the prefrontal cortex. This increase of metabolic activity was associated with hyperactivity in amygdala and abnormalities in the hippocampal circuit.

Recently, in a group of treatment-resistant patients with depression in addition to decreased prefrontal activity an increase of metabolic activity (measured by PET) in the subgenual gyrus cingulate (a part of the limbic system) was observed (Mayberg et al., 2005). This is the same area that demonstrates increased blood flow in healthy subjects when sadness is induced. This is also an area that responds to antidepressant pharmacological treatment.

B. QEEG Asymmetry

EEG correlates explore the idea of laterality of emotional reactions with negative emotions having a bias in activating the right hemisphere and positive emotions activating in more extent the left hemisphere[7]. Frontal alpha asymmetry is often used for these purposes. Given that a major characteristic of depressed persons is their increased sensitivity to negative stimuli and their withdrawal from positive stimuli, asymmetrical distribution of positive and negative emotions in the prefrontal cortex may have important implications for diagnostics and treatment of depression. Indeed, some findings of prefrontal cortex asymmetry (see Chapter 13) suggest that frontal EEG asymmetry may represent a predisposition that underlies individual differences in reactivity to valence stimuli[8]. The idea of asymmetry of the affective system comes from clinical observations that associated left frontal lesions and subsequent depression.

Taken into account the relative temporal stability of alpha asymmetry (Tomarken et al., 1992) and its potential relation to deficits in approach behavior, one would expect to observe evidence of left frontal hypoactivation in depressed persons as well as in individuals who are at elevated risk for experiencing this disorder. Indeed Henriques and Davidson (1991) assessed anterior EEG asymmetry[9] in currently depressed and never depressed subjects, and found elevated left midfrontal alpha power (F3/F4) in the currently depressed subjects. Several investigators have observed that individual differences in frontal asymmetry emerge early in life and are associated with individual differences in infants' behavior along the approach-withdrawal[10]. Taken together, these findings suggest that frontal asymmetry might be

---

[7]The hypothesis of asymmetrical representation of positive and negative emotions (and probably of rewards and punishers) is supported by clinical evidence. In the stroke patients lesions in the left frontal areas are more often associated with depression than lesions at the right side.

[8]More specifically, individuals who exhibit hypoactivation of the left frontal region and who, therefore also demonstrate elevated responsivity to negative stimuli, may be at increased risk for experiencing episodes of depression.

[9]Recall that frontal hemispheric asymmetry of the EEG spectral power is usually calculated as $((L - R)/[(L + R)/2]) \times 100\%$, where L and R are square root power values at the homologous left and right hemisphere sites (F3 and F4, F7 and F8).

[10]For example, these studies found left frontal hypoactivation in children of depressed mothers and in behaviorally inhibited children.

a biological marker of familial and, possibly, genetic risk for mood disorders, which can potentially have important implications for psychiatric genetic research[11].

It should be stressed that values of frontal asymmetry are very small with average in healthy group of about 1 per cent and with standard deviations of about 5 per cent[12]. In line with these results is a study from University of Pittsburgh (Vuga et al., 2006). Using EEG recordings in 1–3 year intervals in individuals with history of depression and healthy controls the authors were able to show that the resting frontal EEG asymmetry reflects a moderately stable (interclass correlation between 0.4 and 0.6) individual difference in adults, irrespective of sex and history of depression. Taken together these data show that that frontal asymmetry might be associated with only one (relatively small) subtype of depression making the results quite inconsistent depending on the procedure of selecting the patients.

C. ERP Asymmetry

Recent studies show that cognitive event-related potentials (ERPs) might serve as endophenotypes for discriminating depressed patients from healthy individuals. A study of a group of researchers from Centre for Neuroimaging Science in London (Sumich et al., 2006) shows that healthy subjects but not sub-clinically depressed participants had asymmetry (R > L) of amplitude of N200 component of ERPs recorded in an auditory oddball task[13].

D. QEEG/ERPs Assessment in a Depressed Patient

An example of application of the Human Brain Institute Normative Database for assessment of one patient with depression is shown in Fig. 21.1. Two types of asymmetry were observed. One type of asymmetry was observed in spectra recorded in eyes open condition. The other type of asymmetry was found in ERPs recorded in the two stimulus GO/NOGO task. For comparison spectra and ERPs computed for symmetrical frontal areas (F7 and F8) are presented. Note larger amplitude

---

[11]However, a recent study in Washington University School of Medicine (Anokhin et al., 2006), with a sample of 246 young adult female twins found very low (although statistically significant) heritability of frontal asymmetry parameter measured at F3/F4 locations, suggesting that only 27 per cent of the observed variance can be accounted for by genetic factors. In contrast, alpha band power was highly heritable at all four frontal sites (85–87 per cent).

[12]Also recall, that the index of frontal asymmetry presumes calculation of a ratio while the standard deviation for the ratio is a sum of standard deviations of two parts of the ratio. This creates difficulties in obtaining robust estimation of this index in a particular subject.

[13]The data were taken from seven world-wide Brain-Resource Company (BRC) clinics. These clinics are located in London, Nijmegen, Sydney, Adelaide, Melbourne, New York, and Rhode Island. BRC clinics operate with a standardized protocol and high interlab reliability which is not affected by age or sex (for details see www.brainresource.com).

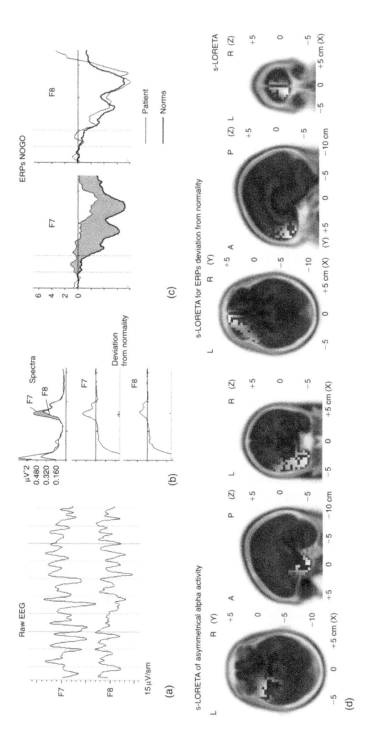

FIGURE 21.1 Spectra and ERP asymmetries in a patient with depression. (a) Fragment of raw EEG in the local average montage at F7, F8. (b) Superposition of EEG spectra for electrodes F7 and F8 and deviations from normality at these sites. (c) ERPs to NOGO cues in the visual two stimulus GO/NOGO task. (d) s-LORETA images of the asymmetrical alpha activity and of deviation from the normative mean in ERPs to NOGO cues.

of alpha oscillations at the frontal left side (F7) in comparison to the right side (F8) in this patient in eyes open condition. s-LORETA images indicate generators of this abnormal[14] alpha rhythm in the left ventro-lateral prefrontal cortex and superior temporal areas. Knowing that the presence of alpha rhythm is the cortical area is associated with hypofunction (idling) of this area we can conclude that the left ventro-lateral prefrontal cortex in this patient is hypoactivated. In line with the quantitative electroencephalography (QEEG) assessment, analysis of ERP components shows asymmetrical activation of frontal areas in response to GO and NOGO stimuli. As one can see from Fig. 21.1 ERPs evoked by NOGO stimulus[15] are suppressed in comparison to healthy subjects at the left side (F7) but not at symmetrical right side (F8). This fact indicates hypofunction of the left medial and ventro-lateral prefrontal cortical areas and matches the alpha asymmetry.

E. QEEG Predictors of Response to Antidepressants

QEEG and ERP indexes can be used in patients with major depression as predictors of their response to antidepressants. This is an important issue because 50–75 per cent of the efficacy of antidepressant medication represents the placebo effect, since many depressed patients improve when treated with either medication or placebo. In a recent study from the Quantitative EEG Laboratory of UCLA School of Medicine, Los Angeles (Leuchter et al., 2002) the researchers examined brain function in depressed subjects receiving either active medication or placebo and sought to determine whether QEEG could detect differences in brain function between medication and placebo responders. Both QEEG power and cordance[16], a new measure that seems to reflect cerebral perfusion better than EEG spectra, were used. The authors showed that cordance exhibited early decreases in prefrontal areas in medication responders, while it increased in placebo responders. The data show that the cordance can be served not only as measure for discriminating medication responders from non-responders, but also as measure to discriminate them from placebo responders.

III. NEURONAL MODEL

A. Monoamine Hypothesis of Depression

The monoamine hypothesis of depression was an early milestone in attempt of understanding brain mechanisms of this disorder. According to the monoamine

---

[14]Note that the power of this rhythm is significantly ($p < 0.01$) higher than the corresponding power in age matching healthy controls.

[15]Presented as an example while ERPs to GO stimuli are not shown.

[16]The cordance reflects a deviation from an average both in relative and absolute power in a type of local average montage (for more details see Methods of Part I).

hypothesis, depression was postulated to reflect a deficiency or imbalance in the mediator noradrenaline (or serotonin) of the brain. The hypothesis were based on observations that several antidepressant drugs increased synaptic concentrations of noradrenaline or serotonin, and that reserpine, a catecholamine depleting drug, could cause depression-like symptoms.

Drugs that target monoamines affect the corresponding neurotransmitter systems within an hour or less after administrating drugs. However positive changes can be seen only after few weeks of medication! One of the theories that try to explain this discrepancy postulates slowly adjusting changes in the brain stem autoreceptor synaptic efficiency resulted in the final desensitization of the autoreceptors[17]. Another hypothesis postulates that depression is caused by impairment in neuronal circuits of the affective system, but not mediators themselves. Reorganizing these pathologically altered circuits requires long-term modifications similar to those involved in acquiring procedural memories.

B. Brain Circuitry of Depressed Mood

Imaging experimental evidence indicates that depression as a multi-symptom disorder involves elements of both affective and executive systems of the brain[18]. The elements of the affective system involved in major depression include the orbito-frontal and medial cortical areas, the insular, the amygdala, and the structures of the hypothalamic–pituitary axis (HPA). The elements of the executive system include the anterior cingulate cortex (ACC) and the corresponding basal ganglia thalamo-cortical loop. Let us describe the circuit that is responsible for depressed mood (Fig. 21.2). Recall that depressed mood is the most widely recognized symptom of depression and is the most often targeted by pharmacological treatment.

Numerous neuroimaging studies show that sadness and depressed mood are associated with abnormal neuronal activation in the medial prefrontal cortex, including the ACC and orbito-frontal cortex. These areas in the cortex receive inputs through the anterior nucleus of the thalamus from the hippocampus, amygdala, and mammilary bodies of the hypothalamus. The activity in these areas is mediated mostly by serotoninergic enervation from the midbrain raphe nucleus, and partly by noradrenergic enervation from the locus coeruleus. Antidepressants

---

[17]The point is that systemic introduction of the drug effects not only the target structures in the affective system, but also autoreceptors in the brainstem nuclei that in turn regulate mediator production in the target structures. So, the net effect of the initial systemic drug administration could be very small or even zero. Slowly evolving desensitization of autoreceptors in the brain stem has been postulated to explain delayed effects of drugs in depression.

[18]This fits well the fact that symptoms of affective disorders besides affective have also cognitive, motor, and neuroendocrinologic components. Each of these components of depression is associated with its own specific neural circuit.

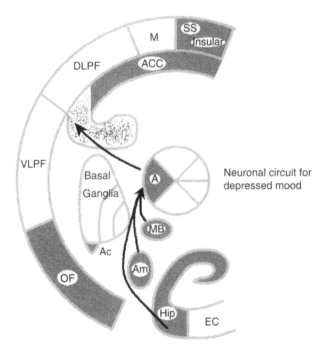

FIGURE 21.2   Neuronal circuitry of depressed mood. Outputs from the amygdala (Am), mammillary bodies of the hypothalamus (MB), and hippocampus (Hip) are projected via the anterior nucleus of the thalamus to the insula, orbito-frontal cortex (OF), and the anterior cingulate cortex (ACC). Sad events are probably mapped into the subgenual gyrus cingulus (depicted by dotted pattern) so that hypoactivation of this area produces a depressed mood.

that improve sadness and depressed mood act on these mediator systems and normalize activity in these areas. Chronic deep brain stimulation (DBS) [19] of the subgenual part in the ACC produces similar effect.

In contrast to hyperactivity of the medial frontal cortex and associated depressed mood, executive dysfunction in major depression is probably reflected in hypoactivity in the dorso-lateral prefrontal cortex. This hypoactivity might be a result of mutual inhibition between affective system and the executive system. Neuronal basis for this inhibition can be given by lateral long distance inhibitory connections within the striatum. Recall that areas in the striatum that receive inputs from the cortical areas of the affective system are located in areas distinct from those that receive inputs from the executive system[20]. As we know, the executive system controls a wide range of cognitive operations including working

---

[19]Recall that deep brain stimulation at high frequencies and large currents suppresses activity in the stimulated area.

[20]This is reflected in the parallel basal ganglia thalamo-cortical circuits of cognitive and limbic origin.

memory, attention, and social motivation. So, cognitive symptoms of depression are associated mostly with dopaminergic innervations in the executive system and may be targeted by the corresponding medication. The suppression of the executive system effects mainly the dominant hemisphere and is reflected in alpha asymmetry in background EEG (more alpha activity at the left side) and in decrease of ERP components associated with the executive system.

IV. TREATMENT

A. Cognitive Behavioral Therapy

Cognitive behavioral therapy is a psychological treatment with roots going back to the times of Sigmund Freid. Psychotherapies are now generally recommended as treatment of milder depression or as an adjunct to antidepressant drugs in more severe illness. The main idea behind this type of treatment is that depressive symptoms arise from dysfunctional beliefs and thoughts developed in early learning experiences. These schemata are activated by a situation or an event that has a specific meaning for the individual. So, the main focus of cognitive behavioral therapy is to identify and challenge negative automatic schemata. Several studies have shown the advantage of cognitive-behavioral therapy over other psychological therapies and placebo[21].

B. ECT and Psychosurgery

Currently accepted methods of physical treatment of depression have been described as early as 1937, with the introduction of electroconvulsive therapy (ECT). ECT despite public and professional worries remains the most effective treatment for depression[22]. The main objection to ECT has been its liability to cause cognitive impairment. However a recent meta-analysis by ECT Review Group in the United Kingdom published in *Lancet* in 2003 indicates that cognitive impairment after ECT consists mostly of short-lasting anterograde and retrograde amnesia.

In 1940–1950s psychosurgery, and more specifically frontal lobotomy, began to be used for the treatment of depression. Later in 1960s the first drugs that could lessen symptoms of major depression were incidentally discovered. This discovery of antidepressant drugs and the study of their pharmacology have revolutionized

---

[21]The results of meta-analysis of the effects of cognitive therapy in depressed patients are present in paper by (Gloaguen et al., 1998).

[22]Note that ECT is also applied for treatment of schizophrenia implying that ECT is the most efficient if depression is combined with psychotic symptoms, such as delusions and hallucinations.

the field[23]. In addition, the massively destructive psychosurgery was replaced by
the modern stereotactic approach allowing precise insertion of electrodes and providing a tool for DBS[24]. A group of researchers from Toronto University in Canada
(Mayberg et al., 2005) recently treated six patients with severe refractory depressive disorder[25]. In this study electrodes were implanted in the white matter lateral
to the subgenual anterior cingulate. The authors reported striking and sustained
remission of depression in four of the six patients. PET images showed a reduction
of metabolism in the subgenual area which was initially elevated in those patients
in comparison to healthy controls.

C. Antidepressants

Antidepressants are in fact a heterogenous group of drugs that act primarily by
increasing the availability of monoamines at the synaptic cleft. Understanding
their pharmacology has provided the means for the formulation of the monoamine hypothesis of depression. It has also broadened the approach of developing
new drugs, such as the selective serotonin reuptake inhibitors.

Each of the many antidepressant drugs has a success rate of about 60 per cent.
At present, there are no reliable predictors of clinical response to specific antidepressants. So, when patients do not respond to one drug, they are switched to
another one, usually of a different class, until various classes of antidepressants are
tried. Because a clinical response occurs after 6–8 weeks, a patient can undergo
several months of trials and errors until an effective antidepressant is identified. This
process is expensive and time consuming. Moreover it leads to increased likelihood
of suicide because patients can have partial responses that improve psychomotor
state but not depressive feelings. And finally, in spite of trail-and-error method of
pharmacological treatment of depression, quite many patients remain unresponsive
to any of known drugs.

A lack of effective pharmacological treatment forced medical science to seek
for alternative forms of treatment, such as EEG-based neurofeedback, transcranial
direct current stimulation (tDCS), deep brain stimulation (DBS), transcranial magnetic stimulation (TMS). All these approaches (together with traditional ones) need
reliable objective measures of disease for diagnosis and monitoring the course of
treatment.

Table 21.1 summarizes most of the currently available treatments of major
depression.

[23]There are now dozens of approved drugs, which belong to four different classes – tricyclic drugs,
selective serotonin reuptake inhibitors, MAO inhibitors, and miscellaneous antidepressants.

[24]Deep brain stimulation as a currently experimental treatment offers an intervention similar to
neurosurgery but, in contrast to it, is reversible and enable placebo control for a particular patient.

[25]Those were patients who had failed to respond to antidepressant, psychotherapeutic, and electroconvulsive therapies.

TABLE 21.1   Currently available treatments for major depression

Type of intervention	Mechanism of action
Tricyclic antidepressants	Inhibition of serotonin and noradrenaline reuptake
Monoamine oxidase inhibitors (MAOIs)	Inhibition of MAO_A and associated inhibition of biogenic amine reuptake
Lithium	Unknown
Atypical antidepressants	Unknown
Selective serotonin reuptake inhibitors (SSRIs)	Inhibition of serotonin selective reuptake
Noradernaline reuptake inhibitors (NRIs)	Inhibition of noradrenaline selective reuptake
Serotonin and noradrenaline reuptake inhibitors (SNRIs)	Inhibition of mixed serotonin and noradrenaline reuptake
Electroconvulsive therapy (ECT)	Global electrical activation of neuronal circuits with intensive releasing of various mediators
Transcranial magnetic stimulation (TMS)	Aftereffects of local electromagnetic activation of neuronal circuits
Deep brain stimulation (DBS)	Chronic stimulation of the subgenual cingulate cortex
Cognitive-behavioral therapy	Unknown
Intrapersonal therapy	Unknown

D. TMS

Transcranial magnetic stimulation (TMS) as a potential method for treatment of depression was first applied in the end of 1990s. However, after initial enthusiasm the current assessment of the method is more moderate. The meta-analysis of all available data made in 2006 by Klaus Ebmeier and colleagues (Ebmeier et al., 2006) indicates a trend with size effects substantially decreasing from 1996 to 2004.

E. Neurofeedback

Neurofeedback for treatment of depression is based mainly on Davidson theory of asymmetrical alpha activity in the lateral frontal areas. On the basis of this theory Rosenfeld developed a neurofeedback protocol with the goal to normalize the abnormal asymmetry in depression. The so-called ALAY protocol (which stands for alpha asymmetry) uses the ratio $(F4 - F3)/(F3 + F4)$ as a biofeedback parameter. It has been used in case studies with encouraging preliminary results, but no controlled research has been conducted. For example, Baehr et al. (1997) carried out 1–5-year follow-ups on patients treated with the ALAY protocol and documented that the changes in depression were enduring and that the frontal alpha asymmetry not only had changed at the end of treatment but that this physiologic asymmetry continued to be reversed on long-term follow-ups. Unfortunately, no placebo control double-blind studies that are usually performed to prove efficacy of pharmacological treatment were conducted.

V. SUMMARY

Major depression is characterized by a triad of symptoms: (1) low or depressed mood, (2) anhedonia (loss of interest or pleasure in almost all activities), and (3) low energy or fatigue. It is a common understanding that there is no one brain structure that is responsible for depression symptoms and that there are several subtypes of depression depending on the structures involved. The heterogeneity of brain structures is expressed in diversity of symptoms, variability of the course, and highly individual responses to available treatments. EEG correlates of depression explore the idea of laterality of emotional reactions with negative emotions having a bias in activating the right hemisphere and positive emotions activating in more extent the left hemisphere. Some findings of frontal alpha asymmetry suggest that his parameter may represent a predisposition in reactivity to valence stimuli. Numerous neuroimaging studies associate sadness and depressed mood with increased neuronal activation in the medial prefrontal cortex. In contrast to hyperactivity of the medial frontal cortex executive dysfunction in major depression is reflected in hypoactivity in the dorso-lateral prefrontal cortex. According to the monoamine hypothesis, depression was postulated to reflect a deficiency in regulation of mediators noradrenaline and serotonin. In line with this hypothesis several antidepressant drugs increase synaptic concentrations of noradrenaline or serotonin. ECT remains the most effective treatment for depression. Antidepressant drugs has a success rate of about 60 per cent that forced the medical science to seek for alternative forms of treatment, such as EEG-based neurofeedback, tDCS, DBS, TMS. A so-called ALAY protocol has been invented to normalize the alpha asymmetry in depression.

CHAPTER 22

Alzheimer's Disease

I. DESCRIPTION OF BEHAVIOR

A. Symptoms

Neuronal cells are slowly dying with age. But in some, fortunately rare, cases this normal slow process turns into abnormally fast degenerative process. In 1906 a German physician Alois Alzheimer published his study on a 51 year old woman with severe dementia. He described behavioral symptoms and associated them with abnormalities found in this patient in the cerebral cortex and the limbic system. Now we are aware of two basic neuronal changes that occur in Alzheimer's disease: a loss of cholinergic cells in the basal forebrain and the development of neuritic plaques in the cerebral cortex located mostly in the temporal lobe areas[1].

II. MEDIATORS

A. Association with Cholinergic/GABA Septal-Hippocampal Circuits

As we learnt earlier, episodic memory is associated with cholinergic/GABA septal-hippocampal circuits. These circuits apparently are responsible for chunking

---

[1]The plaque consists of a central core of a homogeneous protein material known as amyloid, surrounded by degenerative cellular fragments.

information processing in the hippocampus and related structures. This hypothetical chunking is made at short bursts of the theta rhythm generated in the hippocampal circuits. The bursts of the hippocampal theta rhythm can be impaired by means of damage of the septum either due to anatomical destruction or due to physiological interventions by antagonists of acetylcholine. In line with the hypothesis of theta chunking of information encoding, the suppression of the limbic theta rhythm is associated with impairment of episodic memory.

B. Cholinergic Hypothesis of Alzheimer's Disease

The idea that some of the symptoms of Alzheimer's disease are due to a deficiency of the neurotransmitter acetylcholine in the brain first appeared in 1976, when Davies and Maloney published their paper in *Lancet*. Subsequent studies have confirmed their findings. The cholinergic hypothesis of Alzheimer's disease postulates that some of the cognitive decline experienced by patients with Alzheimer's disease results from a deficiency in cholinergic neurotransmission. This hypothesis stimulated a great deal of effort in experimental pharmacology. Most drugs approved for Alzheimer's disease treatment by the Food and Drug Administration (FDA) increase the availability of acetylcholine by reducing its breakdown.

III. NEURAL NET MODEL

A. Theta Bursts in Healthy Brain

Figure 22.1 depicts a hypothetical neuronal network that is responsible for consolidation of episodic memory and that might be impaired in Alzheimer's disease. As we know from Part II, episodic memory is formed by long-term potentiation in the hippocampal circuits by repetitive bursts of activation of hippocampal neurons. These bursts follow each other with 120–200 ms periods. Short lasting activations of hippocampal neurons during salient events are reflected in bursts of the theta rhythm in the hippocampus. This rhythmic activity is transported to the anterior cingulate cortex through the mammillary-thalamic tract and is seen at electroencephalogram (EEG) in a form of the frontal midline theta rhythm. The hippocampal theta rhythm is driven by the input from the septum so that the amplitude of theta bursts strongly depends on the activation of cholinergic neurons in the septum. The mechanism of theta generation involves inhibitory interconnections between septum and hippocampus.

B. Increase of Spontaneous Theta Activity in Diseased Brain

In Alzheimer's disease degeneration of septal neurons appears to decrease the septal inhibitory control of the hippocampal neurons and, as a consequence, dysinhibits

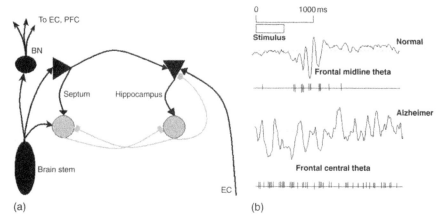

FIGURE 22.1 Neuronal network of Alzheimer's disease. (a) Neuronal network involved in generation of hippocampal theta rhythm. (b) Responses in EEG (recorded at Fz) and hypothetical impulse activity of neurons recorded in the hippocampus in a healthy subject (top) and in patient with Alzheimer's disease.

hippocampal neurons[2]. The dysinhibition leads to increase of spontaneous neuronal activity in the hippocampus (Fig. 22.1). The increased hippocampal activity appears to be grouped into slow fluctuations. These slow oscillations are seen at Fz in a form of fluctuations of frontally recorded cortical potentials in the range of theta–delta bands. These oscillations are quite different from the normal hippocampal theta rhythm because they are not time locked to silent stimuli and are not related to consolidation of episodic memory. Moreover, the lost of inhibitory control from the septal region could cause epileptiform activity in the hippocampus and, in some cases, even epileptic seizures[3]. In addition, degeneration of cholinergic cells of the basal nucleus (BN in Fig. 22.1) in Alzheimer's disease is expressed in decrease of the cholinergic input of the activating ascending system to the prefrontal cortex which in turn may be expressed in increase of slow activity and decrease of beta activity in prefrontal areas.

IV. IMAGING CORRELATES

A. QEEG

In a study at the University of Tübingen, Andreas Stevens and his colleagues (Stevens et al., 2001) recorded 19 channel EEG during eyes open, eyes closed

---

[2]For experimental evidence and for theoretical background see paper by Luis V. Colom from University of Texas at Brownsville.

[3]Indeed, in Alzheimer's disease, 10–22 per cent of patients suffer seizures that eventually necessitates anticonvulsant treatment (Mendez and Lim, 2003).

conditions as well as during watching pendulum condition[4] in patients with mild probable Alzheimer's disease and age/sex-matched controls[5]. A significant effect for discriminating two groups in absolute power and coherence was found only in the theta band that manifested an increased power and decreased coherence in patients. The most reliable parameter yielding the best results in discriminating patients was the coherence in the eyes open condition.

In a recent study by Roy John's laboratory in *New York University School of Medicine* (Prichep et al., 2006) the focus was made on normal elderly people with subjective cognitive complains to assess the utility of quantitative electroencephalography (QEEG) in predicting future decline within the next 7 years[6]. Spectral characteristics of EEG in decliners differed significantly ($p < 0.0001$) from non-decliners. QEEG of decliners was characterized by increases in theta power both in absolute and relative values, slowing of mean frequency, and changes in covariance among regions.

B. ERPs

Components of cognitive event-related potentials (ERPs) can also be used for discriminating patients with Alzheimer's disease from healthy controls. In a recent study from Stanford University, age- and dementia-related changes in ERPs were assessed during a picture–name verification task (Mathalon et al., 2003). The authors used response-synchronized ERPs as markers of response monitoring. Aging was associated with *slower behavioral responses* and decreased amplitude of error-related negativity (ERN) while dementia was associated with decreased accuracy and decreased ERN as compared with healthy controls of the corresponding age.

C. Principle Component Analysis of ERPs

An attempt for using principle component analysis of ERP components for discriminating Alzheimer's disease from normal population was made recently in a study from University of Rochester in USA (Chapman et al., 2007). The authors used a number–letter task. In addition to the well-known P3b, contingent negative variation (CNV), and slow wave (SW) the authors were able to separate other ERP components, including relatively early ones peaking at 145 and 250 ms (memory

---

[4]The last was designed to keep the subjects' attention engaged and the gaze fixed.

[5]Group differences in the EEG power spectra and coherence were largest during resting with eyes open, yielding almost 80 per cent correct classification result. Already in early stages of Alzheimer's disease EEG changes were topographically wide-spread.

[6]Forty-four normal elderly received extensive clinical, neurocognitive, and QEEG examinations at baseline. All subjects had only subjective complaints but no objective evidence of cognitive deficit.

storage component). The ERP component scores to relevant and irrelevant stimuli were used in discriminant analyses to develop functions that successfully classified individuals as belonging to an early-stage Alzheimer's disease group or a like-aged control group. Applying the discriminant function to the half of the data showed that about 90 per cent of the subjects were correctly classified into either the Alzheimer's disease group or the control group with a sensitivity of 1.00[7].

V. TREATMENT

A. Acetylcholinesterase Inhibitors

The main idea of current pharmacotherapy for Alzheimer's disease is to increase the levels of acetylcholine in the brain. It's usually implemented through inhibition of the cholinesterases. These drugs, known as acetylcholinesterase inhibitors (AChEIs), were first approved by the US FDA in 1995 based on clinical trials showing modest symptomatic benefit on cognitive, behavioral, and global measures[8].

B. Neurofeedback

Search for two items "Alzheimer's disease" and neurofeedback in the PubMed did not reveal any papers regarding the use of neurofeedback in correcting symptoms of Alzheimer's disease.

VI. SUMMARY

Alzheimer's disease is a degenerative brain disorder that starts with progressive memory loss. The loss of cholinergic cells in the basal forebrain appears to be responsible for the first stage in developing of the disease. The cholinergic hypothesis of Alzheimer's disease postulates that some of the cognitive decline experienced by patients with Alzheimer's disease results from a deficiency in cholinergic neurotransmission. Most drugs approved for the Alzheimer's disease treatment by the FDA increase the availability of acetylcholine by reducing its breakdown.

---

[7]The two cross-validation results were good with sensitivities of 0.83 and classification accuracies of 0.75–0.79.

[8]In 2004 the FDA approved memantine, an NMDA antagonist, for treating dementia symptoms in moderate to severe Alzheimer's disease cases. In clinical practice, memantine may be co-administered with an AChEI, although neither drug individually or in combination affects the underlying pathophysiology of dementia.

In Alzheimer's disease degeneration of septal neurons appears to decrease the inhibitory control of the hippocampal neurons and, as a consequence, increases the background activity in the hippocampus. This spontaneous hippocampal activity is seen at the frontal leads in a form of theta oscillations which are quite different from the frontal midline theta rhythm. QEEG of Alzheimer's patients is characterized by increases in theta power both in absolute and relative values.

CHAPTER 23

Methods of Neurotherapy

I. PLACEBO

A. Placebo as Expectation of Results

The first time when this problem faced me was the beginning of my carrier in 1970s. In those days we were working with Parkinsonian patients to whom electrodes were implanted for diagnostic and therapeutical purposes[1]. A colleague of mine (Vladimir M. Smirnov) was making deep brain electrical stimulations in the patients while I was recording impulse activity of neurons and slow electric potentials from the same patients and the same implanted electrodes. One day we were scheduled to demonstrate the results of our studies to the Head of Department Professor Natalia Bechtereva. Because we worked with the same patient we had to switch our machines (recording and stimulating) to show our results. First, I demonstrated the effect of motor action on multi-unit activity of neurons recorded by one of the electrodes. Then the colleague was going to demonstrate

---

[1]The author was working on his PhD thesis of application of slow processes for assessment of local metabolic processes in the patients of the Clinic of the Institute of Experimental medicine in Leningrad.

the effect of electrical stimulation at the same electrode and I was supposed to switch the machines. I was distracted by questions and forgot to do it. The colleague and the patient who were not aware of my fault demonstrated the effect quite well – the patient's tremor was inhibited when V.M Smirnov pressed the stimulation button. The point was the patient expected the effect and when he saw that the doctor was pressing a bottom it triggered the expectation. The sham showed its effect!

B. Neuronal Basis of Placebo

Figure 23.1 schematically simulates the placebo effect observed in the above mentioned case. The simulation is implemented by a two stimulus task with warning and trigger stimuli followed each with 2 s intervals. Recording are made in a patient with Parkinson's disease to whom multiple electrodes were implanted for diagnosis and therapy. An electrode was found, high frequency electrical stimulation of which suppressed tremor in the patient. Impulse activity of multi-neurons was recorded from the implanted electrodes. As one can see the warning stimulus alone increase the neuronal background activity and enhances neuronal reaction to the motor action. The deep brain stimulation (DBS) through this electrode increases the background activity and the reaction to action, but does not alter the preparatory

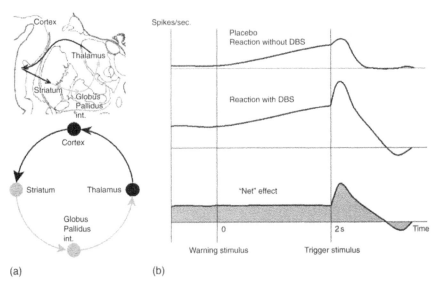

(a)   (b)

FIGURE 23.1   The placebo effect (a model). (a) A scheme of the position of the implanted electrode in a Parkinsonian patient. (b) Poststimulus time histograms (Y-axis – averaged discharge rate, X-axis – time). The poststimulus time histograms are computed for two cases: (1) for placebo, that is, no DBS, (top), (2) for DBS (middle). The net effect is depicted as the difference between the two histograms.

activity between the warning and the trigger stimulus. The reactions that precede the DBS are depicted at the top of Fig. 23.1, while reactions that immediately followed the DBS are shown in the middle. The "net" effect of stimulation that expressed as the difference between the two reactions is presented at the bottom. Note that the placebo induces preparatory activity similar to the one induced by the DBS – a so-called placebo effect, but the DBS evokes a larger response to the motor action. The net effect of the DBS is seen as the increase of the background activity and as well as the increase of reactivity of the thalamic neuron.

This simple observation was repeated 30 years later in a study of Benedetti et al. (2004). The authors recorded impulse activity of neurons in the subthalamic nucleus of Parkinsonian patients who had electrodes implanted for DBS. The activity from single neurons was recorded before and after placebo administration to see whether neuronal changes were linked to the clinical placebo response. The placebo consisted of a saline solution that was given to patients along with the suggestion that it was an antiparkinsonian drug. This procedure was performed intraoperatively after preoperative pharmacological conditioning with apomorphine, a powerful antiparkinsonian drug. It was found that the placebo responders showed a significant decrease of neuronal discharge and a reduction of bursting activity of subthalamic neurons, whereas the placebo non-responders did not. Remarkably, there was a nice correlation between the subjective reports of the patients, the clinical assessment of the neurologist, and the electrical activity of single neurons.

C. Need for Double-Blind Placebo-Controlled Studies

These observations demonstrate that any medical treatment (including DBS, pharmacological, and neurofeedback) encloses a psychological expectation that might affect the therapeutic outcome. The effect of expectation is called placebo (or sham) effect. Recall from Chapter 12, that during preparatory operations the widely distributed executive system (including the dorso-lateral prefrontal cortex and the basal ganglia) is activated. Moreover, neuronal reactions during motor preparatory set in some cases are similar to reactions to motor actions per se[2].

In the context of this book we pose the problem of placebo effects for two reasons. First, the placebo effects show a power of human ability for self-regulation. These effects have a real neurophysiological basis that can be revealed by electroencephalogram (EEG) and other imaging methods. Second, the placebo effect must be excluded in order to prove the efficiency of any new therapeutic method. For this reason, any new method must be tested in placebo-controlled double-blind studies. Double-blind means that neither subjects nor experimenters know whether

---

[2]Classical Pavlovian reflex may be considered as another example of placebo effect. Indeed, after multiple association of a conditional stimulus with the reward the dog reacts to the conditional stimulus as to the reward.

the testing is a real one or a sham. In such studies a sham treatment (the placebo) is given, but the patient believes it is effective and expects a clinical improvement. The placebo effect is the outcome after the sham treatment. A review on the placebo effect is given by Fabrizio Benedetti and colleagues in *The Journal of Neuroscience* in 2005 (Benedetti et al., 2005).

II. NEUROFEEDBACK

> These are still the early days of neurofeedback. Every day we are learning new ways of thinking about brain dis-regulation and new ways of training the brain to self-regulate more effectively... This is in flux. It has always been in flux. It will continue to be in flux.
>
> Sue Othmar in her note on 8th of August 2001

A. History

The *main* events in the history of neurofeedback are briefly presented in Table 23.1. The first attempt to present large review of the studies in the field was made in the book "Introduction to Quantitative EEG and Neurofeedback" edited by Evans, J.R., Abarbanel A. in 1999.

Physiology of conditioned reflexes forms an objective background for neurofeedback[3]. The experiments on conditioned reflexes were carried out by Ivan Pavlov in the Institute of Experimental Medicine in St. Petersburg. The institute was founded in 1990 by prince Odenburgsky – a member of the Russian Royal family[4]. The fruitful ideas of Pavlov's were further developed by his pupils. In the end of 1940s, Petr Kupalov, a former student of Pavlov, invented a methodology of situational conditioned reflexes. In the west this method was coined as the method of operant conditioning. In the method animal behavioral reactions but not external stimuli served as unconditioned stimuli. In times of Pavlov those reactions

---

[3]We presume that the readers are familiar with the Pavlovian method of conditioned reflexes. A famous Russian psychologist Ivan Pavlov was the first who in the beginning of 20th century used this method to study physiological mechanisms of psychological functions. In the Pavlovian method, some conditioned stimulus initially having little behavioral significance for an animal is associated in time with some reinforcement or reward (in Pavlovian terminology, unconditioned stimulus). The conditioned stimulus could be a visual or an auditory stimulus. The unconditioned stimulus could be a piece of meat for dogs, or a small amount of juice for monkeys. The reward having a vital significance for the animal induced essential changes in its behavior and physiological reactions (salivation, for example). Now, if feeding the dog has been many times accompanied with the metronome sound, some time later the dog will salivate in response to the sound itself – conditioned reflex has been established in the animal.

[4]Our laboratory is located just 200 m from the laboratory in the Institute of Experimental Medicine where Ivan Pavlov carried out his research on conditioned reflexes. In a museum after his name there is a harmony – an old musical instrument similar to organ – that Ivan Pavlov used for his experiments to generate conditioned stimuli.

TABLE 23.1 History of Neurofeedback

Year	Event
Beginning of XX century	Ivan P. Pavlov developed the method of studying conditioned reflexes in dogs
End of 1940s	Petr S. Kupalov developed the method of situational conditioned reflexes in animals
1930–1940s	Norbert Wiener and Petr K. Anokhin formulated the idea of feedback in self-regulation of live organisms
1960s	Barry Sterman (US) carried out experiments on conditioned reflexes in cats and used the results for the treatment of epilepsy
1962	Joe Kamiya (US) showed that a person can control his/her own alpha rhythm in the presence of feedback
1960–1970s	Nikolay N. Vasilevsky and Natalia V. Chernigovskaya (USSR) formed theoretical and practical basis for the modern biofeedback method
1970s	Niels Biermbaum (Germany) used slow brain electric processes for biological feedback and began to use this method successfully for epilepsy treatment
1970–1980s	Joel Lubar (US) proved efficiency of beta training for ADHD treatment
Mid-1980s	Application of neurometrics (Roy John, USA) for constructing protocols of EEG-biofeedback
Present	LORETA based and fMRI biofeedback protocols were initiated. In 2006, the *International Journal for Neurotherapy* celebrated its 10th anniversary.

were usually the motor ones such as the animal runs into a specific section of an experimental room. In 1930 an American mathematician Norbert Wiener in collaboration with a Mexican psychologist Arturo Rosenblueth introduced concept of feedback in relation to biological systems. This concept was further on evolved into a new science coined by Wiener "Cybernetics" in his book published in 1948. About the same time, a Russian scientist Petr K. Anokhin, a student of Pavlov and Bechterev, in 1935 developed a theory of functional systems. The key element of this theory was neuronal feedback – an interaction between a so-called "acceptor of actions" and behavioral adjustment of the animal.

Following these traditions of the Russian school of physiological science, Nikolay Vasilevsky, Professor of the Institute of Experimental Medicine, started his studies of cellular mechanisms of neurofeedback regulation in late 1960s and early 1970s. Natalia Chernigovskaya who worked in the department of human physiology of the same institute in those years started using the method of biological feedback for treating some neurological and psychiatric diseases. The idea was simple: to train the brain or muscles (as in the case of cerebral palsy) by using physiological parameters as a feedback. EEG patterns, electric activity of muscles, and slow metabolic processes were used for biofeedback. Approximately at the same time Joe Camiya, an American researcher observed that subjects could learn to voluntarily control their alpha waves. To achieve this goal, every time, when a subject generated the alpha rhythm, the researcher reported this fact. Thus, though Norbert Wiener and Petr Anokhin formulated the idea of feedback in 1930–1940s, only in 1960 it was shown for the first time that EEG parameters can serve as feedback for self-regulating the brain. Further Barry Sterman in his studies with cats introduced a rhythm associated with the sensory-motor system and therefore named as "sensory-motor rhythm." Using operant conditioning, cats were trained to produce this rhythm for food reward. It was also discovered that overtraining protected these animals from experimentally induced seizures. Shortly after that, training of sensory-motor rhythm was applied to epileptic patients. In these studies EEG biofeedback significantly reduced seizures and normalized the EEG.

In 1969, the method of brain self-regulation by means of EEG and other physiological parameters was officially named biological feedback (biofeedback). EEG biofeedback was implemented for treating neuroses and epilepsy neurofeedback as well as an antistress rehabilitation therapy for Vietnam veterans[5]. In 1970s, Niels Biermbaum and his colleagues in Germany started using slow brain electric activity for biofeedback treatment of epilepsy and schizophrenia.

That was a period of euphoria when biofeedback seemed to be a possible panacea for all brain diseases. However, in 1974, an article by Linch et al. showed that the subjects who learned to control their own alpha rhythm with eyes open were not able to increase it more than they could do with eyes closed. The article showed limitations of human abilities in EEG biofeedback, but the constraints were treated too literally and neurofeedback became unpopular[6]. However, a few enthusiasts continued to work with EEG biofeedback. Studies of Joel Lubar from University of Tennessee, USA played an important role in 1970–1980s. He proved that sessions with training beta rhythm UP and simultaneously theta rhythm

---

[5]The antistress rehabilitation neurofeedback includes training of the theta rhythms in EEG with the aim to bring a subject into a changed state of consciousness.

[6]There seemed to be many reasons why neurofeedback got a bad reputation in those years. One of them is misusing this approach in clinical applications. Note that it easy to perform neurofeedback in a wrong way for many reasons: (1) because of the lack of experience, (2) because of the lack of objective criteria for selection of an appropriate protocol (recall that in those years QEEG was seldom used before neurofeedback treatment), and (3) because of the lack of solid experimental support and validation of the selected protocol. So, a transition from laboratory experiments to clinical practice was too fast. The obvious limitations of neurofeedback were used by its opponents against this approach. One should also remember that EEG equipment in those days was rather expensive. Moreover, the method itself is quite sensitive to artifacts and therefore very demanding and time-consuming. It was quite easier for a clinician to use drugs in his/her practice than to invest time and money in this sophisticated and rather unproven approach.

DOWN significantly reduced hyperactivity and improved attention in attention deficit hyperactivity disorder (ADHD) patients (Lubar et al., 1995; Lubar, 1997). However these years were mostly associated with trial and error approach without using of any reliable scientific theory of neurofeedback.

In the same time (in early 1970s) a new approach in the field of EEG was developed. It was coined by Roy John from New York University Medical Center as neurometrics (John et al., 1977)[7]. The idea behind neurometrics was to quantitatively compare parameters of individual EEG with those computed for a normal group. It was a revolutionary idea because up to these years only visual inspection of raw EEG signals had been considered as a gold standard in electroencepalography.

In mid-1980s, the two approaches, EEG biofeedback and neurometics, merged forming a new direction that is now named neurotherapy[8]. An American company Lexicor was the first to produce neurotherapeutic devices. At present, the new approach is actively developing and extending. New views for the genesis of EEG rhythms made it possible to form a theoretical basis for neurotherapeutic approach. Several companies are now specialized in EEG analysis and in development of individual neurotherapeutic protocols.

B. Bulldozer Principle of Neurofeedback

Neurofeedback is based on two facts: (1) the brain state (including any dysfunction or dysregulation) is objectively reflected in parameters of EEG recorded from the scalp, (2) the human brain has plasticity to memorize the desired (and thereby, rewarded) state of the brain. In the neurofeedback technique, some current parameters of EEG recorded from a subject's scalp (such as an EEG power in a given frequency band, or a ratio of EEG powers in different frequency bands) are presented to the subject through visual, auditory, or tactile modality with the task to voluntarily alter these parameters in a desired (leading to a more efficient mode of brain functioning) direction. The position of electrodes and EEG parameters (called neurofeedback parameters) vary depending on the goals of neurofeedback. Altogether, the position of electrodes and the neurofeedback parameter define a so-called protocol of neurofeedback. For medical applications, most of neurofeedback practitioners implicitly or explicitly use a bulldozer principle of neurofeedback. According to this principle the aim of neurofeedback is to normalize a pathologically abnormal EEG pattern. So, if there is an excess of some EEG parameter in a particular patient and in particular location in the cortex, the aim of the neurofeedback is to train this parameter DOWN, if there is a lack of some other EEG characteristic,

---

[7]He gave this name in analogy to psychometrics which is a branch of psychology that studies differences of psychological measures between patients and control groups.

[8]In the present book we are using the concept of neurotherapy in a broader sense, including in it all other neurophysiologically based techniques, such as fMRI-biofeedback, tDCS, TMS, DBS.

the corresponding neurofeedback parameter is trained UP. The method works like a bulldozer filling in the cavities and excavating the bumps.

C. Comparison with the Database

The current practice of neurofeedback in clinical applications presumes several steps for its implementation. The *first step* includes constructing neurofeedback protocol on the basis of quantitative electroencephalogram (QEEG)[9] assessment. As we showed in this book a tremendous amount of empirical knowledge in EEG analysis reveals some abnormal QEEG patterns associated with various medical and psychiatric disorders. For example, a group of ADHD population is character-ized by excess of the theta beta ratio in parietal–central–frontal (depending on age) locations[10].

Placement of at least 19 electrodes is usually required[11] for QEEG analysis. Spectral characteristics of EEG in eyes open, eyes closed conditions, and in some psychological tasks (such as oddball task or arithmetic task) are compared statisti-cally to a normative database. The comparison to the normative data provides sci-entifically objective information on how the patient's spontaneous brain activity differs from age-matching healthy subjects. The statistically significant deviations from normality at spectra or coherence difference curves define the parameters of neurofeedback procedure such as position of electrodes (e.g., Fz, Cz) and the neu-rofeedback parameter (e.g., beta theta ratio). This step is schematically depicted in Fig. 23.2.

D. Defining Electrodes' Position

A fragment of raw EEG in an ADHD girl of 13 years old is presented on the top left of Fig. 23.2. EEG spectra in the whole epoch of eyes open condition was calculated (not shown) and compared with the normative spectra. The difference spectra (patient-norm) together with Z-scores are presented at the middle of Fig. 23.2. Note an excess ($p < 0.001$) of slow activity at Cz electrode. In line with the excess of slow activity, the theta beta ratio (inattention index) computed for Cz[12]

---

[9]In the last few years in addition to QEEG assessment some laboratories and neurofeedback practi-tioners started to use independent component analysis (ICA) of cognitive ERPs. It looks like that this approach will soon become a gold standard because it gives an entirely new data regarding stages of information processing in the human brain.

[10]The theta beta ratio was labeled as inattention index.

[11]Nineteen seems to be is a minimal number of electrodes that enables the user to make 2D maps and s-LORETA images with reasonable (for practical purposes) spatial resolution.

[12]Note, that the theta beta ratio was computed for local average (according to Lemos) montage and therefore is slightly different from the one computed by Monastra et al. in their paper (Monastra et al., 1999).

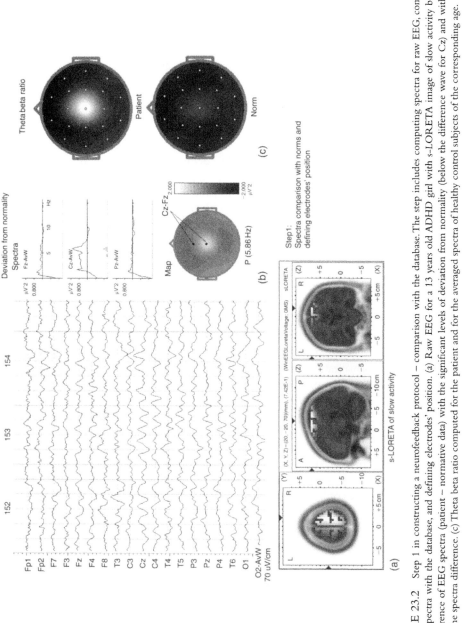

FIGURE 23.2 Step 1 in constructing a neurofeedback protocol – comparison with the database. The step includes computing spectra for raw EEG, comparing the spectra with the database, and defining electrodes' position. (a) Raw EEG for a 13 years old ADHD girl with s-LORETA image of slow activity below. (b) Difference of EEG spectra (patient – normative data) with the significant levels of deviation from normality (below the difference wave for Cz) and with the map of the spectra difference. (c) Theta beta ratio computed for the patient and for the averaged spectra of healthy control subjects of the corresponding age.

in this patient is 2.5 times higher than the corresponding parameter in a group of healthy subjects of the matching age. This fact indicates location of one electrode for neurofeedback protocol, namely Cz. The second electrode can be defined on the basis of the gradient of the spectral parameter. The gradient of the map of deviation from normality in theta (6 Hz) frequency range shows that the difference wave sharply decreases at Fz. This observation indicates location of the second electrode for neurofeedback protocol[13].

E. Defining Neurofeedback Parameter

After defining electrodes' position we need to define a neurofeedback parameter – a spectral characteristic of EEG that we are going to train. For this reason, we need to reconstruct the raw EEG pattern in the patient using the electrodes' location that we already defined. In the Human Brain Normative Database for remontaging we are using the EEG recorded in the patient in eyes open condition. This enables us to reconstruct what the EEG pattern in this particular patient will look like in the selected montage of the two electrodes. The result of remontaging is presented in Fig. 23.3 bottom. A spectrum for the total EEG epoch in eyes open condition is in presented at the right. Using this spectrum we can define the frequency bands for computing the neurofeedback parameter. The low frequency band may be between 3 and 7 Hz, while the high frequency band may be from 13 to 21 Hz. To normalize the spectrum (i.e., to make it closer to normative data) of the patient we have to enhance the high frequency activity and to suppress the low frequency activity. The "normalization" procedure can be done by using just only one parameter: the ratio of EEG powers computed for low and high frequency bands[14].

F. Training Procedure

The second step is the training process per se. During neurofeedback training, usually two electrodes are placed on the scalp at locations defined at the first stage. A ground electrode could be placed on any location, but usually one of the earlobes

---

[13]Note that in this example for the neurofeedback procedure we choose a bipolar montage of electrodes. According to our experience the bipolar montage is less sensitive to artifacts (such as eye movements). This montage, however, has one disadvantage – the training area includes a larger cortical area (covered by both electrodes) in comparison to monopolar montage. Still, if the gradient of the deviated parameter is rather sharp the bipolar montage is preferable.

[14]Some neurofeedback systems use two or even more parameters for training. They are based on human ability to follow several parameters simultaneously. However, our practice shows that the neurofeedback procedure with one neurofeedback parameter works at least not worse than a procedure with multiple parameters.

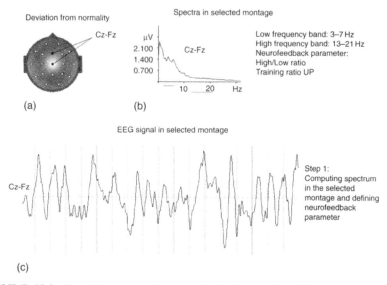

Deviation from normality

Cz-Fz

Spectra in selected montage

μV
2.100
1.400
0.700

Cz-Fz

10   20   Hz

Low frequency band: 3–7 Hz
High frequency band: 13–21 Hz
Neurofeedback parameter:
High/Low ratio
Training ratio UP

(a)   (b)

EEG signal in selected montage

Cz-Fz

Step 1:
Computing spectrum
in the selected
montage and defining
neurofeedback
parameter

(c)

FIGURE 23.3   Step 1 in constructing a neurofeedback protocol – defining a neurofeedback parameter. (a) Map of deviation from normality in spectra at 6 Hz. (b) Spectrum for the montage Cz-Fz for the total EEG epoch in eyes open condition. (c) A fragment of EEG of this patient computed at Cz-Fz montage.

serves as the background electrode. In comparison to other techniques, such as TMS, DBS, and tDCS no electrical current is injected into the brain. The electrodes simply measure the ongoing brain EEG while the computer regularly calculates the neurofeedback parameter and depicts it in some way to the patient. In our daily life without neurofeedback devices we are unable to influence the EEG in a desirable way because humans as probably other animals lack the awareness of the EEG patterns.

There are many neurofeedback systems designed by different manufactures such as Lexiocor, Brain Master, Thought Technology, Brain Inquiry … The critical points of any programmed neurofeedback procedure include two characteristics that describe: (1) how reliable is the computed neurofeedback parameter to reflect the current state of the brain and (2) how frequent the parameter is presented to the subject so that the parameter consistently follows changes in the state of the brain.

The first characteristic is actually the integration period within which the EEG current fluctuations are integrated. This period of integration is also called a sliding window. The second characteristic is the time intervals within which the integrated parameter is presented to the subject. From event-related potential (ERP) studies we know that the state of the brain can be changed in 100 ms time interval while the subject reacts to a stimulus within 300 ms. It gives us a temporal estimation

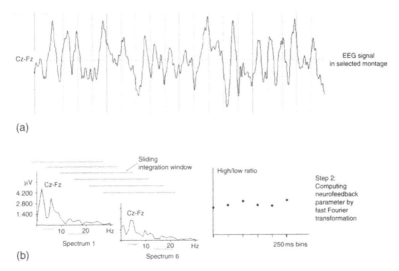

FIGURE 23.4   Step 2 – on-line computing the neurofeedback parameter by FFT. (a) A fragment of raw EEG in the selected montage. (b) Spectra are computed using FFT in 1-s sliding window that shifts every 250 ms. The neurofeedback parameter is computed and presented on the screen (c).

of how fast the computed parameter has to be presented to the subject[15]. In modern computers calculations are very quick so that theoretically the rate of neurofeedback parameter presentation can be rather high. For reliable measuring of EEG spectra we need at least 1 s of recording, that is, 10 cycles of the dominant rhythm. It gives us an estimation of the integration parameter of neurofeedback[16].

G. Computing Neurofeedback Parameters

Different manufactures offer different ways of computing spectral characteristics of neurofeedback parameter. The methods are (1) the Fourier decomposition using fast Fourier transformation – FFT (see Fig. 23.4) and (2) the digital filtration using finite impulse response – FIR (see Fig. 23.5), or (3) infinite impulse response (IIR) digital filters (for details see Methods of Part I). Any of the methods has its advantages and limitations. Not going into technical details, both theoretical considerations and the experience that we got in our laboratory show that IIR filters are preferable.

[15]In example in Fig. 23.3 the "refreshing" interval is selected of 250 ms.
[16]In example in Fig. 23.3 the integration sliding window is equal to 1 s. Note that 1 s is actually the time interval that could be achieved in modern MRI machines. This makes MRI-biofeedback a valuable tool for correcting brain dysfunction.

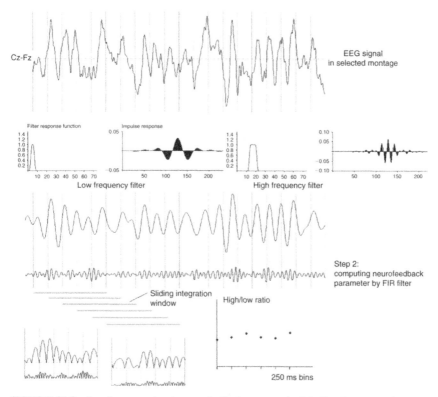

FIGURE 23.5   Step 2 – computing the neurofeedback parameter by FIR filter. From top to bottom – raw EEG, parameters of FIR filters, filtrated EEG, fragments of squared filtered EEG (EEG power in a given frequency band) for 1-s sliding windows. The neurofeedback parameter is defined as the ratio of EEG power in two frequency bands.

So, when subjects get a feedback from their brain, that is, they see or hear representations of neurofeedback parameter, they are supposed to learn how to change this parameter in a desirable direction. The patient is usually placed in front of a computer screen. The computer display may be as simple as possible, for example, a vertical bar on the screen, or can present a kind of complex multi-dimension display with different colors and shapes. The screen could be also a computer game designed by the manufacturing company specifically for neurofeedback, or a commercial computer game (such as Need-for-Speed) in which a parameter of the game (such as the speed of the car) is controlled by the neurofeedback. In our own research and practice we are using a technology that includes computer, video player (it could be also built-in the computer), and TV or computer screen. The subjects watch their favorable movies[17] while the neurofeedback parameter

[17]They are asked to bring a new disk at each session to motivate them to work intensively.

calculated by the computer controls the quality of the video picture: the more "normal" is the parameter, the better is the picture.

In all ways of presenting the neurofeedback parameter the patient concentrates on the feedback and tries to learn the association between the parameter and his/her state. It is not an easy task. Moreover, it can be achieved in different ways. This ambiguity raises a question: how to guide the patient to achieve the task in the most efficient way. Some practitioners prefer not to give any instructions to their patients by simply saying "Just do it." Some practitioners give instructions depending on the type of neurofeedback procedure: relaxation or activation. The learning procedure during neurofeedback training may be compared with the technique how we learn to drive the bicycle. It takes time to learn driving a bicycle!

H. Training Curve

The second step in neurofeedback procedure presumes that after each session the results of training are checked by the practitioner. The point is that not all patients can learn to control a biofeedback parameter. There are several reasons for that: (1) inappropriate selection of the parameter – the practitioner's fault; (2) inability to associate the parameter change with the subjective state – the patient's fault. To assess how well the patient controls the parameter the manufacturing companies supply tools for computing so-called "training curves." The training curve is a smoothed dynamic of the parameter during a single session. If the parameter during the "training" period is statistically different at $p < 0.05$ from that of the "resting" period then the session can be considered as successful (Fig. 23.6). If during 5–7 sessions the practitioner does not see any signs of success the sessions must be interrupted and a new protocol have to be suggested.

I. Learning Curve

The third step in neurofeedback procedure includes the assessment of improvements produced by sequential sessions of neurofeedback. Usually around 5 sessions are required to learn to change the neurofeedback parameter in a desired direction, while 20–35 additional sessions are required to practice this ability in order to "consolidate" the acquired skill. The dynamics of the EEG parameter is reflected in a so-called "learning curve." The learning curve represents dynamics of absolute or relative index of training in each session. Figure 23.6 represents a method of calculating a relative measure of success of the training procedure in a single session. The measure is computed as a ratio of the average neurofeedback parameter during training and resting periods. The confidence level of the difference between two values can be estimated.

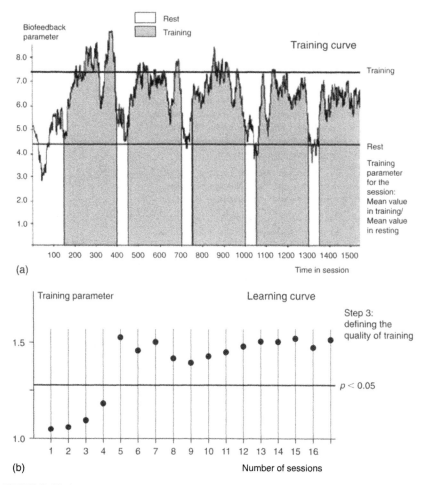

FIGURE 23.6   Step 3 – defining the quality of neurofeedback. (a) Training curve – a smoothed dynamics of the neurofeedback parameter during a single session. The success of the training is defined as the ratio of the mean neurofeedback parameter in the training period divided by the mean neurofeedback parameter in the resting period of the session. This ratio is plotted versus number of session thus giving a so-called learning curve (b).

J. Techniques for Computing Neurofeedback Parameter

It should be stressed here that neurofeedback protocols are not confined by FFT or digital filtration of the current EEG. Other neurofeedback parameters have been suggested. One of those parameters is a measure of correlation between EEG in different cortical locations, such as coherence or co-modulation (suggested by Bary Sterman and David Kaiser in their normative database).

TABLE 23.2   Techniques of Neurofeedback

Name	Neurofeedback parameters	Examples of implementation
EEG spectra	The EEG power in certain frequency bands, or the ratio of EEG powers in two frequency bands of one channel EEG, or the ratio of EEG powers computed in the same frequency band but for different electrodes. FFT, wavelet transformation, or digital filtration are used for extracting these parameters	Sterman, 1989, 1996; Lubar, 1997; Lubar et al., 1995
EEG coherence	The coherence measures reflecting how EEG powers in a given frequency band correlate between distinct scalp electrodes	Horvat, 2004
LORETA	The virtual EEG computed by LORETA for an area of interest and the corresponding spectral characteristics	Congedo et al., 2004
s-LORETA	The intracranial current density computed by means of s-LORETA	Ponomarev and Kropotov, in publication

The other approach is to use low resolution electromagnetic tomography (LORETA or s-LORETA) in order to train a local area in the cortex. The rationale for this approach is the fact that any scalp electrode picks up activity not from the underlying cortex but from widely distributed cortical areas. So, that if we want to use an EEG-feedback from a local cortical area we need to apply tomographic methods that enable us to compute an intracortical EEG on the basis of multiple scalp-recorded EEG. The local intra cortical EEG extracted from the scalp recorded multi-channel EEG is called a virtual EEG. The method of constructing the virtual intracortical EEG for training a local area in the cortex was first applied by Marco Congedo in the laboratory of Joel Lubar (Congedo et al., 2004)[18]. The authors coined this method as LORETA neurofeedback. Recently in our laboratory we developed the software for deriving the local current density of an intracranial area by means of s-LORETA method. The method itself provides no localization error and has been recently developed by Roberto Pascual-Marqui (Pascual-Marqui, 2002). All known EEG-based feedback techniques are listed in Table 23.2.

[18]LORETA provides a tool for computing the current density of generators located on the surface of the cortex including gyri and sulci. The solution is actually a matrix which by multiplication with the multi-channel EEG data gives the result – the current density of cortical micro dipoles. When the area within the cortex is defined, it is feasible to find a so-called inverting matrix. Marco Congedo and his co-workers used LORETA-based neurofeedback to enhance low beta (16–20 Hz) and suppress low alpha (8–10 Hz) current density amplitude (vector length) in a region corresponding approximately to the anterior cingulate cognitive division. The region of interest included 38 voxels encompassing from the total number of 2394 voxels.

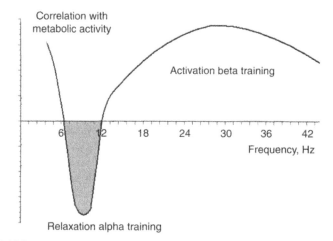

FIGURE 23.7   EEG frequencies for activation and relaxation protocols. A scheme represents relationship between metabolic activity and EEG power in different frequency bands. Note that in the alpha band (8–12 Hz) the correlation is negative which defines the frequency parameter of "relaxation" protocols, while in the beta band the correlation is positive which defines the frequency parameter of "activation" protocols.

K. Types of Neurofeedback Protocols

From physiological point of view neurofeedback protocols can be divided into two big categories: activation and relaxation protocols. This division is made on the basis of the data regarding correlation between EEG activity in different frequency bands and the metabolic activity measured by positron emission tomography (PET) or functional magnetic resonance imaging (fMRI) in the corresponding cortical location[19] (Fig. 23.7). Activating protocols include enhancement of higher (>13 Hz) EEG frequencies, relaxing protocols include enhancement of alpha (8–12 Hz) frequencies and in some specific cases even lower than 8 Hz frequencies of EEG. Although the importance of electrodes' location can not be overestimated, below for didactic purposes we consider the protocols without any reference to electrode location.

1. Activation Protocols

A beta activating training is a common method used for variety of purposes. The protocol is intended to activate the corresponding cortical area. In our experience with relative beta training in ADHD children we sometimes encounter a significant

---

[19]See for example the data from (Cook et al., 1998) where they studied the relationship between local PET perfusion values and relative EEG power.

"aha" phenomenon when the trainee discovers the exact type of mental state that is associated with the production of high amplitude beta activity in the frontal areas. Children used to say: "Aha, now I know what it means to be attentive." Beta is usually trained on the left side, because according to Davidson's theory (see Chapter 13) activating the left side of the brain, especially the frontal lobes, is associated with elevating positive mood and producing positive emotions. Possible negative side effects may include agitation, irritability, or a sense of being "hyper." Therefore, sessions may be as short as 10 min, but usually last for 20–30 min. Often, beta training is used at the end of an EEG session, to bring the trainee into a state of energy and alertness[20].

Another type of activation protocols explores EEG coherence as feedback parameter. Coherence is a QEEG index that reflects correlation between EEG powers in two separate regions (see Methods Part I). Coherence is defined for a certain frequency band. Our studies show that children with ADHD have lower coherence in the alpha band at the frontal–central areas[21]. ADHD as an executive disorder seems to be characterized by poor coordination of the frontal-motor areas of the cortex that is manifested in decrease of coherency of EEG recorded in these areas. The fact that the ADHD population characterized by hypofrontality is described by hypocoherency might give a neurophysiological basis of "coherence" protocols. These protocols appear to be associated with activation of the training areas.

2. Relaxation Protocols

Alpha (8–12 Hz) training is a common method used for many purposes. Taking into account that alpha rhythms are idling rhythms of the brain we can speculate that the neurofeedback protocols oriented to activate alpha rhythms are relaxation protocols, that is, protocols that are intended to deactivate, inhibit the corresponding cortical areas. The relaxation training is often accompanied by presenting auditory stimuli, because visual stimuli activate and desynchronize the brain EEG in a larger extent than auditory stimuli.

3. Peninston-Kulkosky Protocol

The Peninston-Kulkosky protocol is a variant of relaxation protocols. It is designed as follows. Subjects are first taught deep relaxation by skin temperature

[20]Another type of activating protocols is associated with so-called "squash" protocols. The idea of squash training is to suppress the overall production of brain rhythms in wide frequency bands. It is suggested that by training the brain to suppress EEG oscillations (especially of large amplitude), we are reinforcing the desynchronized behavior of neurons – which is associated with activation. A squash protocol may be done on any part of the brain. However, certain practitioners prefer specific locations, such as the frontal areas, or the central area.

[21]The one distinct source of alpha activity at these areas is a family of mu-rhythms reflecting the idling state of the sensory-motor strip of the human cortex.

biofeedback using autogenic phrases and have at least 5 sessions of temperature feedback. In the following sessions they receive neurofeedback, namely while they are in an eyes closed and relaxed condition, they receive auditory signals from EEG apparatus using the O1 site as an area for EEG recording. A standard induction script that uses suggestions to relax and "sink down" into reverie is read. When alpha brain waves exceed a preset threshold, a pleasant tone is heard, and by learning to voluntarily produce this tone, the subject becomes progressively relaxed. When theta brain waves (4–8 Hz) are produced at sufficiently high amplitude, a second tone is heard, and the subject becomes more relaxed and, according to Peninston, enters a hypnagogic state of free reverie and high suggestibility. The transition from the state with dominance of alpha activity to the state with dominance of theta activity is called "crossover." When the trainee spends some time in the theta state, they may be extremely relaxed, even stuporous or languid. It is often necessary to coach or counsel the trainee afterward, to ensure that they do not leave in an excessively sensitive or internally directed state of mind.

L. Neurofeedback and Neurotherapy

In this book we separate the concept of neurofeedback from a more general notion of neurotherapy. Neurotherapy besides neurofeedback includes other electrophysiologically based methods of modulating the state of the brain. These methods are transcranial direct current stimulation (tDCS), AC-stimulation including deep brain stimulation (DBS), trancranial magnetic stimulation (TMS). Neurofeedback in turn can be divided into two subtypes: EEG biofeedback and DC (or infra slow wave) biofeedback. EEG biofeedback (as a sub-type of neurofeedback) is a method for correcting or tuning brain activity by means of electrophysiological feedback. In this feedback, some features of EEG such as EEG power in a given frequency band, intercortical coherence, or beta theta ratio are used as biofeedback parameters.

M. Eastern Self-Regulation Techniques

A parallel can be noticed between neurotherapy and Eastern self-regulation techniques. Ancient eastern arts of self-regulation such as yoga and chi-gun[22] are in

---

[22]Chi Gun is a Chinese meditation technique. Chi (pronounced more like "tsi") means the "life force", and Gun (pronounced more like "goon") means work, the work of chi. Unlike western medical healthcare Chi Gun is focused on relaxation – mental exercises, rather then on muscle exercises. According to Chinese doctrine Chi Gun helps to dysinhibit the "blocks" that prevent the human chi from moving around thus opening "energy channels." In terms of the modern medicine the explanation is not so straightforward. However we can speculate that muscles around our backbone can go to spasm and stay there for a very long time and this spasm can create all sorts of problems, from the

fact based on the human ability to affect internal psychological processes consciously. However, it takes a lot of time and energy to master those arts. Moreover, direct tutor–pupil interaction is often needed. In terms of modern neurofeedback technology, in the eastern self-regulation relaxation technique the tutor (guru) is served as a kind of "feedback" agent. In neurotherapy, learning process takes essentially less time and is directed by feedback going directly from the subject's brain. Moreover, neurofeedback is not confined by relaxation protocols.

N. Sham Effect

Special attention should be paid to placebo effects in neurotherapy (see Methods above). Placebo effect, as we learn from the previous, has distinct neuronal mechanisms, can amount up to 30 per cent from the "pure" effect of a medical drug and it would be no sense to negate its presence in neurofeedback. At early years of neurotherapy development, placebo effect was more than once checked for two protocols, the sensory-motor rhythm training and the beta training. At present, new protocols are compared not with placebo condition but with a situation when a patient takes a medical drug approved and effective for a given disease. This is done due to ethic reasons: it would be inhuman not to treat anyone if an efficient treatment is known.

O. Minimizing Side Effects

Just like a scalpel in surgery, biofeedback can cure but can also harm. The method must not be used without knowledge of what is wrong in a particular brain. Neurotherapy is a method for correcting specific symptoms based on combination of biofeedback with a neurometric diagnostic system. Neurometrics defines the electrophysiological basis of brain dysfunction and the type of EEG biofeedback protocol that should be applied in the particular case[23].

That is why neurotherapy must be performed only by a certified specialist who in turn must follow basic principles of neurotherapy in the practice. Only few

---

headach e to heart conditions. Consequently relaxation of these muscles will be favorable for the subject. Further we can speculate that our emotional state is closely related to our somatic sensations, in other words when we feel happy, we smile, but when we smile – you can also get a feeling of happiness. Consequently, training emotional state will be also favorable for the subject.

[23]Like any other method, biofeedback cannot be used without relevant diagnostic procedures. Though there are quite few reports about negative consequences of biofeedback usage, one should always remember that, if organization of EEG rhythms is changed in a wrong direction, a patient's brain could be dysregulated and symptoms could be elevated.

Universities provide courses in QEEG and neurotherapy. One of them is located in Texas, USA, the other in Trondheim, Norway[24].

One advantage of neurotherapy is that it minimizes side effects. It is not a secret that many pharmacological drugs affect not only the relevant neurotransmission but also other biochemical processes in the brain and in the body. That is why any description of a psychopharmacological drug includes a long list of side effects. In contrary to pharmacological drugs, neurotherapy affects brain processes selectively. Moreover, the subject actively participates in such a correction, avoiding harm effects, consciously or unconsciously, as any self-preserving creature. That is why side effects of neurotherapy are practically not mentioned in the literature, though it does not mean their absolute absence.

P. Stability of Effect

Another advantage of neurotherapy is the stability of effect. A neurotherapeutic procedure is in fact a learning one. The procedure is often compared with a process of acquiring a specific skill – for example, the one to ride a bicycle. One can hardly balance a bike mounting it for the very first time, but after several attempts he or she learns to ride holding the handle bar; while someone, after rather long training, manages even to ride without holding the bar. Similar adjustments happen in neurotherapy: at the beginning, it is difficult for a subject to catch an association between his/her own feelings and indexes of bioelectric activity displayed on the screen. However, as the association becomes gradually understandable, one's mind lights up: "Aha, I know how to do it!" Further, skills are improved and one learns to hold the needed condition for longer time and not only in the laboratory but also at home or in school. After 20–40 sessions the neurotherapy can be ceased but the skill will remain for the rest of the life[25].

Q. Limitations of Neurofeedback

Does all mentioned above mean that neurotherapy has no disadvantages at all? Of course, not. One of the factors restricting usage of neurotherapy is that the sessions of neurotherapy consume about 20–40 h of labor from the clinician and

[24]As was mentioned above the author is currently a Professor in the Norwegian University of Science and Technology in Trondheim teaching a course on QEEG and neurotherapy.

[25]Joel Lubar had a possibility to track histories for more than fifty of his patients for 10 years using objective measurement of behavioral parameters. Positive treatment results appeared to sustain for the whole period in almost all of the patients; however, some of them needed additional series of procedures to refresh their skills, and after one or two procedures the skills returned. Many people said that neurotherapy had changed their lives. In our research, we were able to track neurotherapy effects in children for a year. All children have been keeping brain indices of attention at a high level. If some of them lost skills due to psychic traumas or diseases, one or two additional sessions were enough to recover the skills.

the same amount of intense training from the patient[26]. In addition to that, before starting neurotherapy sessions, individual EEG must be recorded by a technician. Then, the type of brain dysregulation must be assessed by a specially trained person[27] and an individual neurotherapy protocol is to be constructed. This takes 3–5 working hours of the qualified specialists. Up to now, quite a few hardware/software devices for neurotherapy are developed over the whole world[28]. For most of those systems, additional EEG machines for recording multi-channel EEG for diagnostic purposes are needed[29].

Another factor to be considered in neurotherapy is motivation of a patient. Neurotherapy as any learning procedure is based on mood and motivation. The higher is the motivation level, the better are the acquired skills. Some neurotherapeutic centers stimulate children's motivation by prizes like money, toys, or tokens that can be later exchanged for toys or money. Assistance from family also plays an important role in successful neurotherapy. Indeed, during neurotherapy the brain is gradually changing, but to transfer these small changes into behavioral pattern additional efforts are needed. For example, attention is the parameter we are supposed to improve by the relative beta protocol, but attention is not the only parameter that defines behavior. To have good attention is not enough and the children must be able to use this new brain skill to obtain school knowledge, as well as to adapt his/her behavior when contacting with parents or other children. Some ADHD patients may appear not to be able to change established image of a "difficult" child on their own, needing help from the family and teachers. The parents may need special training in order to be able to help their child to get over these social–environmental difficulties.

R. Medical Versus Non-medical Application

Biofeedback is used for both medical and non-medical applications. Currently, in the United States the US Food and Drug Administration (US FDA) recognizes

---

[26]To reduce the waste of time for traveling back and forth the clinic, modern centers for neurotherapy offer so-called home trainers. In these cases, several initial sessions of neurotherapy are performed together with a specialist, and after the patient has developed primary skills, training session are continued at home. The patient can buy or rent a neurotherapeutic device that can be installed at home and connected to a computer or to a TV set.

[27]This person must read not only clinical EEG for detecting spikes and other paroxysms in EEG, but also has to know the QEEG, ERP, and basics of neurotherapy to be able to assess the patient's EEG and to give to the practitioner the recommendations for pharmo- and neuro-therapy. Only few Universities in the world teach students these subjects.

[28]These devices are produced by Thought Technology, Daymed, Brain Inquiry, Brain Master, and some other companies.

[29]In our institute (the Institute of the Human Brain of Russian Academy of Sciences) we developed a multi-functional system that can perform QEEG/ERP/ERD assessment as well as sessions of neurotherapy. The system has been tested in the Center for Neurotherapy of the Institute and is sold by a Russian manufacturing company "Mitsar, Ltd." (Saint Petersburg).

only relaxation training as an accepted use of EEG biofeedback. Medical applications, for example, protocols for treatment depression, seizures, headaches, autism, are considered either experimental or unproven. However, non-medical applications of neurofeedback protocols for general improvement in concentration and attention and for peak performance do not meet objections[30].

Any EEG-based biofeedback equipment may be provided in two versions, addressing both the medical and the non-medical communities. When it is marketed for clinical purposes, specific claims are made, and these claims must be reviewed and cleared by the US FDA or equivalent agencies in other countries. In the non-clinical embodiment the equipment is regarded as an educational and recreational device[31].

So far, published clinical studies deal with the following brain dysfunctions such as ADD/ADHD, conduct disorders, learning disabilities, anxiety, depression, chronic fatigue syndrome, epilepsy, autistic spectrum disorders. Neurotherapy has been also applied for helping drug addicts to relax; for rehabilitating after stroke and traumatic brain injury; as well as enhancing cognitive functions in aging. For non-medical application neurofeedback is used for improvement of attention, concentration, and for peak performance, assistance in meditation and relaxation techniques, improvement of personal awareness and mental fitness.

S. Types of Neurofeedback

The term EEG-feedback presumes using EEG parameters such as spectral indexes, coherence measures, intracranial current density derived by means of LORETA or s-LORETA. Theoretically any physiological parameter measured within the brain can be fed back to the patient and used for shaping the brain activity in a desired way. The list of physiological parameters used in neurofeedback is presented in Table 23.3.

1. ERP-Based Neurofeedback

A priori, ERP components as indexes of information flow might be applied for brain–computer interface (BCI). However, technical hurdles such as a small signal to noise ratio, the absence of normative databases for ERP components have precluded application of the ERP-based BCI. Recently in our laboratory we developed the first version of the ERP-based BCI software (Kropotov and Murashev, in preparation). A starting point for this approach is decomposition

---

[30]Any EEG system designed to enable the user to train for recreational, educational, or entertainment purposes is not a medical instrument. The FDA or an equivalent agency in other countries allows such devices to be produced and marketed freely, as long as they pose no undue health risk to the user.

[31]This is like a scalpel being marketed for surgical use, and for use in a science lab. The same instrument is being provided in both cases, but with different intent.

TABLE 23.3   Parameters of Neurofeedback

Name	Neurofeedback parameters	Examples of implementation
ERD-based neurofeedback	The relative changes of EEG power in a given frequency in response to either real or imagery actions are used as feedback parameters.	Pfurtscheller and Neuper, 2006
ERP-based neurofeedback	The ERP of a group of healthy subjects are decomposed into independent components characterized by topographies and time dynamics. The topographies serve for constructing spatial filters to extract the components from the individual ERPs. The amplitude or latency of the patient's individual components are compared with the normative data and further used as feedback parameters	Kropotov and Murashev, in preparation
Self-regulation of evoked SCP (slow cortical potentials)	Negative or positive shift of slow cortical potential in response to warning stimuli	Strehl et al., 2006
Self-regulation of fMRI (functional magnetic resonance imaging)	Hemodynamic brain activity as indexed by BOLD (blood oxygen level dependent) response	Weiskopf et al., 2004
Self-regulation of HEG (hemoencephalography)	Oxygenation of local blood flow measured by active or passive near infrared spectrophotometry	Toomim and Carmen, 1999

of ERPs into independent components[32]. The components are characterized by topography[33] and time dynamics. The topographies serve for constructing spatial filters to extract the components from the individual ERPs. The next step of the approach is to compare the amplitude or latency of the patient's individual components with the normative data. Statistically significant deviation from normality in a certain component is used as indication for impairment of information flow in the corresponding cortical location defined by s-LORETA. The component can be further extracted from the multi-channel raw EEG in each separate trial

---

[32]Note ICA can be reliably performed only on a large number of single ERPs which assumes that the normative database must include at least several hundreds of healthy subjects.

[33]The topography of the component is transferred into s-LORETA image giving the 3D representation of the cortical area that is responsible for generation of the component.

and can be fed back to the subject. In the next few years we are going to experimentally test this method on ADHD children.

2. Self-regulation of Slow Cortical Potentials

As we learn from Chapter 17 surface-negative slow shifts of potentials originate in the apical dendritic layer of the cortex reflecting synchronized depolarization of apical dendrites of cortical neurons. These negative slow shifts of potential are associated with increase of excitability of cortical neurons[34]. Rockstroh et al. (1993) were the first to hypothesize that patients with intractable epilepsy were characterized by an impaired ability to regulate their level of cortical excitability in the cortico-thalamic feedback loops. Studies with healthy subjects demonstrated the ability of humans to learn the self-regulation of slow cortical potentials. This led to the idea that epilepsy patients can acquire cortical self-regulation during learning. According to this hypothesis, a neurofeedback method was developed in which actual changes of slow cortical potentials are presented to epilepsy patients in the form of a moving object on a screen. In fact, using this method, most patients with drug-resistant epilepsy could learn to control their slow cortical potentials, resulting in a significant and lasting decrement of the seizure rate (Rockstroh et al., 1993).

A similar idea was developed by the same group in a so-called "thought translation device" that was designed to re-establish communication in severely paralyzed patients. The device relies on the self-regulation of slow cortical potentials, that is, the voluntary production of negative and positive potential shifts. After a patient has achieved reliable control over his or her slow cortical potentials, the responses can be used to select items presented on a computer screen. A spelling program allows patients to select single letters by sequential selection of blocks of letters presented in a dichotomic structure with five levels. Several completely paralyzed patients diagnosed with amyotrophic lateral sclerosis were able to write messages of considerable length using their brain potentials[35].

---

[34]Recall that these negativities are recorded during preparations to receive a stimulus and to make a movement.

[35]In a study by the Tuebingen group (Hinterberge et al., 2005) the relationship between negative and positive slow cortical potentials and changes in the BOLD signal of the fMRI were examined in subjects who were trained to successfully self-regulate their slow potentials. fMRI revealed that the generation of negativity (increased cortical excitation) was accompanied by widespread activation in central, pre-frontal, and parietal brain regions as well as the basal ganglia. Positivity (decreased cortical excitation) was associated with widespread deactivations in several cortical sites as well as some activation, primarily in frontal and parietal structures as well as insula and putamen. Regression analyses revealed that cortical positivity was predicted by pallidum and putamen activation and supplementary motor area (SMA) and motor cortex deactivation, while differentiation between cortical negativity and positivity was revealed primarily in parahippocampal regions. These data suggest that negative and positive electrocortical potential shifts in the EEG are related to distinct and widespread differences in cerebral activation/deactivation pattern.

3. fMRI-Based Neurofeedback

In a recent study of the Tuebingen group (Weiskopf et al., 2005) a new neurofeedback method was implemented. The method performs fMRI data processing and feedback of the hemodynamic brain activity within 1.3 s. Using this technique, differential feedback and self-regulation is feasible as exemplified by the supplementary motor area and parahippocampal area. The methodology allows for studying behavioral effects and strategies of local self-regulation in healthy and diseased subjects.

4. HEG-Based Neurofeedback

The term hemoencephalography (HEG) was first used by Hershel Toomim in 1997 in his description of a system for near infrared spectrophotometry. Another implementation of the system, the passive infrared HEG system, evolved from Carmen's application of infrared technology to peripheral thermal biofeedback (Carmen, 2002). Both systems respond to blood flow dynamics as a source of data. The passive infrared HEG system was specifically developed as a potential intervention technique for migraine headaches. The conceptualization for training cerebrovascular regulation to produce migraine control was based on the tentative assumption that if a person could learn to control cerebrovascular activity (especially control over excessive vasodilation) relief from migraine would follow. Unfortunately, training a person to directly constrict excessively dilated cerebrovascular structures did not work. Most people could easily learn to increase the passive infrared HEG signal, but few could reduce it. So, the procedure was modified to train increases instead of decreases in the HEG parameters. The effects of HEG-based neurofeedback were positive on both migraine prophylaxis and actual abortion of migraine headaches.

T. BCI

If the process of modulating brain activity is directed to control of external devices the approach is named "brain–computer interface" (BCI). Sometimes it is called a direct neural interface or a brain–machine interface[36]. In this definition, the word *brain* means the brain or nervous system while *computer* (machine) means any processing or computational device, from simple circuits to sophisticated computers.

---

[36]In general terms BCI can be defined as a direct communication pathway between a human or animal brain (or brain cell culture) and an external device. In one-way BCIs, computers either accept commands from the brain (e.g., to move a prosthesis) or send signals to the barin (e.g., to send visual information to cortical neurons of blind people). Two-way BCIs would allow brains and external devices to exchange information in both directions.

Research on BCIs began in the 1970s, but the first working experimental implants in humans appeared only in the mid-1990s. Working implants in humans now exist, designed to restore damaged hearing, sight, and movement. The common idea behind this research is similar to the basics of neurofeedback, namely the remarkable cortical plasticity of the brain. As in the neurofeedback approach any physiological parameter can be used in BCIs. Electrical scalp recorded potentials are the most studied parameters. For example, Niels Birbaumer of the University of Tuebingen in Germany used EEG recordings of slow cortical potentials to give paralyzed patients control over a computer cursor (Birbaumer, 2006). Jessica Bayliss at the University of Rochester showed that volunteers wearing virtual reality helmets could control elements in a virtual world using their P300 components of ERPs (Beyliss et al., 2004). Gerd Pfurtscheller from Graz University of Technology in Austria used various parameters of EEG to control prostheses in paraplegic patients or to walk through a virtual city in healthy subjects (Leeb and Pfurtscheller, 2004).

III. DEEP BRAIN STIMULATION

A. Psychosurgery

When psychosurgery as a surgical procedure for treatment of severe psychiatric conditions emerged in the mid-20th century, the only method available to neurosurgeons for modulating the brain was through destruction of targeted neural tissue. From Burckhardt to Fulton to Moniz and Freeman came the experience of ablation of frontal lobe tissue for the treatment of psychiatric disorders. However, the indiscriminate use of crude and large surgical interventions often led to dreadful consequences such as radical personality changes and cognitive decline[37]. The discovery of effective pharmacotherapy in 1960s seemed to become a panacea. Alas, it turned out not to be the case. There remain a large number of patients suffering from psychiatric disease without hope for improvement other than through surgical means. It is for this reason that the impetus for psychiatric surgery still remains.

B. Stereotactic Neurosurgery

While the development of stereotaxis in the latter half of the 20th century enabled neurosurgeons to refine their lesions with more precise interventions, ultimately

---

[37]By the mid-1950s, over 20,000 frontal lobotomies had been performed in the United States alone. Although some patients benefited, many patients suffered. So, many countries throughout the world outlawed the practice. Thus, the birth and subsequent demise of the first stage of psychiatric neurosurgery in the early and mid-20th century serve to caution the current attempts to intervene into the brain to improve the symptoms of intractable psychiatric illness.

ablation was still the only means of altering nervous system function. The stereo-tactic lesion, while effective, is permanent in nature and therefore associated with the potential for permanent side effects. There is little room for error in terms of the placement, and once done, there is no means of adjusting the effect except by creating another or larger lesion[38].

C. Deep Brain Stimulation as Reversible Destruction

The experimental search for methods of reversible switching off the local brain activity was started in 1960s. In the Department of Human Neurophysiology of the Institute for Experimental Medicine in St. Petersburg (where the author worked in 1970–1980) we were using methods of direct current stimulation and high frequency stimulation for temporal switching off activity of neurons located around the electrodes implanted for diagnostic and therapeutic purposes in neurological patients[39]. However, only recently due to developing new electronic technology DBS was introduced into routine clinical practice and revolutionized the methods of neurosurgery (see Fig. 23.8). DBS started with treatment of movement disorders and is now applied in the treatment of refractory psychiatric disease.

DBS has advantages over lesioning procedures of neurosurgery. First, the effects produced by DBS are fully reversible. Second, stimulation parameters can be adjusted according to a patient's changing symptoms and disease progression. Third, the stimulation can generally be turned on or off without the patient's awareness, which provides a unique opportunity for double-blind studies. Along with advantages, DBS has some disadvantages, primarily associated with the need for permanent keeping the implant within the brain thus producing a danger for infection.

IV. TRANSCRANIAL MAGNETIC STIMULATION

A. Physics of TMS

Transcranial magnetic stimulation (TMS) was introduced by Anthony Barker at the University of Sheffield, UK in 1985. TMS was then used as non-invasive, safe, and painless method of activating the human motor cortex and assessing the

---

[38]Once made a destruction, the surgeon and, more importantly, the patient must live with the consequences, both good and bad. Nevertheless, the results and side effect profiles of modern lesion procedures have generally been favorable.

[39]Surgical interventions for neurological and psychiatric diseases must use an extremely rigorous gauntlet of safety measures to ensure proper execution. In case of psychiatric disease, a patient must meet DSM-IV or ICD-10 criteria for a particular psychiatric disease such as OCD or major depression. Further, the candidate must meet strictly defined criteria for severity, chronicity, disability, and treatment refractoriness. For example, a patient must fail several rounds of treatment with multiple medications combined with appropriate psychotherapy before he/she is considered for surgical treatment.

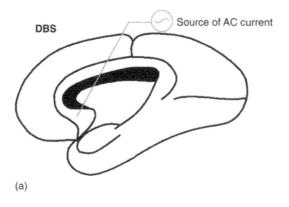

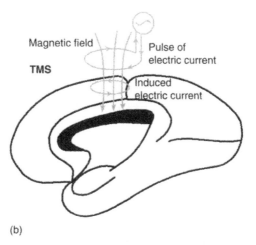

FIGURE 23.8   Deep brain stimulation (DBS) and transcranial magnetic stimulation (TMS). (a) DBS – the AC current is applied through the implanted electrodes with the goal to switch off or on (depending on the current frequency) neuronal activity near the electrode. (b) The electric pulse in the coil generates a changing magnetic field that induces an electric current in the tissue, in the opposite direction.

integrity of the central motor pathways. Since its introduction, the use of TMS in clinical neurophysiology, neurology, and psychiatry has spread widely, mostly in research applications, but increasingly with clinical aims in mind. However, studies to date have not provided enough data to establish the objective indication for a systematic application of TMS as a therapeutic tool.

TMS is based on the principle of electromagnetic induction, as discovered by Michael Faraday in 1838. If a pulse of electric current passing through a coil placed over a subject's head has sufficient strength and short duration it generates rapidly changing magnetic pulses that penetrate scalp and skull to reach the brain with negligible attenuation. These magnetic pulses in their turn induce a secondary ionic current in the brain[40] (Fig. 23.8).

B. Diagnostic and Therapeutic Applications

TMS delivered to different levels of the motor system can provide information about the excitability of the motor cortex, the functional integrity of intracortical neuronal structures, the conduction along corticospinal, corticonuclear, and callosal fibers, as well as the function of nerve roots and peripheral motor pathway to the muscles[41]. The patterns of findings in these studies can help to localize the level of a lesion within the nervous system, distinguish between a predominantly demyelinating or axonal lesion in the motor tracts, or predict the functional motor outcome after an injury.

To enhance the effects of magnetic stimulation, TMS can be applied repeatedly with frequencies from 1 pulse to more than 20 pulses per second. The effect of repetitive TMS may range from inhibition to facilitation, depending on the stimulation variables. TMS at lower frequencies can suppress excitability of the motor cortex, while 20 Hz stimulation trains seem to lead to a temporary increase in cortical excitability. The effect of low frequency repetitive TMS is robust and long lasting. This finding raises the possibility of therapeutic applications of repetitive TMS to "normalize" pathologically decreased or increased levels of cortical activity.

V. TRANSCRANIAL DIRECT CURRENT STIMULATION

A. History

From basic neurophysiology we know that a constant DC[42] shifts membrane potential of neurons toward either hypo or hyperpolarization depending on the direction

---

[40]The capacity of TMS to depolarize neurons depends on the "activating function," which causes transmembrane current to flow and can be described mathematically as the spatial derivative of the electric field along the nerve. Depending on the orientation of the current induced in the brain, TMS will preferentially activate the pyramidal cells indirectly (i.e., trans-synaptically) to evoke indirect waves, or directly at their axon hillocks to cause direct waves. For TMS, fast conducting axons (>75 m/s) have a lower threshold for direct waves, whereas slow-conducting axons (<55 m/s) have a lower threshold for indirect waves.

[41]When TMS is applied to the motor cortex at appropriate stimulation intensity, motor evoked potentials (MEPs) can be recorded from contralateral extremity muscles. Motor threshold refers to the lowest TMS intensity necessary to evoke MEPs in the target muscle when single-pulse stimuli are applied to the motor cortex. Motor threshold is believed to reflect membrane excitability of corticospinal neurons and interneurons projecting onto these neurons in the motor cortex, as well as the excitability of motor neurons in the spinal cord, neuromuscular junctions, and muscle.

[42]DC is a flow of electric charge that does not change direction. It can be caused simply by applying two poles of an electric battery to the brain tissue.

of the current. Although the effect of electrical currents on living tissues has been known for centuries[43], only in the middle of the 20th century systematic research of this phenomenon has been initiated. The evidence that a week scalp DC can induce prolonged changes in brain excitability opened new approaches to the management of neurological conditions. However, even nowadays whereas ample experimental data are available on brain polarization in animals, little is known about how weak DC applied through the scalp affects brain excitability in humans. Nowadays the procedure is called tDCS.

Week direct currents in tDCS change membrane potentials of cortical neurons only slightly. The currents are much smaller than those used in a so-called electroconvulsive therapy (ECT). ECT was discovered in 1930s by Italian scientists Bini and Cerletti. In those days ECT appeared as a fundamental breakthrough in the management of mental disorders. ECT produced the marked and consistent improvement in patients. ECT fundamentally differs from tDCS. Whereas ECT injects strong currents inducing convulsive activity in the brain, tDCS induces much smaller currents slightly modulating brain function by changing spontaneous neuronal activity[44] without inducing seizures. Available evidence indicates that unlike ECT, tDCS causes no memory disturbance or loss of consciousness, neither does it require the patient to be sedated or receive muscle relaxants. tDCS is so mild that the patients subjectively can not discriminate the feeling produced by tDCS when compared with sham.

B. Procedure

In a conventional tDCS procedure, a small amount of direct electric current is applied to the brain by means of two electrodes: the one is a "stimulating" electrode, localized above the area that is supposed to be stimulated, and the other electrode is a "reference electrode," localized on some "silent" part of the brain or the body such as shoulder or earlobe (Fig. 23.9). Two electrodes, attached correspondingly to positive and negative poles of the DC source (e.g., a battery) and

---

[43]The idea to use electricity for treatment of brain disturbances was so straightforward that its first appearance was dated by 43–48 ACwhen Scribonius Largus observed that placing a live torpedo fish – delivering a strong direct electric current – over the scalp of a patient with headache elicited a sudden, transient stupor with pain relief. Neurophysiologists owe a special respect to the torpedo electric fish because its systematic study initiated by Walsh in 1773 started the science of electrophysiology. Several years later Italian scientists Galvani and Volta stated their work on effects of electricity on the leaving organs. Soon after, galvanic currents (DC) were applied in clinical medicine, particularly in mental disorders. In 1804, Galvani's nephew Aldini reported the successful treatment of patients suffering from melancholia by applying galvanic currents over the head.

[44]Although polarizing currents can not excite a silent cell, they slightly change membrane polarization of neuronal cells which due to the collective and cumulative effects has a power for modulating the spontaneous cell firing.

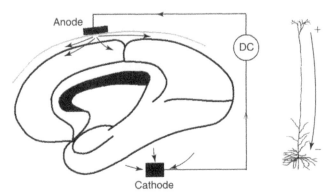

FIGURE 23.9   Transcranial direct current stimulation (tDCS). Left – a scheme of tDCS: two electrodes are attached to the head, the electric current is provided by a battery driven device. The current usually does not exceed 1 mA while only a small part of it goes through the cortical grey matter. In the cortical layers the "anodal" current depolarizes pyramidal cells at their basal membrane (see at right – the current flow of a pyramidal neuron within the cortex).

placed on the scalp, produce electrical field and, according to the Ohm's law, electric currents along this electrical field.

C. Neurophysiological Mechanisms of Membrane Polarization

Only a small part of the electric current passes through the cortex. Neurons in the cortex are oriented perpendicular to the surface, so that apical and basal dendrites are located in different layers. The electric field and corresponding current under the anode electrode induces a lack of positive ions at the basal compartment of the neuronal membrane. The lack of positive ions induces depolarization of the basal part of the neuronal membrane. Depolarization activates voltage gated Ca^{++} and Na^+ channels and is associated with increase of excitability of the neuron. The increase of excitability leads to increase of the overall background activity of depolarized neurons. The net effect is a so-called "anodal activation" of neurons. Vice versa, the current under the cathode electrode induces an excess of positive ions near the external part of the basal membrane. This induces hyperpolarization of this part of the membrane. Hyperpolarization inactivates Ca^{++} and Na^+ channels. The excitability of the neuron reduced and the frequency of the background activity decreases. The net effect is a cathodal suppression of neurons.

Although changes in the basal membrane potential induced by 1 mA DCs are small to generate a spike, they start amplification processes in neuronal networks. These amplification factors eventually induce significant physiological effects. We know at least one amplification factor in the nervous system – collective effect due to recurrent excitatory connections in the cortical areas. In the recurrent networks a small change in membrane potentials can lead to large changes in the overall neuronal spiking. From this point of view, tDCS can be considered as a sub-threshold stimulation technique modulating spontaneous cortical activity and thereby inducing transient functional changes in the human brain. tDCS elicits minimal discomfort and no negative sensations. A recent study (Gandiga et al., 2006) showed that sham (a situation when the researcher pretended to switch on the device, but actually does not inject the current) can not be distinguished from tDCS. This last fact actually implies that tDCS is a nice tool for double-blind placebo-controlled clinical studies.

In early 1970 the author worked together with a group that carried out research on tDCS in the Institute of Experimental Medicine of the Academy of Medical Sciences of the USSR. These studies started in the Department of Human Neurophysiology on patients to whom electrodes were stereotactically implanted for diagnosis and therapy. It was noticed that application of the anodal current increased multi-unit activity while the cathodal current decreased neuronal activity. Cathodal DC was used as a diagnostic procedure for temporal switching off neuronal networks around the electrode before making decision about further lesions in this brain location. In 1970–1980 experiments with polarizing brain tissues were continued on cats and dogs at the Institute of Experimental Medicine. These experiments proved that the anodal currents activate neurons, while the cathodal currents inhibit them. In 1980 the polarization methods were started in a few clinics of Leningrad for treatment of neurological and psychiatric patients. Unfortunately, several tragic events (the death of two principle scientists, collapse of the Soviet Union, and following termination of funding the basic research) led to interruption of these very promising studies. Only in the beginning of the 21st century the research was continued. Nowadays, polarization methods are used with good success in correcting behavior of ADHD children and for treatment of children with speech delay. During the last 5 years the interest to direct current stimulation returned in the western world. This renaissance was partly associated with a search for alternative (non-pharmacological) methods of brain stimulation[45].

D. Physiological Evidence

From neurophysiological studies we know that slow changes of potential recorded from the scalp reflect shifts in the overall membrane potential of the cortical neurons.

---

[45]The research groups that now deal with tDCS are located in: National Institute of Neurological Disorders and Stroke, NIH, Bethesda, USA; Harvard Center for Non-invasive Brain Stimulation, Boston, USA; Institute of Neurology, University College, London, England; University of Occupational and Environmental Health, Japan; Universita di Milano, Italy; and in several universities in Germany – University of Goettingen, University of Luebeck, University of Kiel, Eberhard-Karls University of Tuebingen.

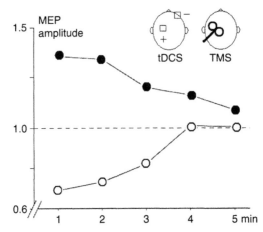

FIGURE 23.10   Polarity-specific effects of tDCS on excitability of the motor cortex. The *y*-axis shows the relative amplitude of the motor potential evoked by TMS after tDCS applied to the motor cortex during 5 min. The *x*-axis shows the time elapsed after the end of tDCS. "Heads" at the top right schematically show the procedures of application of tDCS and TMS. Adapted from Nitsche and Paulus (2001).

The idea that modulation of these slow potentials by simply injecting currents might effect psychological operations of the brain was so obvious that several laboratories in 1960–1970 were testing this suggestion. The question was if the potentials at the level of single neurons had been strong enough to modulate excitability of neurons. Evidence that DC delivered to the human scalp can influence brain excitability was obtained in patients with temporal lobe epilepsy by recording the potential difference from implanted electrodes for presurgical evaluation during scalp DC polarization at intensities up to 1.5 mA (Dymond et al., 1975). At this intensity of the injected current, the potential gradients within the cortex ranged from 6.4 to 16.4 mV/cm. Those gradients are strong enough to modulate spontaneous neuronal firing as was shown in crayfish and lobster experimental preparations by Terzuolo and Bullock (1956).

One of the direct physiological evidences of effects of DC polarization came recently from experiments using changes in the muscle twitch evoked by TMS as indicators of changes in cortical excitability. In these experiments the anode (or cathode) was located over the motor cortex. The effect of tDCS was tested by recording muscle potentials evoked in response to a pulse of TMS (Fig. 23.10). Figure 23.10 shows that changes in excitability of the motor cortex induced by 5 min of tDCS last only for 5 min. Further research shows that longer periods of tDCS lead to prolongation (up to an hour) of the effect. It should be noted that the changes in the cortical excitability turned out to be local. For example, only tDCS of the motor cortex but not occipital or contralateral cortical areas induced activation or inhibition measured selectively in the motor cortex[46].

E. Behavioral Effects

Historically, application of tDCS started in experiments with healthy volunteers. In one of the studies carried out in 1964 (Lippold et al., 1964) DC of 0.5 mA was injected through two frontal electrodes and one electrode over the right knee. The study showed that scalp anodal currents induced an increase in alertness, mood, and motor activity, whereas cathodal polarization produced quietness and apathy. However, it took almost 40 years for the tDCS to re-appear as a research tool. In a recent study of a German group from the University of Goettingen (Antal et al., 2001) cathodal DC stimulation of 1 mA over the occipital cortex significantly decreased contrast sensitivity during and immediately after DC application. It should be noted that in all recent studies the effects of tDCS were compared with effects induced by sham trials[47].

Transcranial direct current stimulation is considered as a quite safe procedure. None of the foregoing studies reported the occurrence of side effects. Nitsche and Paulus (2001) found no changes in serum concentrations of neuron-specific enolase, a sensitive marker of neuronal damage, after the offset of DC. DC stimulation for several minutes, at 1 mA intensity with an electrode area of 35 cm^2, is considered safe by Nitsche and Paulus (2000, 2001)[48].

F. Clinical Applications

In parallel with experiments on healthy subjects studies were performed on patients. In one of the early studies the anodal scalp DC was shown to improve the mood in depressed patients (Costain et al., 1964). In our own studies carried out at the Institute of the Human Brain, tDCS was used to improve symptoms of ADHD.

---

[46]In a study of a group of scientists from University of Goettingen (Antal et al., 2005) the EEG activity in the visual cortex of healthy human subjects after weak tDCS was analyzed. The study showed that cathodal stimulation significantly decreased while the anodal stimulation slightly increased the normalized beta and gamma frequency powers. This observation is in line with speculation that anodal stimulation increases metabolic activity of the corresponding cortical area while cathodal stimulation inhibits the cortex.

[47]The method is ideally suited for these purposes. The application of tDCS evokes only week sensations at the abrupt onset of the current, but if applied with slow increasing intensity no sensations are felt at all. So, in sham control the current usually switches on (to imitate tDCS) for a few seconds and then gradually switches off.

[48]Our own experience shows that tDCS with 0.3–0.7 mA, with electrode area of 4 cm^2 during 20–40 min may produce mild side effects, such as agitation, lack of sleep, or head aches.

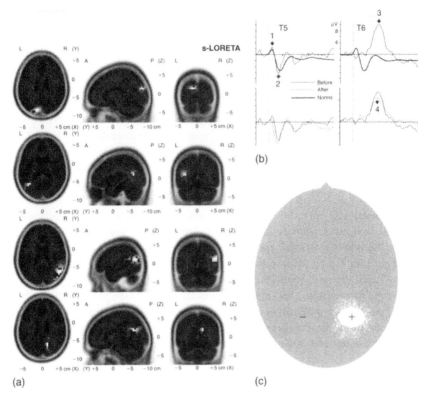

FIGURE 23.11   tDCS in a patient with neglect. (a) From top to bottom – s-LORETA images of evoked potentials taken at different times and at different conditions (before, after) of the patient. (b) ERPs to GO stimuli in the neglect patient before (thin line), after (dotted line) several sessions of tDCS in comparison to ERPs computed for a group of healthy subjects of the same age (thick line). (c) Electrodes location. White area schematically depicts the area of lesion.

The experimental findings on tDCS stimulation of motor areas carried out by the group from the University of Goettingen prompted application of tDCS for rehabilitation of stroke patients. In a recent study by Hummel et al., (2005) tDCS was successfully used in patients with 1–2 year history of stroke compromising motor functions[49]. Improvements in motor performance that appeared during tDCS, persisted beyond the stimulation period for at least 25 min and returned to baseline levels days later.

[49]Direct current was applied through two gel-sponge electrodes (surface area 25 cm²) embedded in a saline-soaked solution. The anode was positioned on the projection of the hand knob area of the primary motor cortex of the affected hemisphere on the patient's scalp, and the cathode on the skin overlying the contralateral supraorbital region. Anodal tDCS was delivered for 20 min in the tDCS session and for up to 30 s in the sham session.

In our own pilot studies[50] we applied tDCS for three patients with the right parietal stroke accompanied by neglect. Figure 23.11 represents results in one of the patients. As one can see, the first component (P1) of ERPs of the patient is generated asymmetrically at the left occipital area with deviations from normality at the right side. The second N1 component is also generated asymmetrically, but more laterally and anterior in the temporal cortex and is absent at the right side. The third late component with latency of 300 ms is dramatically enhanced at the right side[51]. tDCS significantly decreased the latency of the N1 component at the left side and shifted the location of generators of the late positive components. Psychologically after tDCS, patients performed significantly better in lateralized tasks[52]. More clinical studies are needed, but the presented data show possible therapeutic effect of tDCS and advantages of ERP components for monitoring the effect.

[50]The study was performed in Rehabilitation Center in Mokvol, Trondheim, Norway. Neurophsychologists Jan Bruno, Knut Hestad were responsible for psychological assessment and testing of patients before, during, and after 20 min sessions of tDCS.

[51]The increase of the P3 component at the right side is explained by dysinhibition of the cortical areas that surround the area of lesion. Recall that lateral inhibition is one of the common features of cotico-thalamic pathways, so that the lesion of a part of the cortex suppress inhibitory effects of this part and thereby dysinhibit the surrounding parts.

[52]One of the patients received driver license which he was unable to get during 2 years after the stroke.

Conclusion

I. GENERAL PRINCIPLES OF EEG ASSESSMENT AND NEUROTHERAPY

Below we are going to summarize basic principles of the methodology of assessment of brain functions and dysfunctions presented in the book. This methodology was developed in the author's laboratory of the Institute of the Human Brain of Russian Academy of Sciences. The methodology is based on a fundamental and applied research performed in the laboratory during the last 30 years. The methodology was tested in the Center of Neurotherapy of the Institute during assessment and treatment of thousands of patients with different brain dysfunctions such as attention deficit hyperactivity disorder (ADHD), speech delay, obsessive-compulsive disorder (OCD), drug addiction, epilepsy.

A. Principle 1

Electroencephalogram (EEG) oscillations and event-related potentials (ERPs) reflect different and quite independent processes within the brain: (1) EEG oscillations are manifestations of self-regulation of the cortical areas and are associated with modulation of information flow in cortico-subcortical neuronal networks, and (2)ERPs reflect the flow of the signal induced by the external event and associated with the reactions of the brain such as extracting physical, semantic, and emotional features of the stimulus, selection, and execution of actions.

The two independent processes are measured by two different methods. The EEG spontaneous oscillations are usually compressed into the frequency domain by means of the Fourier analysis, while their dynamics in response to tasks is assessed by the wavelet analysis. ERPs are computed by averaging techniques in which the spontaneous oscillations that are not time locked to stimuli cancel each other. Consequently, the averaged potentials are independent of the background activity and reflect the flow of the signal within the neuronal networks of the brain.

B. Principle 2

EEG oscillations and ERPs are decomposed into separate components. The spectral components are associated with different types of EEG rhythms each of them reflecting different neuronal mechanism of cortical regulation. The ERP components are associated with different psychological operations such as processing primary sensory information, extracting semantic meaning and spatial location of the signal, encoding emotional reactions and feelings, detecting physical and semantic changes, selecting and suppressing actions, monitoring the results of executed or suppressed actions.

Different methods can be applied for separation the components of EEG activity and ERPs. One of the modern methods is independent component analysis (ICA).

The ICA can be applied to raw EEG as well as for "whitening" spectra. In the healthy brain the ICA enable us to separate several types of "normal" EEG rhythms, such as parietal and occipital alpha rhythms, mu-rhythms, beta rhythms, and the frontal midline theta rhythm. The normal rhythms are generated by different mechanisms and reflect different modulation properties of neuronal networks. Alpha rhythms are generated by cortico-thalamic reciprocally connected networks and reflect idling states of sensory systems. Beta rhythms are generated by the interplay between excitatory and inhibitory connections in cortical networks and seem to play a reset function for eliminating the traces of the previous cortical activation. The frontal midline theta rhythm is generated in the septo-hippocampal circuits and is associated with enhancement of encoding the episodic memory. Any type of impairment in neuronal circuits can lead to decrease or increase of a normal rhythm, or to emergence of a pathological rhythmicity.

The ICA can be applied to trials of raw EEG as well as to a set of individual ERPs computed for a homogeneous group of subjects or patients. The extracted ERP components reflect stages of sensory processing, comparison operations, engagement, action suppression and monitoring operations as well as some other psychological processes.

C. Principle 3

Brain is decomposed into basic systems: the sensory systems in visual, auditory somato-sensory... modalities, attentional networks, the affective system, the executive system, and the memory systems. Modulation of information flow in each of the systems is characterized by specific rhythms while stages of information processing in these systems are reflected in specific ERP components.

The two Tables C.1 and C.2 represent summaries separately for EEG rhythmic activities and ERP components, their location, mechanisms of generation, functional meaning, and association with brain systems.

D. Principle 4

Varying tasks and modalities it is feasible to test functioning of practically all cortical areas of the brain. For a particular patient the choice of the task is defined on the patient's complains and on the basis of corresponding neuropsychological impairments in the patient.

This principle is illustrated in Fig. C.1. We selected only the largest components that were extracted in response to visual stimuli in three different tasks (the two stimulus GO/NOGO task, the reading task, the mathematic task) from the Human Brain Institute Normative Database. Note that almost the whole cortical mantle is covered by the components' generators distributed over various cortical areas from the occipital cortex to the anterior cingulate cortex. Note also, that the brain is a heavily interconnected neuronal network in which neurons in different cortical areas fire simultaneously to maintain a certain operation. s-LORTEA images presented in Fig. C.1 show only the top of "icebergs" of widely distributed cortical activities.

E. Principle 5

Any of the brain systems obeys to the inverted U-law. The law claims that responses of the system are largest if the activity of the system stays within the normal range and are abnormally smaller if the overall level of activation of the system is below or higher than the normal range.

The level of activation of the system can be assessed by spectral analysis of the spontaneous EEG generated by the cortical part of the system. In general, excess of alpha activity in comparison to the normative range is associated with hypo-activation of the system, while excess of beta activity is associated with hyperac-tivation of the system. The responses of the system are reflected in amplitude and latency of the components generated by cortical areas of the system[1].

---

[1]For example, abnormally high amplitude of beta activity generated in the medial prefrontal cortex indicates overactivation of this part of the executive system while abnormally small P3 monitoring component indicates a reduced response of this system in situations that need monitoring of actions.

TABLE C.1   Normal Rhythms of the Human Brain

Name	Frequency (Hz)	Topography	Mechanism of generation	Function	Brain system
Occipital alpha rhythm	8–12	O1, O2	Ca^{++} spikes following *hyperpolarization* of thalamo-cortical cells of the lateral geniculate body.	Reflects idling state of the first order visual areas. Primary visual information is suppressed but the cortex is ready to promptly process it.	Sensory systems
Parietal alpha rhythm	8–12	Pz	Ca^{++} spikes following *hyperpolarization* of the thalamo-cortical cells in the pulvinar nucleus.	Reflects idling state of the second order visual areas.	Sensory systems
Mu-rhythm	9–13	C3, C4	Ca^{++} spikes following *hyperpolarization* of the thalamo-cortical cells in the ventral-posterior nucleus.	Reflects idling state of the somato-sensory system.	Sensory systems
Beta rhythms	13–30	Frontal or central areas	The interplay between excitatory and inhibitory connections within cortical networks in the state of *depolarization*.	Is associated with resetting the trace of cortical activation	Any system
Frontal midline theta	5–8	Fz	*Depolarization* in the septo-hippocampal circuit in response to a salient stimulus.	Reflects chunking information into episodic memory.	Episodic memory system

F. Principle 6

Brain disorders can be classified in association with impairment of brain systems and diagnosed according to deviations from normality in the corresponding EEG spectral and ERP parameters.
    Any of the currently used classification systems, such as DSM-IV or ICD-10, is based on description of the patient's behavior and, in this respect, is subjective.

TABLE C.2   Main ERP Components

Name	Task	Peak latency (ms)	Topography	Generator	Functional meaning	Brain System
MMN	Auditory oddball	140	Fz	Temporal and frontal cortex.	Automatic comparison of a regularity of acoustic stimulus with the sensory trace.	Sensory system
P1 and N1	Any stimulus presentation	100	Modality specific	In vicinity of primary sensory areas.	Information processing in sensory systems	Sensory system
P3b	Active oddball in any modality	300	Pz	Widely distributed basal ganglia thalamo-cortical circuits.	Activation of posterior anterior regions needed to execution of action.	Executive system
P2 comparison	Discrimination tasks	240–300	T5, T6 visual, F7, F8 auditory	Association areas in visual and auditory modalities.	Activation of neurons that detect a change in physical or semantic characteristics of the repetitive stimulus.	Sensory system
P400 NOGO	GO/NOGO	400	Fz	Anterior gyrus cingulus and medial prefrontal cortex.	Monitoring operation, that is, activation of neurons that compare an executed action with the prepared one.	Executive system
P3a	Three stimulus oddball	260–300	Fz	Widely distributed prefrontal areas	Attention shift.	Executive system

Several components of quantitative electroencephalography (QEEG) and ERPs have been suggested as plausible candidates for objective physiological markers of diseases – endophenotypes. Although more systematic research is required the first results are very promising (see Table C.3).

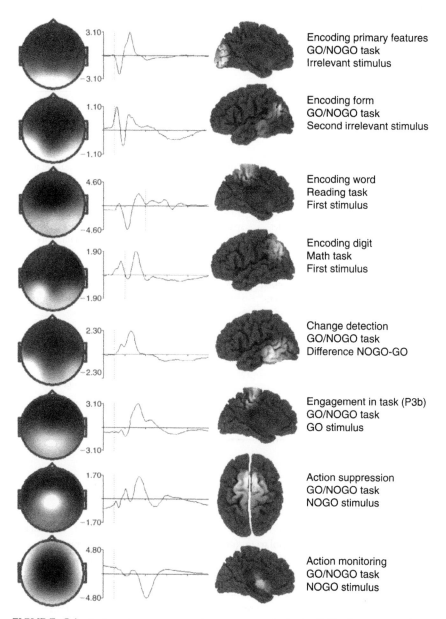

Encoding primary features
GO/NOGO task
Irrelevant stimulus

Encoding form
GO/NOGO task
Second irrelevant stimulus

Encoding word
Reading task
First stimulus

Encoding digit
Math task
First stimulus

Change detection
GO/NOGO task
Difference NOGO-GO

Engagement in task (P3b)
GO/NOGO task
GO stimulus

Action suppression
GO/NOGO task
NOGO stimulus

Action monitoring
GO/NOGO task
NOGO stimulus

FIGURE C.1   Independent components in response to visual stimuli. The largest in amplitude independent components extracted in response to visual stimuli presented in the three tasks of the Human Brain Institute Normative Database. The tasks are the two stimulus visual GO/NOGO task, reading and math tasks. From Left to right – (1) topography of components (2) time courses of components, (3) s-LORETA images of cortical generators of components.

TABLE C.3   Classification of Brain Diseases and Their Endophenotypes

Diagnostic category DSM-IV	Examples of disorders	Brain system	EEG endophenotype	ERP endophenotype
Disorders usually first diagnosed in infancy, childhood, and adolescence	ADHD, autism, learning disorders, conduct disorder	Executive system	Increase of theta beta ratio fronto-centrally	Decrease of P2 comparison, decrease of P4 monitoring
Psychotic disorders	Schizophrenia	Executive system	Increase of beta activity frontally	Decrease of P3b
Mood disorders	Major depression, bipolar disorder	Affective system	Left > Right asymmetry in frontal alpha activity	Elevated ERPs to negative stimuli, Left–Right asymmetry in ERPs
Anxiety disorders	OCD, generalized anxiety disorder, post-traumatic stress disorder	Executive system	Increase of beta activity centrally	Decrease of P4 monitoring
Delirium, dementia, amnestic, and other cognitive disorders	Alzheimer's disease	Episodic memory system	Increase of theta activity fronto-centrally	Decrease of P3b and P4 monitoring components
Substance-related disorders	Heroin addiction, alcoholism	Affective and executive systems	Increase of beta activity centrally	Decrease of P4 monitoring

G. Principle 7

Transcranial direct current stimulation (tDCS) and neurofeedback provide electrophysiologically based tools for activation or suppression of cortical neuronal networks.

tDCS implies injection of small amount of direct currents that depolarize (anodal currents) and hyperpolarize (cathodal currents) cortical pyramidal cells under the stimulation electrode. Neurofeedback implies active involvement of the subject in voluntarily changing the EEG parameters recorded from a given electrode. Our recent studies have shown that the combination of these two techniques might be the best way of activating or suppressing the impaired brain system.

II. TOPICS OF FURTHER RESEARCH

The methods of QEEG/ERPs assessment of brain functions and dysfunctions introduced in the book represent a relatively new but fast developing field of fundamental and clinical research. Electrophysiology-based methods for correcting brain dysfunctions, such as tDCS and neurofeedback, are still in their infancy. They are confined by laboratory settings and are considered mostly as experimental methods. Below we present the topics of the most argent, from our point of view, projects that need to be done within the frames of the filed in a recent future.

A. Topic 1: Constructing Standard Paradigms for Assessment of Affective and Memory Systems

The methods for assessment functioning of the attentional networks and the executive system of the brain presented in the book[2] could serve as a good example of how standardized paradigms for assessment of the affective and memory systems could be designed. For example, using a standard structure of the GO/NOGO paradigm we can suggest a new task for assessing the affective system of the brain. In this task, images of sad, happy, and neutral faces could be presented instead of images of plants, animals, and humans used in the two stimulus GO/NOGO visual task of the Human Brain Institute Database. The patient's task would be to recognize the emotional expression of faces and to press a button in response to two happy faces[3]. Differences of EEG reactions between happy and sad stimuli as well as differences between happy/sad stimuli and neutral ones could serve as indexes of functioning of the affective system of the brain. These indexes might serve as endophenotypes of autism, depression, and other affective disorders.

B. Topic 2: Extracting Independent ERP Components in Behavioral Paradigms

The ICA applied to a set of individual ERPs of a large group of healthy subjects provides a powerful tool for constructing spatial filters for ERP components reflecting basic psychological operations of the human brain. The ICA components extracted in response to visual stimuli in the three tasks of the Human Brain Institute Database (GO/NOGO, math, and reading tasks) are presented in Fig. C.1. Note that the components evoked in the three task conditions are associated with activation of quite different cortical areas. For example, neurons encoding primary visual features, form, arithmetic properties and written words are located in quite different (practically non-overlapping) posterior cortical areas, while neurons responsible for psychological operations with actions (such as action suppression and action monitoring) are located in the frontal–central regions of the brain.

---

[2]They are oddball, three stimulus, and GO/NOGO paradigms, which now could be considered as standard and well studied paradigms.

[3]The other option would be to standardize existing paradigms, such as the old/new and the positive/negative task that were developed for studying the memory and affective systems correspondingly.

Similar approach can be applied to ERPs computed for a homogeneous group of subjects performing other behavioral paradigms[4]. The software of the Human Brain Institute Database provides the users with all computational procedures to implement the methodological approach, including constructing protocols, recording and storing EEG records in the built-in database, automated correcting artifacts, averaging and computing numbers of omission and commission errors, performing ICA on a group of collected ERPs, computing low resolution electromagnetic tomography (LORETA) and s-LORETA images of the extracted components.

C. Topic 3: Using ERPs Independent Components as Endophenotypes in Diagnosis of Different Brain Disorders

In the book we discussed possible ERPs and QEEG markers of different brain disorders such as ADHD, OCD, schizophrenia, depression … However, the methodology presented in the book is still in its infancy. During the last few years after development of the Human Brain Institute Normative Database the EEG spectra and the cognitive independent components in different groups of patients have been collected and analyzed. The data are now continued collecting in different scientific and clinical centers of the world. So, the project has been actually started. It should be noted that the main problem of the project is difficulty in finding medication free patients such as finding patients with depression who had never been treated with medication.[5] Note also, that the number of patients belonging to a separate disease has to be from 100 to 1000, that is, comparable with the number of healthy individuals. So the project on this topic is supposed to unite the efforts in different centers in order to create a Common QEEG/ERP Patient Database which must include several thousands of patients in different categories.

After the Patient Database has been completed, the next step would be to find the endophenotypes that are specific for a disorder or a group of disorders. The endophenotypes must not necessarily be a single QEEG or ERPs[6] parameter. It is quite possible that separation between different disorders may be done by means of so-called discrimination plains in multidimensional space of parameters. Each discrimination plain may represent a linear combination of the parameters with corresponding weights. The first attempt in discriminating a specific disorder from

---

[4]Electrophysiological laboratories all over the world prefer their own behavioral paradigms designed in the laboratories for specific scientific purposes. It seems impossible to force the laboratories to study the same behavioral paradigms but it is quite feasible to provide them with a common tool for using it in studies of the brain.

[5]Note that collecting data in a child population provides better chances of getting medication free patients of ADHD, dyslexia, and learning disabilities.

[6]Even if we will be using independent components both for EEG and ERPs.

the normal population was done by Roy John in 1980s[7]. Later the attempt was continued by Bob Thatcher. Note, however, in all these cases that discriminations were done only for single disorders, such as discrimination of QEEG of patients with traumatic brain injury from QEEG of healthy subjects in the Thatcher's Database. So far there is no possibility to associate the QEEG of a patient with a particular disease.

D. Topic 4: Using ERP Endophenotypes in Pharmacotherapy (Pharmaco-ERP)

The project on this topic is supposed to study the effect of different antipsychotic and neurotrophic drugs on ERP independent components. By using this approach we will get a clue to how different disorders associated with impairment of certain ERP components might be treated by different pharmaceutical agents. The roots of this topic take place in pharmaco-EEG initiated in 1950–1960s. However, big variations of spectral parameters of raw EEG in the normal population imposed certain limitations on this QEEG-based approach. The application of ERPs and especially ERPs independent components open new horizons in using physiological methods for monitoring effects of pharmaceutical agents on the human brain.

E. Topic 5: Using Double-Blind Placebo Controlled Studies to Show Behavioral and Electrophysiological Changes Induced by tDCS and Neurofeedback

Although several attempts have been made in several laboratories with positive results, the studies were carried out on a limited number of patients. Moreover most of the studies were using the same protocol for the same group of patients irrespectively of QEEG/ERPs subtype of the disorder. As we showed in this book protocols of neurofeedback and tDCS must be defined by QEEG/ERP analysis and tailored to a specific pattern of dysfunction. It must be stressed here that tDCS and neurofeedback provide two different approaches aiming the same goal – activation or suppression of the corresponding brain system. It appears that a combination of these two methods may provide better clinical results. Indeed by combining the two methods we explore both (1) the ability of the subject to change voluntarily the state of his/her own brain and (2) the ability of neurons of the brain to undergo plastic changes induced by injected electric currents.

---

[7]Unfortunately the QEEG parameters were limited to few standard bands while EEG was recorded only in eyes closed condition.

References

Alexander, G.E., DeLong, M.R., and Strick, P.L. (1986). Parallel organization of functionally segregated circuits linking basal ganglia and cortex. *Annu. Rev. Neurosci.* Vol. 9, 357–381.

Allan, K. and Rugg, M.D. (1997). An event-related potential study of explicit memory on tests of word-stem cued recall and recognition memory. *Neuropsychologia.* Vol. 35, 387–397.

Anichkov, A.D., Polonsky, J.Z., and Nizkovolos, V.B. (2005). *Stereotactic Systems.* "Nauka" ("Science") Publishing House, Saint-Petersburg. 142 p. (in Russian).

Anokhin, A.P., Heath, A.C., and Myers, E. (2006). Genetic and environmental influences on frontal EEG asymmetry: A twin study. *Biol. Psychol.* 71(3): 289–295.

Antal, A., Nitsche, M.A., and Paulus, W. (2001). External modulation of Visual perception in humans. *Neuroreport.* Vol. 12, 3553–3555.

Aron, A.R., Robbins, T.W., and Poldrack, R.A. (2004). Inhibition and the right inferior frontal cortex. *Trends Cognit. Sci.* 8(4): 170–176.

Asada, H., Fukuda, y., Yamaguchi, M., Tsunoda, S., and Tonoike, M. (1999). Frontal midline theta rhythms reflect alternative activation of prefrontal cortex and anterior cingulate cortex in humans. *Neurosci. Lett.* Vol. 274, 29–32.

Aston-Jones, G. and Cohen, J.D. (2005). An integrative theory of locus coeruleus–norepinephrine function: Adaptive gain and optimal performance. *Annu. Rev. Neurosci.* Vol. 28, 403–450.

Atwater, F.H. (1997). The Hemi-Sync Process. *The Monroe Institute.* http://www.monroeinstitute.com/content.php?content_id=24

Baehr, E., Rosenfeld, J.P. and Baehr, R. (1997). The clinical use of alpha symmetry protocol in the neurofeedback treatment of depression: two case studies. *J. Neurother.* Vol. 2, 10–23.

Baddeley, A. (2003). Working memory: Looking back and looking forward. *Nat. Rev. Neurosci.* Vol. 4, 929–939.

Baddeley, A.D. and Hitch, G.J. (1974). Working memory. In: Recent Advances in Learning and Motivation, Vol. 8, Academic Press, New York.

Ballantine, H.T. and Giriunas, I.E. (1982). Treatment of intractable psychiatric illness and chronic pain by stereotactic cingulotomy. In Schmidek H.H. and Sweet W.H. (eds). *Operative Neurosurgical Techniques.* Grune & Stratton, New York. 1069–1075.

Ballantine, H.T.Jr., Bouckoms, A.J., Thomas, E.K., and Giriunas, I.E. (1987). Treatment of psychiatric illness by stereotactic cingulotomy. *Biol. Psychiatr.* 22(7): 807–819.

Banaschewski, T., Brandeis, D., Heinrich, H., Albrecht, B., Brunner, E., and Rothenberger, A. (2004). Questioning inhibitory control as the specific deficit of ADHD-evidence from brain electrical activity. *J. Neural Transm.* Vol. 111, 841–864.

Barry, R.J., Clarke, A.R., and Johnstone, S.J. (2003a). A review of electrophysiology in attention-deficit/hyperactivity disorder: I. Qualitative and quantitative electroencephalography. *Clin. Neurophysiol.* Vol. 114, 171–183.

Barry, R.J., Clarke, A.R., and Johnstone, S.J. (2003b). A review of electrophysiology in attention-deficit/hyperactivity disorder: I. II. Event-related potentials. *Clin. Neurophysiol.* Vol. 114, 184–198.

Bartfeld, E. and Grinvald, A. (1992). Relationships between orientation-preference pinwheels, cytochrome oxidase blobs, and ocular-dominance columns in primate striate cortex. *Proc. Natl. Acad. Sci. USA* 89(24): 11905–11909.

Bayliss, J.D., Inverso, S.A., and Tentler, A. (2004). Changing the P300 brain computer interface. *Cyberpsychol. Behav.* Vol. 7, (6): 694–704.

Bazhenov, M., Timofeev, I., Steriade, M., and Sejnowski, T.J. (2002). Model of thalamocortical slow-wave sleep oscillations and transitions to activated states. *J. Neurosci.* Vol. 22, 8691–8704.

Beauducel, A., Brocke, B., and Leue, A. (2006). Energetical bases of extraversion: Effort, arousal, EEG, and performance. *Int. J. Psychophysiol.* 62(2): 212–223. Epub 2006 Jan 19.

Bechtereva, N.P. and Kropotov, J.D. (1984). Neurophysiological correlates of visual stimulus recognition in man. *Int. Journal of Psychophysiology.* Vol. 1, 317–324.

Benedetti, F., Colloca, L., Torre, E., Lanotte, M., Melcarne, A., Pesare, M., Bergamasco, B., and Lopiano, L. (2004). Placebo-responsive Parkinson patients show decreased activity in single neurons of subthalamic nucleus. *Nat. Neurosci.* Vol. 7, 587–588.

Benedetti, F., Mayberg, H.S., Wager, T.D., Stohler, C.S., and Zubieta, J-K. (2005). Neurobiological mechanisms of the placebo effect. *J. Neurosci.* 25(45): 10390–10402.

Birbaumer, N. (2006). Breaking the silence: brain-computer interfaces (BCI) for communication and motor control. *Psychophysiology* Vol. 43, (6): 517–532.

Bland, B.H. and Oddie, S.D. (2001). Theta band oscillation and synchrony in the hippocampal formation and associated structures: The case for its role in sensorimotor integration. *Behav. Brain Res.* Vol. 127, 119–136.

Bramon, E., Rabe-Hesketh, S., Sham, P., Murray, R.M., and Frangou, S. (2004). Meta-analysis of the P300 and P50 waveforms in schizophrenia. *Schizophr. Res.* Vol. 70, 315–329.

Broadbent, D.E. (1954). The role of auditory localization in attention and memory span. *J. Exp. Psychol.* 47(3): 191–196.

Bucci, P., Mucci, A., Volpe, U., Merlotti, E., Galderisi, S., and Maj, M. (2004). Executive hypercontrol in obsessive-compulsive disorder: Electrophysiological and neuropsychological indices. *Clin. Neurophysiol.* Vol. 115, 1340–1348.

Buzsáki, G. (1989). Two-stage model of memory formation: A role for noisy brain states. *Neuroscience* Vol. 31, 551–570.

Buzsáki, G. (2006). *Rhythms of the Brain.* Oxford University Press, 448 p.

Calcagnotto, M.E., Paredes, M.F., Tihan, T., Barbaro, N.M., and Baraban, C.S. (2005). Dysfunction of synaptic inhibition in epilepsy associated with focal cortical dysplasia. *J. Neurosci.* 25(42): 9649–9657.

Cantero, J.L., Atienza, M., Stickgold, R., Kahana, M.J., Madsen, J.R., and Kocsis, B. (2003). Sleep-dependent oscillations in the human hippocampus and neocortex. *J. Neurosci.* 23(34): 10897–10903.

Carmen, J.A. (2002). Passive Infrared Hemoencephalography, 4 Years and 100 migraines later. *Presented at* 2002 Society for Neuronal Regulation conference, Scottsdale, AZ.

Castellanos, F.X. and Tannock, R. (2002). Neuroscience of attention-deficit/hyperactivity disorder: The search for endophenotypes. *Nat. Rev.* Vol. 3, 617–628.

Castellanos, F.X., Sharp, W.S., Gottesman, R.F., Greenstein, D.K., Giedd, J.N., and Rapoport, J.L. (2003). Anatomic brain abnormalities in monozygotic twins discordant for attention deficit hyperactivity disorder. *Am. J. Psychiatr.* Vol. 160, 1693–1696.

Chapman, R.M., Nowlis, G.H., McCrary, J.W., Chapman, J.A., Sandoval, T.C., Guillily, M.D., Gardner, M.N., and Reilly, L.A. (2007). Brain event-related potentials: Diagnosing early-stage Alzheimer's disease. *Neurobiol. Aging* 28(2): 194–201. Epub 2006 Jan 20.

Colom, L.V. (2006). Septal networks: Relevance to theta rhythm, epilepsy and Alzheimer's disease. *J. Neurochem.* Vol. 96, 609–623.

Congedo, M., Lubar, J.F., and Joffe, D. (2004). Low-resolution electromagnetic tomography neurofeedback. *IEEE Transactions on Neural Systems and Rehabilitation Engineering* 12(4): 387–397.

Cook, I.A., O'Hara, R., Uijtdehaage, S.H., Mandelkern, M., and Leuchter, A.F. (1998). Assessing the accuracy of topographic EEG mapping for determining local brain function. *Electroencephalogr Clin Neurophysiol.* 107(6): 408–414.

Costain, R., Redfearn, J.W., and Lippold, O.C. (1964). A controlled trial of the therapeutic effects of polarization of the brain in depressive illness. *Br. J. Psychiatr.* Vol. 110, 786–799.

Crawford, H.J. (1994). Brain dynamics and hypnosis: Attentional and disattentional processes. *Int. J. Clin. Exp. Hypn.* 42(3): 204–232.

Creem, S.H. and Proffitt, D.R. (2001). Defining the cortical visual systems: "what", "where", and "how". *Acta Psychol. (Amst.)* Vol. 107, (1–3): 43–68.

Crick, F. (1984). Function of the thalamic reticular complex: the searchlight hypothesis. *Proc. Natl. Acad. Sci. USA* Vol. 81, (14): 4586–4590.

Damasio, A.R. (1999). *The Feeling of What Happens. Body and Emotion in the Making of Consciousness.* Harcourt Brace, New York, NY.

Damasio, A.R., Grabowski, T.J., Bechara, A., Damasio, H., Ponto, L.L., Parvizi, J., and Hichwa, R.D. (2000). Subcortical and cortical brain activity during the feeling of self-generated emotions. *Nat. Neurosci.* Vol. 3, (10): 1049–1056.

Davidson, R.J. (1995). Cerebral asymmetry, emotion, and affective style. In Davidson R.J., and Hugdalh K. (eds). *Brain Asymmetry.* MIT Press, Cambridge, MA. 361–387.

Davidson, R.J. (2004). What does the prefrontal cortex "do" in affect: perspectives on frontal EEG asymmetry research. *Biol. Psychol.* Vol. 67, (1–2): 219–233.

Davies, P. and Maloney, A.J.F. (1976). Selective loss of central cholinergic neurons in Alzheimer's disease. *Lancet* 2(8000): 1403.

Donchin, E. (1981). Surprise! Surprise. *Psychophysiology* 18(5): 493–513.

Donchin, E. and Coles, M.G. (1988). Is the P300 component a manifestation of context updating. *Behav. Brain Sci.* Vol. 11, 357–374.

Douglas, R.J. and Martin, K.A. (1991). A functional microcircuit for cat Visual cortex. *J. Physiol.* Vol. 440, 735–769.

Douglas, R.J., Martin, K.A., and Whitteridge, D. (1989). A canonical microcircuit for neocortex. *Neural Comput.* Vol. 1, 480–488.

Dymond, A.M., Coger, R.W., and Serafetinides, E.A. (1975). Intracerebral current levels in man during electrosleep therapy. *Biol. Psychiatr.* 10(1): 101–104.

Ebmeier, K.P., Donaghey, C., and Steele, J.D. (2006). Recent developments and current controversies in depression. *Lancet.* Vol. 367, 153–167.

Edelman, G.M. (1987). *Neural Darwinism: The Theory of Neuronal Group Selection.* Basic Books, New York.

Edelman, G.M. (1993). Neural Darwinism: Selection and reentrant signaling in higher brain function. *Neuron.* Vol. 10, 115–125.

Ekman, P. and Friesen, W.V. (1976). *Pictures of Facial Affect*. Consulting Psychologists, Palo Alto, CA.

Elston, G.N. (2003). Cortex, cognition and the cell: New insights into the pyramidal neuron and prefrontal function. *Cerebr. Cortex*. Vol. 13, 1124–1138.

Engel, A.K. and Singer, W. (2001). Temporal binding and neuronal correlates of sensory awareness. *Trends Cognit. Sci.* 1(1): 16–25.

Ergenoglu, T., Demiralp, T., Bayraktaroglu, Z., Ergen, M., Beydagi, H., and Uresin, Y. (2004). Alpha rhythm of the EEG modulates Visual detection performance in humans. *Cognit. Brain Res.* Vol. 20, 376–383.

Eriksen, C.W. and Eriksen, B.A. (1979). Target redundancy in Visual search: Do repetitions of the target within the display impair processing? *Percept. Psychophys.* Vol. 26, 195–205.

Evarts, E.V., Shinoda, Y., and Wise, S.P. (1984). *Neurophysiological Approaches to Higher Brain Functions*. Wiley, NY.

Fallgatter, A.J. and Strik, W.K. (1999). The NoGo-anteriorisation as a neurophysiological standard-index for cognitive response control. *Int. J. Psychophysiol.* Vol. 32, 115–120.

Feige, B., Scheffler, K., Esposito, F., Di Salle, F., Hennig, J., and Seifritz, E. (2005). Cortical and subcortical correlates of electroencephalographic alpha rhythm modulation. *J. Neurophysiol.* Vol. 93, (5): 2864–2872.

Fell, J., Klaver, P., Lehnertz, K., Grunwald, T., Schaller, C., Elger, C.E., and Fernández, G. (2001). Human memory formation is accompanied by rhinal–hippocampal coupling and decoupling. *Nat. Neurosci.* Vol. 4, 1259–1264.

Fernández, G., Effern, A., Grunwald, T., Pezer, N., Lehnertz, K., Dümpelmann, M., Van Roost, D., and Elger, C.E. (1999). Real-time tracking of memory formation in the human rhinal cortex and hippocampus. *Science*. Vol. 285, 1582–1585.

Fink, M. and Sackeim, H.A. (1996). Convulsive therapy in schizophrenia? *Schizophr. Bull.* Vol. 22, 27–39.

Ford, J.M. (1999). Schizophrenia: The broken P300 and beyond. *Psychophysiology*. Vol. 36, 667–682.

Forman, S.D., Dougherty, G.G., Casey, B.J., Siegle, G.J., Braver, T.S., Barch, D.M., Stenger, V.A., Wick-Hull, C., Pisarov, L.A., and Lorensen, E. (2004). Opiate addicts lack error-dependent activation of rostral anterior cingulate. *Biol. Psychiatr.* Vol. 55, 531–537.

Fox, M.D. and Raichle, M.E. (2007). Spontaneous fluctuations of brain activity observed with functional magnetic resonance imaging. *Nat. Rev., Neuroscience*. Vol. 8, 700–711.

Foxe, J.J. and Simpson, G.V. (2002). Flow of activation from V1 to frontal cortex in humans: A framework for defining "early" Visual processing. *Exp. Brain Res.* Vol. 142, 139–150.

Fulton, J.F. (1951). *Frontal Lobotomy and Affective Behavior – A Neurophysiological analysis*. WW Norton, New York.

Fuster, J.M. (1990). Inferotemporal units in selective visual attention and short-term memory. *J. Neurophysiol.* Vol. 64, (3): 681–697.

Gallinat, J., Bottlender, R., Juckel, G., Munke-Puchner, A., Stotz, G., and Kuss, H.J. (2000). The loudness dependency of the auditory evoked N1/P2-component as a predictor of the acute SSRI response in depression. *Psychopharmacology* 148(4): 401–411.

Gandiga, P.C., Hummel, F.C., and Cohen, L.G. (2006). Transcranial DC stimulation (tDCS): A tool for double-blind sham-controlled clinical studies in brain stimulation. *Clin. Neurophysiol.* 117(4): 845–850. Epub 2006 Jan 19.

Gemba, H. and Sasaki, K. (1989). Potential related to go/no-go hand movement task with color discrimination in human. *Neurosci. Lett.* Vol. 101, 263–268.

Gemba, H. and Sasaki, K. (1990). Potential related to no-go reaction in go/no-go hand movement with discrimination between tone stimuli of different frequencies in the monkey. *Brain Res.* Vol. 537, (1–2): 340–344.

Gevins, A., Smith, M.E., McEvoy, L., and Yu, D. (1997). High-resolution EEG mapping of cortical activation related to working memory: Effects of task difficulty, type of processing, and practice. *Cerebr. Cortex.* Vol. 7, 374–385.

Gloaguen, V., Cottraux, J., Cucherat, M., and Blackburn, I.M. (1998). A metaanalysis of the effects of cognitive therapy in depressed patients. *J. Affect. Disord.* Vol. 49, 59–72.

Goodglass, H. and Geschwind, N. (1976). Language disorders. In: (eds). Handbook of Perception: Language and Speech, Vol. II, Academic Press, New York.

Gottesman, I.I. and Gould, T.D. (2003). The endophenotype concept in psychiatry: Etymology and Strategic Intentions. *Am. J. Psychiatr.* 160(4): 636–645.

Grechin, V.B. and Kropotov, J.D. (1979). *Slow Non-electrical Processes of the Human Brain.* "Nauka" ("Science") Publishing House, Leningrad. 128 p. (in Russian).

Gruzelier, J., Hardman, E., Wild, J., and Zaman, R. (1999). Learned control of slow potential interhemispheric asymmetry in schizophrenia. *Int. J. Psychophysiol.* 34(3): 341–348.

Guaranha, M.S.B., Garzon, E., Buchpiguel, C.A., Tazima, S., Yacubian, E.M.T., and Sakamoto, A.C. (2005). Hyperventilation revisited: Physiological effects and efficacy on focal seizure activation in the era of Video-EEG monitoring. *Epilepsia* 46(1): 69–75.

Gumenyuk, V., Korzyukov, O., Escera, C., Hamalainen, M., Huotilainen, M., Hayrinen, T., Oksanen, H., Näätänen, R., Von Wendt, L., and Alho, K. (2005). Electrophysiological evidence of enhanced distractibility in ADHD children. *Neurosci. Lett.* 374(3): 212–217. Epub 2004 Nov 24.

Gur, R.E., Turetsky, B.I., Loughead, J., Snyder, W., Kohler, C., Elliott, M., Pratiwadi, R., Ragland, J.D., Bilker, W.B., Siegel, S.J., Kanes, S.J., Arnold, S.E., and Gur, R.C. (2007). Visual attention circuitry in schizophrenia investigated with oddball event-related functional magnetic resonance imaging. *Am. J. Psychiatr.* Vol. 164, (3): 442–449.

Hagemann, D. (2004). Individual differences in anterior EEG asymmetry: Methodological problems and solutions. *Biol. Psychol.* Vol. 67 (1–2), 157–182.

Haider, B., Duque, A., Hasenstaub, A.R., and McCormick, D.A. (2006). Neocortical network activity in Vivo is generated through a dynamic balance of excitation and inhibition. *J. Neurosci.* 26(17): 4535–4545.

Hari, R. and Salmelin, R. (1997). Human cortical oscillations: A neuromagnetic View through the skull. *Trends Neurosci.* 20(1): 44–49.

Hebb, D.O. (1949). *The Organization of Behavior.* Wiley, New York.

Heimer, L. and Van Hoesen, G.W. (2006). The limbic lobe and its output channels: Implications for emotional functions and adaptive behavior. *Neurosci. Biobehav. Rev.* Vol. 30, 126–147.

Henriques, J.B. and Davidson, R.J. (1991). Left frontal hypoactivation in depression. *J. Abnorm. Psychol.* Vol. 100, 535–545.

Hensler, J.G. (2006). Serotonergic modulation of the limbic system. *Neurosci. Biobehav. Rev.* Vol. 30, 203–214.

Herrmann, M.J., Jacob, C., Unterecker, S., and Fallgatter, A.J. (2003). Reduced response-inhibition in obsessive-compulsive disorder measured with topographic evoked potential mapping. *Psychiatr. Res.* Vol. 120, 265–271.

Herskovits, E.H., Megalooikonomou, V., Davatzikos, C., Chen, A., Bryan, R.N., and Gerring, J.P. (1999). Is the spatial distribution of brain lesions associated with closed-head injury predictive of subsequent development of attention-deficit/hyperactivity disorder? Analysis with brain-image database. *Radiology* Vol. 213, (2): 389–394.

Hillyard, S.A. and Anllo-Vento, L. (1998). Event-related brain potentials in the study of Visual selective attention. *Proc. Natl. Acad. Sci. USA.* Vol. 95, 781–787.

Hirvonen, J., Van Erp, T.G.M., Huttunen, J., Aalto, S., Någren, K., Huttunen, M., Lönnqvist, J., Kaprio, J., Hietala, J., and Cannon, T.D. (2005). Increased caudate dopamine D2 receptor availability as a genetic marker for schizophrenia. *Arch. Gen. Psychiatr.* Vol. 62, 271–278.

Huang-Pollock, C.L. and Nigg, J.T. (2003). Searching for the attention deficit in attention deficit hyperactivity disorder: The case of Visuospatial orienting. *Clin. Psychol. Rev.* 23(6): 801–830.

Huang, Z.J., Di Cristo, G., and Ango, F. (2007). Development of GABA innervation in the cerebral and cerebellar cortices. *Nat. Rev. Neurosci.* Vol. 8, (9): 673–686.

Huerta, P.T. and Lisman, J.E. (1993). Heightened synaptic plasticity of hippocampal CA1 neurons during a cholinergically induced rhythmic state. *Nature.* 364(6439): 723–725.

Hughes, S.W., Cope, D.W., Blethyn, K.L., and Crunelli, V. (2002). Cellular mechanisms of the slow (<1 Hz) oscillation in thalamocortical neurons in Vitro. *Neuron.* 33(6): 947–958.

Hughes, S.W., Lorincz, M., Cope, D.W., Blethyn, K.L., Kekesi, K.A., Parri, H.R., Juhasz, G., and Crunelli, V. (2004). Synchronized oscillations at alpha and theta frequencies in the lateral geniculate nucleus. *Neuron.* 42(2): 253–268.

Hummel, F., Celnik, P., Giraux, P., Floel, A., Wu, W.H., Gerloff, C., and Cohen, L.G. (2005). Effects of non-invasive cortical stimulation on skilled motor function in chronic stroke. *Brain* Vol. 128, (Pt 3): 490–499.

Inanaga, K. (1998). Frontal midline theta rhythm and mental activity. *Psychiatr. Clin. Neurosci.* 52(6): 555–566.

Ingvar, D.H. (1985). "Memory of the future": an essay on the temporal organization of conscious awareness. *Hum. Neurobiol.* Vol. 4, (3): 127–136.

Itier, R.J. and Taylor, M.J. (2004). N170 or N1? Spatiotemporal differences between object and face processing using ERPs. *Cerebr. Cortex.* Vol. 14, 132–142.

Jasper, H., Solomon, P., and Bradley, C. (1938). Electroencephalographic analyses of behaviour problem children. *Am. J. Psychiatr.* Vol. 95, 641–658.

Jenike, M.A., Baer, L., Ballantine, H.T., Martuza, R.L., Tynes, S., Giriunas, I., Buttolph, M.L., and Cassem, N.H. (1991). Cingulotomy for refractory obsessive compulsive disorder. A long term follow-up of 33 patients. *Arch. Gen. Psychiatr.* Vol. 48, 548–555.

Jensen, O., Goel, P., Kopell, N., Pohja, M., Hari, R., and Ermentrout, B., (2005). On the human sensorimotor-cortex beta rhythm: sources and modeling. *Neuroimage* Vol. 26, (2): 347–355.

John, E.R., Karmel, B.Z., Corning, W.C., Easton, P., Brown, D., Ahn, H., John, M., Harmony, T., Prichep, L., Toro, A., Gerson, I., Bartlett, F., Thatcher, F., Kaye, H., Valdes, P., and Schwartz, E. (1977). Neurometrics. *Science* Vol. 196 (4297): 1393–1410.

Johnson, M.D. and Ojemann, G.A. (2000). The role of the human thalamus in language and memory: Evidence from electrophysiological studies. *Brain Cognit.* 42(2): 218–230.

Jonkman, L.M., Kemner, C., Verbaten, M.N., Van Engeland, H., Camfferman, G., Buitelaar, J.K., and Koelega, H.S. (2000). Attentional capacity, a probe ERP study: Differences between children with attention-deficit hyperactivity disorder and normal control children and effects of methylphenidate. *Psychophysiology.* Vol. 37, 334–346.

Jonkman, L.M., Kenemans, J.L., Kemner, C., Verbaten, M.N., and van Engeland, H. (2004). Dipole source localization of event-related brain activity indicative of an early visual selective attention deficit in ADHD children. *Clin. Neurophysiol.* Vol. 115, (7): 1537–1549.

Jung, T.-P., Makeig, S., Westerfield, M., Townsend, J., Courchesne, E., and Sejnowski, T.J. (2001). Analysis and Visualization of single-trial event-related potentials. *Hum. Brain Mapp.* Vol. 14, 166–185.

Kalivas, P.W. and Volkow, N.D. (2005). The neural basis of addiction: A pathology of motivation and choice. *Am. J. Psychiatr.* 162(8): 1403–1413.

Kandel, E., Schwartz, J., and Jessel, T. (2000). *Principles of Neural Science.* McGraw-Hill, New York. (*Also*: http://www.en.wikipedia.org/wiki/Principles_of_Neural_Science)

Kastner, S. and Ungerleider, L.G. (2000). Mechanisms of Visual attention in the human cortex. *Annu. Rev. Neurosci.* Vol. 23, 315–341.

Keedwell, P.A., Andrew, C., Williams, S.C.R., Brammer, M.J., and Phillips, M.L. (2005). A double dissociation of Ventromedial prefrontal cortical responses to sad and happy stimuli in depressed and healthy individuals. *Biol. Psychiatr.* Vol. 58, 495–503.

Kilts, C.D., Schweitzer, J.B., Quinn, C.K., Gross, R.E., Faber, T.L., Muhammad, F., Ely, T.D., Hoffman, J.M., and Drexler, K.P. (2001). Neural activity related to drug craving in cocaine addiction. *Arch. Gen. Psychiatr.* 58(4): 334–341.

Kimura, M., Katayama, J., and Murohashi, H. (2006). An ERP study of Visual change detection: Effects of magnitude of spatial frequency changes on the change-related posterior positivity. *Int. J. Psychophysiol.* Vol. 62, 14–23.

Kitabatake, Y., Hikida, T., Watanabe, D., Pastan, I., and Nakanishi, S. (2003). Impairment of reward-related learning by cholinergic cell ablation in the striatum. *Proc. Natl. Acad. Sci. USA* 100(13): 7965–7970.

Klein, C., Rockstroh, B., Cohen, R., and Berg, P. (1996). Contingent negative variation (CNV) and determinants of the post-imperative negative variation (PINV) in schizophrenic patients and healthy controls. *Schizophr. Res.* Vol. 23, (21(2)): 97–110.

Klimesch, W. (1999). EEG alpha and theta oscillations reflect cognitive and memory performance: A review and analysis. *Brain Res. Rev.* Vol. 29, 169–195.

Kolb, B. and Whishaw, I.Q. (2001). *An introduction to brain and behavior.* Worth Publishers, New York. 601 pp.

Kramis, R., Vanderwolf, C.H., and Bland, B.H. (1975). Two types of hippocampal rhythmical slow activity in both the rabbit and the rat: Relations to behavior and effects of atropine, diethyl ether, urethane, and pentobarbital. *Exp. Neurol.* 49(1 Pt 1): 58–85.

Krause, K.-H., Dresel, S.H., Krause, J., Kung, H.F., and Tatsch, K. (2000). Increased striatal dopamine transporter in adult patients with attention deficit hyperactivity disorder: Effects of methylphenidate as measured by single photon emission computed tomography. *Neurosci. Lett.* Vol. 285, 107–110.

Kringelbach, M.L. and Rolls, E.T. (2004). The functional neuroanatomy of the human orbitofrontal cortex: Evidence from neuroimaging and neuropsychology. *Prog. Neurobiol.* Vol. 72, 341–372.

Kropotov, J.D. (1989). Brain organization of perception and memory: Hypothesis for action programming. *Hum. Physiol.* 15(3): 19–27 (in Russian).

Kropotov, J.D. and Gretchin, A. (1979). Phase dynamics of slow oscillations of local oxygen during Verbal processing. *Hum. Physiol.* 1(6): 14–24 (in Russian).

Kropotov, J.D. and Etlinger, S.C. (1999). Selection of actions in the basal ganglia-thalamocortical circuits: Review and model. *Int. J. Psychophysiol.* 31(3): 197–217.

Kropotov, J.D. and Kremen, I.Z. (1999). Canonical cortical module as a spatial-frequency filter. *J. Opt. Technol.* 66(9): 832–835 (in Russian).

Kropotov, J.D., Etlinger, S.C., and Ponomarev, V.A. (1997). Human multiunit activity related to attention and preparatory set. *Psychophysiology.* Vol. 34, 495–500.

Kropotov, J.D., Kropotova, O.V., Ponomarev, V.A., Polyakov Yu, I., and Nechaev, V.B. (1999). Neurophysiological mechanisms of action selection and its impairment in ADHD. *Hum. Physiol.* 25(1): 143–152 (in Russian).

Kropotov, J.D., Alho, K., Näätänen, R., Ponomarev, V.A., Kropotova, O.V., Anichkov, A.D., and Nechaev, V.B. (2000). Human auditory-cortex mechanisms of preattentive sound discrimination. *Neurosci. Lett.* Vol. 280, 87–90.

Kropotov, J.D., Chutko, L.S., Yakovenko, E.A., Grin-Yatsenko, V.A. (2002). Application of transcranial micro-polarization for treatment of ADHD children. *J. Neurol. Psychiatr.* after Korsakov, S.S. N.5: 26–28 (in Russian).

Kropotov, J.D., Grin-Yatsenko, V.A., Ponomarev, V.A., Chutko, L.S., Yakovenko, E.A., and Nikishina, I. (2005). ERPs correlates of EEG relative beta training in ADHD children. *Int. J. Psychophysiol.* 55(1): 23–34.

Ktonas, P.Y. (1987). Automated spike and sharp wave (SSW) detection. In Gevins A.S., and Remond A., (eds). *Methods of Analysis of Bysis of Brain Electrical and Magnetic signals. EEG handbook* (revised series, Vol 1). Elsevier Science Publishers B. V. 211–241.

Lashley, K.S. (1950). In Search of the Engram // Psychological mechanisms in animal behavior. *Soc. Exp. Biol. N.Y.* 454–482.

Laukka, S.J., Järvilehto, T., Alexandrov, Yu.I., and Lindqvist, J. (1995). Frontal midline theta related to learning in a simulated driving task. *Biol. Psychol.* 40(3): 313–320.

Lee, S.H., Wynn, J.K., Green, M.F., Kim, H., Lee, K.J., Nam, M., Park, J.K., and Chung, Y.C. (2006). Quantitative EEG and low resolution electromagnetic tomography (LORETA) imaging of patients with persistent auditory hallucinations. *Schizophr. Res.* 83(2–3): 111–119. Epub 2006 Mar 9.

Leeb, R. and Pfurtscheller, G. (2004). Walking through a virtual city by thought. *Conf. Proc. IEEE Eng. Med. Biol. Soc.* Vol. 6, 4503–4506.

Lenroot, R.K. and Giedd, J.N. (2006). Brain development in children and adolescents: insights from anatomical magnetic resonance imaging. *Neurosci. Biobehav. Rev.* Vol. 30, (6): 718–729.

Leuchter, A.F., Sebastian, U., Uijtdehaageb, H.J., Cook, I.A., O'Harae, R., and Mandelkernd, M. (1999). Relationship between brain electrical activity and cortical perfusion in normal subjects. *Psychiatr. Res.: Neuroimaging Section.* Vol. 90, 125–140.

Leuchter, A.F., Cook, I.A., Witte, E.A., Morgan, M., and Abrams, M. (2002). Changes in brain function of depressed subjects during treatment with placebo. *Am. J. Psychiatr.* 159, 122–129.

Lippold, O.C. and Redfearn, J.W. (1964). Mental changes resulting from the passage of small direct currents through the human brain. *Br. J. Psychiatr.* 110, 768–772.

Lubar, J.F. (1997). Neocortical dynamics: implications for understanding the role of neurofeedback and related techniques for the enhancement of attention. *Appl. Psychophysiol. Biofeedback* Vol. 22, (2): 111–126.

Lubar, J.F., Swartwood, M.O., Swartwood, J.N., and O'Donnell, P.H. (1995). Evaluation of the effectiveness of EEG neurofeedback training for ADHD in a clinical setting as measured by changes in T.O.V.A. scores, behavioral ratings, and WISC-R performance. *Biofeedback Self Regul.* Vol. 20, (1): 83–99.

Llinás, R.R., Ribary, U., Jeanmonod, D., Kronberg, E., and Mitra, P.P. (1999). Thalamocortical dysrhythmia: A neurological and neuropsychiatric syndrome characterized by magnetoencephalography. *Proc. Natl. Acad. Sci. USA* Vol. 96, (26): 11527–15222.

Lømo, T. (2003). The discovery of long-term potentiation. *Philos. Trans. R. Soc. Lond. B Biol. Sci.* Vol. 358, (1432): 617–620.

Luck, S.J. (2005). *An Introduction to the Event-Related Potential Technique.* The MIT Press, Cambridge, MA. 374 p.

Lynch, J.L., Paskewitz, D., and Orne, M.T. (1974). Some factors in the neurofeedback control of the human alpha rhythm. *Psychosomatic Med.* Vol. 36, 399–410.

Maltez, J., Hyllienmark, L., Nikulin, V.V., and Brismar, T. (2004). Time course and variability of power in different frequency bands of EEG during resting conditions. *Neurophysiol. Clin.* Vol. 34, (5): 195–202.

Makeig, S., Jung, T.-P., Bell, A.J., Ghahreman, D., and Sejnowski, T.J. (1997). Blind separation of auditory event-related brain responses into independent components. *Proc. Natl. Acad. Sci. USA* Vol. 94, 10979–10984.

Makeig, S., Bell, A.J., Jung, T.-P., and Sejnowski, T.J. (1996). Independent component analysis of electroencephalographic data. *Adv. Neural Inf. Process. Syst.* Vol. 8, 145–151.

Malach, R., Levy, I., and Hasson, U. (2002). The topography of high-order human object areas. *Trends Cogn. Sci.* Vol. 6, (4): 176–184.

Marshal, M.P. and Molina, B.S. (2006). Antisocial behaviors moderate the deviant peer pathway to substance use in children with ADHD. *J. Clin. Child Adolesc. Psychol.* 35(2): 216–226.

Marshall, L., Molle, M., Hallschmid, M., and Born, J. (2004). Transcranial direct current stimulation during sleep improves declarative memory. *J. Neurosci.* 24(44): 9985–9992. Erratum in: *J Neurosci.* (2005), 25(2): 1 p following 531.

Mathalon, D.H., Bennett, A., Askari, N., Gray, E.M., Rosenbloom, M.J., and Ford, J.M. (2003). Response-monitoring dysfunction in aging and Alzheimer's disease: An event-related potential study. *Neurobiol. Aging* Vol. 24, 675–685.

Mayberg, H.S., Lozano, A.M., Voon, V., McNeely, H.E., Seminowicz, D., Hamani, C., Schwalb, J.M., and Kennedy, S.H. (2005). Deep brain stimulation for treatment-resistant depression. *Neuron* Vol. 45, 651–660.

McCarley, R.W., O'Donnell, B.F., Niznikiewicz, M.A., Salisbury, D.F., Potts, G.F., Hirayasu, Y., Nestor, P.G., and Shenton, M.E. (1997). Update on electrophysiology in schizophrenia. *Int. Rev. Psychiatr.* Vol. 9, 373–386.

McCormick, D.A. and Pape, H.C. (1990). Properties of a hyperpolarization-activated cation current and its role in rhythmic oscillation in thalamic relay neurones. *J. Physiol.* Vol. 431, 291–318.

McCulloch, W. and Pitts, W. (1943). A logical calculus of the ideas immanent in nervous activity. *Bull. Math. Biophys.* Vol. 7, 115–133.

McNaughton, BL. (1989). The neurobiology of spatial computation and learning. In and Stein D.J. (eds). *Lectures on Complexity: Santa Fe Institute Studies in the Sciences of Complexity.* Addison-Wesley, Redwood, CA. 389–437.

Mendez, M. and Lim, G. (2003). Seizures in elderly patients with dementia: Epidemiology and Management. *Drugs Aging.* Vol. 20, 791–803.

Meyer-Lindenberg, A. and Weinberger, D.R. (2006). Intermediate phenotypes and genetic mechanisms of psychiatric disorders. *Nat. Rev. Neurosci.* 7(10): 818–827.

Monastra, V., Lubar, J., Linden, M., VanDeusen, P., Green, G., Wing, W., Phillips, A., and Fenger, T. (1999). Assessing attention deficit hyperactivity disorder Via quantitative electroencephalography: An initial Validation study. *Neuropsychology.* Vol. 13, 424–433.

Monastra, V.J., Lynn, S., Linden, M., Lubar, J.F., Gruzelier, J., and LaVaque, T.J. (2005). Electroencephalographic biofeedback in the treatment of attention-deficit/hyperactivity disorder. *Appl. Psychophysiol. Biofeedback.* 30(2): 95–114.

Moore, N.C. (2000). A review of EEG biofeedback treatment of anxiety disorders. *Clin. Electroencephalogr.* 31(1): 1–6.

Morris, P.L., Robinson, R.G., Raphael, B., and Hopwood, M.J. (1996). Lesion location and poststroke depression. *J. Neuropsychiatr. Clin. Neurosci.* Vol. 8, 399–403.

Mountcastle, V.B. (1978). Brain mechanisms for directed attention. *J. R. Soc. Med.* Vol. 71, (1): 14–28.

Näätänen, R. (2003). Mismatch negativity: Clinical research and possible applications. *Int. J. Psychophysiol.* Vol. 48, 179–188.

Näätänen, R., Gaillard, A.W.K., and Mäntysalo, S. (1978). Early selective-attention effect reinterpreted. *Acta Physiol.* Vol. 42, 313–329.

Näätänen, R. (1992). *Attention and Brain Function.* Lawrence Erlbaum Associates, Hillsdale, NJ. 517 pp.

Neuper, C., Wörtz, M., and Pfurtscheller, G. (2006). ERD/ERS patterns reflecting sensorimotor activation and deactivation. *Prog. Brain Res.* Vol. 159, 211–222.

Neisser, U. (1978). Anticipations, images, and introspection. *Cognition* Vol. 6, (2): 169–174.

Niedermeyer, E. (1997). Alpha rhythms as physiological and abnormal phenomena. *Int. J. Psychophysiol.* 26(1–3): 31–49. Review.

Niki, H. and Watanabe, M. (1979). Prefrontal and cingulate unit activity during timing behaviour in the macaque. *Brain Res.* Vol. 171, 213–224.

Nishiyama, N., and Yamaguchi, Y. (2001). Human EEG theta in the spatial recognition task, *Proceedings of 5th World Multiconference. on Systemics, Cybernetics and Informatics (SCI 2001), 7th Int. Conf. on Information Systems, Analysis and Synthesis (ISAS 2001)*, pp. 497–500.

Nitsche, M.A. and Paulus, W. (2000). Excitability changes induced in the human motor cortex by weak transcranial direct current stimulation. *J. Physiol.* 527(Pt 3): 633–639.

Nitsche, M.A. and Paulus, W. (2001). Sustained excitability elevations induced by transcranial DC motor cortex stimulation in humans. *Neurology* 57(10): 1899–1901.

O'Keefe, J. and Recce, M.L. (1993). Phase relationship between hippocampal place units and the EEG theta rhythm. *Hippocampus* 3(3): 317–330.

Olbrich, H.M., Maes, H., Valerius, G., Langosch, J.M., and Feige, B. (2005). Event-related potential correlates selectively reflect cognitive dysfunction in schizophrenics. *J. Neural Transm.* Vol. 112, 283–295.

Onton, J. and Makeig, S. (2006). Information-based modeling of event-related brain dynamics. *In* Neuper, K. (Eds.). *Progress in Brain Research,* Vol. 159, 99–120.

Pascual-Marqui, R.D. (2002). Standardized low-resolution brain electromagnetic tomography (sLORETA): technical details. *Meth. Find. Exp. Clin. Pharmacol.* Vol. 24, 5–12.

Pascual-Marqui, R.D., Michel, C.M., and Lehmann, D. (1994). Low resolution electromagnetic tomography: a new method for localizing electrical activity in the brain. *Int. J. Psychophysiol.* Vol. 18, 49–65.

Pascual-Marqui, R.D., Esslen, M., Kochi, K., and Lehmann, D. (2002). Functional imaging with low resolution brain electromagnetic tomography (LORETA): a review. *Meth. Find. Exp. Clin. Pharmacol.* Vol. 24C, 91–95.

Penfield, W. and Perot, P. (1963). The brain's record of auditory and Visual experience. *Brain.* Vol. 86, 595–696.

Peniston, E.G. and Kulkosky, P.J. (1989). Alpha–theta brainwave training and beta-endorphin levels in alcoholics. *Alcohol. Clin. Exp. Res.* 13(2): 271–279.

Pfurtscheller, G. (2003). Induced oscillations in the alpha band: functional meaning. *Epilepsia* Vol. 44, (Suppl 12): 2–8.

Pfurtscheller, G. and Lopes Da Silva, F.H. (1999). Event-related EEG/MEG synchronization and desynchronization: Basic principles. *Clin. Neurophysiol.* Vol. 110, 1842–1857.

Pfurtscheller, G. and Neuper, C. (2006). Future prospects of ERD/ERS in the context of brain-computer interface (BCI) developments. *Prog. Brain Res.* Vol. 159, 433–437.

Pfurtscheller, G., Neuper, C., Andrew, C., and Edlinger, G. (1997). Foot and hand area mu rhythms. *Int. J. Psychophysiol.* Vol. 26, (1–3): 121–135.

Pfurtscheller, G., Neuper, C., and Krausz, G. (2000). Functional dissociation of lower and upper frequency mu rhythms in relation to voluntary limb movement. *Clin. Neurophysiol.* Vol. 111, (10): 1873–1879.

Pineda, J.A., Foote, S.L., and Neville, H.J. (1989). Effects of locus coeruleus lesions on auditory, long latency, event-related potentials in monkey. *J. Neurosci.* Vol. 9, 81–93.

Pizzagalli, D.A., Oakes, T.R., and Davidson, R.J. (2003). Coupling of theta activity and glucose metabolism in the human rostral anterior cingulate cortex: An EEG/PET study of normal and depressed subjects. *Psychophysiology* Vol. 40, 939–949.

Pliszka, S.R., Liotti, M., and Woldorff, M.G. (2000). Inhibitory control in children with attention-deficit/hyperactivity disorder: Event-related potentials identify the processing component and timing of an impaired right-frontal response–inhibition mechanism. *Biol. Psychiatr.* Vol. 48, 238–246.

Pogarell, O., Mulert, C., and Hegerl, U. (2006). Event related potentials and fMRI in neuropsychopharmacology. *J. Clin. EEG Neurosci.* 37(2): 99–107.

Porjesz, B., Rangaswamy, M., Kamarajan, C., Jones, K.A., Padmanabhapillai, A., and Begleiter, H. (2005). The utility of neurophysiological markers in the study of alcoholism. *Clin. Neurophysiol.* Vol. 116, 993–1018.

Posner, M.I., Petersen, S.E., Fox, P.T., and Raichle, M.E. (1988). Localization of cognitive operations in the human brain. *Science* Vol. 240, 1627–1631.

Posthuma, D., Neale, M.C., Boomsma, D.I. and de Geus, E.J. (2001). Are smarter brains running faster? Heritability of alpha peak frequency, IQ, and their interrelation. *Behav. Genet.* Vol. 31, (6): 567–579.

Prichep, L.S., John, E.R., Ferris, S.H., Rausch, L., Fang, Z., Cancro, R., Torossian, C., and Reisberg, B. (2006). Prediction of longitudinal cognitive decline in normal elderly with subjective complaints using electrophysiological imaging. *Neurobiol. Aging* 27(3): 471–481.Epub 2005 Oct 6.

Reynolds, J.H., Chelazzi, L., and Desimone, R. (1999). Competitive mechanisms subserve attention in macaque areas V2 and V4. *J. Neurosci.* 19(5): 1736–1753.

Robinson, D.L. and Petersen, S.E. (1992). The pulvinar and Visual salience. *Trends Neurosci.* 15(4): 127–132.

Robinson, T.E. and Berridge, K.C. (1993). The neural basis of drug craving: An incentive-sensitization theory of addiction. *Brain Res. Rev.* 18(3): 247–291.

Rockstroh, B., Elbert, T., Birbaumer, N., Wolf, P., Düchting-Röth, A., Reker, M., Daum, I., Lutzenberger, W., and Dichgans, J. (1993). Cortical self-regulation in patients with epilepsies. *Epilepsy Res.* Vol. 14, (1): 63–72.

Romo, R. and Salinas, S. (2003). Flutter discrimination: Neural codes, perception, memory and decision making. *Nat. Rev., Neuroscience* Vol. 4, 203–218.

Ropohl, A., Sperling, W., Elstner, S., Tomand, B., Reulbach, U., Kalten, Kornhuber, J., and Maihöfner, C. (2004). Cortical activity associated with auditory hallucinations. *Neuroreport* 15(3): 523–526.

Roth, W.T. and Cannon, E.H. (1972). Some features of the auditory evoked response in schizophrenics. *Arch. Gen. Psychiatr.* Vol. 27, 466–471.

Rothenberger, A., Banaschewski, T., Heinrich, H., Moll, G.H., Schmidt, M.H., and Van't Klooster, B. (2000). Comorbidity in ADHD-children: Effects of coexisting conduct disorder or tic disorder on event-related brain potentials in an auditory selective-attention task. *Eur. Arch. Psychiatr. Clin. Neurosci.* Vol. 250, 101–110.

Rugg, M.D. and Yonelinas, A.P. (2003). Human recognition memory: A cognitive neuroscience perspective. *Trends Cognit. Sci.* 7(7): 313–319.

Sasaki, K., Tsujimoto, T., Nishikawa, S., Nishitani, N., and Ishihara, T. (1996). Frontal mental theta wave recorded simultaneously with magnetoencephalography and electroencephalography. *Neurosci. Res.* Vol. 26, (1): 79–81.

Satterfield, J.H., Cantwell, D.P., Lesser, L.I., and Podosin, R.L. (1972). Physiological studies of the hyperkinetic child. *Am. J. Psychiatr.* Vol. 128, 102–108.

Schmolesky, M.T., Wang, Y.C., Hanes, D.P., Thompson, K.G., Leutgeb, S., Schall, J.D., and Leventhal, A.G. (1998). Signal timing across the macaque Visual system. *J. Neurophysiol.* Vol. 79, 3272–3278.

Schneider, F., Heimann, H., Mattes, R., Lutzenberger, W., and Birbaumer, N. (1992a). Self-regulation of slow cortical potentials in psychiatric patients: Depression. *Biofeedback Self Regul.* Vol. 17, 203–214.

Schneider, F., Rockstroh, B., Heimann, H., Lutzenberger, W., Mattes, R., Elbert, T., Birbaumer, N., and Bartels, M. (1992). Self-regulation of slow cortical potentials in psychiatric patients: Schizophrenia. *Biofeedback Self Regul.* 17(4): 277–292.

Schulte-Körne, G., Deimel, W., Bartling, J., and Remschmidt, H. (1998). Auditory processing and dyslexia: Evidence for a specific speech processing deficit. *Neuroreport* 9(2): 337–340.

Seeman, P., Chau-Wong, M., Tedesco, J., and Wong, K. (1975). Brain receptors for antipsychotic drugs and dopamine: Direct binding assays. *Proc. Natl. Acad. Sci. USA* 72(11): 4376–4380.

Seeman, P., Lee, T., Chau-Wong, M., and Wong, K. (1976). Antipsychotic drug doses and neuroleptic/dopamine receptors. *Nature* 261(5562): 717–719.

Sherlin, L. and Congedo, M. (2005). Obsessive-compulsive dimension localized using low-resolution brain electromagnetic tomography (LORETA). *Neurosci. Lett.* Vol. 387, 72–74.

Sherman, S.M. and Guillery, R.W. (2006). *Exploring the Thalamus and its Role in Cortical Function.* MIT Press. 484 p.

Shima, K. and Tanji, J. (1998). Role for cingulate motor area cells in Voluntary movement selection based on reward. *Science* Vol. 282, 1335–1338.

Singh, K.D., Barnes, G.R., Hillebrand, A., Forde, E.M., and Williams, A.L. (2002). Task-related changes in cortical synchronization are spatially coincident with the hemodynamic response. *NeuroImage* Vol. 16, 103–114.

Smirnov, V.M. (1976). *Stereotactic Neurology.* Medicina, Moscow. 264 p. (in Russian)

Smit, D.J., Posthuma, D., Boomsma, D.I., and Geus, E.J. (2005). Heritability of background EEG across the power spectrum. *Psychophysiology* 42(6): 691–697.

Smith, E.E. and Jonides, J. (1999). Storage and executive processes in the frontal lobes. *Science* 283(5408): 1657–1661.

Sterman, M.B. (1989). Future perspectives for applied psychophysiology and biofeedback. *Biofeedback Self Regul.* Vol. 14 (2): 83–88.

Sterman, M.B. (1996). Physiological origins and functional correlates of EEG rhythmic activities: Implications for self-regulation. *Biofeedback Self Regul.* Vol. 21, 3–33.

Sterman, M.B. and Egner, T. (2006). Foundation and practice of neurofeedback for the treatment of epilepsy. *Appl. Psychophysiol. Biofeedback* Vol. 31 (1): 21–35.

Stevens, A., Kircher, T., Nickola, M., Bartels, M., Rosellen, N., and Wormstall, H. (2001). Dynamic regulation of EEG power and coherence is lost early and globally in probable DAT. *J. Neurochem.* Vol. 96, 609–623.

Strehl, U., Leins, U., Goth, G., Klinger, C., Hinterberger, T., and Birbaumer, N. (2006). Self-regulation of slow cortical potentials: a new treatment for children with attention-deficit/hyperactivity disorder. *Pediatrics* Vol. 118 (5): 1530–1540.

Suetsugi, M., Mizuki, Y., Ushijima, I., Kobayashi, T., Tsuchiya, K., Aoki, T., and Watanabe, Y. (2000). Appearance of frontal midline theta activity in patients with generalized anxiety disorder. *Neuropsychobiology* Vol. 41, 108–112.

Sumich, A.L., Kumari, V., Heasman, B.C., Gordon, E., and Brammer, M. (2006). Abnormal asymmetry of N200 and P300 event-related potentials in subclinical depression. *J. Affect. Disord.* 92(2–3): 171–183. Epub 2006 Mar 9.

Takahashi, T., Murata, T., Hamada, T., Omori, M., Kosaka, H., Kikuchi, M., Yoshida, H., and Wada, Y. (2005). Changes in EEG and autonomic nervous activity during meditation and their association with personality traits. *Int. J. Psychophysiol.* Vol. 55, (2): 199–207.

Talairach, J., Bancaud, J., Geier, S., Bordas-Ferrer, M., Bonis, A., Szikla, G., and Rusu, M. (1973). The cingulate gyrus and human behaviour. *Electroencephalogr. Clin. Neurophysiol.* Vol. 34, 45–52.

Tallon-Baudry, C. and Bertrand, O. (1999). Oscillatory gamma activity in humans and its role in object representation. *Trends Cognit. Sci.* 3(4): 151–162.

Tallon-Baudry, C., Bertrand, O., Hernaff, M.-A., Isnard, J., and Fischer, C. (2005). Attention modulates gamma-band oscillations differently in the human lateral occipital cortex and fusiform gyrus. *Cerebral Cortex.* Vol. 15, 654–662.

Tamm, L., Menon, V., Ringel, J., and Reiss, A.L. (2004). Event-related fMRI evidence of frontotemporal involvement in aberrant response inhibition and task switching in attention-deficit/hyperactivity disorder. *J. Am. Acad. Child Adolesc. Psychiatr.* 43(11): 1430–1440.

Terzuolo, C.A. and Bullock, T.H. (1956). Measurement of imposed Voltage gradient adequate to modulate neuronal firing. *Proc. Natl. Acad. Sci. USA* 42(9): 687–694.

Thatcher, R.W., North, D., and Biver, C. (2005). EEG and intelligence: relations between EEG coherence, EEG phase delay and power. *Clin. Neurophysiol.* Vol. 116 (9): 2129–2141.

Thatcher, R.W., North, D.M., Curtin, R.T., Walker, R.A., Biver, C.J., Gomez, J.F., and Salazar, A.M. (2001). An EEG severity index of traumatic brain injury. *J. Neuropsychiatr. Clin. Neurosci.* Vol. 13, (1): 77–87.

Toga, A.W. and Thompson, P.M. (2003). Mapping brain asymmetry. *Nat. Rev. Neurosci.* Vol. 4, 37–48.

Tomarken, A.J., Davidson, R.J., Wheeler, R.E., and Kinney, L. (1992). Psychometric properties of resting anterior EEG asymmetry: Temporal stability and internal consistency. *Psychophysiology* Vol. 29, 576–592.

Toomim, H. and Carmen, J. (1999). Hemoencephalography (HEG). *Biofeedback* 27(4): 10–14.

Tsai, A.C., Liou, M., Jung, T.P., Onton, J.A., Cheng, P.E., Huang, C.-C., Duann, J.-R., and Makeig, S. (2006). Mapping single-trial EEG records on the cortical surface through a spatiotemporal modality. *NeuroImage.* Vol. 32, 195–207.

UK ECT Review Group (2003). Efficacy and safety of electroconvulsive therapy in depressive disorders: A systematic review and metaanalysis. *Lancet.* Vol. 361, 799–808.

Umbricht, D.S.G., Bates, J.A., Lieberman, J.A., Kane, J.M., and Javitt, D.C. (2006). Electrophysiological indices of automatic and controlled auditory information processing in first-episode, recent-onset and chronic schizophrenia. *Biol. Psychiatr.* 59(8): 762–772. Epub 2006 Feb 21.

van Veen, V. and Carter, C.S. (2002). The anterior cingulate as a conflict monitor: fMRI and ERP studies. *Physiol. Behav.* Vol. 77, 477–482.

Vanhatalo, S., Palva, J.M., Holmes, M.D., Miller, J.W., Voipio, J., and Kaila, K. (2004). Infraslow oscillations modulate excitability and interictal epileptic activity in the human cortex during sleep. *Proc. Natl. Acad. Sci. USA* 101(14): 5053–5057. Epub 2004 Mar 24.

Verleger, R. (1988). Event related potentials and cognition: A critique of context updating hypothesis and alternative interpretation of P3. *Behav. Brain Sci.* Vol. 11, 343–427.

Vuga, M., Fox, N.A., Cohn, J.F., George, C.J., Levenstein, R.M., and Kovacs, M. (2006). Long-term stability of frontal electroencephalographic asymmetry in adults with a history of depression and controls. *Int. J. Psychophysiol.* Vol. 59, 107–115.

Walter, G. (1964). Contingent negative Variation: An electrical sign of sensorimotor association and expectancy in the human brain. *Nature* Vol. 203, 380–384.

Walter, W.G. (1967). The analysis, synthesis and identification of evoked responses and contigent negative variation (CNV). *Electroencephalogr. Clin. Neurophysiol.* Vol. 5, 489.

Weiskopf, N., Scharnowski, F., Veit, R., Goebel, R., Birbaumer, N., and Mathiak, K. (2004). Self-regulation of local brain activity using real-time functional magnetic resonance imaging (fMRI). *J. Physiol. Paris* Vol. 98 (4–6): 357–373.

Weiskopf, N., Mathiak, K., Bock, S.W., Scharnowski, F., Veit, R., Grodd, W., Goebel, R., and Birbaumer, N. (2004). Principles of a brain-computer interface (BCI) based on real-time functional magnetic resonance imaging (fMRI). *IEEE Trans. Biomed. Eng.* 51(6): 966–970.

Wheeler, M.E., Petersen, S.E., and Buckner, R.L. (2000). Memory's echo: Vivid remembering reactivates sensory-specific cortex. *Proc. Natl. Acad. Sci. USA* Vol. 97, 11125–11129.

Wheeler, R.E., Davidson, R.J., and Tomarken, A.J. (1993). Frontal brain asymmetry and emotional reactivity: a biological substrate of affective style. *Psychophysiology* Vol. 30, (1): 82–89.

Whittle, S., Allen, N.B., Lubman, D.I., and Yücel, M. (2006). The neurobiological basis of temperament: towards a better understanding of psychopathology. *Neurosci. Biobehav. Rev.* Vol. 30 (4): 511–525.

Wickelgren, W.A. (1979). Chunking and consolidation: A theoretical synthesis of semantic networks, configuring in conditioning, S–R Versus cognitive learning, normal forgetting, the amnesic syndrome, and the hippocampal arousal system. *Psychol. Rev.* 86(1): 44–60.

Wiersema, J.R., Van der Meere, J.J., and Roeyers, H. (2005). ERP correlates of impaired error monitoring in children with ADHD. *J. Neural. Transm.* 112(10): 1417–1430. Epub 2005 Feb 22.

Wong-Riley, M.T., Hevner, R.F., Cutlan, R., Earnest, M., Egan, R., Frost, J., and Nguyen, T. (1993). Cytochrome oxidase in the human visual cortex: distribution in the developing and the adult brain. *Vis. Neurosci.* Vol. 10 (1): 41–58.

Yarbus, A. (1967). *Eye Movements and Vision.* Plenum Press

Yerkes, R.M. and Dodson, J.D. (1908). The relation of strength of stimulus to rapidity of habit-formation. *J. Comp. Neurol. Psychol.* Vol. 18, 459–482.

Zatorre, R.J., Bouffard, M., Ahad, P., and Belin, P. (2002). Where is 'where' in the human auditory cortex? *Nat. Neurosci.* Vol. 5, 905–909.

Index

A

ACC. *See* Anterior cingulate cortex
Acetylcholine, 315–317
Action potential, xxxii
Action selection
 in basal ganglia, 258–260
 executive functions' association with, 254–255
Action suppression, 272–273
Addiction
 definition of, 389
 MRI/PET studies on, 434
 nucleus accumbens' dopamine level increased
  through, 434–435
 stages of, 435–438
  consolidation, 436
  expectation, 435
  habituation/sensitization, 436
  neural net model, 437–438
 substances of abuse for, 433
 symptoms of, 432–433
 tolerance/dependence/withdrawal, 433–444
 treatment for, 438–440
  neurofeedback, 439–440
  stereotactic neurosurgery, 438, 439f
ADHD. *See* Attention deficit hyperactivity disorder
Affective state, 184
Affective system
 anatomy of, 294–297
  cortical/subcortical elements, 295–297
  Papez circuit, 295, 296f
 ERPs, paradigms involving, 364–365
 limbic system compared to, 294–295
 physiology of, 297–305
  ACC, 304
  amygdala, 302–303
  emotion, frontal midline theta rhythm, 305
  emotion patterns in neuroimaging, 304–305
  hypothalamus, 303–304
  positive/negative reinforcers, monitoring
   characteristics, 299–301
  thalamus, 303
 psychology of, 292–294
  emotions v. reasoning, 292–293
  motivation/drive, 293–294

negative reinforcer/positive reinforcer,
 293, 294t
reaction stages of, 305–307
serotonin mediating, 307–309
Agnosia, 184
Akinetic mutism, 279–280
Alpha rhythms. *See also* Mu-rhythms; Occipital
 alpha rhythms; Parietal alpha rhythm
 abnormality of, 52–57
  absence, 52
  anterior alpha asymmetry, 55, 56f, 57
  unusual sites, 52–53, 54f
 definition of, 4
 frontal midline theta rhythm's independence
  from, 79, 80f
 history of, 29–30
 as idling EEG activity, 50, 51f
 lateral inhibition in activation of,
  50–52
 sleep spindles compared to, 42
 types of, 30–36
 of wakefulness, 42–43
Alpha ringing, 351, 352f
Alzheimer's disease
 definition of, 390
 ERP studies for, 466–467
 mediators for, 463–464
 neural net model for, 464–465
 QEEG studies for, 465–466
 symptoms of, 463
 treatment for, 467
Amplifier
 characteristics of, 121
 definition of, 4
Amygdala
 affective system physiology and, 302–303
 definition of, 184
Anhedonia, 390
Anterior alpha asymmetry, 55, 56f, 57
Anterior cingulate cortex (ACC)
 affective system physiology and, 304
 akinetic mutism in, 279–280
 function of, 278–279
 monitoring concept in, 280–281

531

Printed and bound by CPI Group (UK) Ltd, Croydon, CR0 4YY

03/10/2024

01040418-0013